Exercise and Sport Sciences Reviews

Volume 23, 1995

EXERCISE AND SPORT SCIENCES REVIEWS

Volume 23, 1995

Editor

JOHN O. HOLLOSZY, M.D.

Professor of Medicine
Department of Internal Medicine
Washington University School of Medicine
St. Louis, Missouri

American College of Sports Medicine Series

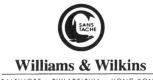

Williams & Wilkins

BALTIMORE • PHILADELPHIA • HONG KONG
LONDON • MUNICH • SYDNEY • TOKYO

A WAVERLY COMPANY

Accurate indications, adverse reactions, and dosage schedules for drugs are provided in this book, but it is possible that they may change. The reader is urged to review the package information data of the manufacturers of the medications mentioned.

Printed in the United States of America
(ISBN 0-683-00037-3)

95 96 97 98
1 2 3 4 5 6 7 8 9 10

Preface

Exercise and Sport Sciences Reviews, an annual publication sponsored by the American College of Sports Medicine, reviews current research concerning behavioral, biochemical, biomechanical, clinical, physiological, and rehabilitational topics involving exercise science. The Editorial Board for this series currently consists of 15 recognized authorities who have assumed responsibility for one of the following general topics: athletic medicine, biochemistry, biomechanics, environmental physiology, epidemiology, exercise physiology, gerontology, growth and development, metabolism, molecular biology, motor control, physical fitness, psychology, rehabilitation, and sociology. The organization of the Editorial Board should help foster the commitment of the American College of Sports Medicine to publish timely reviews in areas of broad interest to clinicians, educators, exercise scientists, and students. The goal for this Editorial Board is to provide reviews in each of these 15 areas whenever sufficient new information becomes available on topics that are likely to be of interest to the readership of *Exercise and Sport Sciences Reviews.* Further, the Editor selects additional topics to be developed into chapters based on current interest, timeliness, and importance to the above audience. The contributors for each volume are selected by the Editorial Board members and the Editor.

John O. Holloszy, M.D.
Editor

Contributors

Douglas K. Bowles, Ph.D.
Dalton Cardiovascular Research Center
University of Missouri
Columbia, Missouri

Robert C. Cantu, M.D. F.A.C.S., FACSM
Neurosurgery Service
Service of Sports Medicine
Concord, Massachusetts

John R. Claybaugh, Ph.D.
Physiology Section
Tripler Army Medical Center
Honolulu, Hawaii

Edward F. Coyle, Ph.D., FACSM
Department of Physical and Health Education
University of Texas
Austin, Texas

Loretta DiPietro, Ph.D., MPH
The John B. Pierce Laboratory
New Haven, Connecticut

Roger M. Enoka, Ph.D.
Department of Biomedical Engineering
Cleveland Clinic Foundation
Cleveland, Ohio

Scott Going, Ph.D.
Department of Exercise and Sports Sciences
University of Arizona
Tucson, Arizona

Mark D. Grabiner, Ph.D., FACSM
Department of Biomedical Engineering
Cleveland Clinic Foundation
Cleveland, Ohio

William R. Hiatt, M.D.
Department of General Internal Medicine
University of Colorado Health Sciences Center
Denver, Colorado

Li Li Ji, Ph.D., FACSM
Department of Kinesiology
University of Wisconsin–Madison
Madison, Wisconsin

Mitchell Kanter, Ph.D.
Quaker Oats Company
John Stuart Research Lab
Barrington, Illinois

Jane A. Kent-Braun, Ph.D., FACSM
UCSFA/VA Medical Center
Magnetic Resonance Unit
San Francisco, California

Timothy G. Lohman, Ph.D.
Department of Exercise and Sports Sciences
University of Arizona
Tucson, Arizona

Robert G. Miller, M.D.
UCSFA/VA Medical Center
Magnetic Resonance Unit
San Francisco, California

Patrick J. O'Connor, Ph.D., FACSM
Department of Exercise Science
The University of Georgia
Exercise Psychology Lab
Athens, Georgia

Peter P. Purslow, Ph.D.
Department of Veterinary Medicine
University of Bristol Veterinary School
Langford, Bristol, United Kingdom

Judith G. Regensteiner, Ph.D.
Department of General Internal Medicine
University of Colorado Health Sciences Center
Denver, Colorado

Shawn Rhind, M.Sc.
University of Toronto
School of Physical and Health Education
Toronto, Ontario, Canada

Frances J. R. Richmond, Ph.D.
Department of Psychology
Queen's University
Kingston, Ontario, Canada

Pang N. Shek, Ph.D.
Defense and Civil Institute of Environmental Medicine
Downsview, Ontario, Canada

Roy J. Shephard, M.D. (Lond.), Ph.D., FACSM
University of Toronto
School of Physical and Health Education
Toronto, Ontario, Canada

Keizo Shiraki, M.D., Ph.D.
Department of Physiology
University of Occupational and Environmental Health (UOEH)
Kitakyushu, Japan

Joseph W. Starnes, Ph.D., FACSM
Department of Kinesiology and Health Education
University of Texas
Austin, Texas

John A. Trotter, Ph.D.
Department of Anatomy
The University of New Mexico
Albuquerque, New Mexico

Michael W. Weiner, M.D.
UCSF/VA Medical Center
Magnetic Resonance Unit
San Francisco, California

Jill Whitall, Ph.D.
Department of Physical Therapy
University of Maryland
Baltimore, Maryland

Daniel P. Williams, Ph.D.
Department of Exercise and Sports Sciences
University of Arizona
Tucson, Arizona

Shawn D. Youngstedt, M.A.
Department of Exercise Science
The University of Georgia
Exercise Psychology Lab
Athens, Georgia

Contents

1
Exercise Rehabilitation for Patients with Peripheral Arterial Disease

JUDITH G. REGENSTEINER Ph.D.
WILLIAM R. HIATT, M.D.

Peripheral arterial disease (PAD) is a common manifestation of athero-sclerosis, affecting about 12% of the general population and up to 20% of older people [24, 41]. Because persons with PAD often also have systemic atherosclerosis, there is an associated increase in a mortality from other cardiovascular diseases, including those affecting the coronary and cerebral circulations [23, 25]. In addition, patients with PAD have cardiovascular risk factors similar to those of patients with coronary artery disease.

In the patient with PAD, with walking exercise during usual activities, the limited arterial supply cannot meet the metabolic demand of the muscles in the lower extremity, resulting in muscle ischemia and the symptom of intermittent claudication. Intermittent claudication is defined as pain or aching in the calf, thighs and/or buttocks, which is reproducibly brought on by walking and which subsides upon resting. Patients with PAD are able to walk only short distances before they must rest to relieve the symptom of intermittent claudication. When tested on a treadmill, persons with PAD also have a maximal exercise capacity that is only about 50% of normal [31, 42]. In addition, ability to walk in the community-based setting is impaired [78, 79] and overall habitual physical activity levels are lower than in the non-PAD population [78]. Thus, in symptomatic patients, functional status is markedly impaired by PAD. The limited ability to carry out physical activities, especially those requiring ambulation, represents a disability when persons are unable to carry out their normal personal, social, and occupational activities.

In contrast to persons with coronary artery disease, in which there is often a spontaneous recovery of function after a myocardial infarction or cardiac surgery [38], persons with PAD often remain at the same level of walking impairment for years if not offered specific treatments. Because the symptom of claudication is often relatively stable over a 5-yr period [60, 67], the major goals of treatment are to relieve the symptom of intermittent claudication, improve functional status, and improve walking ability. In the present article, we will focus on the role of exercise rehabilitation as a treatment for claudication.

1

EVALUATION OF CLAUDICATION THERAPIES

Appropriate evaluation of a given therapy for claudication is critical to determining the value of an intervention. Before choosing an evaluation method for this purpose, certain criteria should be applied prospectively to the tests to ensure that they will accomplish the goals of the evaluation process. For the purposes of the present article, the main goal of evaluation is to measure change in functional status due to an intervention.

A useful test to evaluate the benefit of a treatment in the PAD population must have adequate precision and accuracy if it is to be used in an intervention trial. Importantly, evaluation procedures must be able to measure functional status accurately and precisely over a wide range of walking abilities because patients differ in the degree of functional limitation resulting from claudication. A given test's characteristics must also be stable with respect to time in the absence of an intervention. Because repetitive testing over time is often required to follow the progress of a therapy, it is important that a test not introduce a learning effect or bias that would limit the ability to assess an intervention.

The issue of practicality is an important one in several respects. The costs of a test must be considered such that the evaluation procedures do not require prohibitively expensive equipment or be prohibitively expensive to perform. Both patient and investigator time required for the test should be minimized, and acceptability of the test maximized. Finally, a test used in clinical trials should address patient-focused clinical outcomes, including functional status, walking ability, and quality of life.

Tests that can be applied to all treatments for claudication include hemodynamic measures, treadmill testing, and questionnaire assessment. These tests have been developed for the purpose of assessing clinical status both at baseline and after treatment in the PAD population.

Hemodynamic Assessment

The most commonly used noninvasive test of the peripheral circulation is the measurement of resting and postexercise systolic blood pressures in the ankle and arm with a Doppler ultrasonic instrument. At rest, the ratio of ankle-to-arm systolic blood pressure or ankle/brachial index (ABI) is an index of the severity of the underlying vascular disease [14]. The ABI (and other hemodynamic tests such as calf blood flow) is an excellent means to assess vessel patency after a peripheral bypass operation or angioplasty. In addition, these tests are practical in that they are not complicated to perform, are well tolerated by patients, require only simple equipment, and are relatively inexpensive. However, the hemodynamic severity of the vascular disease defined by ABI, or calf blood flow, is not well correlated to treadmill exercise performance [4, 42, 71]. Therefore, these measures should not be used as the main test of the functional effects of interventions whose primary goal is to improve or relieve claudication.

Measurement of Exercise Performance

Most studies that evaluate change in functional status because of a treatment have used treadmill testing as the primary objective measure of changes in exercise performance. The two measures most commonly used to evaluate exercise performance on the treadmill are claudication-free walking time or distance (initial claudication distance) and maximal, claudication-limited walking time or distance (absolute claudication distance). The traditional treadmill protocol for persons with PAD has until recently been a constant-load test, which has generally been conducted at a slow speed of 1.5–2 mph, with the grade fixed at a level typically of 8–12% [58, 69]. Despite the constant workload, most (but not all) persons reach a maximal level of claudication pain, at which point they stop walking. However, constant-load protocols have several potential limitations. For instance, a single workload may not be appropriate for a heterogeneous population of patients with different walking abilities. If the workload remains constant at a low level, some patients may be claudication limited on entry to a program, but never reach a maximal level of claudication pain after an intervention from which they experience a large improvement. A second limitation is that there is a large degree of variability in walking time from test to test when a constant-load protocol is used in this population. Coefficients of variation of 30–45% have been found for constant-load protocols for both initial and absolute walking times [16, 36]. Therefore, repeated testing on entry has been necessitated in individual patients to establish the true baseline walking time or distance [62, 73]. Repetitive testing over a short time engenders other confounding problems in that multiple testing may induce an improved walking performance or placebo response. The placebo response has been seen in some studies, where it was found that the control group increased maximal walking time [12, 16, 61, 73], although not in all studies [26, 48, 59]. Thus, in the absence of a control group, data on an intervention may be uninterpretable if a constant-load protocol is used.

Although the constant-load treadmill test has limitations for measuring change in walking ability in terms of precision and accuracy as well as reproducibility, it has been well accepted by both patients and physicians. The treadmill equipment is widely available at relatively low cost, and testing requires minimal preparation. Finally, the constant-load treadmill test has provided an important historical data base from prior exercise training studies [15, 30, 65], as well as from trials of drug therapy [12, 61, 73] and surgical intervention studies [22, 88]. Thus, this type of treadmill test has been an important tool for clinical research in PAD.

In comparison with the constant-load test, graded treadmill protocols have been developed more recently to test patients with PAD [36, 37]. Two widely used graded protocols maintain the speed of treadmill walking at 2.0 mph. With one protocol, the grade increases 3.5% ever 3 min [42]; with the other, grade increases 2.0% every 2 min [36, 37]. An important feature of the graded protocol is that it is much more reproducible than the constant-load protocol. For example, the coefficient of variation of maximal walking distance for the graded test is 12–13% compared with 30–45% for the constant-load protocol [16, 36, 37, 42]. It was therefore observed that only one graded test would be required to obtain reliable measurements of exercise performance in claudication, whereas three tests may be needed with the constant-load protocol [36, 37]. Additional benefits of the graded protocol are that patients with varying walking distances can be enrolled, and all patients can be analyzed after treatment, regardless of the magnitude of improvement. Thus, precision and accuracy over a range of patient walking capabilities, as well as reproducibility, are superior with the graded treadmill test compared with the constant-load test. Another benefit of the graded test is that exercise performance on a graded protocol correlates with community-based walking ability determined by questionnaire (discussed below) [79].

Performance of graded exercise testing protocols requires somewhat more sophisticated treadmill equipment than does constant-load testing. However, this equipment is widely available at nearly all major health care centers and there is extensive physician, technician, and patient experience with these systems. The test is well tolerated by patients and well accepted by investigators. Time requirements to perform the test are similar to or less than those required for the constant-load test.

For the reasons discussed above, it is recommended that investigators use the graded treadmill protocol for studies in PAD patients where the primary goal is to evaluate change in exercise performance.

Measurement of Oxygen Consumption with Exercise Testing
Measuring oxygen consumption during graded exercise testing provides an additional objective physiological marker of maximal exercise performance as well as of cardiovascular function [39, 94]. Oxygen consumption in the PAD population can be modified through either exercise training or surgical treatment [44, 76], and it is reproducible and has a coefficient of variation of approximately 12% in repeated tests [42].

In contrast to exercise tests based solely on work load, the measurement of oxygen consumption requires expensive equipment and highly trained personnel, and thus accessibility to this technique is limited. In addition, the measurement is not always well tolerated by patients, who may dislike the constrictive feeling imposed by a mouthpiece or mask.

Functional Status Measures
In the PAD population, to evaluate functional status comprehensively, it is important not only to consider laboratory-based measures such as treadmill tests, but also to examine community-based measures such as can be obtained from questionnaires. Only recently have questionnaires been used routinely in clinical trials in persons with PAD. Therefore, in patients with intermittent claudication, relatively little is known about the effects

of a treatment program on community-based walking ability or quality of life. Criteria by which to judge the utility of a questionnaire must therefore be established. To be useful, a questionnaire should be valid, reliable, and sensitive to change [34]. To evaluate validity, questionnaire responses may be correlated to objective measures of treadmill performance. Reliability (or reproducibility) is assessed by evaluating the stability of responses in control patients over time (i.e., at two or more separate time points). Assessment of the questionnaire's sensitivity to change (ability to discern a change in function due to an intervention) is obtained by comparing the mean values obtained at entry and exit. In addition to being valid, reliable, and sensitive to change, another important questionnaire attribute is feasibility. To be feasible, a questionnaire must be easy to administer and evaluate.

To address the need to assess functional status, we developed the Walking Impairment Questionnaire (WIQ) to assess defined walking distances, speeds, stair climbing ability, and claudication severity in this patient population [78, 79]. The WIQ has previously been used in PAD patients to evaluate changes in community-based walking ability resulting from an exercise training program and from peripheral bypass surgery [78, 78, 79]. Validity and sensitivity to change have been established in the PAD population, but reliability is still being evaluated [76, 78, 79]. Feasibility is also good for this questionnaire, which can be administered and scored in 6–8 min. The questionnaire's feasibility adds to its value for use by clinicians, epidemiologists, and health service researchers who are dealing with large populations and limited time to acquire data.

Another questionnaire used in the PAD population is the Physical Activity Recall (PAR) [78]. This questionnaire provides a more general measure of physical activity by assessing the total energy expenditure of the patient at work and during home and leisure-time activities for the preceding week [82]. The PAR has been used primarily in large population studies to evaluate habitual physical activity levels in healthy persons and in persons with diabetes [7, 77, 82, 90]. Although reliability was established in non-PAD patients for the PAR in the Five-City Project (a population study) using test-retest measures in all study sites [82], reliability has not yet been established for PAD patients. For the PAD population, the PAR has been modified to better enable measurement of the lower end of the activity scale because these patients are usually quite sedentary [78]. Sensitivity to change for the PAR has been established in the PAD population [78], whereas reliability and validity are still being evaluated. The PAR must be administered, by an interviewer, but it can be administered and scored in less than 12 min.

The Medical Outcomes Study (MOS) questionnaire evaluates physical, social, and role functioning as well as patients' perception of their general health and well-being [89]. This questionnaire has been used in population studies to evaluate functional status in a number of disease states (including cardiac) and in healthy persons [87, 89]. This self-administered questionnaire has been shown to be valid and reliable in large studies [87] and is also easy to score. We have evaluated sensitivity to change of the MOS in the PAD population; reliability and validity are still being evaluated [78].

Together, these questionnaires can be used to evaluate the impact of a variety of interventions on community-based functional status in the PAD patient with claudication. The information provided by the questionnaires is thus a valuable adjunct to the laboratory-based measures.

Physical Activity Monitors

Questionnaires are limited in that self-assessment of physical activity is subject to bias. Monitoring devices including motion sensors provide a more objective estimate of physical activity because these devices have been validated against indirect calorimetry in the laboratory setting [55, 68]. However, the use of activity monitors requires special equipment that can be costly, and places additional demands on the patient, who must be compliant with monitoring procedures. In selected small-scale trials, an activity monitor may serve to further validate the patient response to a treatment. Such an application is comparable with the use of continuous ambulatory blood pressure devices and Holter monitors in previous clinical trials. One physical activity monitor that has been used in the PAD population is the Vitalog activity monitor [55, 68], which measures activity and heart rate using simultaneous motion sensor and electrocardiogram monitoring [78]. Clearly, such devices will be used primarily in the research rather than the clinical setting given the cost and greater complexity of usage.

Summary

Measures by which to evaluate a given treatment for claudication are available. The use of hemodynamic measures, while important for establishing degree of disease severity, is not an appropriate means of evaluating functional status. The use of a graded treadmill protocol, while requiring more advanced equipment and training than a constant-load treadmill, is preferable for the purpose of measuring functional status in the PAD population because of the much higher levels of precision, accuracy, and reproducibility obtained from this type of test. Finally, specific questionnaires, appropriate for the purpose of evaluating functional status in PAD patients, will provide information on community-based functional status.

AVAILABLE NONEXERCISE TREATMENTS FOR CLAUDICATION

Before focusing discussion on exercise rehabilitation per se, it will be helpful to review briefly the other options used to treat persons with claudication. Currently, available nonexercise treatments for this purpose include risk factor modification, peripheral bypass surgery, percutaneous transluminal angioplasty, and pharmacological interventions.

Risk Factor Modification
The risk factors identified for PAD include cigarette smoking, diabetes mellitus, hypertension, hyperlipidemia (particularly a reduced high-density lipoprotein cholesterol level), abnormalities of hemostatic function and hemorheology, and abnormalities of homocysteine metabolism [9, 18, 28, 56, 57, 72, 91]. To date, the primary purpose of prescribing risk factor modification in the medical management of PAD is to alter the underlying disease process rather than to improve claudication and functional status directly. Modification of most risk factors for PAD is not associated with improving functional status. Of the major risk factors, only smoking cessation appears to improve claudication symptoms [75]. In a nonrandomized study of smokers who quit compared with those who did not, it was found that quitting was associated with a 40% increase in maximal walking distance (measured by a constant-load treadmill). Smokers who continued smoking showed no improvement in walking time.

Interventional Therapies: Surgery and Angioplasty
In patients with ischemic rest pain, ulceration, or gangrene, peripheral bypass surgery or percutaneous transluminal angioplasty is necessary for the relief of symptoms and limb preservation. Patients with incapacitatingly severe claudication that is unresponsive to other medical treatments may also be candidates for revascularization [70].

One of the primary goals of interventional therapy is to improve functional ability. However, as previously discussed, changes in exercise performance and community-based walking ability have not been evaluated extensively in most studies of patients treated with interventional therapy for claudication. In fact, the outcome most often reported for interventional therapy typically has been to achieve and maintain graft patency, as reflected by an improvement in the hemodynamics of the peripheral circulation [21, 81]. However, changes in ankle blood pressure or flow do not adequately reflect the effects of surgery on the ability to walk or to relieve claudication pain [4, 42, 71]. The few previous studies that have measured the benefit of surgery on walking performance generally have shown that exercise duration is improved during constant-load treadmill testing [63, 88]. By using a graded treadmill exercise protocol to evaluate maximal exercise capacity [42], we found an increase of 207% in pain-free walking time and an increase of 96% in maximal walking time after surgery in a group of patients with claudication [76]. Use of the WIQ questionnaire similarly revealed a substantial increase in community-based walking ability after surgical therapy [76]. In contrast, one study evaluating the effects of PTA on walking distance reported that although ABI's improved and remained improved after angioplasty over a 12-mo follow-up period, walking distance in this group was modestly improved at the 3-mo time point only.

Although interventional therapy is associated with improvements in functional status, there is a higher morbidity and mortality rate for both surgery and angioplasty than for that of other therapies [29]. In addition, costs of the interventional therapies are high [51, 93]. Thus, alternative, effective means of therapy are of value in the treatment of claudication, and in fact the majority of patients with intermittent claudication should be managed without an interventional procedure [67, 92].

Pharmacological Interventions
Recent pharmacological advances have increased the interest in the use of drugs to treat claudication with new agents in clinical development. Examples include antiplatelet and anticoagulant drugs, drugs that alter blood rheology [73], drugs that alter muscle metabolism [12, 13], and others [19]. It is outside the scope of this article to address the varying classes of drugs being investigated, so only classes of drugs that appear to alter functional status will be discussed.

Pentoxifylline, a hemorheologic agent that decreases blood viscosity, is currently the only approved drug for treating intermittent claudication. In early controlled clinical trials the drug was associated with a 22% improvement over placebo in pain-free walking distance and a 12% improvement in the maximal walking distance [73]. However, it should be noted that only constant-load testing was used to evaluate pentoxifylline, and interpretation of the results was limited by a large placebo response, as previously discussed.

Antiplatelet and anticoagulant drugs largely have been shown to be ineffective in treating claudication [17, 84, 86]. However, ticlopidine, a potent inhibitor of platelet aggregation with hemorheologic effects, was shown to improve claudication symptoms and increase walking ability by about 67% in one randomized, placebo-controlled trial, compared with an improvement of 25% in the placebo-treated group [5]. As with pentoxifylline, constant-load testing was used.

Patients with PAD not only have a limited arterial blood flow, but also develop metabolic abnormalities in their skeletal muscle. An example of altered muscle metabolism in PAD is illustrated by changes in carnitine metabolism [12, 13, 20]. Carnitine is an important cofactor for skeletal muscle intermediary metabolism during exercise. It has been hypothesized that supplementation of patients with carnitine would improve ischemic muscle metabolism and thereby increase exercise tolerance. Carnitine, and an acyl form of carnitine (propionyl-L-carnitine), are experimental drugs that have been shown to increase exercise performance and improve claudication symptoms in patients with PAD [12, 13]. However, further investigation is necessary to establish fully the role of carnitine supplementation in treating patients with claudication. Trials using graded treadmill protocols and questionnaires have been instituted for this purpose.

Summary
Interventional and pharmacological therapies have been used to treat claudication and improve walking ability. Interventional therapies are effective in increasing walking time as measured by the constant-load and graded treadmill protocols and community-based walking ability as assessed by a questionnaire in one study. However, these therapies carry higher morbidity and mortality rates than other therapies, in addition to higher costs.

Pharmacological therapies to date have been less thoroughly evaluated using the recommended testing procedures. Only recently have graded treadmill protocols and questionnaires become a part of the evaluation process. Future trials incorporating these measures will provide more information about the relative efficacy of the drugs under investigation for improving functional status in the PAD patient.

EXERCISE REHABILITATION

Background and Overview

A supervised exercise rehabilitation program is a highly effective treatment for claudication and for other cardiovascular disease such as coronary artery disease or congestive heart failure [44, 45]. Walking exercise training is associated with well-established changes in treadmill exercise performance and community-based walking ability in the person with claudication [26, 27, 44, 45, 48, 59]. Therefore, exercise training has been recommended in some form for nearly 50 years as a means to help patients with PAD improve their walking ability.

Numerous trials of exercise conditioning in this patient population have been conducted to date [2, 26, 27, 32, 48, 54, 61, 83, 85], of which the vast majority were not randomized or controlled trials. All studies of exercise conditioning in persons with PAD, whether randomized, controlled trials or not, have reported an increase in treadmill exercise performance and a lessening of claudication pain severity during exercise. Most of the previous studies evaluated changes in walking ability with a constant-load treadmill protocol. Unfortunately, data obtained from studies that use this protocol are often difficult to interpret because in some cases a large placebo effect is observed with constant-load testing; in addition, most of the studies did not use control groups. However, studies that performed testing using a graded exercise protocol and that used a control group have also shown an improvement in maximal exercise performance [44, 45]. Thus, both types of treadmill testing protocols were able to detect improvement due to exercise rehabilitation. The improvement in pain-free walking time ranged from 44% to 290%, and the maximal walking time increased from 25% to 183% in the above studies. Therefore, the ability to sustain walking exercise for longer durations with less claudication pain is improved by training. The consistency of findings discussed above demonstrates that exercise training programs have a clinically important impact on functional capacity in persons in whom spontaneous recovery does not occur.

Randomized, Controlled Trials

To date, nine randomized trials have been carried out to evaluate the efficacy of exercise rehabilitation (Table 1.1). Of these, seven had a nonexercising control group and three were randomized trials comparing exercise to an interventional therapy or active drug (where the group receiving the interventional therapy or drug can be considered the control). Seven of these trials used a constant-load treadmill protocol to evaluate walking ability and two used a graded protocol. The latter two trials have used questionnaire assessment to evaluate change in community-based functional status. These studies are reviewed in the following section.

In 1966, in the first randomized, controlled trial of exercise training in patients with PAD, 14 patients were paired and then randomized into exercise and control groups [59]. Entry and exit testing was done using a constant-load protocol with the treadmill speed at 3 mph and elevation set at an individualized grade that gave rise to claudication within 2–3 min. Patients were tested once a month using the same protocol over the 6-mo treatment phase. The exercise group was instructed to take a walk over an hour's time on a daily basis with a pedometer and record distance walked for 6-mo, whereas the placebo group took a lactose tablet twice daily. Maximal walking time increased in the exercise-treated group by 183% and pain-free walking distance by 106%. In contrast, the control group did not change maximal walking distance. In this trial, only one treadmill test was used to establish the baseline values. Because it has been reported that three tests may be required to obtain reliable baseline measurements using constant-load testing [36], the data obtained in this and other trials using constant-load treadmill testing may have some degree of variability and thus be difficult to interpret.

Three studies done in the 1970s evaluated the benefits of a program of "dynamic leg exercises" (including walking, running, dancing, and playing ball games) for improving walking ability in persons with PAD [26, 27, 48]. One of the studies [26] had only a partially randomized design, and the first 10 patients were put into a training program. The remaining 24 patients were randomized into treatment (n = 13) and control groups (n = 11). The training regimen was composed of a supervised program of dynamic leg exercises three times a week, one-half hour per session, over a 4–6 mo period in men and women with claudication. Treadmill testing was with the con-

TABLE 1.1
Summary of Randomized Controlled Trials Evaluating the Efficacy of Exercise Rehabilitation for Patients with Peripheral Arterial Disease

Author	Group	N	Intervention	Treadmill Test	Duration of Program	Functional Assessment	Change in ICD	Change in ACD
Larsen and Lassen, 1966 [59]	T	7	Daily walks	Constant-load	6 mo	No	106%*	183%*
	C	7	Placebo pill				−11%	−6%
Holm et al., 1973 [48]	T	6	Dynamic leg exercise	Constant-load	4 mo	No	220%*	133%*
	C	6	Placebo pill				No change	No change
Dahllof et al., 1974 [27]	T	23	Dynamic leg exercise	Constant-load	6 mo	No	150%*	117%*
	C	11	Placebo pill				No change	No change
Dahllof et al., 1976 [26]	T	10	Dynamic leg exercise	Constant-load	4 mo	No	170%*	135%*
	C	8	Placebo pill				120%*	75%*
Mannarino et al., 191 [64]	T1	10	Dynamic leg exercise + daily walks	Constant-load	6 mo	No	90%*	86%*
	T2	10	Exercise + antiplatelet				120%*	105%*
	T3	10	antiplatelet				35%*	38%
Lundgren et al., 1989 [63]	T1	25	Dynamic leg exercise	Constant-load	6 mo	No	179%*	151%*
	T2	25	surgery + dynamic leg exercise				698%*	263%*
Creasy et al., 1990 [22]	T3	25	Surgery	Constant-load	6 mo treatment (follow-up of 12 mo)	No	376%*	173%*
	T1	20	Exercise				296%*	442%*
Hiatt et al., 1990 [44]	T2	13	Angioplasty				21%	57%
	T	10	Walking exercise	Graded	3 mo	Yes	165%*	123%*
	C	9	Non-exercising control				6%	20%*
Hiatt et al., 1994 [45]	T	10	Walking exercise	Graded	6 mo	Yes	209%*	128%*
	C	8	Non-exercising control		3 mo		−18%	−1%

T, treat; C, control; ICD, initial claudication distance; ACD, absolute claudication distances. Functional assessment = use of questionnaire to evaluate community-based functional status, "No change" = a finding of no improvement is stated but the data are not given. For the Creasy study, the data given are for the 12-mo follow-up time point.
* = P<0.05 compared with baseline.

stant-load protocol every other week for the duration of the studies. In all three studies, treated patients improved their maximal walking distance significantly, with increases ranging from 117% to 135% and pain-free walking distance from 170% to 220%. In one of the studies [27], the control subjects had a significant improvement in maximal walking time of 75%, which was still less than the 135% achieved by the exercising group. In neither of the other two studies did the control subjects improve their exercise performance.

The effect of 6 mo of exercise training alone or combined with antiplatelet therapy (dipyridamole and aspirin) was evaluated in 30 patients with PAD [64]. A single constant-load test was used to establish baseline values and then repeated after the first, third, and sixth months. The exercise training program consisted of walking in the community daily (with increases in walking distance and time prescribed on a weekly basis), combined with a twice-a-week supervised program of dynamic leg exercises. After 6 mo of treatment, the pain-free walking time and maximal walking time improved in all three groups compared with baseline. In the group receiving drug only, maximal walking time improved by 38% and pain-free walking time by 35%. In the group receiving exercise training only, maximal walking time improved by 86% and pain-free walking time by 90%. Finally, in the group receiving both treatments, maximal walking time improved by 105% and pain-free walking time by 120%. The differences in walking time between the group receiving drug only and the two groups receiving exercise therapy were significant, but there were no differences between the two exercise groups. Again, limitations in this study result from a single baseline test, given the high coefficient of variation required to establish reliable results for constant-load testing.

Lundgren et al. [63] conducted a randomized, controlled trial comparing the effects of peripheral bypass surgery, surgery followed by 6 mo of supervised exercise training (dynamic leg exercises), or 6 mo of supervised exercise training alone on 75 patients with claudication. Constant-load treadmill testing was used in this study. It was found that at 13 mo after randomization, walking ability was improved in all three groups. In this study, the most effective treatment to improve functional status was exercise training plus surgery. The changes in maximal walking distance were 173% for the operated group, 263% for the group that received both therapies, and 151% for the exercise-trained group. The authors found that although all surgically treated patients increased their walking distance more than patients who received only exercise training, they also had a greater rate of complications than the exercise group. One problem with the study was that the authors imposed a prospectively determined treadmill distance limit, and after the intervention, the exercise performance of some patients was terminated early relative to their increased walking ability.

Another randomized study compared percutaneous transluminal angioplasty (n = 20) to a supervised program of dynamic leg exercises (n = 16) [22]. Constant-load treadmill testing was performed at 3, 6, 9 and 12 mo to evaluate change in pain-free and maximal walking distances. It was found that after angioplasty, mean ABI values were significantly improved, but only at the 3-mo time point was maximum walking distance improved over baseline. In contrast, in the exercise group, despite no improvement in the ABI, maximal and pain-free walking distances were progressively increased at each follow-up, with significant increases at 6, 9 and 12 mo. For example, pain-free walking distance increased by 296% and maximum walking distance by 442% at the 12-mo time point in the exercise-trained group.

Two randomized, controlled trials of exercise conditioning for patients with PAD have been performed using graded treadmill protocols [44, 45, 78, 79]. To summarize briefly, in the first study [44], 20 patients with walking impairment due to PAD were randomized into an exercising group or a control group. Treadmill testing, using a graded protocol, was conducted at entry, 6 wk, and 12 wk. The exercise program consisted of 3 mo of supervised treadmill walking, and the training intensity was increased progressively on a weekly basis. Each session was 1 hr long and there were three sessions per week. After 12 wk, treated subjects increased their maximal walking time by 123%, $\dot{V}O_2$max by 30%, and pain-free walking time by 165%. Control subjects had a 20% increase in maximal walking time but no change in pain-free walking time, $\dot{V}O_2$max, or any other measures of treadmill exercise performance. On entry to the training study, all patients reported significant difficulty walking defined distances and speeds as assessed by the WIQ [79]. After training, there were significant improvements in walking speed and distance only in the treated group. Thus, the training program also allowed the patients to return to a more active life-style. In addition to our initial findings, we also found that when patients maintained an exercise program, benefits were also maintained over a 9-mo follow-up period [43].

In a more recent trial [45, 78], 29 patients with disabling claudication were randomized to one of two exercise programs or a control group. Both graded and constant-load tests were used. Graded tests were primarily used to evaluate change in functional status, whereas constant-load protocols were used to measure walking efficiency and metabolic parameters (see section on potential mechanisms for improvement). In addition to testing the value of treadmill training, a secondary goal was to investigate strength training as an alternative mode of exercise training in the PAD population. The testing of strength training as a therapeutic mode for PAD was based on the finding of muscle weakness in the legs of PAD patients [80]. The trial was designed to last for a total of 24 wk, with crossover at 12 wk from one treatment to another, based on consideration of the types of training involved. Patients initially received either 12 wk of supervised walking exercise on a treadmill, 12 wk of strength training (3 hr per wk of resistance training) or 12 wk of a nonexercising control group [45]. At the 12-wk time point, the first 12 wk of treadmill training were followed by 12 additional wk of treadmill training. Twelve weeks of strength training were followed by 12 wk of treadmill training, and 12 wk of being a nonexercising control subject were followed by a combined strength and treadmill program for 12 wk.

After the first 12 wk, patients in the treadmill-trained group had a 74 ± 58% increase in maximal walking time as well as improvements in maximal oxygen consumption and a prolonged pain-free walking time. In terms of functional status, the PAR score increased by 31 ± 35% and the MOS score improved from 38 ± 29% to 66 ± 19% (both P<0.05) [78]. After 12 more weeks of treadmill exercise in this group a total 128% increase in maximal walking time had occurred and the Vitalog score had improved. Improvements in the PAR and the MOS scores were maintained, and the ability to walk distances and climb stairs (WIQ) was improved as well.

After 12 wk of strength training, patients improved maximal walking time but no other marker of treadmill exercise performance. Fewer benefits to functional status measured by questionnaire resulted from strength training than with the treadmill-trained group. Treadmill training after 12 wk of strength training resulted in increases in maximal exercise performance similar, but not greater than those observed with 12 wk of treadmill training alone.

Control subjects showed no change in treadmill or community-based functional variables. The combined strength and treadmill training program that the control subjects received after the first 12 wk caused improvements in maximal exercise performance similar to, but not greater than, those observed with 12 wk of treadmill training alone, with minimal benefits to functional status measured by questionnaire.

We concluded that a supervised, treadmill walking exercise program was an effective means to improve exercise performance and functional status in patients with intermittent claudication, with continued improvement over 24 wk of training. In contrast, 12 wk of strength training alone were less effective than 12 wk of supervised treadmill walking exercise. Finally, strength training, whether sequential or concomitant, did not augment the response to a supervised walking exercise program.

The two last trials discussed above illustrate that exercise training is an effective means of improving community-based functional status in the PAD patient with claudication. The value of using questionnaires to assess community-based functional status was also demonstrated. The use of questionnaires allow the clinical investigator to determine whether an intervention has a beneficial impact on the everyday or community-based activities of the patient.

Exercise Training-Specific Methods
In persons with PAD, early descriptions of exercise therapy consisted of advice to take daily walks. This was to be done at an intensity below the thresh-

old of claudication pain, and exercise was to cease at the onset of pain [35]. These basic recommendations for physical activity were never formally evaluated in terms of the potential benefit to the patient, but did serve to increase the awareness of the importance of exercise in these persons. Subsequent studies of exercise training were conducted in a supervised (usually hospital) setting, with the walking exercise performed on a treadmill [26, 27, 48, 83] or under the direction of a physiotherapist [27, 30, 32]. This allowed a specific exercise intensity to be prescribed that was usually sufficient to bring on at least mild to moderate claudication pain [2, 30, 44, 95]. Each bout of exercise lasted from 5 to 10 min, followed by a rest period to allow the claudication pain to subside. These exercise and rest sessions were repeated for 30–60 min, 2–3 times a week for a total duration of 3–6 mo. Training programs lasting up to 1 yr have been described, but there is no evidence that supervised exercise training of this duration produces better results than programs of shorter duration [32, 61]. In addition to treadmill walking exercise, other activities have been incorporated into the training sessions of some programs. Examples include "dynamic" exercises of the leg (combination of walking, running, bicycling, and dancing) [26, 27, 48], isotonic exercise of specific muscle groups [8, 95], bicycle exercise [52, 53, 95], gymnastic exercise [32, 54], stair climbing, and unsupervised walking in the community [2].

In contrast to other types of therapy for claudication, exercise training has the characteristic of being highly participatory for the patient. Patients in an exercise training program must spend considerable blocks of time participating in a training program to derive benefit. This is in contrast to an interventional therapy in which the patient, outside of consenting to the procedure, is more of a passive participant. It is also in contrast to pharmacological therapy, in which the patient's involvement is limited to taking a medication.

The most utilized and effective mode of exercise therapy for PAD to date has been treadmill walking exercise in a hospital-based setting. In our institution, a patient is enrolled in a exercise rehabilitation program after entry assessment of exercise performance and functional status (as described previously) has been completed [44]. Exercise sessions are typically held three times a week for approximately 1 hr each, and 3-mo periods of training are customary. On the initial visit, the patient is instructed in the use of the telemetry monitors if monitoring is desired to evaluate heart rate response, or required, as in the case of the subgroup who have ongoing cardiac ischemia in addition to PAD. A 5-min warm-up period precedes treadmill walking exercise, and a 5-min cool-down follows it to minimize risk of injury. The warm-up period is designed to increase the heart rate slowly and promote flexibility, and should involve the use of large muscle groups, especially those muscles used for walking. The cool-down period is designed to return the heart rate to baseline values and primarily involves stretching of the large muscle groups, particularly those in the legs.

The beginning training work load is determined from the symptom-limited maximal treadmill test on entry, such that the intensity of the treadmill exercise is set to the workload that initially brings on claudication pain in the patient. In subsequent visits, the speed or grade is increased if the patient is able to walk for 8–10 min or longer at the lower workload without reaching moderate claudication pain. Either speed or grade can be increased, but in our program, we increase grade first if the patient can already walk at 2 mph. If the patient's initial speed of walking is less than 2 mph, we increase speed first. One of the goals of our program is to increase patient walking speed up to the normal 3.0 mph, from the average PAD patient walking speed of 1.5–2.0 mph.

The goal of the initial training session is for the patient to spend 35 min performing intermittent treadmill exercise exclusive of the warm-up and cool-down periods, with subsequent increases of 5 min each session until a 50-min exercise session is possible. During the exercise sessions, rest periods (induced by claudication) are interspersed between bouts of treadmill walking. The patient walks on the treadmill until a mild or moderate level of pain is reached (scored as 3 or 4 on a 1 to 5 scale, where 1 equals no pain and 5 is maximal pain). At that point, the patient sits and rests until the pain abates. After the pain is gone, the patient resumes walking until a mild or moderate level of pain is reached again, followed by another rest period. This process is repeated until the 50-min exercise period has elapsed. Our experience has been that (after patients become somewhat conditioned) of the 50-min period, walking on the treadmill comprises about 35 min and rest periods total about 15 min [44].

Precautions
In our previous experience of treadmill training in more than 100 patients, no patient has suffered a cardiovascular complication. Five patients have reported an exacerbation of existing musculoskeletal problems (i.e., knee stiffness). For the most part, patients have tolerated exercise training well. However, the potential for an adverse event exists in any exercise program, especially one in which a diseased group of patients is involved. There are two main types of problems to be concerned with: cardiovascular and musculoskeletal. First, a cardiovascular complication is possible in PAD patients because they have a high prevalence of cardiac disease as well as PAD. To promote safety, all patients in out programs with clinical evidence of comorbid coronary disease are telemetry monitored during exercise sessions to evaluate heart rate and cardiac rhythm during exercise, and blood pressure is recorded before and after each training session.

EXERCISE REHABILITATION—POTENTIAL MECHANISMS FOR IMPROVEMENT

Although recent studies have confirmed the efficacy of a supervised program of graded treadmill walking for persons with claudication, the mechanism(s) through which regular exercise exerts its beneficial effects remain incompletely delineated. Discussed below are the potentially important mechanisms for improvement that are under investigation. These include adaptations in peripheral blood flow or distribution of flow, changes in muscle metabolism, or changes in gait and pain threshold that may account for the improvement in exercise performance with training.

Peripheral Blood Flow

Exercise training in animals with arterial occlusions has been associated with increases in collateral blood flow, and a redistribution of flow toward fast-twitch glycolytic fibers [66]. In human studies, peripheral blood flow primarily has been measured postexercise or with reactive hyperemia. With training, five studies have shown an increase in maximal flow, but in two, the changes in flow were modest and not correlated to changes in exercise performance [2, 3, 32, 44, 63]. Many more studies have not shown an increase in peripheral flow with training [27, 30, 48, 53, 59, 64, 65, 95]. Importantly, these studies show no relationship between any changes in flow and exercise performance. However, in humans, other modifications of flow may occur. For example, a decrease in blood viscosity [33] or an increase in capillary density may alter the exchange of oxygen and substrate at the capillary/muscle fiber interface. Therefore, despite a lack of evidence for a substantive increase in total flow to the lower extremities, changes in the distribution of flow, capillary surface area, and blood hemorheology may improve oxygen delivery.

Muscle Metabolism

In normal subjects, exercise training leads to an improvement in oxidative metabolism of skeletal muscle. Evidence for this adaptation is an increase in aerobic, mitochondrial enzyme activity from muscle biopsy specimens related to an increase in mitochondrial protein content [47]. These changes are associated with an improvement in the extraction of oxygen and substrate during exercise.

In humans, it has been postulated that the presence of a chronic state of arterial insufficiency may lead to changes in the metabolic state of muscle [50]. However, studies that have evaluated the activity of oxidative or glycolytic enzymes in skeletal muscle in these patients have not always shown an increase in enzyme activity [40, 80]. Furthermore, in patients with PAD, it has been seen that enzyme activities do not correlate with changes resulting from exercise training in the PAD population, so that increases or decreases in the activity of a given enzyme may not affect walking ability [80].

Another metabolic adaptation relates to changes in carnitine metabolism with exercise training. Under normal metabolic conditions, carnitine is required for transportation of long-chain fatty acyl groups into mitochondria. Under abnormal metabolic conditions, such as muscle ischemia, carnitine interacts with the cellular acyl-CoA pool to form acylcarnitines and remove a variety of acyl groups derived from the corresponding acyl-CoA intermediates [6]. Under these conditions, the formation of acylcarnitines reflects the underlying metabolic state of the cellular acyl-CoA pool [11], and may serve to maintain normal metabolism by removing potentially toxic acyl groups [10].

Exercise to claudication pain has been associated with an increase in the muscle concentration of acylcarnitines, which reflects the disordered metabolic state of ischemic muscle [46]. We have previously observed that exercise training reduced the plasma concentration of short-chain acylcarnitines, and treated subjects who had the greatest response to training also had the greatest reduction in the plasma short-chain acylcarnitine concentration [44]. Studies are currently in progress to determine whether any training-induced changes in muscle carnitine metabolism are associated with improved functional status in the patient with claudication.

Gait and Pain Perception
An additional possible mechanism of improvement in walking ability with training may be a change in gait or pain threshold. Measurements of patients' walking speed, step frequency, and other aspects of gait have not been made in training studies. However, we found that oxygen consumption for a given *constant* workload decreased after exercise training [44, 45]. If the onset of claudication is due to a mismatch of oxygen delivery to oxygen demand, the lower oxygen consumption per workload may be associated with the ability to walk longer after exercise training. This observation suggests that a change in the biomechanics of walking with training improves walking efficiency and decreases the energy requirements of a given work load in PAD. Although the oxygen consumption/workload relationship is not altered by training in normal elderly people [74], it is altered in a similar way to that observed in PAD patients in cardiac patients [1]. Thus, although the constant-load treadmill is not recommended for measuring change in maximal exercise performance, it remains a valuable research tool for use in measuring exercise efficiency and some metabolic parameters during exercise.

SUMMARY

Intermittent claudication, resulting from PAD, impairs functional status. Reducing the disability resulting from the disease is therefore an important goal of treatment. To evaluate the efficacy of an intervention designed to improve functional status requires that appropriate outcome measures be developed to assess all treatments. Such outcome measures include graded treadmill testing and questionnaire assessment. These methodologies are important because they have a high degree of precision and accuracy and are practical and reproducible. Thus, functional status changes resulting from any intervention can be evaluated, and interventions can be compared with one another using the same methodologies.

Currently, interventional therapies are often used to treat a portion of patients with claudication [49]. Such therapies restore blood flow and improve functional status, but with a high associated cost: morbidity and mortality. Pharmacological therapies currently are being developed, but the role of drugs in the overall management of claudication needs further study. Importantly, exercise therapy has been shown in numerous studies to be efficacious and very well tolerated by patients. Patients improve both their walking ability in the laboratory and their community-based functional status. Because of the efficacy of this treatment, in addition to the low associated morbidity, exercise therapy is recommended as a major treatment option for persons with intermittent claudication due to PAD.

ACKNOWLEDGMENTS

Dr. Hiatt is the recipient of an NIH Academic Award in Vascular Disease. We thank the patients with PAD who have participated in our various studies. Melanie Hargarten and Katherine Barriga conducted the exercise rehabilitation classes for all patients in our trials.

REFERENCES

1. Ades, P.A., M.L. Waldmann, E.T. Poehlman, et al. Exercise conditioning in older coronary patients. Submaximal lactate response and endurance capacity. *Circulation* 88:572–577, 1993.
2. Alpert, J.S., O.A. Larsen, and N.A. Lassen. Exercise and intermittent claudication. Blood flow in the calf-muscle during walking studied by the xenon-133 clearance method. *Circulation* 39:353–359, 1969.
3. Andriessen, M.P.H.M., G.J. Barendsen, A.A. Wouda, and L. de Pater. Changes of walking distance in patients with intermittent claudication during six months intensive physical training. *Vasa* 18:63–68, 1989.
4. Arfvidsson, B., A. Wennmalm, J. Gelin, A.G. Dahllof, B. Hallgren, and K. Lundholm. Co-variation between walking ability and circulatory alterations in patients with intermittent claudication. *Eur. J. Vasc. Surg.* 6:642–646, 1992.
5. Balsano, F., S. Coccheri, A. Libretti, et al. Ticlopidine in the treatment of intermittent claudication: a 21-month double-blind trial. *J. Lab. Clin. Med.* 114:84–91, 1989.
6. Bieber, L.L., R. Emaus, K. Valkner, and S. Farrell. Possible functions of short-chain and medium-chain carnitine acyltransferases. *Fed. Proc.* 41:2858–2862, 1982.
7. Blair, S.N., W.L. Haskell, R.S. Paffenbarger, K.M. Vranizan, J.W. Farquhar, and P.D. Wood.

Assessment of habitual physical activity by a seven-day recall in a community survey and controlled experiments. *Am. J. Epidemiol.* 122:794–804, 1985.

8. Blumchen, G., F. Landry, H. Kiefer, and V. Schlosser. Hemodynamic responses of claudicating extremities. Evaluation of a long range exercise program. *Cardiology* 55:114–127, 1970.

9. Brand, F.N., R.D. Abbott, and W.B. Kannel. Diabetes, intermittent claudication, and risk of cardiovascular events. *Diabetes* 38:504–509, 1989.

10. Brass, E.P., P.V. Fennessey, and L.V. Miller. Inhibition of oxidative metabolism by propionic acid and its reversal by carnitine in isolated rate hepatocytes. *Biochem. J.* 236:131–136, 1986.

11. Brass, E.P., and C.L. Hoppel. Relationship between acid-soluble carnitine and coenzyme A pools in vivo. *Biochem. J.* 190:495–504, 1980.

12. Brevetti, G., M. Chiariello, G. Ferulano, et al. Increases in walking distance in patients with peripheral vascular disease treated with L-carnitine: a double-blind, cross-over study. *Circulation* 77:767–773, 1988.

13. Brevetti, G., S. Perna, C. Sabba, et al. Superiority of L-propionyl carnitine vs L-carnitine in improving walking capacity in patients with peripheral vascular disease: An acute, intravenous, double-blind, cross-over study. *Eur. Heart J.* 13:251–255, 1992.

14. Carter, S.A. Clinical measurement of systolic pressures in limbs with arterial occlusive disease. *J.A.M.A.* 207:1869–1874, 1969.

15. Carter, S.A., E.R., Hamel, J.M. Paterson, C.J. Snow, and D. Mymin. Walking ability and ankle systolic pressures: observations in patients with intermittent claudication in a short-term walking exercise program. *J. Vasc. Surg.* 10:642–649, 1989.

16. Clyne, C.A.C., A. Tripolitis, C.W. Jamieson, R. Gustave, and F. Stuart. The reproducibility of the treadmill walking test for claudication. *Surg. Gynecol. Obstet.* 149:727–728, 1979.

17. Coffman, J.D. Vasodilator drugs in peripheral vascular disease. *N. Engl. J. Med.* 300:713–717, 1979.

18. Coleridge-Smith, P.D., P. Thomas, J.H. Scurr, and J.A. Dormandy. Causes of venous ulceration: a new hypothesis. *Br. Med. J.* 296:1726–1727, 1988.

19. Cook, N.S., M.Rudin, C. Pally, S. Blarer, and U. Quast. Effects of the potassium channel openers SDZ-PCO 400 and cromakalim in an in vivo rat model of occlusive arterial disease assessed by 31P-NMR spectroscopy. *J. Vasc. Med. Biol.* 4:14–22, 1993.

20. Coto, V., L. D'Alessandro, G. Grattarola, et al. Evaluation of the therapeutic efficacy and tolerability of levocarnitine propionyl in the treatment of chronic obstructive arteriopathies of the lower extremities: a multicentre controlled study vs. placebo. *Drugs Exp. Clin. Res.* 18:29–36, 1992.

21. Crawford, E.S., R.A. Bomberger, D.H. Glaeser, S.A. Saleh, and W.L. Russell. Aortoiliac occlusive disease: factors influencing survival and function following reconstructive operation over a twenty-five-year period. *Surgery* 90:1055–1067, 1981.

22. Creasy, T.S., P.J. McMillan, E.W.L. Fletcher, J. Collin, and P.J. Morris. Is percutaneous transluminal angioplasty better than exercise for claudication? Preliminary results from a prospective randomised trial. *Eur. J. Vasc. Surg.* 4:135–140, 1990.

23. Criqui, M.H., S.S. Coughlin, and A. Fronek. Noninvasively diagnosed peripheral arterial disease as a predictor of mortality: results from a prospective study. *Circulation* 72:768–773, 1985.

24. Criqui, M.H., A. Fronek, E. Barrett-Connor, M.R. Klauber, S. Gabriel, and D. Goodman. The prevalence of peripheral arterial disease in a defined population. *Circulation* 71:510–515, 1985.

25. Criqui, M.H., R.D. Langer, A. Fronek, et al. Mortality over a period of 10 years in patients with peripheral arterial disease. *N. Engl. J. Med.* 326:381–386, 1992.

26. Dahllof, A., P. Bjorntorp, J. Holm, and T. Schersten. Metabolic activity of skeletal muscle in patients with peripheral arterial insufficiency. Effect of physical training. *Eur. J. Clin. Invest.* 4:9–15, 1974.

27. Dahllof, A., J. Holm, T. Schersten, and R. Sivertsson. Peripheral arterial insufficiency. Effect of physical training on walking tolerance, calf blood flow, and blood flow resistance. *Scand. J. Rehabil. Med.* 8:19–26, 1976.
28. Dormandy, J.A., E. Hoare, A.H. Khattab, D.E. Arrowsmith, and T.L. Dormandy. Prognostic significance of rheological and biochemical findings in patients with intermittent claudication. *Br. Med. J.* 4:581–583, 1973.
29. Doubilet, P., and H.L. Abrams. The cost of underutilization. Percutaneous transluminal angioplasty for periperal vascular disease. *N. Engl. J. Med.* 310:95–102, 1984.
30. Ekroth, R., A. Dahllof, B. Gundevall, J. Holm, and T. Schersten. Physical training of patients with intermittent claudication: indications, methods, and results. *Surgery* 84:640–643, 1978.
31. Eldridge, J.E., and K.F. Hossack. Patterns of oxygen consumption during exercise testing in peripheral vascular disease. *Cardiology* 74:236–240, 1987.
32. Ericsson, B., K. Haeger, and S.E. Lindell. Effect of physical training on intermittent claudication. *Angiology* 21:188–192, 1970.
33. Ernst, E.E.W., and A. Matrai. Intermittent claudication, exercise, and blood rheology. *Circulation* 76:1110–1114, 1987.
34. Feinstein, A.R. *Clinimetrics.* New Haven: Yale University Press, 1987.
35. Foley, W.T., and I.S. Wright. Medical management of arterial occlusion and thrombophlebitis. *Mod. Concepts, Cardiovasc. Dis.* 22:162–165, 1953.
36. Gardner, A.W., J.S. Skinner, B.W. Cantwell, and L.K. Smith. Progressive vs single-stage treadmill tests for evaluation of claudication. *Med. Sci. Sports Exerc.* 23:402–408, 1991.
37. Gardner, A.W., J.S. Skinner, N.R. Vaughn, C.X. Bryant, and L.K. Smith. Comparison of three progressive exercise protocols in peripheral vascular occlusive disease. *Angiology* 43:661–671, 1992.
38. Greenland, P., and J.S. Chu. Efficacy of cardiac rehabilitation services with emphasis on patients after myocardial infarction. *Ann. Intern. Med.* 109:650–663, 1988.
39. Haskell, W.L., A.S. Leon, C.J. Caspersen, et al. Cardiovascular benefits and assessment of physical activity and physical fitness in adults. *Med. Sci. Sports Exerc.* 24:S201–S220, 1993.
40. Henriksson, J., E. Nygaard, J. Andersson, and B. Eklof. Enzyme activities, fibre types and capillarization in calf muscles of patients with intermittent claudication. *Scand. J. Clin. Lab. Invest.* 40:361–369, 1980
41. Hiatt, W.R., J.A. Marshall, J. Baxter, et al. Diagnostic methods for peripheral arterial disease in the San Luis Valley Diabetes Study. *J. Clin. Epidemiol.* 43:597–606, 1990.
42. Hiatt, W.R., D. Nawaz, J.G. Regensteiner, and K.F. Hossack. The evaluation of exercise performance in patients with peripheral vascular disease. *J. Cardiopulmonary Rehabil.* 12:525–532, 1988.
43. Hiatt, W.R., and J.G. Regensteiner. Exercise rehabilitation in the treatment of patients with peripheral arterial disease. *J. Vasc. Med. Biol.* 2:163–170, 1990.
44. Hiatt, W.R., J.G. Regensteiner, M.E. Hargarten, E.E. Wolfel, and E.P. Brass. Benefit of exercise conditioning for patients with peripheral arterial disease. *Circulation* 81:602–609, 1990.
45. Hiatt, W.R., E.E. Wolfel, R.H. Meier, and J.G. Regensteiner. Superiority of treadmill walking exercise vs. strength training for patients with peripheral arterial disease. Implications for the mechanism of the training response. *Circulation* 1994, in press.
46. Hiatt, W.R., E.E. Wolfel, J.G. Regensteiner, and E.P. Brass. Skeletal muscle carnitine metabolism in patients with unilateral peripheral arterial disease. *J. Appl. Physiol.* 73:346–353, 1992.
47. Holloszy, J.O., and E.F. Coyle. Adaptations of skeletal muscle to endurance exercise and their metabolic consequences. *J. Appl. Physiol.* 56:831–838, 1984.
48. Holm, J., A. Dahllof, P. Bjorntorp, and T. Schersten. Enzyme studies in muscles of patients with intermittent claudication. Effect of training. *Scand. J. Clin. Lab. Invest.* 31 (suppl 128): 201–205, 1973.

49. Isner, J.M., and K. Rosenfield. Redefining the treatment of peripheral artery disease. Role of percutaneous revascularization. *Circulation* 88:1534–1557, 1993.

50. Jansson, E., J. Johansson, C. Sylven, and L. Kaijser. Calf muscle adapatation in intermittent claudication. Side-differences in msucle metabolic characteristics in patients with unilateral arterial disease. *Clin. Physiol.* 8:17–29, 1988.

51. Jeans, W.D., R.M. Danton, R.N. Baird and M. Horrocks. A comparison of the costs of vascular surgery and balloon dilatation in lower limb ischaemic disease. *Br. J. Radiol.* 59:453–456. 1986.

52. Jonason, T., and I. Ringqvist. Prediction of the effect of training on the walking tolerance in patients with intermittent claudication. *Scand. J. Rehabil. Med.* 19:47–50, 1987.

53. Jonason, T., and I. Ringqvist. Effect of training on the post-exercise ankle blood pressure reaction in patients with intermittent claudication. *Clin. Physiol.* 7:63–69, 1987.

54. Jonason, T., I. Ringqvist, and A. Oman-Rydberg. Home-training of patients with intermittent claudication. *Scand. J. Rehabil. Med.* 13:137–141, 198.

55. Juneau, M., F. Rogers, V. de Santos, et al. Effectiveness of self-monitored, home-based, moderate-intensity exercise training in middle-age men and women. *Am. J. Cardiol.* 60:66–70, 1987.

56. Kannel, W.B., and D.L. McGee. Diabetes and cardiovascular disease. The Framingham Study. *J.A.M.A.* 241:2035–2038, 1979.

57. Kannel, W.B., and D.L. McGee. Update on some epidemiologic features of intermittent claudication: The Framingham Study. *J. Am. Geriatr. Soc.* 33:13–18, 1985.

58. Laing, S., and R.M. Greenhalgh. Treadmill testing in the assessment of peripheral arterial disease. *Int. Angiol.* 5:249–252, 1986.

59. Larsen, O.A., and N.A. Lassen. Effect of daily muscular exercise in patients with intermittent claudication. *Lancet* 2:1093–1096, 1966.

60. Lassila, R., M. Lepantalo, and O. Lindfors. Peripheral arterial disease-natural outcome. *Acta Med. Scand.* 220:295–301, 1986.

61. Lepantalo, M., S. Sundberg, and A. Gordin. The effects of physical training and flunarizine on walking capacity in intermittent claudication. *Scand. J. Rehabil. Med.* 16:159–162, 1984.

62. Lindgarde, F., R. Jelnes, H. Bjorkman, et al. Conservative drug treatment in patients with moderately severe chronic occlusive peripheral arterial disease. *Circulation* 80:1549–1556, 1989.

63. Lundgren, F., A. Dahllof, K. Lundholm, T. Schersten, and R. Volkmann. Intermittent claudication–surgical reconstruction or physical training? A prospective randomized trial of treatment efficiency. *Ann. Surg.* 209:346–355, 1989.

64. Mannarino, E., L. Pasqualini, S. Innocente, V. Scricciolo, A. Rignanese, and G. Ciufetti. Physical training and antiplatelet treatment in stage II peripheral arterial occlusive disease: alone or combined? *Angiology* 42:513–521, 1991.

65. Mannarino, E., L. Pasqualini, M. Menna, G. Maragoni, and U. Orlandi. Effects of physical training on peripheral vascular disease: a controlled study. *Angiology* 40:5–10, 1989.

66. Mathien, G.M., and R.L. Terjung. Influence of training following bilateral stenosis of the femoral artery in rats. *Am. J. Physiol.* 250:H1050–H1059, 1986.

67. McAllister, F.F. The fate of patients with intermittent claudication managed nonoperatively. *Am. J. Surg.* 132:593–595, 1976.

68. Mueller, J.K., D. Gossard, F.R. Adams, et al. Assessment of prescibed increases in physical activity: application of a new method for microprocessor analysis of heart rate. *Am. J. Cardiol.* 57:441–445, 1986.

69. Patterson, J.A., J. Naughton, R.J. Pietras, and R.M. Gunnar. Treadmill exercise in assessment of the functional capacity of patients with cardiac disease. *Am. J. Cardiol.* 30:757–762, 1972.

70. Pentecost, M.J., M.H. Criqui, G. Dorros, et al. Guidelines for peripheral percutaneous transluminal angioplasty of the abdominal aorta and lower extremity vessels. *Circulation* 89:511–531, 1994.

71. Pernow, B., and S. Zetterquist. Metabolic evaluation of the leg blood flow in claudicating patients with arterial obstructions at different levels. *Scand. J. Clin. Lab.* Invest. *21:277–287, 1968.*

72. Pomrehn, P., B. Duncan, L. Weissfeld, et al. The association of dyslipoproteinemia with symptoms and signs of peripheral arterial disease. The lipids research clinics program prevalence study. *Circulation* 73(suppl I):1–100–1–107, 1986.

73. Porter, J.M., B.S. Cutler, B.Y. Lee, et al. Pentoxifylline efficacy in the treatment of intermittent claudication: multicenter controlled double-blind trial with objective assessment of chronic occlusive arterial disease patients. *Am. Heart J.* 104:66–72, 1982.

74. Poulin, M.J., D.H. Paterson, D. Govindasamy, and D.A. Cunningham. Endurance training of older men: responses to submaximal exercise. *J. Appl. Physiol.* 73:452–457, 1992.

75. Quick, C.R.G., and L.T. Cotton. The measured effect of stopping smoking on intermittent claudication. *Br. J. Surg.* 69 (suppl):S24–S26, 1982.

76. Regensteiner, J.G., M.E. Hargarten, R.B. Rutherford, and W.R. Hiatt. Functional benefits of peripheral vascular bypass surgery for patients with intermittent claudication. *Angiology* 44:1–10, 1993.

77. Regensteiner, J.G., E.J. Mayer, S.M. Shetterly, et al. Relationship between physical activity and hyperinsulinemia among nondiabetic men and women. The San Luis Valley Diabetes Study. *Diabetes Care* 14:1066–1074, 1991.

78. Regensteiner, J.G., J.F. Steiner, and W.R. Hiatt. Exercise training improves functional status in patients with peripheral arterial disease (PAD). *Clin. Res.* 42:294A, 1994.

79. Regensteiner, J.G., J.F. Steiner, R.J. Panzer, and W.R. Hiatt. Evaluation of walking impairment by questionnaire in patients with peripheral arterial disease. *J. Vasc. Med. Biol.* 2:142–152, 1990.

80. Regensteiner, J.G., E.E. Wolfel, E.P. Brass, et al. Chronic changes in skeletal muscle histology and function in peripheral arterial disease. *Circulation* 87:413–421, 1993.

81. Reichle, R.A., K.P. Rankin, R.R. Tyson, A.S. Finestone, and C.R. Shuman. Long-term results of femoroinfrapopliteal bypass in diabetic patients with severe ischemia of the lower extremity. *Am. J. Surg.* 137:653–656, 1979.

82. Sallis, J.F., W.L. Haskell, P.D. Wood, et al. Physical activity assessment methodology in the five-city project. *Am. J. Epidemiol.* 121:91–106, 1985.

83. Skinner, J.S. and D.E. Strandness. Exercise and intermittent claudication. II. Effect of physical training. *Circulation* 36:23–29, 1967.

84. Solomon, S.A., L.E. Ramsay, W.W. Yeo, L. Parnell, and W. Morris-Jones. B blockade and intermittent claudication: placebo-controlled trial of atenolol and nifedipine and their combination. *Br. Med. J.* 303:1100–1104, 1991.

85. Sorlie, D., and K. Myhre. Effects of physical training in intermittent claudication. *Scand. J. Clin. Lab. Invest.* 38:217–222, 1978.

86. Spence, J.D., J.M.O. Arnold, C.E. Munoz, et al. Angiotensin-converting enzyme inhibition with cliazapril does not improve blood flow, walking time, or plasma lipids in patients with intermittent claudication. *J. Vasc. Med. Biol.* 4:23–28, 1993.

87. Stewart, A.L., S. Greenfield, R.D. Hays, et al. Functional status and well-being of patients with chronic conditions: results from the Medical Outcomes Study. *J.A.M.A.* 262:907–913, 1989.

88. Strandness, D.E. Functional results after revascularization of the profunda femoris artery. *Am. J. Surg.* 119:240–245, 1970.

89. Tarlov, A.R., J.E. Ware, S. Greenfield, E.C. Nelson, E. Perrin, and M. Zubkoff. The medical outcomes study. An application of methods for monitoring the results of medical care. *J.A.M.A.* 262:925–930, 1989.

90. Taylor, C.B., T. Coffey, K. Berra, R. Iaffaldano, K. Casey, and W.L. Haskell. Seven day activity and self-report compared to a direct measure of physical activity. *Am. J. Epidemiol.* 120:818–824, 1984.

91. Taylor, L.M., R.D. DeFrang, E.J. Harris, and J.M. Porter. The association of elevated

plasma homocyst(e)ine with progression of symptomatic peripheral arterial disease. *J. Vasc. Surg.* 13:128–136, 1991.

92. Thompson, J.E., and W.V. Garrett. Peripheral-arterial surgery. *N. Engl. J. Med.* 302:491–503, 1980.

93. Tunis, S.R., E.B. Bass, and E.P. Steinberg. The use of angioplasty, bypass surgery, and amputation in the management of peripheral vascular disease. *N. Engl. J. Med.* 325:556–562, 1991.

94. Whipp, B.J., J.A. Davis, F. Torres, and K. Wasserman. A test to determine parameters of aerobic function during exercise. *J. Appl. Physiol.* 50:217–221, 1981.

95. Zetterquist, S. The effect of active training on the nutritive blood flow in exercising ischemic legs. *Scand. J. Clin. Lab. Invest.* 25:101–111, 1970.

2
Integration of the Physiological Factors Determining Endurance Performance Ability

EDWARD F. COYLE, Ph.D.

This chapter presents a model of the physiological factors that determine endurance performance ability in sports such as distance running, bicycling, and race-walking. The objective is to integrate the many physiological variables that individually have been correlated with endurance performance ability to a reasonable model. This model has developed from a series of eight studies performed by the author and his laboratory colleagues over the course of the last two decades [11, 13–15, 19, 25, 31, 38]. This chapter is not meant to be a comprehensive review of the vast literature and information in this area, which has been recently summarized [36, 55]. The positive aspect of following one group's approach is that their data can be used as the framework to develop an integrated model. The negative aspect is that it presents a limited and inherently biased view.

This review will first introduce the model and define its terminology. Thereafter, it will generally take a chronological approach in integrating the sequential research findings, with the goal of providing students with insights not normally obtained from separate papers. The model centers around two very important functional abilities, and we think we have identified certain previously unrecognized morphological components that exert important influence on these abilities. First, we think that the degree of muscle and blood lactate accumulation during cycling is influenced by the amount of muscle mass sharing in the distribution of power output [13]. Second, the oxygen cost or *Economy* of movement as well as gross mechanical efficiency appears to be determined largely by muscle fiber type composition, with Type I fibers being much more efficient than Type II fibers [15]. *Endurance Performance Ability* is the sum and interaction of these many factors and every person is unique in his or her pattern of physiological attributes.

THE INTEGRATED MODEL

Figure 2.1 presents the model of the interrelationship of the physiological factors that determine endurance *Performance Ability,* which can be assessed in several ways. In athletics, success is determined by the *Performance Velocity* maintained for a given distance. With the instrumentation provided by lab-

FIGURE 2.1.

Hypothetical model of the interrelationships of the physiological factors determining endurance performance ability. Terms are defined in the text.

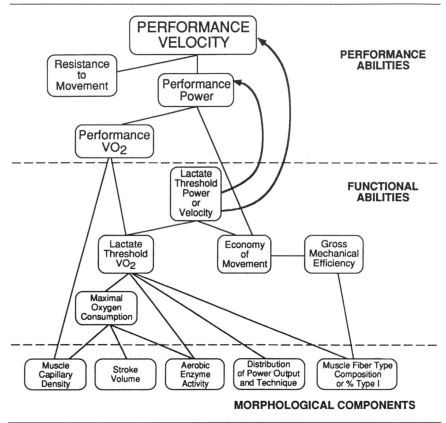

oratory studies, performance can also be assessed by the *Performance Power* output maintained for a given time or by the energy expenditure determined from oxygen consumption (i.e., *Performance VO_2*).

These *Performance Abilities* are the product of certain discrete *Functional Abilities*. One ability is characterized by identifying the degree of muscular metabolic stress from measurements of the *Lactate Threshold* and another by measuring *Maximal Oxygen Consumption*. The other *Functional Ability* relates to *Economy of Movement* as defined by the oxygen cost for a given activity, which can also be termed *Gross Mechanical Efficiency* when power is quantified. These *Functional Abilities* displayed by people during exercise are made possible by the possession of certain physical characteristics, termed *Morphological Components*. Generally, these are anatomical factors describing the structure of muscle, as well as the cardiovascular system. The lines connecting the boxes in Fig. 2.1, and thus suggesting a cause-and-effect relationship, will be supported with direct data from the various studies. The components of this model are displayed in *italic* typeface throughout the text.

DEFINITIONS

Performance Abilities

PERFORMANCE VELOCITY. This is simply the average speed that an athlete maintains for a given racing distance (i.e., velocity = distance/time). *Performance Velocity* is a function of the *Performance Power* of propulsion and the forces that present *Resistance to Movement* (e.g., drag).

RESISTANCE TO MOVEMENT. This is the drag encountered by the athlete and equipment while moving through the environment. The nature of the resistance or drag or friction on the athlete will vary according to the environmental medium and velocity achieved. For example, when bicycling at 40 km/hr, approximately 90% of the power generated is used to overcome air drag [44]. Therefore, the more aerodynamic the bicyclist and equipment, the faster the velocity for a given power production. Sports such as running and race-walking are performed at lower velocities and air resistance is much reduced and not as important. It is beyond the scope of this review to discuss the factors offering *Resistance to Movement*.

PERFORMANCE POWER. This is the rate of energy output or power production that a person is capable of generating for the specific period of time. Power output is typically expressed in watts (i.e., joules per second or work per unit time). Power production can be measured accurately using ergometers during activities such as cycling and rowing, where physical work is performed. *Performance Power* during these prolonged aerobic activities is a function of the *Performance* $\dot{V}O_2$ (i.e., energy expenditure) and *Economy of Movement*. In sports such as running, it is not possible to measure actual work accomplished and therefore power [63]. In these cases, *Performance Velocity* is a function of *Performance* $\dot{V}O_2$ and *Economy of Movement*. (This relationship is not shown in Fig. 2.1).

PERFORMANCE OXYGEN CONSUMPTION ($\dot{V}O_2$). This represents the highest rate of whole body aerobic energy expenditure, as measured by oxygen consumption ($\dot{V}O_2$), possible for the athlete to maintain over the given duration of the event. During prolonged steady-state exercise, this measure, along with measurement of the respiratory exchange ratio to determine the caloric equivalent for each liter of oxygen consumption, provides a measure of energy expenditure. *Performance* $\dot{V}O_2$ is a function of *Lactate Threshold* $\dot{V}O_2$ and *Muscle Capillary Density*.

Functional Abilities

ECONOMY OF MOVEMENT. This is a measure of the power or velocity generated relative to the energy expenditure measured from $\dot{V}O_2$. It is most common to use the term *Economy* in describing activities such as running, where power is not quantified. In this case, *Economy* can be expressed either as the velocity achieved for a given rate of $\dot{V}O_2$ or the $\dot{V}O_2$ needed to maintain a given velocity of movement. When cycling, *Economy* is the watts produced per liter per minute oxygen consumed.

LACTATE THRESHOLD $\dot{V}O_2$ (LT $\dot{V}O_2$). This is the $\dot{V}O_2$ (rate of bodily energy expenditure) that elicits a 1 mM increase in lactic acid within the blood. This intensity is the approximate $\dot{V}O_2$ that athletes maintain during a marathon or 3-hr cycling event. As discussed below, it provides an index of muscle fatigue. *LT $\dot{V}O_2$* is shown to be a function of *$\dot{V}O_2$max, Aerobic Enzyme Activity,* and *Distribution of Power Output and Technique* as well as muscle fiber type composition.

LACTATE THRESHOLD VELOCITY OR POWER (LT VELOCITY OR LT POWER). This is the velocity of movement or power output corresponding to the LT. *LT Velocity* or *LT Power* is a central component of this model because it incorporates both *LT $\dot{V}O_2$* and *Economy.* For these reasons it is an excellent predictor of *Performance Velocity* or *Power,* as indicated by the bold line in Figure 1 and as discussed below.

GROSS MECHANICAL EFFICIENCY. This is the percentage of power produced relative to the energy expended. The energy expenditure in Kilocalories per minute can be calculated from steady-state $\dot{V}O_2$ and respiratory exchange ratio. The power production is directly measured by the ergometer. Simply, this is the percentage of chemical energy converted to mechanical work, with the remainder lost as heat. *Gross Mechanical Efficiency* will influence *Economy* when cycling at 80 rpm and it is largely related to *Muscle Fiber Type Composition (% Type I).*

MAXIMAL OXYGEN CONSUMPTION ($\dot{V}O_2$MAX). This is a measure of maximal aerobic power defined as the highest rate of O_2 consumption possible during large muscle mass activity. $\dot{V}O_2$max is largely a function of myocardial stroke volume, *Aerobic Enzyme Activity,* and *Muscle Capillary Density.*

Morphological Components

MUSCLE CAPILLARY DENSITY. This is the number of capillaries per square millimeter of muscle cross-sectional area determined from histochemical analysis of a biopsy sample.

STROKE VOLUME. This is the volume of blood pumped per heartbeat. It is a primary determinant of $\dot{V}O_2$max.

AEROBIC ENZYME ACTIVITY. This is a measure of mitochondrial aerobic activity in the trained muscles. It is typically related to the activity of certain TCA-cycle enzymes such as citrate synthase.

DISTRIBUTION OF POWER OUTPUT AND TECHNIQUE. This is a new concept that revolves around the idea that the amount of muscle mass that shares in the power production influences the relative work rate per muscle fiber. As discussed, this seems to exert an influence on the *LT $\dot{V}O_2$* when cycling.

The *Technique* of coordinating muscular contractions may also be involved in these processes.

MUSCLE FIBER TYPE COMPOSITION (% TYPE I FIBERS). This is the percentage of muscle fibers that are Type I (i.e., slow twitch), determined from histochemical analysis of a biopsy sample. This appears to exert a large influence on *Gross Mechanical Efficiency* and *Economy* when cycling.

EXPRESSION OF POWER. Power can be expressed in absolute terms or made relative to some factors with the idea that this normalization equalizes the degree of stress on the athlete. When bicycling on a level road in an aerodynamic position or on a stationary ergometer, the $\dot{V}O_2$ needed to maintain a give power varies little with alterations in body weight [41]. Therefore, when cycling, the power output is expressed in absolute watts and energy expenditure or $\dot{V}O_2$ in liters per minute. When running and walking, however, the energy expenditure or $\dot{V}O_2$ needed to maintain a given velocity increases with increasing body weight. Therefore, to better normalize different body size, $\dot{V}O_2$ is usually expressed per kilogram of body weight (ml/kg/min). These expressions of power will be followed throughout the review. There may be situations when scaling to body weight that it is best to raise body weight to a power of less than one [1].

CENTRAL ROLE OF THE LACTATE THRESHOLD CONCEPT

This model revolves around the concept that measurement of the blood lactate threshold (LT) provides information that is most indicative of the stress experienced by the exercising person as it relates to *Performance Velocity*. It had been recognized since the 1933 study of Margaria et al. [42] that the production of lactic acid by muscle is indicative of metabolic stress.

Our first study using blood lactate concentration to predict endurance performance ability was published by Farrell et al. in 1979 [19]. At that time it was already understood that blood lactate concentration represents the balance between lactate production by muscle, its diffusion into blood, and its removal [27]. It was also clear that as exercise intensity increases to moderate intensities (i.e., 60–75% $\dot{V}O_2$max), there exists a certain intensity above which muscle glycogenolysis is markedly stimulated and lactate concentration begins to accumulate exponentially in active muscle and blood [26, 27, 30, 46, 49, 53, 58]. It was also recognized that there was a limited diffusion rate of lactate from muscle into blood and as a result there was not a constant ratio difference between the two compartments. Thus, blood levels did not always reflect muscle concentration [18, 26, 27, 35, 37, 64]. However, it was generally thought that the exercise intensity at which lactate began to accumulate at an exponential rate in blood was due to an exponential increase in muscle production, which has been more recently verified by Ivy et al. [33].

As others had done before [8, 46], Farrell et al. [19] plotted the relationship between blood lactate concentrations and exercise intensity. They identified the intensity just before the exponential increase in blood lactate concentration and termed it the "onset of plasma lactate accumulation" (OPLA).

Costill et al. [8] established that, on average, lactate begins to accumulate in blood when marathoners exercise at 70% $\dot{V}O_2$max, whereas Costill and Fox [7] demonstrated that marathon runners maintain approximately 75% $\dot{V}O_2$max during the race. Therefore, this suggested that marathon runners set a pace that is slightly faster than the intensity of the OPLA. This is exactly what was observed by Farrell et al. [19], with OPLA occurring at 70% $\dot{V}O_2$max, whereas marathon pace appeared to be at 75% $\dot{V}O_2$max. The thinking was that pace was selected according to the sensation of stress in the running musculature that is proportional to muscle and blood lactate concentration and indicative of the rate of muscle glycogenolysis.

In a heterogeneous population of 18 distance runners, Farrell et al. [19] correlated running *Performance Velocity* with several of the *Morphological Components* and *Functional Abilities,* as now defined in Fig. 2.1. Running *Economy* was defined as the VO_2 in ml/kg/min required to maintain a pace of 268 m/min, with lower values indicative of better *Economy*. From another perspective, superior *Economy* allows a runner to maintain a faster velocity for a given $\dot{V}O_2$. The $\dot{V}O_2$ (ml/kg/min) and velocity corresponding to OBLA (analogous to lactate threshold in Fig. 2.1) was also determined, as was the estimated $\dot{V}O_2$ during the performance of a race (i.e., *Performance* $\dot{V}O_2$).

As indicated in Table 2.1, *Performance Velocity* was most highly correlated (r=0.97) with the velocity of running corresponding to the accumulation of lactate in blood (i.e, OPLA velocity or generally *LT Velocity*), which accounted for 94% of the variance in performance. Other variables were also significantly correlated with *Performance Velocity* with values ranging from 0.54 to 0.94. More importantly, a multiple regression analysis was performed and it was found that the prediction of race pace from OPLA velocity was not improved by the addition of other physiological variables. This suggests that this measure of OPLA velocity (or *LT Velocity* in Fig. 2.1) contains within it the predictive ability of the other factors. This is exhibited by Fig. 2.1, which indicates that *LT Velocity* is a function of the LT $\dot{V}O_2$ and *Economy*. That is, runners select a given rate of energy expenditure that can be maintained during the race relative to *LT* $\dot{V}O_2$ and their running *Economy* dictates the actual velocity corresponding to this $\dot{V}O_2$. By itself, *Economy* was correlated 10.5 with *Performance Velocity*, agreeing with the idea at that time that it is an important component to performance [17, 22]. Interestingly, although the components $\dot{V}O_2$*max* and *Muscle Fiber Type Composition* were correlated with *Performance Velocity*, they also did not contribute added predictive value, which agrees with the Fig. 2.1 portrayal of them being incorporated into the respective measures of *LT* $\dot{V}O_2$ and *Economy*.

TABLE 2.1.
Correlations Observed in Farrell et al. [19] Between 15 km Race Pace (Performance Velocity) and Physiological Variables.

	OPLA Velocity (m/min)	$\dot{V}O_2$ at Race Pace (ml/kg/min)	OPLA $\dot{V}O_2$ (ml/kg/min)	$\dot{V}O_2$ max (ml/kg/min)	Running Economy ($\dot{V}O_2$ at 268 m/min)	% Type I Muscle Fibers
15 km Race Velocity	0.97	0.94	0.91	0.89	−0.59	0.54

All correlations were statistically significant; P<0.05. In order, these variables correspond to the following terminology used in the *LT Velocity, Performance, $\dot{V}O_2$, LT $\dot{V}O_2$, $\dot{V}O_2$ max, economy,* and *% Type I Muscle Fibers.* OPLA, onset of plasma lactate accumulation.

Although Farrell et al. [19] observed *Performance Velocity* to be best correlated with OPLA velocity (0.97) (e.g., *LT Velocity*), it was also observed that $\dot{V}O_2$max was significantly correlated 0.89 with 15 km *Performance Velocity* (Table 2.1). Therefore, this study could not be interpreted as providing evidence to indicate that measures incorporating the blood lactate profile or economy were significantly better than just $\dot{V}O_2$max in predicting performance. The studies described below were designed to dissect those difference [11, 13]. However, a few comments about the confusing terminology in this area seem appropriate.

CONFUSION OF TERMINOLOGY DESCRIBING THE LACTATE VERSUS INTENSITY PROFILE

In the mid-1970s the concept of the "anaerobic threshold" was already firmly entrenched [61, 62]. It maintained that during an exercise test with increases in intensity every minute, sudden (i.e., threshold) hyperventilation is due to the increase in blood lactate concentration and that this reflects muscle hypoxia and thus energy production from anaerobic pathways [61, 62]. We did not think lactate production was due to lack of oxygen, and thus the term "anaerobic" was inappropriate. Therefore, we decided to use a term that simply described the phenomenon, which was the onset of plasma lactate accumulation (OPLA) [19]. However, we went too far in our attempt to describe this phenomenon most accurately by specifying the accumulation of lactate in "plasma" rather than "blood." It is correct that lactate produced by muscle will first diffuse into the plasma and then eventually into the red cells and thus throughout the blood. However, it is impractical to measure lactate in plasma, which must first be separated from whole blood. It is easier to simply measure lactate concentration on whole blood. In this case the term O*B*LA should be used to signify the onset of *blood* lactate accumulation.

To confuse the definitions and methodology even more, in 1981 Sjodin and Jacobs [56] published a paper using the term "Onset of *Blood* Lactate Accumulation" (O*B*LA). The problem is that they defined the OBLA as the exercise intensity at which blood lactate concentration reached 4 mM. This definition of OBLA was at a much higher intensity and blood lactate concentration than the previous classification of OPLA and LT, which generally corresponded to blood lactate concentrations of 1.5–3.0 mM. The usefulness of comparing people at the fixed blood lactate level of 4 mM is questionable in light of the fact that muscle lactate concentration can differ widely at this fixed blood level [60]. In addition, this classification also implied that 4 mM is the maximal steady-state blood lactate concentration at which people can exercise for prolonged periods [39]. We have found this idea to be without basis, and as described below, most of the athletes we test can exercise for 1 hr with a blood lactate of 6–10 mM.

In any event, since 1983 we resorted to using the term lactate threshold (LT) with measurements made on whole blood. In our opinion, blood lactate concentration is best collected after at least 5 min of steady-state exercise at approximately 5–6 different work rates (i.e., 55, 60, 65, 70, 75, and 80% $\dot{V}O_2$max for a person with an LT of about 70% $\dot{V}O_2$max). By first determining $\dot{V}O_2max$ and then estimating LT, the goal is to set the work rates so that three points are measured below the LT and 2–3 points above LT. We have defined the LT as the intensity at which blood lactate is increased 1 mM above baseline, as shown in Fig. 2.2. Baseline is established by the straight line connecting the 3 points obtained at the lowest intensities and by extending this line through the high intensities. Typically, this baseline slopes upward in untrained people and less so as fitness is increased. Our first reason for identifying LT as the 1 mM increase above baseline is that this increase can be measured reliably from the plotted values of only 5–6 points. Second, this intensity occurs at about a 5% higher intensity than the intensity at which lactate first increases above baseline (e.g., OPLA) and as a result, this definition of LT coincides closely with pace selected by marathon runners [7, 8, 10, 19]. In cyclists, we have also found that this intensity results in a remarkably similar rate of muscle glycogenolysis among subjects and as a result these athletes uniformly fatigue due to carbohydrate depletion after approximately 3 hr at an intensity equal to their LT [4].

APPLICATION TO COMPETITIVE RACE-WALKERS

To better describe the practical application of these concepts on an individual basis, Hagberg and Coyle [25] compared the responses of eight competitive race-walkers, as shown in Fig. 2.3. These endurance athletes were ranked from 1 to 8 according to their pace for a 20-km race. *LT Velocity* correlated 0.94 with *Performance Velocity* (i.e., race pace) and these two velocities were almost identical (Fig. 2.3A). $\dot{V}O_2max$ was only moderately corre-

FIGURE 2.2.

Example of the method used to identify a person's blood "lactate threshold" (LT), from analysis of the blood lactate concentration versus exercise intensity relationship. Each point represents a data point obtained during steady-state exercise after 5–10 min of either discontinuous exercise or continuous exercise progressing from low to high intensity. The dotted line represents the "baseline" drawn through three points collected during relatively low intensity exercise (40%, 50%, 60% $\dot{V}O_2$max) and extended beyond that range. The LT is identified as the intensity of exercise at which blood lactate concentration is 1 mM above baseline.

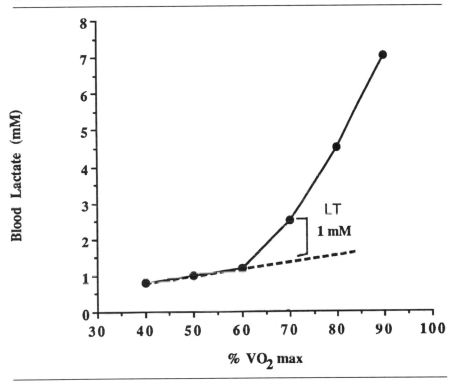

lated with race pace (0.62) and it was observed that the top six athletes all possessed a $\dot{V}O_2$max while race-walking of about 60 ml/kg/min, with a slightly higher value observed in Subject 2 (Fig. 2.3D). This was despite the fact that their *Performance Velocity* differed by more than 30%. LT $\dot{V}O_2$ displayed a better correlation with *Performance Velocity* (0.83; Fig. 2.3B), but again it was observed that the top three athletes had a similar LT $\dot{V}O_2$ (i.e., 51 ml/kg/min). The superior performance of Subject 1 compared with 2 and 3 was due to his *Economy* (Fig. 2.3C). Although the *Performance $\dot{V}O_2$* maintained during competition were comparable in Subjects 1, 2, and 3, Subject 1 was able to translate that $\dot{V}O_2$ into an 11% faster velocity because

FIGURE 2.3.

Relationship between race-walking Performance Velocity *(race pace for 20 km) versus* A, Lactate Threshold Velocity; B, Lactate Threshold $\dot{V}O_2$, C, $\dot{V}O_2$ *at a velocity of 10 km/hr, a measure of* Economy; *and* D, $\dot{V}O_2$max. *The numbers refer to the individual subjects ranked from the fastest (1) to the slowest (8) performer. The solid line is the regression of best fit and r corresponds to the correlation. All values are statistically significant, P<0.05. Reproduced from ref. 25.*

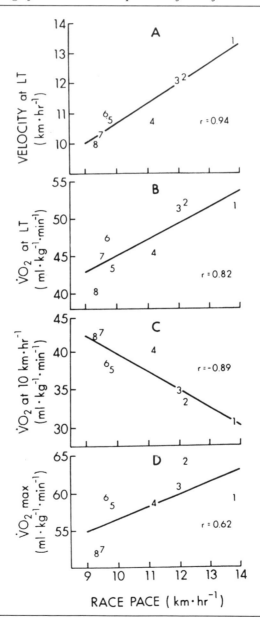

of his superior *Economy*. In the group of race-walkers, *Economy* was correlated 0.89 with *Performance Velocity* (Fig. 2.3C). These observations support
the model that *LT Velocity* provides the best prediction of *Performance Velocity* and that it is determined by the integration of *LT $\dot{V}O_2$* and *Economy*. In
this case, *Economy* appeared to be the factor that in this case distinguished
the top three race-walkers, which is similar to an observation made previously in a group of homogenous and highly trained runners [6, 16].

RELATIONSHIP BETWEEN *LT $\dot{V}O_2$* AND *AEROBIC ENZYME ACTIVITY*

There is much evidence supporting the idea introduced by Holloszy et al.
[28] that mitochondrial or *Aerobic Enzyme Activity* is a major determinant of
the degree of muscle stress during exercise [3, 9, 29, 30, 32, 57]. Muscle
glycogenolysis and lactate production are stimulated with increasing exercise intensity as a result of disturbances in muscle cell homeostasis, such as
increases in ADP and AMP concentration with reductions in ATP [29, 30].
These disturbances stimulate mitochondrial respiration to increase ATP
production from oxidative phosphorylation within the mitochondria, to
supply the ATP turnover needed to exercise. With relatively low mitochondrial activity in muscle, each mitochondria must be stimulated at high rates
to meet the ATP requirements for exercise at a given intensity, $\dot{V}O_2$, and
given rate of ATP turnover. This increase in ADP and AMP also has the effect of stimulating muscle glycogenolysis and lactate production. Increases
in the number of mitochondria and thus *Aerobic Enzyme Activity*, for example, as a result of endurance training, provide more mitochondria to share
in the oxidative resynthesis of ATP during exercise at a given intensity. As
a result, each mitochondria does not have to be stimulated to respire as
much and the disturbance of cellular homeostasis is less, thus reducing the
extent to which glycogenolysis is stimulated and lactate produced [29, 30].

Ivy et al. [32] found that muscle respiratory capacity, which reflects mitochondrial enzyme activity, is highly related to the *LT $\dot{V}O_2$* when examining a heterogeneous group of people. In addition, we have found that the
time course with which *Aerobic Enzyme Activity* (i.e., citrate synthase) declines
over the course of 84 days of detraining is closely paralleled by reductions
in *LT $\dot{V}O_2$* as shown in Fig. 2.4 [12]. Therefore, there is strong theoretical
and direct support for the idea that mitochondrial *Aerobic Enzyme Activity* is
a major determinant of *LT $\dot{V}O_2$*. The concept is that as energy expenditure
is increased, that the $\dot{V}O_2$ eliciting LT represents the rate of energy expenditure at which muscle cell homeostasis is disturbed sufficiently to more
markedly stimulate glycogenolysis and lactate production. The more mitochondria sharing in the power output, the higher the absolute $\dot{V}O_2$ needed
to elicit LT. As discussed below, methods for increasing the number of mitochondria sharing in the oxidative power output include not only increasing the number of mitochondria in a given muscle mass, but also increasing the amount of muscle mass sharing in the power output.

FIGURE 2.4.

Time course of decline during 84 days of detraining. Day 0 corresponds to values measured in well-trained endurance athletes exercising daily, with values set at 100%. The Lactate Threshold $\dot{V}O_2$ is denoted $\dot{V}O_2$ *at LT.* Aerobic Enzyme Activity *is reflected by citrate synthase activity* (Cit. Syn.). *Reproduced from ref. 12.*

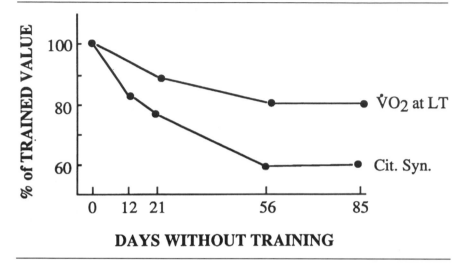

SEPARATING THE PREDICTIVE VALUE OF *LT* $\dot{V}O_2$ FROM $\dot{V}O_2$MAX

Patients with Ischemic Heart Disease

Although these empirical observations suggested that performance is related more to *LT* $\dot{V}O_2$ than it is to $\dot{V}O_2max$, this point had not yet been proven definitively in the early 1980s. The challenge was to find groups who were similar in one of these variables but different in the other and then to determine which factor was related to performance ability.

About this time, we observed that endurance-trained ischemic heart disease patients (age 55 yr) who had been training 5 days per week at the highest intensity they could tolerate, were able to run at an unusually fast pace relative to their $\dot{V}O_2max$ [11]. An unusually high running *Economy* in these patients was ruled out by examining their $\dot{V}O_2$ to different speeds of treadmill running. In the process, it was observed that these endurance-trained patients appeared able to run for prolonged periods (>35 min) at intensities that were very close to their $\dot{V}O_2max$. Interestingly, blood lactate concentration in these patients did not increase until the exercise intensity elicited $\dot{V}O_2max$. As shown in Fig. 2.5, LT occurred at a $\dot{V}O_2$ of 37 ml/kg/min in these trained patients, which corresponded to their $\dot{V}O_2max$ (i.e., LT occurred at 100% $\dot{V}O_2max$). This unusual response appeared to be due to their ischemic heart disease, which prevented their cardiac output and $\dot{V}O_2$ from increasing when heart rate was increased above 153 beats per minute, despite increasing exercise intensity. Apparently their hearts failed to pump more blood and oxygen at intensities above this level, thus limiting their $\dot{V}_{O_2}max$.

These trained patients were matched to normal men of the same age and who had been performing identical training in terms of distance and pace. These trained normal men were found to have a $\dot{V}_{O_2}max$ that was 18% higher than the trained patients. This was because the trained normal men were able to increase their $\dot{V}_{O_2}$ when heart rate was increased from 153 to 175 beats per minute, at which point their $\dot{V}_{O_2}max$ was 45 ml/kg/min. The most important observation of this study was that the $LT\ \dot{V}_{O_2}$ was identical in the two groups (i.e., 37 ml/kg/min) which represented 84% $\dot{V}_{O_2}max$ for

FIGURE 2.5.
Blood lactate threshold (LT) relative to $\dot{V}_{O_2}max$ in "untrained patients" with ischemic heart disease, endurance-"trained ischemic heart disease patients," and healthy "trained normal" subjects matched to the endurance-trained patients. The absolute $\dot{V}_{O_2}$ corresponding to the LT is identified by the dotted line and it was identical in the two trained groups (37 ml/kg/min). LT occurred at 84% $\dot{V}_{O_2}max$ in the "trained normal" subjects and at 100% $\dot{V}_{O_2}max$ in the trained patients. Reproduced from ref. 11.

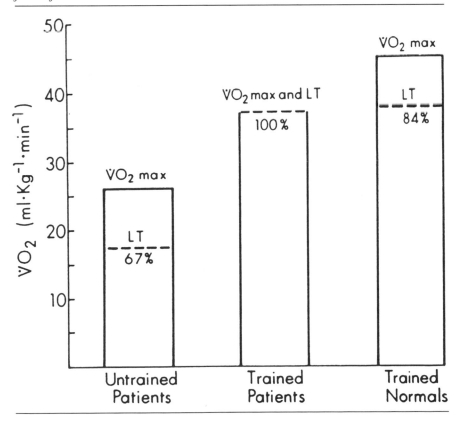

the trained normal subject compared with 100% $\dot{V}O_2max$ for the trained patients (Fig. 2.5). Therefore, the unique situation was that we had two groups with identical $LT\ \dot{V}O_2$ (i.e., 37 ml/kg/min) yet with big differences in $\dot{V}O_2max$.

Despite the large difference in $\dot{V}O_2$max, these two groups had identical *Performance Velocity* when competing in a 8-km race. Their running *Economy* was also identical, indicating that the two groups performed at a similar $\dot{V}O_2$. Therefore, in this unusual situation, performance was a function of *LT* $\dot{V}O_2$ and not $\dot{V}O_2max,$ per se. This does not indicate that $\dot{V}O_2max$ is unimportant to *Performance* $\dot{V}O_2$ because it sets the upper limits for prolonged steady-state exercise, which was clearly and uniquely demonstrated by the trained patients' ability to run for prolonged periods at $\dot{V}O_2max,$ but not at speeds much higher.

It is likely that because of the similarity of the training program in the two groups, the patients and normal subjects had similar adaptive increases in *Aerobic Enzyme Activity* in their running muscles and therefore started to accumulate lactate at the same $\dot{V}O_2$ and running speed. However, we did not perform muscle biopsies to measure *Aerobic Enzyme Activity*. Therefore, we were not able to discount the possibility that the trained patients underwent greater muscle adaptation and that in their case, LT was not determined by the *Aerobic Enzyme Activity* per se, but occurred at the intensity of cardiac dysfunction that prevented a further increase in cardiac output and oxygen delivery to muscle. In this case, the increase in blood lactate could be due to hypoxia and therefore truly an "anaerobic threshold."

With this study design it was possible to determine definitively that $LV\ \dot{V}O_2$ is more relevant to performance than is $\dot{V}O_2max$. Furthermore, as shown in Fig. 2.1, $\dot{V}O_2max$ should be viewed as a *Functional Ability* contributing to performance during prolonged exercise through its influence on $LT\ \dot{V}O_2$. However, these patients clearly are not normal. Therefore, we conducted another study on normal endurance-trained subjects.

Endurance Trained Cyclists with Similar $\dot{V}O_2max$
In this next study [13] we examined 14 cyclists, all of whom had been training intensely for 3–12 yr and who possessed similarly high values for $\dot{V}O_2max$ of approximately 4.8 liters/min. However, these subjects differed tremendously in $LT\ \dot{V}O_2$ with values ranging from 61% to 86% $\dot{V}O_2max$. Performance was determined as the length of time that these athletes could maintain 88% $\dot{V}O_2$max on a cycle ergometer. We did not report the power output or determine the racing velocity that could be maintained. Instead, performance was defined as the length of time that a given *Performance* $\dot{V}O_2$ could be maintained. This *Performance* $\dot{V}O_2$ elicited approximately 88% $\dot{V}O_2$max in each subject, which also elicited a very homogeneous absolute $\dot{V}O_2$ (i.e., 4.2–4.3 liters/min). Fig. 2.6 displays the cycling time to fatigue in

the 14 subjects in relation to their individual percent $\dot{V}O_2$max at LT. (Each subject is identified by a number according to their rank order in time to fatigue.) In these subjects, all of whom cycled at 88% $\dot{V}O_2$max, which was also at approximately the same absolute *Performance $\dot{V}O_2$*, time to fatigue varied more than 6-fold with values ranging from 12 to 75 min. However, there was a strong relationship in the entire group (r=0.90) between time to fatigue and percent $\dot{V}O_2$ at LT (Fig. 2.6). *Performance $\dot{V}O_2$* time was most closely related to *LT $\dot{V}O_2$* (i.e., the same as with percent $\dot{V}O_2$max at LT in this case). Therefore, we showed in the heart disease patients that performance can be similar when $\dot{V}O_2$max varies greatly, and in this study of competitive cyclists, performance varied greatly although $\dot{V}O_2$max was similar. However, in both studies, performance was highly related to the *LT $\dot{V}O_2$*.

FIGURE 2.6.
Relationship between cycling time to fatigue at 88% $\dot{V}O_2$max and Lactate Threshold $\dot{V}O_2$ *(identified in this case as percent $\dot{V}O_2$max at LT). The 14 subjects are numbered 1–14 based upon their time to fatigue. One group of subjects (1, 2, 7, and 8) possessed a high* Muscle Capillary Density *(high cap/mm2) and are identified by arrows. They displayed a longer exercise "time to fatigue" when compared at a given exercise intensity (percent $\dot{V}O_2$max at LT) to subjects with a lower* Muscle Capillary Density. *Reproduced from ref. 13.*

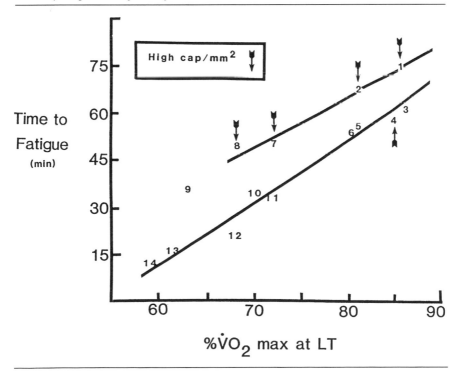

MUSCLE CAPILLARY DENSITY AND PERFORMANCE

In these endurance-trained cyclists, exercise time to fatigue was also related to *Muscle Capillary Density* (0.74). Apparently, capillary density (i.e., capillaries per square millimeter) interacted with percent $\dot{V}O_2$max at LT and together these two factors accounted for more than 92% of the variance in time to fatigue (e.g., multiple regression with these two factors yield a correlation of 0.96, indicating that 92% of the variance in *Performance* was accounted for by these two variables). The responses of the individual subjects, displayed in Fig. 2.6, tended to cluster about two lines. Subjects 1, 2, 7, and 8 formed one line that predicted an approximately 12-min longer cycling time to fatigue for a given percent $\dot{V}O_2$max at LT compared with the subjects on the line below, who had a lower *Muscle Capillary Density*. The subjects along the top line possessed the first, second, third and fifth highest *Muscle Capillary Density*. A high *Muscle Capillary Density* has been postulated to increase muscle perfusion by reducing diffusing distances and thus aid in removing lactate from muscle [59]. We interpret this relationship to indicate that time to fatigue during exercise at an intensity above the LT is related to both lactate production (as reflected by $LT\,\dot{V}O_2$ or percent $\dot{V}O_2$max at LT) and removal from muscle (as related to *Muscle Capillary Density*). It is likely that the reason that subjects with a high *Muscle Capillary Density* exercised longer than subjects with the same percent $\dot{V}O_2$max at LT, but lower *Muscle Capillary Density,* was because lactate accumulated in muscle at a slower rate. Therefore, Fig. 2.1 indicates that *Performance* $\dot{V}O_2$, at least during exercise at intensities well above LT, is a function of both $LT\,\dot{V}O_2$ and *Muscle Capillary Density*.

MUSCLE GLYCOGEN USE AND OTHER INDICES OF METABOLIC STRESS ARE INFLUENCED BY THE LACTATE THRESHOLD

When establishing a common exercise intensity at which to compare people's response to exercise, it is customary to make it relative to $\dot{V}O_2max$ (i.e., at a given percent $\dot{V}O_2$max) because to some extent this normalizes the general cardiovascular stress. However, it must be realized that this often does not guarantee that all the responses to exercise will be uniform in a given population, particularly if the population is heterogeneous in factors such as age, acute state of physical training, years of participation in endurance training, etc. This point is demonstrated quite well by our observation that glycogen use during 30 min of cycling at 79% $\dot{V}O_2$max varied 3–4 fold in our population of cyclists who were heterogeneous in percent $\dot{V}O_2$max at LT [13]. However, glycogen use was found to be directly related (r=0.90) to $LT\,\dot{V}O_2$. Therefore, if an experiment is designed to determine the effect of a certain treatment on glycogen utilization, it is more appropriate to establish the work rate relative to each subject's LT, rather than their $\dot{V}O_2max$.

This will better normalize the rate of glycogen utilization. This is how we have conducted our studies of carbohydrate feeding and glycogen use and, as mentioned earlier, this normalizes the rate of glycogen use and results in a more uniform time to fatigue and thus better control of the variable to be studied [4].

Interestingly, the cardiovascular responses to exercise appeared to be influenced by the degree of muscle stress. Although maximal heart rate was identical in the group of subjects with a low compared with a high LT (i.e., 185 beats per minute) during exercise at 79% $\dot{V}O_2$max, the low LT group displayed a significantly higher percentage of maximal heart rate compared with the high LT group (i.e., 90% vs. 85% maximum heart rate). (The distinction of low and high LT is presented below.) This agrees with the idea that the degree of muscle stress during exercise is sensed by the afferent nerves and integrated into the efferent response and thus the cardiovascular adjustments to exercise [44].

LACTATE THRESHOLD SPECIFIC TO CYCLING

A major reason for conducting the study of cyclists with similar $\dot{V}O_2max$ yet differing $LT \dot{V}O_2$ was to identify the factors related to the LT. We expected muscle *Aerobic Enzyme Activity* as reflected by the mitochondrial marker citrate synthase to explain much of the variance in LT. However, in fact, we observed no relationship (r=0.08) between citrate synthase and percent $\dot{V}O_2$max at LT [13] and we were perplexed. These cyclists turned out to be relatively homogeneous in terms of citrate synthase activity in their vastus lateralis, probably because they were all training intensely and had been following the similar regimented interval training program (3 days/wk) for the 2 mo before the study. We implemented this program to familiarize them with laboratory performance and in some cases to raise $\dot{V}O_2max$ to the level required of the study. Therefore, we unwittingly created a population who was homogeneous in muscle *Aerobic Enzyme Activity*. This was somewhat fortuitous because it seems to have allowed us to identify other factors besides aerobic enzyme activity that determines LT.

Our approach was to split the 14 cyclists into two groups, based upon their percent $\dot{V}O_2$max at LT. Therefore, one group of 7 had a low LT (i.e., 66% $\dot{V}O_2$max); the other group had a high LT (i.e., 81% $\dot{V}O_2$max). [13]. Although both groups had been performing endurance training (e.g., swimming, rowing, running) for 7–8 yr, the low LT group had been cycling for only 2.7 ± 0.7 yr compared with 5.1 ± 0.9 yr for the high LT group. We hypothesized that the high LT group had developed some skill or technique of cycling. Our first thought was that the high LT subjects may have learned to "pull up" during the cycling up-stroke by somehow using their cleated shoes and toe straps. However, that did not appear to be the case because we found that their LT and exercise tolerance were not reduced much when we had them cycle while wearing tennis shoes without fixing the foot onto the pedal, so it was impossible to pull up. That suggested to us that if some cycling skill or technique had been developed in the high LT group, it must occur during the cycling down-stroke.

We thought that if indeed these two groups (high and low LT when cycling) possessed similar mitochondrial *Aerobic Enzyme Activity* in the vastus lateralis, it would be interesting to determine whether their lactate responses to running up a 10% grade were different. This exercise has been shown to rely heavily on the vastus lateralis [10]. Running and cycling $\dot{V}O_2max$ were not different in the two groups and therefore work rate can again be expressed as percent $\dot{V}O_2max$. As shown in Fig. 2.7, the group with a high LT when cycling had an equally high LT when running (i.e., 81–84% $\dot{V}O_2max$). However, the subjects with the low LT when cycling (i.e., 66% $\dot{V}O_2max$) displayed a high LT when running that occurred at 82% $\dot{V}O_2max$. Therefore, the low LT in these endurance athletes was specific to cycling. Apparently they possessed the high $\dot{V}O_2max$ and muscle *Aerobic Enzyme Activity* to be considered very well trained, but they lacked the ability to reduce the rate of glycogenolysis in the vastus lateralis and lactate production during intense cycling. We interpreted this to mean that they had not yet learned the technique of cycling in a manner that reduces the stress on the quadriceps muscle.

LACTATE THRESHOLD APPEARS ALSO TO BE RELATED TO THE AMOUNT OF MUSCLE MASS SHARING IN THE POWER OUTPUT

Careful analysis of the sources of carbohydrate metabolism suggests that the low and high LT groups displayed relatively large differences in the amount of muscle mass used when cycling (Table 2.2). The amount of muscle mass active when cycling can be estimated as the quotient of the total millimoles of glycogen oxidized and the millimoles of glycogen used per kilogram of muscle (i.e., vastus lateralis) during 30 min of cycling at 79% $\dot{V}O_2max$. The total amount (i.e., millimoles) of carbohydrate oxidized was calculated from open circuit spirometry, which we have shown recently to be valid during exercise at these intensities [50]. In addition, during exercise at these intensities in very similar populations of cyclists, we have also shown recently that the amount of blood glucose disappearance and oxidation is approximately 84 mmol in 30 min [51, 52]. We have used this estimate of blood glucose oxidation for both groups, although it is probably actually slightly higher in the low LT group [5], which would have the effect of decreasing the estimated muscle mass in the low LT group and magnifying the difference between groups even more. Therefore, our current estimate is conservative. Because muscle glycogen and blood glucose are the sources for total carbohydrate oxidation, glycogen oxidation can be estimated as

FIGURE 2.7.
Blood lactate responses to cycling and running up a 10% grade in subjects with a low lactate threshold (LT) when cycling ("low LT Group") with subjects with a high LT when cycling ("high LT Group"). Asterisks (*) indicate that blood lactate responses and LT of "Low LT group" while cycling are significantly different (P<0.001) from their responses while running and also significantly different from responses of "high LT Group" while cycling or running. Reproduced from ref. 13.

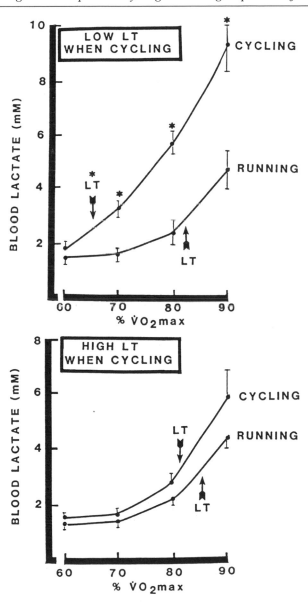

the differences between the total carbohydrate and blood glocuse oxidation [50, 51]. Glycogen oxidation divided by the glycogen use per kilogram of muscle provides an estimate of the mass of muscle used when cycling, with the assumption that the relative glycogen use in the vastus lateralis is generally representative of the cycling musculature.

From this comparison, as shown in Table 2.2, the high LT group appeared to be spreading the power production over a 22% greater muscle mass (i.e., 9.8 vs. 8.0 kg for the high and low LT groups, respectively). Interestingly, LT was elicited at a 24% higher $LT \dot{V}O_2$ in the high versus low LT group. This observation, that the amount of muscle mass used and the $LT \dot{V}O_2$ were proportionally greater (i.e., 22–24%) in the high compared with low LT Group, agrees with the idea that the higher LT was in large part due to having more muscle mass sharing in the power production. This implies that there is little difference in muscle *Aerobic Enzyme Activity* (e.g., mitochondrial enzyme activity) between the two groups, which is what we observed.

As discussed below, we think the high LT group has developed the ability to better utilize their hip extensors muscles for powering the cycling down-stroke, possibly as a result of their greater number of years spent training for cycling. Our concept is that with a larger amount of muscle mass to share in the power output, the average fibers that are active are allowed to maintain a lower relative work rate. In essence, the power output is "spread over a larger muscle mass." As a result of the reduction in work rate per muscle fiber during cycling at a given intensity, the individual fibers experience a reduction in their individual requirement for oxidative resynthesis of ATP from their individual mitochondria. As a result, disturbance of cellular homeostasis is reduced, as are glycogenolysis and lactate production.

TABLE 2.2.
Calculation of the Estimated Amount of Muscle Mass Sharing in the Distribution of Power Output During 30 min of Cycling at 79% $\dot{V}O_2$max (from ref. 13)

	Total Carbohydrate Oxidized (mmol)	Blood Glucose Oxidized (mmol)[a]	Glycogen Oxidized (mmol)	Glycogen Used/kg of Muscle (mmol/kg)	Estimated Muscle Mass Sharing in Work (kg)
High LT Group	358 ± 24[b]	84 ± 14	274 ± 18[b]	27.9 ± 3.0[b]	9.8 ± 1.4[b]
Low LT Group	605 ± 20	84 ± 14	521 ± 17	65.4 ± 5.6	8.0 ± 0.7

Values are mean ± SE. Total carbohydrate oxidation is measured using open cicuit spirometry [50] and the amount of glycogen used per kilogram of muscle was determined from analysis of biopsy samples [13]. The estimated amount of muscle mass sharing in the work is calculated by dividing total carbohydrate oxidation by the measured use of glycogen per kilogram of muscle. Estimated muscle mass (kg) = glycogen oxidized (mmol) glycogen use/kg (mmol/kg). Glycogen oxidation = total carbohydrate oxidized (mmol) − blood glucose oxidized (mmol).
[a] Blood glucose oxidation calculated from refs. 51 and 52.
[b] Significantly different. P<0.01.

The amount of muscle mass that is used during exercise and thus the *Distribution of Power Output* and therefore the relative stress this distribution places on individual muscle fibers is a factor that has not been given much attention when discussing the physiological factors determining endurance performance. In Fig. 2.1 we indicate that this phenomenon of *Distribution of Power Output and Technique* influences LT $\dot{V}O_2$. We have no direct information about the neurological patterns that accomplish this phenomenon. As discussed below, it seems most likely to us that greater muscle fiber recruitment will result in higher peak muscle force and that the reduction in work rate at the fiber level would be due to a reduced frequency of activation (e.g., more recovery time). Our pedal torque data support this interpretation. An obvious reason this factor has not received much attention is because it is a very difficult factor to measure. However, our present calculations seem reasonable in absolute terms and at the very least they demonstrate convincingly that these athletes display sizable differences in the amount of muscle mass sharing in the power output. Undoubtedly this has much potential for influencing performance by greatly reducing the stress on individual fibers, which seems to be reflected by improvements in LT.

CYCLING TECHNIQUE

In our next study [14] we used an "instrumented pedal dynamometer" to measure the forces and torque developed while cycling to gain information as to whether the cyclists with superior LT and performance display a characteristic technique that is consistent with use of a larger muscle mass. We assembled a group of 15 competitive cyclists whose specialized race was the 40-km time-trial. During competition, these athletes bicycle 40 km as fast as possible (i.e., *Performance Velocity*), without drafting other riders. Performance times in this group ranged from 51.0 min to 65.0 min, and the use of aerodynamic equipment at this time was limited and uniform. To collect biomechanical and physiological data under conditions similar to a 40-km time-trial race, we designed a laboratory cycling performance test. The performance criteria were the average power output generated over a duration of exactly 1 hr. A laboratory ergometer was modified to place each cyclist in a position similar to when on their own bicycle. By varying their cadence and flywheel resistance they were able to select their power outputs during the 1-hr test.

These men were split into two groups based upon 40-km performance (more or less than 56 min). Group 1 was composed of "Elite" bicyclists, who included the best amateurs in the United States at that time, several of whom eventually became professionals and succeeded in international competition. Group 2 comprised cyclists with "Good" performances as evidenced by their placing in races within Texas. A detailed comparison of these groups is presented below (Table 2.3). However, for the purpose of comparing their technique, these groups were identical in lean body weight (i.e., 65 kg) and

$\dot{V}O_2max$ (69 ml/kg/min) and therefore, cycling at a given absolute power output elicited very comparable stress relative to their muscle mass and aerobic power. In addition, all measures of pedaling technique were obtained at 90 rpm, which was the chosen cadence for most of these athletes. Group 1 (Elite) possessed an $LT\ \dot{V}O_2$ that was 8.7% higher compared with Group 2 (3.99 vs.

TABLE 2.3.
Comparison of the Various Components of the Model (Figs. 1 and 11) in the Three Populations of Competitive Cyclists Presented in Refs. 13 and 14.

	Novice, Low LT	Good, Group 2	Elite, Group 1	% Differences, Group 1 and 2
History				
Age (yr)	25 ± 1	23 ± 1	24 ± 4	
Endurance Training (yr)	7.0 ± 0.8	5.0 ± 3.0	8.8 ± 0.9	+76%
Cycling Training (yr)	2.7 ± 0.7	4.2 ± 0.9	5.7 ± 1.0	+36%
Performance Abilities				
40-km time trial performance (min)		60.0 ± 1.1	53.9 ± 0.5[a]	+10.1%[a]
1-h performance power (watts)		311 ± 12	346 ± 7[a]	+11.2[a]
Performance $\dot{V}O_2$ (liters/min)		4.18 ± 0.15	4.54 ± 0.09[a]	+8.6%[a]
Performance percent $\dot{V}O_2$ max		85.8 ± 1.6	89.7 ± 1.1[a]	+4.5%
Functional Abilities				
Lactate threshold power (watts)		273	311[a]	11.1%[a]
Lactate threshold $\dot{V}O_2$ (liters/min)	3.12 ± 0.15	3.67 ± 0.17	3.99 ± 0.10[a]	+8.7%[a]
% $\dot{V}O_2$max at lactate threshold	65.8 ± 1.7	74.3 ± 1.4	79.2 ± 1.1[a]	+6.6%[a]
Economy (watts/liter $\dot{V}O_2$/min)		74.3 ± 1.4	76.3 ± 1.0	+2.7%
Maximal oxygen uptake (liters/min)	4.75 ± 0.03	4.88 ± 0.19	5.07 ± 0.11[a]	+3.9%
Maximal oxygen uptake (ml/kg/min)	66.0 ± 1.2	69.3 ± 1.2	69.6 ± 1.2	0%
Morphological components				
% Type I muscle fibers	46.9 ± 3.8	52.9 ± 5.7	66.5 ± 3.7[a]	+13.6%[a]
Muscle capillary density (cap/mm²)	327 ± 36	377 ± 22	464 ± 25[a]	+23%[a]
Aerobic enzyme activity-citrate synthase (mol/kg/p/hr)	9.8 ± 1.5	9.3 ± 1.1	11.2 ± 0.9[a]	+20%[a]

Values are means ± SE. The "low LT Group" of ref. 13 are considered novice because they had only been cycling for 2–3 years and they did not have the ability to reduce glycogenolysis in the vastus lateralis when cycling. The "Good, Group 2" and "Elite, Group 1" displayed relatively high LT. However, the differences between these two groups are indicated ([a]).
[a] P<0.05.

3.67 liters min; Table 2.3; Good). In agreement with this, during the 1-hr performance test, Group 1 maintained an 8.6% higher average *Performance* $\dot{V}O_2$ and an 11.2% higher average 1-hr *Performance Power* (346 vs. 311 watts; Table 2.3). What about their technique allowed them to accomplish this?

Figure 2.8 shows the information gained from the pedal dynamometer, in particular the torque generated at the crank and the vertical and horizontal forces on the pedal. The average pattern of torque development of Group 1 compared with Group 2 at the *Performance Power* is displayed in Fig. 2.9. The area under the curves represents the amount of work performed per pedal revolution, which was 9% higher in Group 1 (Fig. 2.9). First of all, it is clear that almost all of the propulsive torque is generated during the cycling down-stroke (i.e., 0–180°; top dead-center to bottom dead-center). The only minor difference between the groups during the cycling up-stroke (180–360°) was that Group 2 pulled up with slightly more torque, whereas Group 1 generated no torque and thus just appeared to just prevent the weight of their leg from loading the pedal. Clearly, the greater work performed over an entire pedal revolution by Group 1 had nothing to do with the cycling up-stroke and, contrary to some popular notions, Group 1 cyclists actually pull up less.

More importantly, Group 1 maintained an 11.2% higher power output during the 1-hr performance (i.e., *Performance Power*) test by generating more torque during the cycling down-stroke. This was accomplished by generating 22% more peak torque compared with Group 2 (i.e., 76.8 vs. 62.8 N/m), with peak torque occurring slightly before the crank was horizontal in both groups (i.e., 86–90°) (Fig. 2.9). Finally, Fig. 2.9*B* indicates that greater peak torque was generated by Group 1 simply by producing 24% higher vertical force directed downward and 14% higher horizontal force directed forward. Simply put, they pushed down harder.

Group 1's ability to generate more torque and power in the down-stroke was not accomplished by adopting a pedaling technique that was more effective (defined as the percent of the force applied to the pedal that actually creates propulsive torque throughout the pedal revolution). They actually tended to be less effective. This indicates that they had not developed a skill that more effectively transferred muscle force into torque at the cranks. Therefore it is likely that the larger peak torque represents a muscular phenomenon. Interestingly, Group 1 display the characteristic of higher peak torque development even when cycling at the same power output as Group 2 (i.e., 324 watts for two legs and 162 for a single leg) (Fig. 2.9*B*). Group 1 also displayed the pattern of pushing down harder and pulling up less when pedaling at this given absolute power output.

FACTORS RELATED TO HIGHER PEAK TORQUE PRODUCTION

We think that the characteristic pattern of developing higher peak torque and downward force when pedaling is in agreement with our observation

FIGURE 2.8.

A, Diagram of the measurements obtained from the pedal dynamometer, used to cal-
culate torque at the center of the crank. B, Comparison of the pedaling technique of
the "Elite Group 1" cyclists with the "Good Group 2" cyclists. As shown, Group 1 pro-
duced 22% greater peak torque at the cranks by generating 24% more vertical force
and 14% more horizontal force compared with Group 2. B, displays the technique
used during the 1-hr performance test by Group 1 to produce greater power and it cor-
responds to the top of Fig. 2.9.

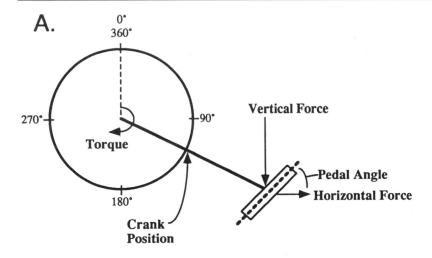

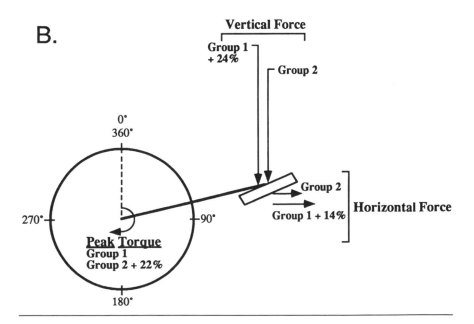

FIGURE 2.9.

Comparison of the average torque production versus crank orientation in the two groups. The crank orientation is expressed in degrees from top dead-center (0°) to bottom dead-center (180°) and back up, as shown in Fig. 2.8. The upper panel displays the technique used when cycling at the power output maintained during the 1-hr performance test. The lower panel displays the torque patterns when both groups cycled at the same power output. Redrawn from ref. 14.

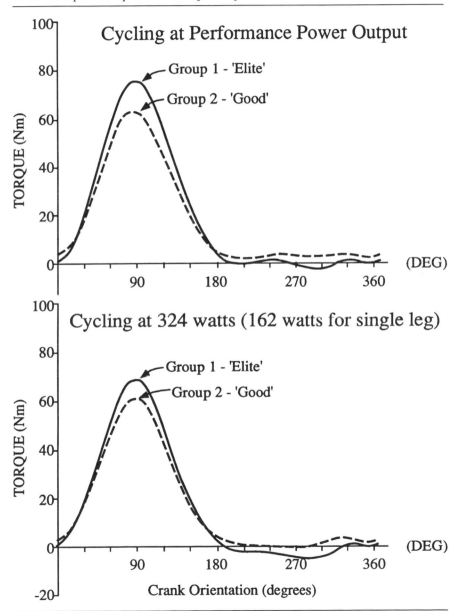

that cyclists with superior LT and performance are able to activate more muscle mass during the cycling down-stroke. It would seem that the methods for producing higher pedal force and torque are by (a) recruiting a greater cross-sectional area of muscle, or (b) obtaining more force output per cross-sectional area. It seems possible that both of these may be operative to some extent.

Recruitment of a Larger Muscle Mass and Area
A cyclist's position on the bicycle, particularly the relationships of pedal and crank axis relative to the center of rotation about the knee and hip joint, alters the relative amount of torque generated about the hip and knee. We attempted to calculate joint torque in these subjects, but did not publish these data because of technical difficulties (movement) in measuring certain segment lengths during cycling itself. Despite these difficulties, we noted that the Group 1 cyclists, especially the top riders, generally adopted a seat position that theoretically would allow more hip torque development compared with Group 2. Indeed, the joint torque data collected were of sufficient accuracy to agree with this qualitative assessment. The best "time trialists" also seemed to rely more heavily on their gluteus muscles, which extend the hip during the cycling down-stroke. They also commented that they consciously try to use these muscles for added power and they indicated that these gluteus muscles were quite fatigued after the performance test. We think this draws the general picture that part of the phenomenon we have seen as being increased recruitment or the ability to spread the power output over a larger muscle mass, probably involves, to some extent, increasing the participation of the hip extensor muscles.

Greater Force and Power Output Relative to Muscle Area and Mass
It is also possible that Group 1 was able to generate higher peak torque and greater power throughout the 1-h performance test because their muscles were less fatigable. As shown in Table 2.3, the vastus lateralis muscle of Group 1 possessed a 20–23% higher *Muscle Capillary Density* and *Aerobic Enzyme Activity* compared with Group 2. These factors undoubtedly played a role in the 8.6% higher *Performance* $\dot{V}O_2$ of Group 1 compared with Group 2 (Table 2.3). However, this does not explain the strategy of their producing higher peak torque and forces when cycling at the given intensity (Fig. 2.8*B*).

Group 1 also possessed higher *% Type I Fibers* in their vastus lateralis (66.5 vs 52.9% Type I; $P<0.05$) and a nonsignificant trend for greater *Economy* (defined as the watts of power production per liter of oxygen consumed per minute). As discussed below, *% Type I Fibers* has great potential to influence performance when all other factors are comparable, by increasing muscle efficiency and cycling *Economy*. People most commonly have about 50% *Type I Fibers* in their vastus lateralis [34]. Five of the nine subjects in Group

1 and three of six subjects in Group 2 displayed more than 60% *Type I Fibers,* whereas only four subjects, all in Group 1, had more than 70% *Type I Fibers.* Another reflection of the trend for the greater *Economy* of Type I fibers to influence power output was the observation that Group 1 displayed in 8.6% higher *Performance* $\dot{V}O_2$ yet 11.2% greater *Performance Power* during the 1-hr test (Table 3) (i.e., they produced more power than expected relative to the increase in $\dot{V}O_2$). Therefore, part of the reason Group 1 generated greater torque and force in the down-stroke and power may reflect the greater efficiency of Type I fibers, which would be manifested during the cycling down-stroke.

CYCLING EFFICIENCY IS RELATED TO THE PERCENTAGE OF TYPE I MUSCLE FIBERS

In the course of these studies, we observed that when cycling at a given power output, two cyclists could vary by as much as 15–20% in their absolute $\dot{V}O_2$ (liters/minute). This seemed to be related to *Muscle Fiber Type Composition* (i.e., *% Type I Fibers*) [15]. Therefore, we performed another study on 19 competitive cyclists who ranged from 32 to 76% *Type I Fibers* (i.e., slow twitch) [15]. In addition to measuring *Efficiency* when cycling at 80 rpm, *Efficiency* was also measured while performing the novel task of two-legged knee extension. Both cycling at 80 rpm and knee extension elicited knee extension velocities of approximately 200°/s. *Gross Mechanical Efficiency* was calculated simply as the ratio of worked accomplished per minute relative to energy expenditure per minute. Delta efficiency, which is the ratio of the relative change in these parameters with increasing work rate, was also calculated because it provides a better reflection of true muscular *Efficiency* [48].

As shown in Fig. 2.10A, *Gross Mechanical Efficiency* when cycling ranged from 18.3 to 22.6% in this population and it was significantly correlated with *% Type I Muscle Fibers* (r = 0.75). *% Type I Muscle Fibers* was also related to the *Gross Mechanical Efficiency* with which the subjects performed two-legged knee extension (Fig. 2.10B). The observation that *% Type I Fibers* was correlated with *Efficiency* during both activities suggests that *Efficiency* is a phenomenon of the muscle itself when contracting at these velocities and that it is not just a skill manifested when cycling. In addition, our pedal dynamometer measures of pedaling "effectiveness" were not related to *% Type I Muscle Fibers* or *Gross Mechanical Efficiency* when cycling. Finally, delta *Efficiency* when cycling was also directly and highly related to *% Type I Fibers* (r = 0.85), which most convincingly supports our hypothesis that it is a muscular phenomenon (Fig. 2.10B). It should also be realized that *Economy* may be related to other properties of muscle (2).

Our findings that *Gross Mechanical Efficiency* when cycling is directly re-

FIGURE 2.10.

The relationship between % Type I Muscle Fibers *and efficiency expressed as A,* Gross Mechanical Efficiency *when cycling at 80 rpm, defined as the ratio of work accomplished to energy expenditure; B, Delta efficiency when cycling at 80 rpm, defined as the ratio of the change in work accomplished and the change in energy expended; C,* Gross Mechanical Efficiency *when performing two-legged knee extension at a velocity of 200°/s. All correlations are significant with P<0.05. Reproduced from ref. 15.*

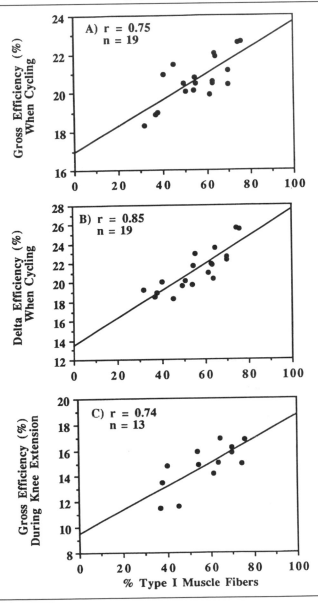

lated to % *Type I Muscle Fibers* should be interpreted in light of the velocities of contraction employed. Peak muscular efficiency generally occurs at a velocity of approximately one-third of the maximal shortening velocity ($\dot{V}$ max) in both Type I and Type II fibers [21, 24, 40]. It is likely that Type I fibers were found to be more efficient during knee extension at 200°/s because this velocity is closer to their velocity of peak efficiency compared with Type II fibers [23, 40]. We attempted to illustrate this theoretical point by calculating the estimated velocity of fiber shortening in the vastus lateralis under these experimental conditions and indeed found that it seemed surprisingly close to the velocity of peak efficiency for Type fibers [15].

Higher muscular efficiency would be manifested as a lower rate of ATP utilization and turnover, and thus lower $\dot{V}O_2$, during exercise at a given submaximal power output. From another perspective, when cycling at a given $\dot{V}O_2$, people with a high muscular efficiency would display higher power output and greater pedal force development and crank torque during the down-stroke [38]. This indicates that during relatively slow velocity contractions, Type I muscle fibers appear more efficient at converting chemical energy (e.g., ATP) into mechanical work compared with Type II fibers. These observations agree with previous work using in vitro muscle preparations [24, 40] and indicate it is a phenomenon of the contractile proteins themselves [65, 66].

It is well recognized that *Economy* of movement in running is an important determinant of performance [6, 17, 22, 45, 47]. Indeed, studies generally have found correlations of approximately 0.5 between *Economy* and performance [19]. Despite great interest, the physiological and biomechanical factors that determine *Economy* when running remain unknown [43, 45]. It is possible, and we think likely, that *Muscle Fiber Type Composition* also influences running *Economy*. However, the mechanics of running are complex and the most appropriate factor for normalizing the scaling may not be simple body weight [1]. Williams and Cavanagh [67] found nonsignificant trends for groups with high, medium, and low running *Economy* to differ in % *Type I Fibers* with the best *Economy* in the high % *Type I Fiber* group.

HIGH EFFICIENCY OF TYPE I MUSCLE FIBERS IMPROVES PERFORMANCE

The influence on *Performance Power* or *Gross Efficiency* when cycling is illustrated by comparison of subjects listed in Table 2.4. These competitive cyclists were divided into two groups of seven according to their % *Type I Muscle Fibers* [31]. Subjects with more than 56% Type I fibers were considered the *High % Type I* group, whereas subjects with less than 56% *Type I Fibers* were considered to be the *Normal % Type I* group. Each subject was paired with a member of the other group according to their similarity in $\dot{V}O_2max$, $LT \dot{V}O_2$, and *Performance* $\dot{V}O_2$ during a 1-hr laboratory test. As shown in Table 2.4, the

TABLE 2.4.
Comparison of Subjects with "High % Type I" Fibers versus "Normal % Type I" Fibers. Variable Presented are % Type I Muscle Fiber Composition, Average Oxygen Consumption ($\dot{V}O_2$), and Average Power (watts) during the 1-hr Performance Bout (Performance $\dot{V}O_2$ and Performance Power).

| Subject Pair | Muscle Fiber Composition (% Type I Fibers) | | Performance $\dot{V}O_2$ (liters/min) | | Performance Power (watts) | |
	High % Type I	Normal % Type I	High % Type I	Normal % Type I	High % Type I	Normal % Type I
1 + 8	83	46	4.62	4.67	357	335
2 + 9	77	54	4.39	4.38	336	293
3 + 10	76	49	4.59	4.54	363	336
4 + 11	76	55	4.12	4.065	325	287
5 + 12	70	38	4.61	4.66	324	314
6 + 13	64	45	4.00	4.01	313	287
7 + 14	62	52	5.00	4.91	376	359
Mean ± SE	73 ± 3[a]	48 ± 2	4.48 ± 0.13	4.46 ± 0.13	342 ± 9[a]	315 ± 11

High % Type I Group (Subjects 1–7) possessed more than 56% Type I fibers, whereas the Normal % Type I Group possessed 38–55% Type I fibers (subjects 8–14). The subjects were paired according to the criteria in methods section. For each variable, the values for Subjects 1–7 are listed on left and next to it are the values for the paired subject, 8–14.
[a] = Significantly greater than Normal % Type I Group (P<0.002). (By design, the groups differed in % Type I muscle fibers).

Normal % Type I group was indeed similar to the average composition of the general population with a mean of 48% Type I and a distribution of 38–54%. The mean value of 73% in the *High Type I* group also represents values reported in some exceptional endurance athletes [20].

Despite having almost identical *Performance $\dot{V}O_2$*, each subject in the *High % Type I* group generated between 3 to 15% more *Performance Power* compared with his pair in the *Normal % Type I* group. As a result, the average *Performance Power* of the *High % Type I* group was 9% higher compared with the *Normal % Type I* group (342 vs. 315 watts). It should be realized that during the 1-hr performance test, not only were the subject pairs and groups identical in *Performance $\dot{V}O_2$*, they were also identical in other parameters of cardiovascular and metabolic stress such as heart rate, blood lactate, percent $\dot{V}O_2$max, and even perceived exertion. The only measurable difference was in their *Performance Power*. The most striking examples were Subject Pair 2 and 9, who both averaged slightly less than 4.4 liters/min for *Performance $\dot{V}O_2$*, but who differed by 15% in *Performance Power* (i.e., 336 vs. 293 watts). In addition, Subject Pair 4 and 11 differed by 13% in *Performance Power* (i.e., 325 vs. 287 watts). As discussed below, the differences in *Performance Power* translate directly into differences in *Performance Velocity* in an actual time trial race.

From another perspective, a relatively high *% Type I Fibers* and superior *Gross Mechanical Efficiency* can allow cyclists with a below-average *LT* $\dot{V}O_2$ and *Performance* $\dot{V}O_2$ to perform as well as athletes with much higher *LT* $\dot{V}O_2$ and *Performance-* $\dot{V}O_2$, yet only normal *% Type I Fibers*. For example, subjects 6 and 12 both had a *Performance Power* of 313–314 watts despite the fact that their *Performance* $\dot{V}O_2$ differed by more than 16% (i.e., 4.00 vs. 4.66 liters/min). Subject 6 possessed 64% *Type I Fibers*, whereas Subject 12 had only 38% *Type I Fibers*. A very similar analogy can be made by comparing Subjects 4 and 8, who also performed comparably (i.e., 325–335 watts) despite a 13% higher *Performance* $\dot{V}O_2$ in Subject 8 (i.e., 4.67 vs. 4.12 liters/min), who had a normal fiber type (i.e., 46% *Type I Fibers*), whereas Subject 4 possessed 76% *Type I Fibers*. Therefore, a high *% Type I Fibers* and thus superior *Efficiency* can compensate quite well for shortcomings in *LT* $\dot{V}O_2$ and *Performance* $\dot{V}O_2$.

Table 4 indicates that the cyclist with the best *Performance Power* (i.e., Subject 7, 376 watts), which was 4% greater than second place, distinguished himself from his competitors by possessing a *Performance* $\dot{V}O_2$ that was 7% higher than any other cyclist. His *% Type I Fibers* and *Efficiency* were toward the low end of the *High % Type I* group. Obviously, *Performance Power* is a function of both *Performance* $\dot{V}O_2$ and *Economy*, as shown in Figure 1. In this case, superior *Economy* when cycling is due to superior *Gross Mechanical Efficiency*, which in turn is highly related to *% Type I Fibers* in the vastus lateralis. Of course, having a high *Economy* with a low *LT* $\dot{V}O_2$ would not allow superior performance. On the other hand, poor *Economy* can be combined with superior *LT* $\dot{V}O_2$ to produce better than average *Performance Power*. Obviously both factors must be considered. We have seen that the coefficient of variation (SD/mean) for *Efficiency* and *Gross Mechanical Efficiency* is approximately 4–6% in competitive cyclists. However, the coefficient of variation in other *Functional Abilities (i.e., LT* $\dot{V}O_2$ *and Performance* $\dot{V}O_2$) is relatively greater, averaging 8–10%. This greater variability in *LT* $\dot{V}O_2$ and *Performance* $\dot{V}O_2$ is probably because it is composed of more *Morphological Components* compared with *Economy*.

VALIDITY OF THE MODEL IN A HOMOGENOUS GROUP OF COMPETITIVE CYCLISTS

Having discussed the theoretical basis for the model presented in Figure 1 and the individual studies designed to distinguish the various components, the next step is to determine the model's validity when applied to a population. We have applied this model to the group of 15 Elite and Good competitive cyclists (Groups 1 and 2, respectively) [14], who were very homogeneous in that they all had been training for several years and all possessed a high $\dot{V}O_2$max (> 64 ml/kg/min) and raced 40 km faster than 65 min. Therefore, high correlations in a homogeneous group indicate good predictive ability. See Table 2.3 for comparison of the Good and Elite groups.

The model is redrawn in Fig. 2.11 and the variances are displayed. The lines connecting the boxes indicate a relationship between the two variables, and the percentage of variance in the upper box that is accounted for by the lower box is listed next to the line. Variance is simply the correlation squared (r^2). Inside the boxes of the *Performance* and *Functional Abil-*

FIGURE 2.11.

Validation of the model presented in Fig. 2.1. The relationship between the variables in the boxes are denoted by lines, and the percent of variance in the variable in the upper box that is explained by the lower box is denoted next to the line. Variance is calculated simply as r^2. At the bottom of the boxes, the percent of variance explained by the specified multiple factors (identified from forward multiple regression) are shown. See text for explanation.

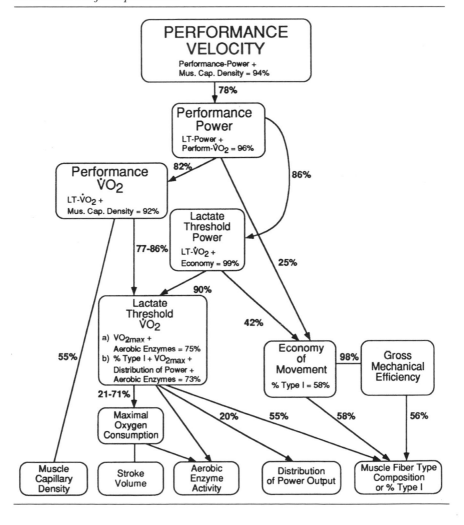

ities are listed the variables identified by forward multiple regression and the amount of variance they account for when combined.

Performance Velocity when bicycling for 40 km had 78% of its variance predicted by *Performance Power* with 94% predicted when *Muscle Capillary Density* was also considered (Fig. 2.11). The Elite cyclists had 10–11% greater *Performance Velocity* and *Performance Power* compared with the Good cyclists, while also having a 23% higher *Muscle Capillary Density* (Table 2.3).

Performance Power had 82% of its variance related to *Performance* $\dot{V}O_2$ and 25% of its variance related to *Economy*. This does not indicate that *Economy* is not important for the reasons discussed when comparing the subjects in Table 2.4. *Performance Power* was also highly related to *Lactate Threshold Power* (r^2 = 86%). In addition, 96% of the variance in *Performance Power* was accounted for by the combination of *LT Power* and *Performance* $\dot{V}O_2$.

LT Power was a function of *LT* $\dot{V}O_2$ (90% of variance) and *Economy* (42% of variance). The combination of both these two factors accounted for 99% of the variance in *LT Power*. The 11.1% higher *LT Power* of the Elite compared to Good group was because of an 8.6% higher *LT* $\dot{V}O_2$ and a 2.7% higher *Economy* (Table 2.3).

Performance $\dot{V}O_2$ was also highly related to *LT* $\dot{V}O_2$ in the Elite and Good cyclists (r^2 = 0.77) [14], as it was in the comparison of cyclists with low and high LT (r^2 = 0.86) [13]. In this latter study [13], we also found *Muscle Capillary Density* to account for 55% of the variance in *Performance*, as shown in Fig. 2.11. In addition, 92% of the variance in *Performance* $\dot{V}O_2$ was accounted for by the combination of *LT* $\dot{V}O_2$ and *Muscle Capillary Density*.

LT $\dot{V}O_2$ is an important *Functional Ability* that appears to be composed of several factors. $\dot{V}O_2max$ is certainly important and it, of course, sets the upper limit for *LT* $\dot{V}O_2$. However, the amount of variance it accounts for can vary from 21% in a population with a homogeneous $\dot{V}O_2max$ [13] to 71% in Good and Elite cyclists [14] and to 74% in heterogeneous runners [19]. In the Elite and Good cyclists, 75% of the variance in *LT* $\dot{V}O_2$ (see "a)" in Fig. 11) was accounted for by the combination of $\dot{V}O_2max$ and *Aerobic Enzyme Activity* [14]. In a population homogeneous in $\dot{V}O_2max$ (i.e., low and high LT from ref. 13), approximately 20% of the variance in *LT* $\dot{V}O_2$ was accounted for by the estimation of the amount of active muscle mass sharing in the *Distribution of Power Output*. An additional 30% of the variance in *LT* $\dot{V}O_2$ is accounted for by *% Type I Fibers*, which may be related to the fact that glycolytic enzyme activity and glycogenolysis are lower in Type I compared with Type II fibers. Therefore, muscular factors that reduce glycolytic stimuli account for much of the variance in *LT* $\dot{V}O_2$ when variance in $\dot{V}O_2max$ is reduced. The combination of all four factors (*% Type I, $\dot{V}O_2max$, Distribution Power Output,* and *Aerobic Enzyme Activity*) accounted for 73% of the variance (see "b)" in Fig. 2.11). Along these lines, the 8.7% higher *LT* $\dot{V}O_2$ in the Elite group was associated with a 3.9% higher $\dot{V}O_2max$, as well as higher *% Type I Fibers* and *Aerobic Enzyme Activity* (P=0.18), compared with the Good group. The Elite group also displayed possible characteristics of increased

Distribution of Power Output, as reflected by their higher peak down-stroke torque, as previously discussed (Fig. 2.9).

Aerobic Enzyme Activity in the vastus lateralis, by itself, did not account for much variance in $LT \dot{V}o_2$, although it did improve the multiple correlation. It also displayed substantial variability in the Elite and Good group, possibly for the following reasons. We found that some of the subjects with exceptionally high citrate synthase activity in the vastus lateralis displayed a pedaling technique that classified them as generating a relatively high amount of knee torque and thus overloading the vastus lateralis more than other cyclists. Although we did not study their carbohydrate metabolism sufficiently to calculate their *Distribution of Power Output,* they did display more glycogen depletion in their vastus lateralis after the performance test (unpublished data obtained from histochemical staining of muscle sections using the periodic acid-Schiff reagent for glycogen). This suggests that they activated a relatively small amount of muscle, as we had seen with the low LT cyclists, although not to that degree. This heavier reliance on the vastus lateralis when training and racing probably stimulated a high *Aerobic Enzyme Activity* in that muscle. However, this increase would be limited in how much it could increase $LT \dot{V}o_2$ without also developing the ability to *Distribute Power Output* to a larger muscle mass. Therefore, when relating *Aerobic Enzyme Activity* of the cycling musculature to $LT \dot{V}o_2$, it seems necessary to factor the total amount of muscle mass when cycling. The analogy is that the measurement of mitochondrial concentration per kilogram of muscle does not indicate how many total mitochondria are sharing in the work, without an estimation of the active muscle mass.

Economy and *Gross Mechanical Efficiency* were, of course, highly related to each other ($r^2 = 0.98$). Approximately 56–58% of their variance was accounted for by *Muscle Fiber Type Composition (% Type I)*. The *% Type I Fibers* were 66.5% and 52.9% in the Elite and Good group, respectively and *Economy* was 2.7% higher in the Elite group (Table 2.3).

$\dot{V}o_2max$ is the most basic *Functional Ability* listed in the model. For bicycling a 40-km time trial, it is most appropriate to compare athletes by using absolute $\dot{V}o_2max$ in liters per minute. Obviously, when other components are equal, the bigger person will have the advantage of a higher $\dot{V}o_2max$. Figure 2.11 indicates that 21–71% of the variance in $LT \dot{V}o_2$ is indeed related to $\dot{V}o_2max$. In this model, $\dot{V}o_2max$ is the variable that will carry with it the influence of body size.

SUMMARY

This model is used to understand the interrelationships of the physiological factors determining endurance performance ability during prolonged exercise. Early studies found that marathon runners maintain a velocity in competition that corresponds to the intensity at which lactate begins to accumulate in blood and muscle [7, 8, 19]. From this observation, the concept developed that this blood lactate threshold ($LT\ \dot{V}O_2$) reflects the degree of muscular stress, glycogenolysis and fatigue. However, it was not clear whether the lactate accumulation was a result of cardiovascular limitations linked to oxygen delivery, as reflected by $\dot{V}O_2max$ [54], as opposed to metabolic factors in the exercising muscle related to the extent to which mitochondrial respiration is disturbed to maintain a given rate of O_2 consumption [29, 30]. Two studies were performed to determine whether $LT\ \dot{V}O_2$ was tightly coupled to $\dot{V}O_2max$. In one study, endurance-trained ischemic heart disease patients were observed to possess a $\dot{V}O_2max$ that was 18% below that of normal master athletes who followed the patient's training program and who displayed the same performance ability as the patients. Both the patients and the normal men displayed an identical $LT\ \dot{V}O_2$ (i.e., 37 ml/kg/min) (Fig. 2.5). Therefore, performance was determined primarily by $LT\ \dot{V}O_2$ instead of $\dot{V}O_2max$ in this situation, albeit with abnormal subjects. In a second study we assembled two groups of competitive cyclists who were identical in $\dot{V}O_2max$ but differed by having a high or low $LT\ \dot{V}O_2$ (82% vs. 66% $\dot{V}O_2max$) [13]. When cycling at 80–88% $\dot{V}O_2max$, the low LT group displayed more than a 2-fold higher rate of muscle glycogen use and blood lactate concentration, and as a result were able to exercise only one-half as long as the high LT group. Performance time for a given $\dot{V}O_2$ was clearly related to $LT\ \dot{V}O_2$ instead of $\dot{V}O_2max$ (Fig. 2.6). This is not to say that $\dot{V}O_2max$ plays no role in determining $LT\ \dot{V}O_2$, because as in heart disease patients, it clearly sets the upper limit. Indeed, we have seen that much of the variance (i.e., 31–72%) in $LT\ \dot{V}O_2$ is related to $\dot{V}O_2max$. (Fig. 2.11.) However, improvements in performance after the first 2–3 yr of intense training are associated with improvements in $LT\ \dot{V}O_2$, whereas $\dot{V}O_2max$ generally increases very little thereafter (Table 2.3). The next question concerns the factors responsible for further increases in $LT\ \dot{V}O_2$ and *Performance*.

Another major factor determining $LT\ \dot{V}O_2$ is the muscle's *Aerobic Enzyme Activity* or mitochondrial respiratory capacity, as discussed in previous reviews [29, 30]. To support this, we have seen an identical rate of decline in $LT\ \dot{V}O_2$ and *Aerobic Enzyme Activity* with detraining (Fig. 2.4). However, by studying cyclists who were very homogeneous in both $\dot{V}O_2max$ and *Aerobic Enzyme Activity*, we were able to identify a new and important factor. Cyclists with a high $LT\ \dot{V}O_2$ when cycling appeared to be using approximately 20% more muscle mass when cycling at the same absolute work rate and percent $\dot{V}O_2max$ as subjects with a low $LT\ \dot{V}O_2$. The active muscle mass was estimated by comparing whole body carbohydrate metabolism to that of an exercising muscle. Although this estimate is not without limitations, we think that it introduces the important point that the degree of stress placed on individual muscle fibers during exercise has potential to be influenced by the amount of muscle sharing in the *Distribution of Power Output*. This concept is an extension of that introduced by Holloszy [28, 30] indicating that increases in the muscle mitochondrial number sharing in the work reduce glycogenolysis and lactate production. This new concept emphasizes that mitochondrial number sharing in the work can also be increased by using more muscle fibers, provided they can be adequately perfused.

Having established that $LT\ \dot{V}O_2$ is the most important determinant of the energy expenditure maintained during performance (i.e., *Performance* $\dot{V}O_2$), the other factor determining how well this translates into actual athletic *Performance Velocity* is the *Economy of Movement,* as has been long recognized [17]. This is best demonstrated by comparing individual athletes as we did with race-walkers (Fig. 2.3) and cyclists (Table 2.4). The important new finding is that *Economy* and *Gross Mechanical Efficiency* are highly related to % *Type I Muscle Fibers,* at least when cycling at 80 rpm. This has great potential to distinguish top competitive cyclists as evidenced by our demonstration that cyclists with 73% *Type I Fibers* produce 9% more *Performance Power* compared with cyclists with 48% *Type I Fibers,* despite the fact that they have an identical $LT\ \dot{V}O_2$ and *Performance* $\dot{V}O_2$ (Table 2.4).

The main purpose of this review was to summarize these observations into the usable model introduced in Fig. 2.1 and validated in Fig. 2.11. This indicates that 92–96% of the variance in the three *Performance Abilities* can be accounted for by the *Functional Abilities.* Furthermore, these appear to be related to discrete *Morphological Components* that have a reasonably good theoretical and experimental basis.

ACKNOWLEDGMENTS

About 20 years ago, my undergraduate teachers, Frank Katch and Bill McArdle, had me write a paper on the "Physiology of Marathon Running." In struggling through that paper, I got "hooked" on this area and have enjoyed trying to answer that question, "what physiological factors determine endurance performance?" In the process, I've had the good fortune being able to work in the labs of Dave Costill, Jack Wilmore, and John Holloszy, and I appreciate their support and many contributions. I've also thoroughly enjoyed working with and learning from my friends and colleagues Peter Farrell, Jim Hagberg, Ali Ehsani, and John Ivy, to name just a few. Special thanks to my University of Texas collaborators Larry Abrahams, Andy Coggan, Mike Feltner, Marc Hamilton, Jeff Horowitz, Steve Kautz, Scott Montain, as well as my current students, Paul Below, Ricardo Mora-Rodriquez, and Ricardo Fritzsche for their review of this manuscript.

REFERENCES

1. Bergh, U., B. Sjodin, A. Forsberg, J. Svedenhag. The relationship between body mass and oxygen uptake during running in humans. *Med. Sci. Sports Exerc.* 23:205–211, 1991.
2. Bosco, C., G. Montanari, R. Ribacchi, et al. Relationship between the efficiency of muscular work during jumping and the energetics of running. *Eur. J. Appl. Physiol.* 56:138–143, 1987.

3. Burke, E. R., F. Cerny, D. Costill, and W. Fink. Characteristics of skeletal muscle in competitive cyclists. *Med. Sci. Sports* 9:109–112, 1977.
4. Coggan, A. R., and E. F. Coyle. Carbohydrate ingestion during prolonged exercise: Effects on metabolism and performance. *Exerc. Sport Sci. Rev.* 19:1–40, 1991.
5. Coggan, A. R., W. M. Kohrt, R. J. Spina, J. P. Kirwan, D. M. Bier, and J. O. Holloszy. Plasma glucose kinetics during exercise in subjects with high and low lactate thresholds. *J. Appl. Physiol.* 73:1873–1880, 1992.
6. Conley, D. L., and G. S. Krahenbuhl. Running economy and distance running performance of highly trained athletes. *Med. Sci. Sports Exerc.* 12:357–360, 1980.
7. Costill, D. L., and E. L. Fox. Energetics of marathon running. *Med. Sci. Sports* 1:81–86, 1969.
8. Costill, D. L. H. Thomason, and E. Roberts. Fractional utilization of the aerobic capacity during distance running. *Med. Sci. Sports* 5:248–252, 1973.
9. Costill, D. L., J. Daniels, W. Evans, W. Fink, G. Krahenbuhl, and B. Saltin. Skeletal muscle enzymes and fiber composition in male and female track athletes. *J. Appl. Physiol.* 40:149–154, 1976.
10. Costill, D. L., E. Jansson, P. D. Gollnick, and B. Saltin. Glycogen utilization in leg muscles of men during level and uphill running. *Acta Physiol. Scand.* 91:475–481, 1974.
11. Coyle, E. F., W. H. Martin, A. A. Ehsani, et al. Blood lactate threshold in some well-trained ischemic heart disease patients. *J. Appl. Physiol.* 54:18–23, 1983.
12. Coyle, E. F., W. H. Martin III, S. A. Bloomfield, O. H. Lowry, and J. O. Holloszy. Effects of detraining on responses to submaximal exercise. *J. Appl. Physiol.* 59:853–859, 1985.
13. Coyle, E. F., A. R. Coggan, M. K. Hopper, T. J. Walters. Determinants of endurance in well trained cyclists. *J. Appl. Physiol.* 64:2622–2630, 1988.
14. Coyle, E. F., M. E. Feltner, S. A. Kautz, M. T. Hamilton, S. J. Montain, A. M. Baylor, L. D. Abraham and G. W. Petrek. Physiological and biomechanical factors associated with elite endurance cycling performance. *Med. Sci. Sports Exerc.* 23:93–107, 1991.
15. Coyle, E. F., L.S. Sidossis, J. F. Horowitz, J. D. Beltz. Cycling efficiency is related to the percentage of Type I muscle fibers. *Med. Sci. Sports Exerc.* 24:782–788, 1992.
16. Daniels, J. Physiological characteristics of champion male athletes. *Res. Q.* 43:342–348, 1974.
17. Diamant, B., J. Karlsson, and B. Saltin. Muscle tissue lactate after maximal exercise in man. *Acta Physiol. Scand.* 72:383–384, 1968.
18. Essen, B., and T. Häggmark. Lactate concentration in type I and II muscle fibers during muscular contraction in man. *Acta Physiol. Scand.* 95:344–346, 1975.
19. Farrell, P. A., J. H. Wilmore, E. F. Coyle, J. E. Billing, D. L. Costill Plasma lactate accumulation and distance running performance. *Med. Sci. Sports Exerc.* 11:338–344, 1979.
20. Fink. W. J., D. L. Costill, M. J. Pollock. Submaximal and maximal working capacity of elite distance runners. Part II. Muscle fiber composition and enzyme activity. *Ann. N. Y. Acad. Sci.* 301:323–327, 1977.
21. Fitts, R. H., D. L. Costill, and P. R. Gardetto. Effect of swim exercise training on human muscle fiber function. *J. Appl. Physiol.* 66:465–475, 1989.
22. Foster, C., D. L.Costill, J. T. Daniels, and W. J. Fink. Skeletal muscle enzyme activity, fiber composition and VO_2max in relation to distance running performance. *Eur. J. Appl. Physiol. Occup. Physiol.* 39:73–80, 1978.
23. Gibbs, C. L., and W. R. Gibson. Energy production of rat soleus muscle. *Am. J. Physiol.* 223:864–871, 1972.
24. Goldspink, G. Energy turnover during contraction of different types of muscle. E. Asmussen and K. Jørgensen (eds). *Biomechnics VI-A*, Baltimore: University Park Press, 1978, pp. 27–39.
25. Hagberg, J. M., and E. F. Coyle. Physiological determinants of endurance performance as studied in competitive racewalkers. *Med. Sci. Sports. Exerc.* 15:287–289, 1983.
26. Hermansen, L., E. Hultman, and B. Saltin. Muscle glycogen during prolonged severe exercise. *Acta Physiol. Scand.* 71:129–139, 1967.

27. Hermansen, L., and I. Stensvold. Production and removal of lactate during exercise in man. *Acta Physiol. Scand.* 86:191–201, 1972.
28. Holloszy, J. O. Biochemical adaptations in muscle. Effects of exercise on mitochondrial oxygen uptake and respiratory enzyme activity in skeletal muscle. *J. Biol. Chem.* 242:2278–2282, 1967.
29. Holloszy, J. O., and F. W. Booth. Biochemical adaptations to endurance training in muscle. *Annu. Rev. Physiol.* 38:273–291, 1976.
30. Holloszy, J. O., and E. F. Coyle. Adaptations of skeletal muscle to endurance exercise and their metabolic consequences. *J. Appl. Physiol.* 56:831–838, 1984.
31. Horowitz, J. F., L. S. Sidossis, and E. F. Coyle. High efficiency of Type I muscle fibers improves performance. *Int. J. Sports Med.* 15:152–157, 1993.
32. Ivy, J. L., R. T. Withers, P. J. Van Handel, D. H. Elger, D. L. Costill. Muscle respiratory capacity and fiber type as determinants of the lactate threshold. *J. Appl. Physiol.* 48:523–527, 1980.
33. Ivy, J. L., M. M.-Y. Chi, C. S. Hintz, W. M. Sherman, R. P. Hellendall, and O. H. Lowry. Progresive metabolite changes in individual human muscle fibers with increasing work rates. *Am. J. Physiol. 252 (Cell Physiol 21):* C630–C639, 1987.
34. Johnson, M. A., J. Polgar, D. Weightman, and D. Appleton. Data on the distribution of fiber types in thirty-six human muscles. *J. Neurol. Sci.* 18:111–129, 1973.
35. Jorfeldt, L. Turnover of 14C-1 (+)-lactate in human skeletal muscle during exercise. B. Pernow and B. Saltin (eds.) *Muscle Metabolism During Exercise.* New York: Plenum Press, 1971, pp. 409–417.
36. Joyner, M.J. Physiological limiting factors and distance running: influence of gender and age on record performance. *Exerc. Sports Sci. Rev.* 21:103–134, 1993.
37. Karlsson, J. Lactate in working muscles after prolonged exercise. *Acta Physiol. Scand.* 82:123–130, 1971.
38. Kautz, S. A., M. E. Feltner, E. F. Coyle, A. M. Baylor. The pedaling technique of elite endurance cyclists: changes with increasing workload at constant cadence. *Int. J. Sport Biomech.* 7:29–53, 1991.
39. Kindermann, W., G. Simon, and J. Keul. The significance of the aerobic-anaerobic transition for the determination of work load intensities during endurance training. *Eur. J. Appl. Physiol.* 42:25–34, 1979.
40. Kusherick, M. J. Energetics of muscle contraction. L. E. Peachey, R. H., Adrian, S. R. Geiger (eds). *Handbook of Physiology, Section 10: Skeletal Muscle.* Bethesda, MD: American Physiological Society, 1983, pp. 189–236.
41. Kyle, C. R. Ergogenics of bicycling. D. R. Lamb and M. H. Williams (eds). *Perspectives in Exercise Science and Sports Medicine.* Vol 4. *Ergogenics: Enhancement of Performance in Exercise and Sport.* Brown & Benchmark, 1991.
42. Margaria, R., H. T. Edwards, and D. B. Dill. The possible mechanisms of contracting and paying the oxygen debt and role of lactic acid in muscle contraction. *Am. J. Physiol.* 106:689–715, 1933.
43. Martin, P. E., Morgan, D. W. Biomechanical considerations for economical walking and running. *Med. Sci. Sports Exerc.* 24:467–474, 1992.
44. Mitchell, J. H. Neural control of the circulation during exercise. *Med. Sci. Sports Exerc.* 22:141–154, 1990.
45. Morgan, D. W., Craib, M. Physiological aspects of running economy. *Med. Sci. Sports Exerc.* 24:456–461, 1992.
46. Nagle, F., D. Robinhold, E. Howley, J. Daniels, G. Baptista, and K. Stoedefalke. Lactic acid accumulation during running at submaximal aerobic demands. *Med. Sci. Sports* 2:182–186, 1970.
47. Pollock, M. L. Submaximal and maximal working capacity of elite distance runnrs. Part I: Cardiorespiratory aspects. *Ann. N. Y. Acad. Sci.* 301:310–322, 1977.

48. Poole, D. C., G. A. Gaesser, M. C. Hogan, D. R. Knight, P. D. Wagner. Pulmonary and leg VO_2 during submaximal exercise: implication for muscular efficiency. *J. Appl. Physiol.* 72:805–810, 1992.

49. Poortmans, J. R., J. Bossche, and R. Leclercq. Lactate uptake by inactive forearm during progressive leg exercise. *J. Appl. Physiol.* 45:835–839, 1978.

50. Romijn, J. A., E. F. Coyle, J. Hibbert, R. R. Wolfe. Comparison of indirect calorimetry and a new breath $^{13}C/^{12}C$ ratio method during strenuous exercise. *Am. J. Physiol.* (Endocrinol. Metab. 26):E64–E71, 1992.

51. Romijn J.A., E. F. Coyle, L. Sidossis, et al. Regulation of endogenous fat and carbohydrate metabolism in relation to exercise intensity. *Am. J. Physiol.* 265(Endocrinol. Metab. 28) 263:E380–E391, 1993.

52. Romijn, J. A., E. F. Coyle, X.-J. Zhang, L. S. Sidossis, R. R. Wolfe. Relationship between fatty acid delivery and fatty acid oxidation during exercise. *Am. J. Physiol.* (Endocrinol. Metab.): in press.

53. Saltin, B., and J. Karlsson. Muscle ATP, CP, and lactate during exercise after physical conditioning. B. Pernow and B. Saltin (eds). *Muscle Metabolism During Exercise.* New York: Plenum Press, 1971, pp. 395–399.

54. Saltin, B., S. Strange. Maximal oxygen uptake: "old" and "new" arguments for a cardiovascular limitation. *Med. Sci. Sports Exerc.* 24:30–37, 1992.

55. Shepard, R. J., and P.-O. Astrand. *Endurance In Sport.* Oxford: Blackwell Scientific Publications, 1992.

56. Sjodin, B., and I. Jacobs. Onset of blood lactate accumulation and marathoning running performance. *Int. J. Sports Med.* 2:23–26, 1981.

57. Sjodin, B., I. Jacobs, and J. Karlsson. Onset of blood lactate accumulation and enzyme activities in m. vastus lateralis in man. *Int. J. Sports Med.* 2:166–170, 1981.

58. Stainsby, W. N., and H. G. Welch. Lactate metabolism of contracting dog skeletal muscle in situ. *Am. J. Physiol.* 211:177–183, 1966.

59. Tesch, P. A., and J. E. Wright. Recovery from short term exercise: its relation to capillary supply and blood lactate concentration. *Eur. J. Appl. Physiol. Occup. Physiol.* 52:98–103, 1983.

60. Tesch, P. A., and W. L. Daniels, and D. S. Sharp. Lactate accumulation in muscle and blood during submaximal exercise. *Acta Physiol. Scand.* 114:441–446.

61. Wasserman, K., B. J. Whipp, S. N. Koyal, and W. L. Beaver. Anaerobic threshold and respiratory gas exchange during exercise. *J. Appl. Physiol.* 35:235–243, 1973.

62. Wasserman, K., and B. J. Whipp. Exercise physiology in health and disease. *Am. Rev. Respir. Dis.* 112:219–249, 1975.

63. Webb, P. The work of walking: a calorimetric study. *Med. Sci. Sports Exerc.* 20:331–337, 1988.

64. Welltman, A., D. Snead, P. Stein, R. Schurrer, R. Ruth, and J. Weltman. Reliability and validity of a continuous incremental treadmill protocol for the determination of lactate threshold, fixed blood lactate concentrations, and VO_2max. *Int. J. Sports Med.* 11:26–32, 1990.

65. Wendt, I. R., and C. L. Gibbs. Energy production of rate extensor digitorum longus muscle. *Am. J. Physiol.* 224:1081–1086, 1973.

66. Wendt, I. R., and C. L. Gibbs. Energy production of mammalian fast- and slow-twitch muscles during developments. *Am. J. Physiol.* 226:642–647, 1974.

67. Williams, K. R., and P. R. Cavanagh. Relationship between distance running mechanics, running economy, and performance. *J. Appl. Physiol.* 63:1236–1245, 1987.

3
Changes in Movement Capabilities
with Aging

MARK D. GRABINER, Ph.D.
ROGER M. ENOKA, Ph.D.

It is evident, even to the casual observer, that movement capabilities decline with age. For example, world record performances for numerous athletic events exhibit a parabolic relationship with peak values occurring about the second or third decade of life [104]. Identification of the mechanisms underlying these reduced capabilities, however, is not a simple matter. There are a number of confounding variables, such as differences among subjects due to ethnicity, gender, and health status [65, 103, 169, 173], differences among studies in the complexity of the experimental task, and a reliance on cross-sectional rather than longitudinal studies [7, 84, 143, 184]. These differences can impede the development of general principles on aging, including those related to changes in movement capabilities.

Despite these constraints, the challenge of this chapter is to review how the aging process affects the motor system and the ability of humans to move about their environment. There are at least two experimental strategies that can be used to address this question. One approach is to select a movement from among the repertoire of daily activities (e.g., grasp control, sit-to-stand movement, stumbling reaction), to perform a complete biomechanical analysis of the selected movement, and then to deduce the physiological adaptations that might underlie the change in performance with age. Alternatively, an investigator might select a component of many movements (e.g., reaction time, reflexes, balance control, strength, fatigability), characterize how this component is affected by age, and then extrapolate to describe how these changes might affect movement capabilities. This chapter will review selected examples of both experimental strategies, beginning with changes in strength and fatigability and then examining the effects of age on such tasks as the precision grip, maintenance of a static posture, and recovery from large postural perturbations. Furthermore, because this chapter addresses changes in movement capabilities, there is a greater emphasis on results from studies on human subjects.

MUSCLE STRENGTH

In the exercise physiology literature, the assessment of muscle strength is typically regarded as an index of the quantity of contractile protein available to move the musculoskeletal system. When muscle strength involves measurement of the maximum voluntary contraction (MVC) force, however, the exerted force is the product of a learned skill and is not necessarily proportional to muscle size. The task of exerting an MVC force is afforded this status because it is possible to increase MVC force without an increase in muscle size; that is, the increase in strength (MVC force) occurs because of adaptations that occur within the nervous system. Indeed, it is possible to increase MVC force without an increase in the quantity of contractile protein but not without an adaptation within the nervous system.

There are several lines of evidence to support this conclusion. First, numerous authors have reported that the increase in muscle strength, especially for naive subjects, precedes observable increases in muscle size [56, 102, 176, 186]. For example, an 8-wk strength training for the knee extensor muscles produced an increase in strength but no increase in the cross-sectional area of Type I, IIa, or IIb muscle fibers [196]. Second, although the maximal force that a muscle can exert is proportional to its cross-sectional area [203], there is a poor correlation between increases in MVC force and muscle size [102, 154, 166, 227]. This poor correlation has been observed for both young and elderly subjects [89, 109, 229]. Third, increases in muscle strength are specific to the type of exercises performed during training. For example, Rutherford and Jones [185] found that subjects who trained with isometric exercises for 12 wk had a 40% increase in MVC force (isometric), whereas subjects who trained with anisometric exercises experienced a 15–20% increase in MVC force but a 170–200% increase in the load that could be lifted during the anisometric exercises. These effects were interpreted as a training-induced improvement in coordination of the muscles involved in the task. Fourth, Carolan and Cafarelli [26] found that 8 wk of strength training produced an increase in MVC force for the knee extensor muscles and that this was associated with a reduction in activation of the antagonist muscles (hamstrings) during the MVC task. The decrease in coactivation would cause an increase in the net knee extensor torque. Fifth, it appears that for large muscle groups (e.g., quadriceps femoris) the entire volume of muscle may not be activated during an MVC. For example, Narici et al. [154] reported that 60 days of training produced differential increases in muscle cross-sectional area both among the four quadriceps femoris muscles and along the length of each muscle. Furthermore, Adams et al. [1] used T2-weighted magnetic resonance images to estimate that electrical stimulation of 71% of the cross-sectional area of the quadriceps femoris was sufficient to elicit a force equivalent to the MVC force. This suggests that in these subjects an MVC did not involve activation of the entire volume of this muscle. Taken together, these observations suggest that changes in strength with training are probably due to adaptations that occur in both the musculoskeletal and nervous system.

Decline in Strength with Aging

One of the most frequently observed consequences of aging is a loss of muscle mass and strength [50, 180]. For example, a cross-sectional study of men indicated that the MVC force of the knee extensor muscles increased up to age 27 yr, remained stable until about age 45 yr, and then began to decline [117]. For 50–70-yr-olds, the loss of strength is about 15% per decade [180]. Longitudinal studies have reported quite different rates of decline for the same muscle group. Greig et al. [84] found over an 8-yr period that MVC force for the knee extensors of 80-yr-olds had declined at a rate of −0.3% per annum. In contrast, Aniansson et al. [4] reported a 35% decrease in MVC force for the knee extensors of 80-yr-old men over an 11-yr period. However, the rate of decline varies among individuals and muscle groups, and there is an effect due to gender [88]. In a cross-sectional study on the decline in strength of women, Christ et al. [30] found that MVC force began to decline for the wrist and finger flexor muscles at 45–49 yr, for the plantar flexor muscles at 65–74 yr, and for the wrist extensor muscles at 65–69 yr. The gender effect occurs largely because of the changes that accompany menopause. When the strength of a hand muscle (adductor pollicis) was normalized to its cross-sectional area, Phillips et al. [173] observed a marked decrease in MVC force among women at the time of and subsequent to menopause. This decline, however, was prevented by hormone replacement therapy.

Accompanying the reduction in strength is a marked decline in muscle mass in elderly subjects. Although some studies have found a parallel decrease in MVC force and muscle cross-sectional area [225], most have reported that the loss of MVC force is greater than the reduction in cross-sectional area [22, 111, 213, 226]. Thus, the decrease in MVC force is due to both a loss of muscle mass and some other factor, such as a reduced ability to activate muscle or a change in specific tension. It seems well established that the decline in muscle mass is partly due to smaller muscle fiber diameters, more so for Type II fibers, but is mainly caused by a decrease in the number of muscle fibers [5, 111, 116, 124, 163].

Frequently the dissociation between the change in MVC force and cross-sectional area is expressed as specific tension, which is defined as the ratio of these two variables (N/cm^2). In human subjects, specific tension is typically estimated by measuring the MVC force and using imaging techniques such as computed tomography or magnetic resonance imaging to determine the cross-sectional area of a whole muscle. Under these conditions, there have been some reports of a decline in specific tension with age [22, 42, 111, 172, 227] and other reports of no change [66, 229]. There are at least two factors that contribute to this discrepancy. First, the imaging procedures provide information on the anatomical cross-sectional area of the muscle but not its physiological cross-sectional area. This limitation causes the calculation of specific tension to ignore the effect of muscle architecture on the maximum force the muscle can exert. When muscle architecture is considered, as in measurements on isolated muscle, there is a deficit of about 20% in the specific tension of muscle from old mice and rats [15, 25, 171]. Second, because the quantity of noncontractile protein in a cross-sectional image of a muscle can vary with age [164], this measurement of specific tension based on cross-sectional area does not provide a valid index of the force-generating capacity of muscle. Rather, it is necessary to express the maximum force relative to the quantity of myofibrillar protein [203]. This measurement has not been undertaken systematically in aged muscle. However, Brooks and Faulkner [17] propose that there is a decrease in specific tension with age and that this decline is due to a decrease in either the number of crossbridges per unit area or in the average force exerted by each crossbridge.

Similarly, the effects of age on the ability to activate a muscle maximally during a strength maneuver are uncertain [50]. Based on the interpolated twitch, some evidence suggests that elderly human subjects remain as capable of activating a muscle maximally during a voluntary contraction as younger subjects [18, 212]. In these experiments, 1–5 supramaximal shocks are delivered to the test muscle during a maximal contraction and the investigators assess whether the stimuli elicit additional force. The absence of an added force is interpreted as evidence of maximal activation during the voluntary contraction. In contrast, observations on the maximum force exerted during lengthening (eccentric) contractions suggest that there may be some changes in activation capabilities as a function of age. Despite substantial effort, human subjects are generally unable to activate a muscle maximally during an eccentric contraction. This is made evident by a submaximal electromyogram (EMG) during an eccentric contraction compared with that associated with a concentric contraction [204] and by the possibility of eliciting a greater force during an eccentric contraction when electrical stimulation is superimposed on a maximum voluntary activation [215]. In older subjects, there is less of a decline in the maximum force during eccentric contractions compared with concentric contractions, with the result that there is an increase in the difference between the maximum eccentric and concentric forces during voluntary contractions [175, 212]. The role of a diminished ability to activate muscle maximally by voluntary commands in this disproportionate decline is strength (concentric and eccentric) is unknown. Furthermore, aging is accompanied by a decline in the safety factor associated with neuromuscular transmission, which increases the likelihood that an action potential may not be transmitted across a neuromuscular junction and hence impairs the ability to activate muscle maximally [98, 110].

Despite the uncertainty over the contributions of changes in specific tension and activation capabilities to the decline in muscle strength, it is apparent that aging can be associated with a substantial decline in muscle mass and loss of strength [13, 17, 27, 50, 180]. One adaptation that contributes to the decline in muscle mass is a reduction in the number of muscle fibers secondary to the death of α motor neurons [124]. The loss of ventral horn cells in the human lumbosacral spinal cord appears to begin at around age 60 yr and to occur at a rate of about 10% per decade [71, 108, 147, 208]. In rats, the largest motor neurons with the lowest oxidative capability seem to be preferentially lost with age [97]. As expected with a loss of α motor neurons, there is also a decline in the number of motor units in a muscle that also begins at about age 60 yr [24, 123]. The reduction in muscle mass, however, is not directly related to motor neuron death because some of the surviving motor units develop collateral sprouts to reinnervate some, but not all, of the abandoned muscle fibers [19, 21]. As a consequence, aged muscles contain fewer motor units but these have greater innervation ratios, especially the slow-twitch (Type S) motor units [97, 106]. This reorganization is also evident electrophysiologically by an increase in the amplitude of motor unit action potentials as a function of age [44, 194, 195].

Although the loss of motor neurons is a significant contributor to the decline in muscle mass with age, other factors must be involved in this loss of contractile protein. The literature on recovery of motor function has demonstrated that after a partial lesion of a muscle nerve the surviving motor units develop collateral sprouts and reinnervate many of the denervated muscle fibers. Apparently all the motor unit types within a pool are able to compensate for these types of nerve injuries by collateral sprouting [55, 178]. The number of additional fibers reinnervated depends on the size of the motor unit, with motor units capable of enlarging to about 5 times the original size [78]. The extent of the sprouting, and hence the innervation ratio, depends on the number of muscle fibers that are denervated [209]. In adult mammals, collateral sprouting can recover the maximum force capability of muscle with a loss of up to 80% of the motor neurons [78]. Given this recuperative ability in adults, the inability of the aging nervous system to reinnervate all of the abandoned muscle fibers suggests that this collateral-sprouting capability is also reduced with age [60, 85, 98, 99].

Neuromuscular Responses to Strength Training
Although aging human muscle can be characterized by a loss of mass and a decline in strength, two features associated with this adaptation are noteworthy. First, there is marked variability across subjects in the extent of these adaptations such that some elderly people retain strength capabilities that are comparable with young subjects [84, 111, 153]. Second, the neuromuscular system in even the frail elderly remains responsive to the stressors associated with strength training [63]. Given these observations, there has been considerable interest in the neuromuscular responses to strength training, and numerous studies have documented the ability of the system to increase strength with short- and long-term training programs [50, 180].

Most studies have employed 8–12-wk training programs and have found that substantial increases in strength are accompanied by modest increases in muscle size [28, 67]. For example, Keen et al. [109] had young (23 yr, n = 10) and elderly (65 yr, n = 11) subjects perform a 12-wk strength training program (3 times/wk, 6 sets of 10 repetitions) with the first dorsal interosseus muscle. The training program caused similar increases (% initial) in the training load (137%), twitch force (23%), and MVC force (39%) for the young and elderly subjects. The increase in strength was associated with a modest increase in magnetic resonance imaging-determined muscle volume (9% for the young, 4% for the elderly) and a nonmonotonic increase in the surface-recorded EMG that, with respect to week 0, was significantly greater at week 8 but not at week 12. The similarity of the increase in muscle volume for the young and elderly subjects is consistent with the observation that strength training appears to increase the fractional rate of protein synthesis (percent of muscle mass synthesized per hour) to similar levels in young and elderly subjects [222, 224]. However, the relative contribution of the different fiber types to the increase in muscle size has been inconsistent, with some reports indicating a selective increase in the cross-sectional area of Type II fibers [28, 182] and others reporting an increase for both Type I and II fibers [18, 67, 176]. In general, it appears that the increase in cross-sectional area is greater in Type II muscle fibers. Undoubtedly, this discrepancy is due to differences in the subjects across studies, in the muscles examined, and in the details of the strength-training protocols.

Such results suggest that some of the increase in strength can be attributed to an increase in muscle size but that other factors are also important. This interpretation is underscored by the observation that the increase in strength precedes the increase in muscle size [59, 87, 176, 185], by the finding that strength training can cause an increase in the cross-sectional area of muscle but without an increase in the maximum isometric force [18], and by the different effects of a given training program on various strength tasks [18, 109, 185]. One class of factors that can contribute to these dissociations is the so-called "neural factors." As described previously, these factors include such possibilities as a reduction in the level of coactivation, differences in the distribution of activity among synergist muscles, an improvement in the coordination among muscles involved in the task, and alterations in the recruitment and discharge (rate and pattern) of motor units. However, the finding by Keen et al. [109] of a nonmonotonic change in the surface EMG over the course of a 12-wk strength training program suggests that the interaction among these mechanisms is nonlinear and therefore difficult to determine. There remains much to be learned about the relative contribution of these various mechanisms to the change in strength with age and to the response of the neuromuscular system to strength training.

Functional Consequences of Strength Training

As stated in the Introduction, the reason for studying changes in strength with aging is 2-fold: to determine the associated physiological adaptations and to identify the functional consequences of changes in muscle strength. Most studies on this topic, however, have focused on the physiological mechanisms and have not addressed the effects of changes in strength on the activities of daily living. This issue clearly needs more attention. One example of a study that did consider the relationship between changes in strength and motor performance was performed on a group of frail 90-yr-old volunteers who were institutionalized. In this study, Fiatarone et al. [63] had the subjects perform an 8-wk training program for the knee extensor muscles that involved 3 sessions per week and 3 sets of 8 repetitions with a load that was 80% of maximum in each session. The average increase in the one repetition-maximum load was 174%, which was accompanied by an increase in midthigh muscle cross-sectional area in 5 of the 7 subjects who were given computed tomography scan. However, even the subjects who did not experience an increase in muscle area demonstrated an increase in strength. For this group of subjects, the cross-sectional area of the quadriceps femoris increased an average of 11% over the 8 wk, but this was not correlated with the strength gains. The clinical outcomes of the training program were that thigh girth and skinfold measurements did not change, habitual gait speed did not change, one subject improved in the ability to rise from a chair, two subjects were able to discard the use of a cane while walking, and there was a significant decrease in walking time during tandem gait. Such outcomes have been used to emphasize the importance of strength in the activities of daily living.

An alternative strategy used by some groups to determine the importance of strength for the activities of daily living has been to compare the biomechanical requirements of various tasks to the capabilities of elderly subjects. Based on such a comparison, some tasks have been found to be within the capabilities of even frail older adults (e.g., rising from a chair at a comfortable speed, resisting small postural disturbances with a sway or stepping response [3, 134, 188], some tasks require certain levels of strength (e.g., trunk flexion strength in rising from a bed, ankle strength in single-leg balance [214], and performance on other tasks covaries with strength (e.g., walking speed [6, 9]. For example, sway responses to small postural disturbances required mean joint movements of force of about 30 N·m, which are well below the maximum torques available at the ankle, knee, and hip joints of older adults [33]. More substantial postural disturbances, such as those that produce up to 3° of initial body lean, require a stepping response and although the number and sizes of the steps differ with age, the mean peak torques were only 20, 18, and 24 N·m for the ankle, knee, and hip of the stepping leg and 32, 19, and 22 N·m for the support leg [131, 132]. Differences in muscle strength (peak torque) does not appear to distinguish between young and older subjects in performance on these tasks. However, the rate of force development appears to be an important determinant in time-critical tasks such as the ability of subjects to recover from a trip [29] and to maintain single-leg balance [119], and it is significantly decreased with age [203]. Because some strength-training protocols can increase the rate of force development [186], it would be informative to determine the effect of these protocols on the ability of elderly subjects to perform these tasks.

MUSCLE FATIGUE

Because aging is associated with a loss of low-oxidative motor neurons, a reduction in the number and size of Type IIb muscle fibers, and a reorganization of surviving motor units, it is probable that the mechanisms limiting performance under various conditions change as a function of age. Despite substantial literature on muscle fatigue [58, 64, 187], little attention has been directed toward the interaction between aging and muscle fatigue. A few studies have measured fatigability in older humans under various conditions, but these results have provided only a cursory description of the changes that occur with age.

Voluntary Activation and Neuromuscular Electrical Stimulation
A number of fatigue protocols have been used to assess the effect of age on the fatigability of human muscle. The studies that have used voluntary activation of muscle generally have found no change in fatigability with age [43, 91, 114]. These studies have involved submaximal and maximal voluntary contractions, isometric and dynamic contractions, and continuous and intermittent contractions as performed by hand and leg muscles. When fatigue is assessed with tasks that involve absolute rather than normalized (% MVC) levels of muscle force (eg., % body weight), endurance capabilities decline with age because of the reduction in muscle mass [152]. Under these conditions, elderly subjects perform the task at an absolute force that corresponds to a higher normalized force and consequently fatigue more rapidly. The absence of an effect due to age on fatigability involving normalized forces is surprising because it implies that the changes in fiber-type proportions and the reorganization of motor unit territories does not influence the mechanisms that limit performance in these different tasks. Furthermore, these findings suggest that the decline in muscle mass, maximum force capabilities, and fatigue mechanisms scale linearly as a function of age. This possibility seems inconsistent with the report by Hagberg et al. [86] that elderly men undergo less physiological stress than young untrained men during submaximal exercise at the same relative exercise intensity.

In contrast, the activation of muscle by electrical stimulation has provided equivocal conclusions on changes in fatigability with age. There have been reports of no change in fatigability as well as reports of an increase or a decrease in fatigability. For example, 30 s of ulnar-nerve stimulation at 20 Hz [122] resulted in an increased fatigability (greater decline in force) of the adductor pollicis muscle in elderly men (67 yr) but not elderly women (63 yr), whereas stimulation at 30 Hz [153] resulted in a decrease in fatigability with age (70 male subjects, 20–91 yr). In both studies, a fatigue index was computed as the force at 30 s relative to the initial force. With the 20-Hz stimulation protocol [122], the young male subjects (34 yr) experienced a 5% decline in force, whereas for the older men (67 yr), the force declined by 8%. With the 30-Hz stimulation protocol [153], the reduction in force after 30 s of stimulation was 29% for subjects in their 20s but only 10% for those in their 70s. The relative difference in fatigability for the 30-Hz stimulation was consistent with a leftward shift of the force-frequency relationship for the adductor pollicis muscle in the older subjects [153]. The greatest difference between these two studies was in the amount of fatigability (force reduction) measured for the young subjects; the results were similar (8–10%) for the elderly subjects. However, Cupido et al. [40] found no effect of age on the fatigability of the tibialis anterior muscle with stimulation rates of 20, 30, and 40 Hz. Similarly varied results have been obtained with electrical stimulation in studies on rodent muscle [27].

Task Specificity
One of the prominent themes emerging in the study of muscle fatigue is the concept that the mechanisms limiting performance depend on the details of the task [68, 144]. The task variables that influence this relationship include subject motivation, the pattern of muscle activation, the intensity and duration of activity, and the extent to which activity is sustained continuously [58]. The literature contains a rich and imaginative set of protocols that have been used to study muscle fatigue. From these studies, it is apparent that an experimental protocol can be designed to impair any process in the sequence of physiological events from the generation of the motor command to the activity of the crossbridges. The critical issue, however, is to determine which mechanisms are functionally important for the various conditions encountered in the repertoire of human capabilities.

Only a few studies have addressed this issue with regard to aging. One example involved changes in the median power frequency of the EMG during a fatiguing contraction. Merletti et al. [142] had young (18–43 yr) and elderly (65–84 yr) subjects perform several types of 20-s contractions with the tibialis anterior muscle: voluntary contractions at 20 and 80% MVC or contractions elicited with high and low levels of electrical stimulation. For the 80% MVC task, the decline in muscle conduction velocity and the median power frequency was less for the elderly subjects. Because aging is associated with a decline in the number of Type II muscle fibers, this finding can be explained by a reduced reliance on glycolytic metabolism and the accompanying accumulation of metabolites that will influence conduction velocity and median frequency. In contrast, there was no difference between the young and elderly subjects in the effects of high-level electrical stimulation on the conduction velocity and spectral variables of the EMG. Similarly, Enoka et al. [57] found less of a decline in the mean frequency of the EMG for the first dorsal interosseus muscle when elderly subjects sustained an abduction force at 35% MVC; mean power frequency declined by 27% for the elderly subjects (67 yr) and 39% for the young subjects (28 yr). However, the young and elderly subjects were able to sustain the submaximal force for similar durations (212 ± 29 s and 183 ± 22 s, respectively), which suggests that the difference in the median frequency was not functionally significant.

Because the fatigue mechanisms vary with the task requirements, some investigators have examined the effect of age on the ability to sustain power production. In contrast to the absence of an effect of age on the decline in force during sustained contractions, the ability to sustain power production does decline with age [16, 43]. For example, Brooks and Faulkner [16] measured the power produced by the extensor digitorum muscle of mice during shortening contractions for which the duty cycle increased continuously. When the maximum sustained power was normalized to body mass, power production of adult mice (5.8 W/kg) was only 55% of that produced by young mice (10.5 W/kg) and power production of old mice (4.7 W/kg) was 45% of that produced by young mice. Furthermore, the duty cycle at which the maximum power was sustained was 0.22 for the young mice, 0.13 for the adult mice, and 0.07 for the old mice. These findings suggest that the mechanisms limiting performance during isometric contractions are different from those for nonisometric contractions and that these two sets of mechanisms are affected differently by age.

CONTROL OF THE PRECISION GRIP

Many activities of daily living, such as fastening buttons, tying laces, eating a meal, and combing hair, rely on the dextrous manipulation of objects by the hands. At an anatomical level, the hand movements that enable these activities comprise sequences of digit flexion-extension, abduction-adduction, and opposition of the thumb and index finger. At a functional level, the many different combinations of digit movements that can be performed are generally constrained to one of two sets, either a power grip or a precision grip. The power grip is a whole-hand grasp of an object, whereas the precision grip refers to the pinch of an object by the thumb and index finger. The ability of humans to explore and shape their world relies extensively on the sensorimotor capabilities of the hand, especially the thumb and index finger, and the unique interaction between the hand and the brain [148, 170].

Hand dexterity is impaired with age. For example, performance on such tasks as card turning, and hand writing, spirography, and target tracking indicate that the time required to manipulate small objects increases by 25–40% of initial by 70 years of age [100]. To explore this effect, Cole [35] utilized a simple task to assess performance and then attempted to identify the mechanisms associated with the changes that occur in performance due to age. The task involved the vertical lift (5 cm) of a small object (160 g) using a precision grip. The object was designed to measure the horizontal pinch force and the contact surfaces were changeable so that the slipperiness of the surface could be varied. Each subject performed 252 lifts and the contact surface was changed frequently (sandpaper, leather, rayon) to assess grip-force adjustments. Although all 9 young subjects (mean age, 22 yr) and 10 elderly subjects (mean age, 81 yr) were able to perform the task and not drop the object, many of the elderly subjects executed the task with an excessive grip force that varied over the course of the lift (Fig. 3.1).

The grip force can be considered to be composed of two components, one to prevent the object from slipping (the slip force) and another that adds a margin of safety above the slip force to accommodate uncertainties in the lifting task (e.g., slipperiness of the contact, estimated weight of the object). Whether the contact surface was rayon (most slippery) or sandpaper, both the slip force and the safety margin force (N and %) were greater for the elderly subjects. Differences in the slip force between subject groups is attributable to differences in hand slipperiness and the associated coefficient of static friction [37]. However, the larger grip forces used by the elderly subjects were not solely due to differences in hand slipperiness because the elderly subjects also used a greater safety margin in the performance of the lift. Furthermore, because the safety margin force was not a constant percentage of the total grip force, the greater grip force used by the elderly subjects could not be ascribed totally to differences in hand slipperiness. As expected, these differences in forces were associated with both a reduced two-point discrimination ability on the thumb and index finger (300% increase for each) and an increased duration (62% increase) for a standardized card-turning task for the elderly subjects. The increased grip forces used by the elderly subjects may have been related to their impaired tactile sensibility that affected the signaling of frictional conditions.

One feature of the protocol used by Cole [35] was to have subjects perform three lifts with a sandpaper surface followed by three lifts with a rayon surface. By examining the first lift with the rayon surface (dashed line in Fig. 3.1), it was possible to determine the adjustments used by the subjects to accommodate unexpected changes in slipperiness. On the first rayon trial, the young subjects increased the force rapidly and gradually reduced the force over the course of the first trial and for subsequent rayon trials (dotted line in Fig. 3.1). In contrast, elderly subjects increased grip force on the first and subsequent rayon trials (Fig. 3.1). These differences in grip-

FIGURE 3.1.

Pinch forces exerted by a young subject (top) and elderly subject (bottom) during three trials of the precision grip. The sides of the object were either covered with rayon (slippery) or sandpaper. Both subjects lifted the same object. The force used by the elderly subject was greater and more variable. From ref. 35. Adapted by permission of Heldref Publications.

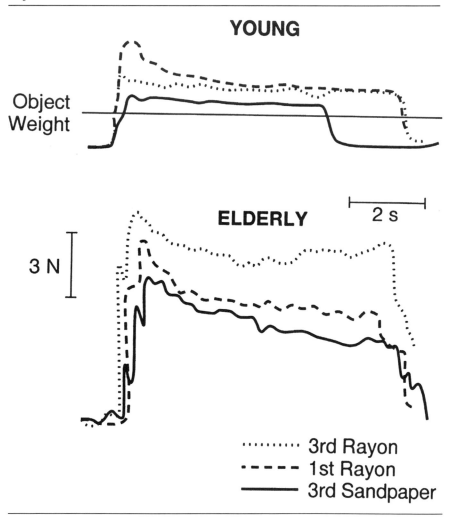

force adjustment suggest that age affects the automatic sensory control of grasping and manipulation activities. This control appears to be accomplished by the use of feedforward mechanisms to integrate somatosensory and visual signals with sensorimotor and memory systems [101].

An alternative explanation for the excessive grip forces used by the elderly subjects is that they use such a strategy to compensate for the force fluctuations that occur with increasing pinch force. Despite attempts to the contrary, the force exerted by muscle is never constant but rather the amplitude varies over time. Furthermore, the magnitude of the force fluctuations increases with an increase in the sustained force [89, 140, 160, 192, 202]. Perhaps the strategy used by these elderly subjects was to exert a greater grip force so that the minimum force during the fluctuations was always greater than the slip force. To assess this possibility, Cole and Beck [36] examined force stability (standard deviation of the force fluctuations) while subjects exerted a precision grip (thumb and index finger) at three submaximum levels (the highest forces were 13–24% of MVC force). When the arm and hand were supported during the precision grip (pinch) and no visual feedback was provided on force stability, Cole and Beck found that the standard deviations of the force fluctuations increased with the target force but that the young subjects were more variable at the highest force. However, when the subjects lifted an object with the precision grip, the older subjects exerted a greater and more variable force. The force fluctuations exhibited by the elderly subjects during the lifting task were greater than would be expected at an equivalent force during the supported-arm pinch. Furthermore, there was no correlation between the size of the force fluctuations (standard deviations) and the safety margin, which led Cole and Beck to conclude that elderly subjects do not use excessive grip forces to compensate for greater force fluctuations.

Others have found similarly that there is no difference between young and elderly subjects in the standard deviations of the force fluctuations (force stability) during submaximal isometric contractions [23, 70, 109, 200]. Furthermore, when the force fluctuations are quantified in the frequency domain, the energy in the power spectra of the force records in the range of physiological tremor (4–12 Hz) increased with target force and by comparable amounts for young (18–27 yr) and elderly (59–74 yr) subjects (Fig. 3.2). Although some reports have suggested that the peak amplitude in the power density spectrum occurs at slightly lower frequencies (6 Hz) for elderly subjects [138, 139], others have found no difference (7 Hz for both young and elderly) due to age [70].

Because strength declines as a function of age, there is a difference between young and elderly subjects when the force fluctuations are normalized to the target force (coefficient of variation). The coefficient of variation for the force fluctuations during submaximal isometric contractions is greater for the elderly subjects (60–75 yr) and greatest for the low forces [70, 109]. For example, when subjects exerted submaximal abduction forces with the index finger, the coefficient of variation (%) was 6.6 ± 0.5 (mean $\pm$ SE) for the young subjects and 11.0 ± 1.8 for the elderly subjects at a target of 5% of MVC compared with 2.9 ± 0.2 and 3.9 ± 0.2, respec-

FIGURE 3.2.

Fluctuations in the abduction force exerted by the index finger of young and elderly subjects. The forces were held at 2.5, 5, and 20% of maximum for 20 s. The fluctuations (mean ± SE) are characterized in the time domain (A) and in the frequency domain (B, C). The power density spectrum of the force record was analyzed over the frequency range of 4–12 Hz. The standard deviation of the force fluctuations was greatest at the 20% MVC force and greater for the elderly subjects. Both the peak amplitude and the energy in the 4–12 Hz spectrum increased with target force, but similarly for young and elderly subjects.

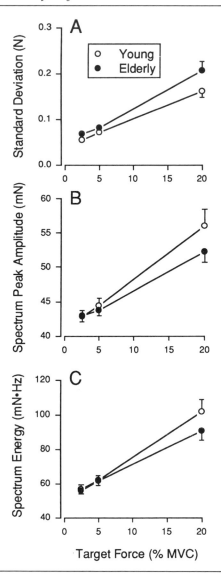

tively, for a target force of 50% of MVC [70]. At both target forces, the coefficient was significantly greater for the elderly subjects.

Mechanisms Underlying Force Fluctuations
This difference in the normalized force fluctuations raises the issue of how muscle activation might differ between young and elderly subjects to produce such an effect. Christakos [32] has shown that for low-to-moderate forces the peak in the power density spectrum is the result of two effects: newly recruited motor units producing unfused contractions and the low-pass filtering property of muscle. These effects result in the force record being dominated by low-frequency components. When these factors are combined with the known reorganization of motor units that occurs with age [20, 24, 106, 195], it seems that differences in motor unit size might account for the greater normalized force fluctuations of elderly subjects. Indeed, Galganski et al. [70] found that the amplitude of the spike-triggered average force of motor units discharging near their repetitive-discharge threshold was greater (67%) for the elderly subjects who also exhibited greater coefficients of variation. Furthermore, there were fewer low-threshold motor units in the first dorsal interosseus muscle of elderly subjects. The greater motor unit forces are probably due, at least in part, to an increase in the innervation ratio of the motor units [106, 195] and perhaps also to an increase in the short-term synchronization of motor unit discharge.

To test the possibility that differences in motor unit size (force) are responsible for the greater normalized force fluctuations of the elderly subjects, Keen et al. [109] had subjects perform a strength-training program for the purpose of assessing the relationship between changes in motor unit size and force fluctuations. Young (18–27 yr) and elderly (59–74 yr) subjects performed 12 wk of strength training with the first dorsal interosseus muscle and progress was evaluated at weeks 0, 4, 8, and 12. The training program caused similar increases in strength for the young and elderly subjects. Furthermore, the elderly subjects exhibited a decrease in the normalized force fluctuations for isometric contractions sustained at target forces of 2.5, 5, and 20% MVC but not at 50% MVC. The normalized force fluctuations did not change with training for the young subjects. However, the reduction in the fluctuations occurred in the first 4 wk of training and was not associated with changes in the amplitude of the spike-triggered average motor unit force (n = 668). This finding suggests that the greater normalized force fluctuations present in the submaximal contractions of elderly subjects are not primarily due to differences in motor unit force.

It seems unlikely that other features of motor unit behavior influence the normalized force fluctuations. When motor units in the first dorsal interosseus muscle discharged action potentials at rates slightly greater than the repetitive-discharge threshold, there was no difference between young (20–37 yr) and elderly (60–75 yr) subjects in the distribution of interimpulse intervals (normality, skewness, or kurtosis) or in the variability of discharge [70]. The coefficient of variation for interimpulse interval (mean ± SE) was 22.4 ± 0.72% for the young subjects and 23.6 ± 0.78% for the elderly subjects. These data are similar to coefficients of variation reported for the biceps brachii [72] and masseter muscles [162]. Nelson et al. [158] also found no difference among motor units in discharge rate or variability due to age (60–90 yr) at low forces (5–10% MVC force) for the abductor digiti minimi muscle. Other features of motor unit discharge, such as synchronization, double discharges, and motor unit rotation, have not been examined systematically to determine whether they might contribute to the greater normalized force fluctuations of elderly subjects for such tasks as the precision grip.

As with the basic elements of motor unit discharge (viz., rate and variability), age does not appear to affect the recruitment order of motor units over the range of forces used in the precision grip studies [105]. Galganski et al. [70] reported a linear relationship for both young ($r^2 = 0.49$) and elderly ($r^2 = 0.28$) subjects between the amplitude of the spike-triggered average force for motor units discharging at near-minimum rates and the force at which the motor units in first dorsal interosseus were recruited. This observation suggests that motor units in the first dorsal interosseus muscle were recruited in order of increasing twitch force, which is consistent with the Size Principle [11]. However, more of the variability in the motor unit threshold–spike-triggered average force relationship, especially for elderly subjects, could be explained by the use of the force at which the motor unit began to discharge action potentials repetitively (repetitive-discharge threshold, $r^2 = 0.44$) rather than the force at which the first action potential appeared (ramp-force threshold, $r^2 = 0.12$) as the index of motor unit threshold [193].

In contrast to recruitment, Kamen and De Luca [105] found that some elderly subjects (mean age, 75 yr) exhibited unusual patterns of motor unit derecruitment in the first dorsal interosseus and tibialis anterior muscles. The normal sequence of motor unit derecruitment is from largest to smallest; that is, from the last recruited to the first recruited. The unusual derecruitment patterns involved the concurrent derecruitment of many motor units and the derecruitment of smaller motor units before larger ones. In the records provided by Kamen and De Luca [105, their Fig. 3.1], the concurrent derecruitment of motor units occurred at the end of the isometric ramp contraction and in two of three examples produced a step decrease in force. However, the absence of a sequential derecruitment order did not appear to cause an increase in the force fluctuations. Similarly, the relationship between the recruitment force and the derecruitment force of a motor unit appears to be affected by age. Spiegel et al. [193] examined this relationship for low threshold motor units in the first dorsal interosseus muscle and found it to be more variable ($r^2 = 0.34$ vs. 0.13) for elderly subjects (60–81 yr). The variability was greatest among the motor units with recruitment thresholds less than 10% MVC force.

The data available to date suggest that for such tasks as the precision grip and the ramp change in isometric force both the recruitment and discharge (rate and variability) of motor units are unaffected by age. Although there are some effects of age on the derecruitment of motor units, these effects do not seem to impair performance substantially. Nonetheless, when elderly subjects are asked to perform such tasks, especially the ramp decrease in isometric force, they find the task much more difficult than do younger adults. This is evident by increased attention during the performance, the need to practice the task, greater variability in measured variables, and a reduced ability to match timing requirements. However, elderly subjects do not display a greater amount of agonist-antagonist coactivation during the ramp decrease in isometric force, as might be expected for a more difficult task [78].

The lack of an effect of motor unit properties (size, recruitment, discharge rate, and variability) on the difference in normalized force fluctuations as a function of age suggests that alternative mechanisms are important. One possibility is the behavior of populations of motor units rather than single motor units. There are at least two ways to assess population behavior: motor unit synchronization and frequency domain analysis (EMG or force). The calculation of an index for motor unit synchronization provides information about the activating neural input to a group of motor units. When the index is high, there is an increased level of common input to the motor units. An index can be calculated by comparing the discharge of pairs of motor units (cross-correlogram; 41, 149, 161, 189) or by correlating the discharge of a single motor unit to the discharge of a population [31, 145, 146, 228]. However, these techniques have not yet been applied systematically to elderly subjects.

The other approach to study motor unit population behavior is to perform a frequency domain analysis of its output (EMG or force). As mentioned previously, the peak frequency of the power spectrum for force fluctuations during isometric contractions was similar (about 7 Hz) for young and elderly subjects, and the amplitude increased with the target force. Similarly, when young subjects performed slow finger movements involving rotation about the metacarpophalangeal joint, the acceleration-time profiles were dominated by peaks in the power spectrum of 8–10 Hz [210]. Each cycle in the acceleration record included an acceleration phase followed by a deceleration phase, with the peak deceleration greater than the acceleration. These cycles were produced by the biphasic activation of the agonist-antagonist muscles, were larger for movements than for isometric contractions, were more pronounced in the extensor muscles, and were present in movements of widely varying velocity (4–62°/s). For this task, Vallbo and Wessberg [210] demonstrated that the acceleration (force) fluctuations were caused by the alternating activity of populations of motor units in the agonist and antagonist muscles. Perhaps the excessive grip force observed by Cole [35] and the greater normalized force fluctuations reported by Galganski et al. [70] are the result of differences due to age in the control strategy used for these types of movements. Consistent with this suggestion, Glendinning et al. [77] found that elderly subjects use a greater amount of agonist-antagonist (first dorsal interosseus-second palmar interosseus) coactivation than young subjects when the index finger exerted submaximal, isometric abduction forces.

POSTURAL STABILITY

Age-related changes in skeletal muscle organization and subsequent central nervous system adaptations, shown to affect the control of simple tasks such as the precision grip, also influence the performance of more complex motor skills. Perhaps the most pernicious of age-related musculoskeletal limitations and impairments are those that affect mobility. Mobility limitations affecting postural stability and the ability to walk without assistance are a primary cause of institutionalization in the elderly, accounting for 40% of nursing home admissions [188, 214]. Mobility limitations also contribute to the high incidence of falling, injury, and mortality in the elderly. It is commonly estimated that more than 30% of persons older than 75 years of age experience a fall. Tinetti and colleagues [205, 207] reported that during the course of a 1-year prospective study, there were 26 serious fall-related injuries in a group of 336 subjects; 5 of the injuries were fractures.

Figure 3.3 presents a conceptual model that has been implemented to study the mechanisms governing the ability to recover from postural perturbations [80]. The model, which has an information-processing basis, comprises stimulus detection and response selection times and response execution parameters. These parameters reflect the ability to (a) perceive the threat of an impending fall (stimulus detection), (b) process the information contained in the stimulus and select an appropriate corrective or protective motor response (response selection), and (c) properly execute the motor response (response execution). Although conceptually useful, these models do not identify the specific age-related deficits and the individual variability that contribute to falling symptoms. The sequence of events that characterize a recovery, or failure to recover from a perturbation, is initiated with a disturbance that decreases postural stability. The decreased stability produces afferent feedback containing information related to the characteristics of the instability, such as magnitude and direction. Before postural corrections are executed, the central nervous system must integrate the afferent information in such a way that it recognizes that a corrective, or protective, action is required to preserve stability. The ability of persons to detect the stimuli (mechanical, audio, visual) associated with the loss of stability is often measured using *simple* reaction time experiments involving a single stimulus and a single response. A commonly extracted variable in such paradigms is the latency between the onset of the

FIGURE 3.3.

A model of the components proposed to underlie recovery from a posturally destabilizing force. Both the cause (environmental stress) and the effects of the postural disturbance give rise to sensory information that is processed by the central nervous system, which then selects a response and formulates the motor commands to generate the automatic and/or voluntary responses. The biomechanical characterization of the response execution dictates the response efficacy that results in either a recovery of stability or a fall. The success or failure of the recovery attempt is a function of all of the components.

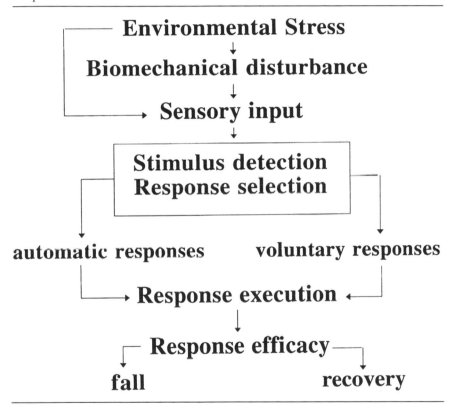

stimulus and the activation of a muscle associated with the task execution. This latency is referred to as the premotor reaction time. Simple premotor reaction time generally demonstrates an age-related increase, although the increase may be functionally insubstantial [34, 79, 96, 201].

Once the stimulus in a loss of stability condition has been detected, an appropriate response must be selected and the motor commands that drive the musculoskeletal system must be formulated. Measurement of response selection time is often performed using a *choice* reaction time paradigm in which multiple stimuli are associated with multiple possible responses. The difference between the simple and choice premotor reaction time is associated with the response selection latency. Notably, age-related increases in choice reaction time become more marked with increased movement complexity [125]. The response selection may involve both automatic and voluntary components. Ultimately, assuming that the correct response has been selected and programmed, it is the response execution that determines the success or failure of the recovery. The response execution must match the biomechanical requisites of the recovery and do so in the appropriate time frame.

One of the primary functions of the central nervous system is to maintain both static and dynamic *postural stability*. Broadly, the body has static postural stability when the center of pressure of the body is maintained within the area defined by the base of support in the absence of externally applied forces other than gravity. However, it is clear that as the center of pressure approaches a boundary of the base of support, although by definition the body still has postural stability, the postural stability is directionally reduced to a minimum. The mathematical characterization of dynamic postural stability is troublesome because the biomechanical criteria reflective of dynamic stability are difficult to validate [223]. Conceptually, dynamic stability exists when the joint moments required for goal-directed motion are sufficient to counteract destabilizing forces.

Postural stability is maintained by the *postural control* system. The postural control system comprises redundant, converging neural feedback from the visual, vestibular, and somatosensory systems. These systems experience significant age-related deterioration that influences the control of posture. Vision may be the single most important contributor to the regulation of posture, and degradation of the visual system with aging is well recognized. For example, Pyykko et al. [177] have suggested that elderly persons rely more on visual information, particularly peripheral vision [168], for maintenance of posture because of the age-related degeneration of the vestibular and somatosensory systems. This reliance on visual information becomes problematic because of the reduced ability to accommodate, poorer depth perception, decreased visual acuity, and reduced visual field, that is, peripheral vision [53, 190, 201]. These changes undoubtedly compromise postural stability by increasing postural sway, although they do not necessarily lead to a predisposition to falling.

The vestibular system directly modulates postural reflexes that maintain the head and neck vertically oriented, thereby providing a stable platform for the visual system. The vestibular system may resolve conflicting afferent information from the visual and somatosensory systems [12]. The vestibular system reportedly demonstrates a 40% reduction in sensory cells after age 70 [183]. However, these age-related changes may not necessarily result in an obligatory increase in measures of static postural sway.

The somatosensory system, too, demonstrates age-related degradation of function. Laidlaw and Hamilton [115] and Kokmen [112] reported that the detection of unloaded passive motion of lower extremity joints was substantially larger in subjects older than 50 yr of age compared with subjects younger than 40 yr. The upper extremities, however, demonstrated no such trends. The effects of age on the threshold to detect active motion, in contrast to passive motion, has been less consistent. Impaired vibration sense, affecting primarily the lower extremities, is commonly reported in elderly subjects. Notably, reduced vibration sense has been associated with increased postural sway [14]. Gilsing et al [76] have reported a 3-fold-age-related deterioration in the threshold with which elderly subjects, relative to young subjects, can detect ankle inversion or eversion rotations with 75% reliability. Even so, the threshold for ankle proprioception (at 75% reliability of detection) in the stance limb loaded by half or full body weight is remarkably good at less than half a degree [76]. Peripheral neuropathy has been found to reduce this threshold 4–6-fold relative to age-matched elderly subjects. [211].

Postural Control and Postural Stability

Two pressing issues related to changes in mobility with aging are the problems of postural control and postural stability, and the relationships between postural control, postural stability, and the predisposition to falling. Although it has been well documented that postural sway of elderly subjects is generally larger than that of younger subjects, and although it is clear that the predisposition to falling increases with age, the relationship between increased postural sway and falling behavior is unclear.

The environmental stresses presented in Figure 3.3 include those that range from the effects of gravity, the postural effects of which can generally be controlled without steps, to the maintenance of an upright posture during motion of body segments and recovery of postural stability after large postural perturbations that require stepping responses. The postural control system may be realized by closed-loop and open-loop mechanisms [135]. Closed-loop control involves the use of feedback whereby differences between actual and desired posture are detected and subsequently corrected, whereas open-loop control utilizes feedforward strategies that involve the generation of a command based on prior experience rather than on feedback. An example of open-loop control is the anticipatory postural adjustments that precede goal-directed movements.

Control of anterior-posterior postural sway has been characterized by three motor strategies: an ankle strategy, a hip strategy, and, if those do not suffice, a stepping strategy [93]. While standing on a moving surface, the strategy selected in a given condition depends on the surface upon which the subject stands and the amplitude of the perturbation of the surface. The ankle strategy, observed during reasonably slow and small perturbations that occur on firm surfaces large enough to accommodate plantar and dorsiflexion moments, consists of the anterior-posterior position of the center of pressure being controlled with ankle moments and minimum knee and hip joint involvement. In contrast, the hip strategy, involving hip and trunk flexion-extension, occurs with larger amplitude perturbations that are rapidly applied when the subject stands on compliant (but not slippery) surfaces or when the support surfaces are smaller than the size of the foot. Stepping strategies are those that require repositioning of the lower extremities to establish a new base of support. Stepping strategies are used when ankle or hip strategies are inappropriate because of the amplitude of the perturbation.

Automatic responses associated with closed- and open-loop of posture have been examined extensively in clinical and laboratory environments. The postural disturbances have usually been delivered by linearly or angularly accelerating platforms upon which the subjects stand. The activation (EMG) amplitude and timing of postural muscles have been recorded before and after the perturbation. Nashner et al. [155, 157] observed that a posturally destabilizing perturbation that elicits an ankle strategy involves the sequential activation of stretched muscles from those most distal to those most proximal. In contrast, the hip strategy is initiated with activation of proximal muscles acting at the hip followed by activation of thigh musculature [92]. These strategies also involve automatic activation of the neck and trunk muscles.

Voluntary movement, which can destabilize posture, is consistently preceded by activation of postural muscles (anticipatory postural adjustment). Anticipatory adjustment compensates, in advance, for the postural disturbances associated with the primary motor task. For example, Belen'kii et al. [8] reported that in young subjects who rapidly flexed the shoulder joint, anterior deltoid activation was preceded by activation of the ipsilateral biceps femoris and contralateral paraspinal muscles by 40 to 60 ms. Similarly, Cordo and Nashner [38] reported that gastrocnemius activation consistently preceded biceps brachii activation during a task in which the standing subjects were required to pull on a handle. Lee et al. [121] demonstrated that the timing of anticipatory activation of lower extremity muscles, before a bilateral handle-pulling task, was a function of the magnitude of the pulling force.

The slowness that elderly subjects often demonstrate in both initiation and execution of movement has been attributed to disruption of the coordination between anticipatory adjustments and voluntary activation [150, 198, 199]. Man'kovskii et al. [137] compared anticipatory activation of young and elderly adults for a task in which subjects, standing upright, were required to flex the knee of one leg as fast as possible. They found that elderly subjects demonstrated a shorter latency between the anticipatory adjustment and the voluntary activation. These observations were not found during conditions in which the knee was flexed at a slow speed. Inglin and

Woollacott [96] investigated the anticipatory adjustment of calf muscles associated with a push and pull task performed with the upper extremity. The anticipatory adjustment latencies of the leg muscles were significantly longer than those of younger subjects and the voluntary activation latency of the upper extremity muscles was significantly increased, but to a greater extent, than that of the anticipatory adjustment. Rogers et al. [181] reported that the anticipatory activation of thigh and trunk muscles occurred closer to the time of shoulder muscle activation in elderly subjects. Woollacott and Manchester [221] concluded that aging was associated with diminished anticipatory responses rather than reduced movement speeds of the elderly, precluding the need for anticipatory adjustments. However, the effect of age on the time between the anticipatory adjustment and the subsequent voluntary activation seems variable and may depend critically on the experimental task and the details of the perturbation. For example, Lee et al. [120] proposed that varying mechanical disturbances may induce subtle differences in motor programs that are responsible for maintaining stability.

The muscle activation patterns of postural control strategies become somewhat less stereotyped in the elderly subject. Whereas Woollacott et al. [219, 220] have reported that the timing of lower extremity activation demonstrated age-related differences, Manchester et al. [136] reported that the differences between young and elderly subjects did not differ significantly although elderly subjects did show more antagonist coactivation of leg and thigh muscles than did young subjects. Stelmach et al. [198] reported that older adults demonstrated diminished coordination between postural reflexes and voluntary movement and that stabilizing responses to postural disturbances during postural sway were slower and demonstrated less bilateral coupling than younger subjects. It is therefore not surprising that Lee [119] has shown that healthy elderly subjects employ 20% larger ankle movements than young subjects to effect unipedal balance and this may be the reason they can only stand half as long as young subjects.

Postural Control, Postural Stability, and the Predisposition to Falling
The methods and variables by which predisposition to falling may be characterized have been scientific and clinical issues for decades but a unified opinion remains elusive. Relationships between falling and a number of variables have been reported: leg press strength and lower extremity flexibility [74], dorsiflexor weakness [216], hip weakness [179], impaired gait [151, 218], decreased proprioception [107], decreased reaction time [2, 126], abnormal plantar reflex [69], impaired position sense [128], and difficulty in rising from a chair [159] or in turning 360°, while standing [128]. However, given the multifactorial nature of recovery from large postural perturbations, it seems unlikely that a univariate approach will identify a sensitive discriminator.

A performance variable that has most often been associated with falling in the elderly is increased postural sway [39, 90, 127, 179]. However, the increased incidence of falling in the elderly and its relationship to increased postural sway is arguable. An alternative suggestion links increased postural sway to increased probability of larger postural disturbances. The previous section reviewed some of the literature related to automatic activation of skeletal muscle after postural perturbations administered during static upright posture. This area of research has contributed much to our understanding of how the central nervous system organizes and controls the return to a stable upright posture. However, the extrapolation of these principles to the increased incidence of falling in the elderly has been the subject of some criticism. For example, most falls that occur in elderly people occur during motion, whether walking, ascending or descending stairs, or transferring from one support surface to another. Winter et al. [217] have argued that the demands of stability during dynamic activities are of greater complexity than those of static upright posture. For example, the center of mass falls within the confines of the base of support, which is the minimum requirement for static stability, for only 20% of the stride.

From a motor control standpoint, there are many differences between static upright posture and dynamic activities such as locomotion that will affect stability. For example, the optical flow provided by focal and peripheral vision, which is critical to many types of goal-directed locomotion control [118], is absent during static posture. Similarly, Dietz et al. [48] have reported that the vestibulospinal reflexes, which play a large role in balance recovery from perturbed upright posture, play only a minor role in balance recovery during locomotion. Furthermore, there is phase- (stance vs. swing) and task-dependent modulation of lower limb reflexes during locomotor activities [47, 54, 129, 198]. In addition, the sterotypical distal-to-proximal activation sequence observed during perturbed static posture is reversed during swing leg clearance of obstacles during locomotion [167].

The commonly observed, age-related increase in postural sway is interpreted as a decrease in postural stability, and there exists a widespread consensus that increased postural sway increases the predisposition to, and incidence of, falling in the elderly. Sheldon [191] appears to have been one of the early supporters of a relationship between diminished postural control and increased incidence of falling. Subsequently, Overstall et al. [165] reported that anterior-posterior postural sway, measured using an ataxiameter, was significantly larger in subjects who reported five or more falls in the 12-mo period preceding the test than in subjects with fewer than five falls. Notably, increased postural sway was not greater in subjects who had fallen because of trips compared with subjects who had not fallen, but the "tripping fallers" did sway less than those who had fallen for other reasons. Fernie et al. [61] reported contradictory conclusions in the same paper; "postural sway [mean sway velocity] was an indicator of a tendency to fall" but that "no increasing postural sway correlating with increased frequency of falls was found."

The relationship between postural sway and predisposition to falling that is promulgated in the literature has an imbedded and implicit relationship between static postural stability and dynamic postural stability. However, whereas static postural stability is easily defined and measured, dynamic postural stability is neither. Imms and Edholm [95] reported a significant relationship between static postural sway and performance on a sequence of dynamic activities including rising from and sitting into a chair, walking, climbing stairs, and turning around. However, the performance of dynamic activities was measured somewhat qualitatively and the correlation coefficient of 0.48 between the two raises some question as to its functional significance. Nonetheless, these results have been corroborated recently. Posiadlo and Richardson [174] modified the "up and go" test [141], which comprises standing from and sitting into a chair, walking, and turning around, and found that the time required to complete the test was correlated to the Berg Balance Scale (a 14-item, quasiqualitatively scored test, r = −0.72) for frail elderly subjects. Lichtenstein et al. [127] reported significant correlations (r = 0.59) between a measure of static postural stability during one-legged stance (measured as center of pressure excursion) and performance on the Tinetti mobility index [207].

Two recent experiments examined the relationship between measures of static postural sway and the ability to perform mobility-related tasks (J. E. Kasprisin and M.D. Grabiner, unpublished data). One experiment implemented clinically derived tests of postural stability (the Functional Reach Test [51, 52] and a modification of the timed "up-and-go test" [173]. The modifications to the test included the addition of a step up and down from a platform and the fractionation of the test into the elapsed times to perform the component tasks. The component tasks, and sequence, of the up and go test were rising from a chair, walking 3 m, stepping up (30.5 cm) onto, across (91.5 cm), and down from a platform, walking 3 m, turning around, and sitting down into a chair. The functional reach was assessed as the difference between arm length and the maximum voluntary distance the subject reached anteriorly. The second experiment consisted of quantitatively measuring postural sway as center of pressure excursions on an instrumented platform [82] and a locomotor task that required subjects to step over a foam obstacle (30.5 × 45.5 × 30.5 cm) placed between two force plates. The data obtained for the locomotor task included the braking, propulsion, and vertical impulses measured by two force plates. Seventeen elderly subjects (>70 yr) participated in the first experiment and 9 young (<30 yr) and 11 elderly subjects (>70 yr) participated in the second study. No significant correlations were found between performance on the Functional Reach Test and any of the fractionated up-and-go test components (−0.56 <r<0.04). Similarly, there were no significant correlations between static postural sway and the variables extracted from the force plates for the locomotor task ($-0.75 < r < 0.54$). Whereas others have reported statistically significant correlations, often accounting for less than 30% of shared variance between variables, Kasprisin and Grabiner (unpublished data) concluded that the relationship between measures of static postural stability and dynamic performance are tenuous and that the use of static postural sway to infer dynamic (in)stability and predisposition to falls is questionable.

There have been few systematic investigations of the biomechanics of recovery from large postural perturbations that require stepping responses, and fewer still that have focused on elderly people. One particular classification of large postural perturbations is the trip. Garrett and Luckwill [73] and Ghori and Luckwill [75] used a copper wire attached to the ankle of the subject to provide momentary resistance to the swing leg during gait on a treadmill. Dietz et al. [45, 46] and Berger et al. [10] used a suddenly accelerating or decelerating treadmill to produce postural perturbations during gait. This method affects the support leg rather than the swing leg and, thus, is functionally different than the perturbation that typically occurs as a result of a trip. Nashner [156] used a moveable platform to deliver a perturbation to subjects walking across the platform, which, similar to the work of Dietz et al., affects the support leg. Broadly, these studies have suggested that the initial part of the response is invariant [45] and that muscle activation patterns associated with perturbed gait appear to reinforce ongoing muscle activity [75, 156]. However, the potential application of these studies to the problem of falling in the elderly is restricted because the primary analyses were directed at the organization of automatic activation of the lower extremity muscles.

A number of biomechanical analyses have reported on stepping strategies associated with postural perturbations. Do et al. [49] described the *temporal* aspects of the stepping responses of subjects who, while leaning forward and restrained by a cable, were suddenly released. Recovery was reported to consist of two phases. The duration of the initial phase, which corresponded to the reaction time, was invariant and ended when the toe of the recovery foot left the supporting surface. The second phase comprised the stepping response. It was reported that as the angle of inclination increased, both the stride length and execution speed increased in parallel.

The temporal results of Do et al. [49] were confirmed by Feuerbach and Grabiner [62], who also examined the kinematics and kinetics of the stepping responses. Subjects were released from initial inclinations of 5°, 10°, 15°, 20°, and 25° from the vertical. Of interest was a variable called *relative foot position*, which was defined as the horizontal distance between the recovery foot center of gravity and the whole body center of gravity at the time of recovery foot touchdown. Similar to Do et al., the step length of a successful recovery from an impending forward fall varied as a function of inclination angle, reflecting the adaptability of the recovery phase. However, the relative foot position was *invariant*, regardless of the inclination angle (Table 3.1). Based upon its invariant characteristic, relative foot position was suggested as a control parameter specified by the central nervous system.

Luchies et al. [130] compared the stepping responses of young and elderly (>70 yr) subjects following posteriorly directed postural perturbations applied to the pelvis. Elderly subjects tended to use a multiple-step strategy compared with the single-step strategies used by younger subjects. Notably, elderly subjects initiated recovery sooner after the perturbation than did young subjects. However, the results may be different from anteriorly directed perturbations. Zhang et al. [230] used a similar method to examine stepping responses to laterally directed perturbations. Four different recovery patterns were identified but there were no age-related differences in the selected strategy. Interestingly, there were no age-related differences in the distance stepped to recover, which is in contrast to the results of Luchies et al. [130], who studied posteriorly directed perturbations. However, the findings of Zhang et al. [230] did support the premise that age-related differences in stepping strategies are dependent upon direction of the perturbation.

There have been few experimental or modeling studies emphasizing recovery from trips. Grabiner et al. [81] used a mechanical obstacle to trip young subjects by obstructing the motion of the swing leg during gait. These types of trips account for about 17% of falls by elderly people (W. C. Hayes, personal communication). They found two recovery phases: positioning and support phases of recovery. The former is composed the period during which the recovery leg is positioned to establish a new base of support in accordance to the mechanical demands of the recovery task. The support phase begins at recovery foot touchdown. Compared with normal walking trials, recovery from the trip was associated with significantly larger maximum knee and hip flexion angles and substantial increases in maximum hip flexion and knee extension velocities. A notable effect of the perturbation was a large trunk flexion (18.3° compared to the 4.3° of normal gait, p = 0.057) that was significantly related to the preperturbation walking

TABLE 3.1.
Mean (± SD) of Relative Foot Position and Step Length Normalized to Height

Lean Angle (degrees)	Foot Position (% Height)	Step Length (% Height)
5	11.9 (2.4)	26.7 (0.8)
10	13.1 (2.8)	32.6 (2.7)
15	12.8 (3.0)	34.5 (2.8)
20	14.6 (3.0)	40.63 (3.1)
25	13.0 (2.2)	44.9 (2.5)

velocity. Krebs et al. [113] and MacKinnon and Winter [134] addressed the importance of trunk control during normal locomotor tasks such as walking, ascending and descending stairs, and rising from a chair. Based upon proposed mechanical, intersegment interactions the authors proposed that control of trunk flexion during the recovery from a trip may be an important criterion underlying successful recovery.

To examine this possibility, Grabiner et al. [83] tested the hypothesis that subjects with greater eccentric trunk extension strength and faster paraspinal automatic latencies and voluntary reaction times would demonstrate less trunk flexion during the positioning phase of recovery from a trip. However, because of a lack of substantive associations, the hypotheses were rejected. In the study by Feuerbach and Grabiner [62], in which subjects were released from statically inclined positions, EMG data revealed that the paraspinal musculature was essentially quiescent during the initial part of the positioning phase. The paraspinal muscles did become active before recovery foot touchdown. Not surprisingly, the largest trunk/hip extension moment observed during recovery was just after recovery foot touchdown. For the larger initial inclination angles, the trunk extension moment required a trunk extension force up to 80% of body weight; a value that exceeds the capability of most normal elderly women [133]. Furthermore, the plantar flexion movements of the propulsion leg approached values that may exceed the ability of elderly people, especially women. Although the release experiment was conducted from initially static conditions, it seems reasonable that the ability to generate a reasonably large trunk extension movement would be an important performance criterion during the support phase of recovery. Biomechanical modeling studies showed that the rate of developing plantar flexion force in the stance limb and hip flexion force in the swing limb hip are key determinants underlying successful recovery from a trip [29]. In 24 healthy elderly subjects, rates of developing ankle joint force were indeed significantly (25–36%) lower than those of 24 healthy young subjects. Thus, the impaired rate of developing muscle force, and thereby joints movements, would appear to be an important determinant in recovering from a trip (D. G. Thelen, A. B. Schultz, N. B. Alexander, and J. A. Ashton-Miller, unpublished data).

There remain many unanswered questions related to postural control, locomotion, and falling in the elderly. From a practical standpoint it is reasonable to pose the question of whether the age-related decrease in postural stability can be reduced or reversed. Although there is presently some agreement that training programs that target specific deficits in physiological systems subserving postural control, i.e., somatosensory, visual, or vestibular, are effective in improving postural control [94], it is not yet clear whether these types of programs are more effective than traditional programs that address generalized balance skills [93]. Perhaps more importantly, the relationship between static postural stability and dynamic stability needs to be systematically addressed and, by extension, it is crucially important to determine whether the predisposition to falling in the elderly can be reduced or reversed. Ultimately, solutions to these questions will determine whether much of the related research will have an impact on the quality of life of the elderly population.

CONCLUSIONS

Despite the intense interest in aging research, remarkably little is known about the effects of aging on movement capabilities. Some information is available on the elements of movement (e.g., muscle strength, fatigability), but the functional consequences of those changes due to aging are uncertain. Furthermore, even less is known about performance on specific tasks and the adaptations that mediate the changes that occur with age. Based upon the literature reviewed in this chapter, the following conclusions seem warranted:

- The decline in maximum voluntary contraction force with age is due to a loss of muscle mass and probably also a decline in the specific tension and a reduced ability to activate the muscle maximally.
- The muscle atrophy observed in older subjects is largely due to the death of α motor neurons and a reduced ability of surviving motor units to develop collateral sprouts and to reinnervate abandoned muscle fibers.
- Strength training programs produce modest increases in muscle size but substantial increases in the strength of elderly subjects.
- Except for the frail elderly, the functional consequences of increased strength for activities of daily living are uncertain.
- The fatigability of human muscle during voluntary contractions does not change with age. However, the use of neuromuscular stimulation has produced variable results for the effects of age on muscle fatigue.
- The absence of an effect due to age on fatigability implies that the changes in fiber-type proportions and the reorganization of motor unit territories do not influence the mechanisms that limit performance during fatiguing contractions.
- Control of the precision grip by elderly subjects is characterized by the use of an excessive and variable pinch force. There is no difference between young and elderly subjects in the absolute amplitude of the force fluctuations, but the normalized fluctuations (coefficient of variation) are larger for elderly subjects, especially at low forces.
- The greater normalized force fluctuations for elderly subjects, however, are not primarily due to differences in motor unit force.
- For both the precision grip and ramp change in isometric force, motor unit recruitment order and discharge (rate and variability) are unaffected by age.

- The effect of age on the pinch force exerted during the precision grip may reflect differences in the neural strategy (quality of the central command) used for this task.
- The degradation of the various systems through which postural stability is controlled (visual, vestibular, somatosensory) that occurs with aging does not necessarily lead to increased postural sway.
- The increased postural sway commonly associated with aging increases the probability of a postural perturbation requiring a stepping response to recover stability, but this may not predispose an elderly person to falling.
- Most falls in elderly people occur during activities including locomotion, ascending and descending stairs, and transferring from one support surface to another. The statistical relationships between measures of static postural sway and performance of these types of activities have been only weak and nonsystematic.
- The increased predisposition to falling in elderly people may be less related to increased postural sway than to the inability to generate and coordinate the joint power necessary to execute the recovery task. The diminished ability to generate and coordinate these joint powers relates to the decrease in muscle mass, specific tension, and ability to activate muscle.

ACKNOWLEDGMENTS

We acknowledge the support received from the National Institutes of Health (Grant AG 09000, to R. M. E.) and the American Federation for Aging Research to M. D. G.) We also gratefully acknowledge the scholarly review of the manuscript by James Aston-Miller, Ph.D.

REFERENCES

1. Adams, G. R., R. T. Harris, D. Woodward, and G. A. Dudley. Mapping of electrical muscle stimulation using MRI. *J. Appl. Physiol.* 74:532–537, 1993.
2. Adelsberg S., M. Pitman, and H. Alexander. Lower extremity fractures: relationship to reaction time and coordination time. *Arch. Phys. Med. Rehabil.* 70:737–739, 1989.
3. Alexander, N. B., A. B. Schultz, and D. N. Warwick. Rising from a chair: effects of age and functional ability on performance biomechanics. *J. Gerontol.* 46:M91–M99, 1991.
4. Aniansson, A., G. Grimby, and M. Hedberg. Compensatory muscle fiber hypertrophy in elderly men. *J. Appl. Physiol.* 73:812–816, 1992.
5. Aniansson, A., M. Hedberg, G.-B. Henning, and G. Grimby. Muscle morphology, enzymatic activity, and muscle strength in elderly men: a follow-up study. *Muscle Nerve* 9:585–591, 1986.
6. Bassey, E. J., M. J. Bendall, and M. Pearson. Muscle strength in the triceps surae and objectively measured customary walking activity in men and women over 65 years of age. *Clin. Sci.* 74:85–89, 1988.
7. Bassey, E. J., and U. J. Harris. Normal values for handgrip strength in 920 men and women aged over 65 years, and longitudinal changes over 4 years in 620 survivors. *Clin. Sci.* 84:331–337, 1993.

8. Belen'kii, V. Y., V. S. Gurfinkel, and Y. I. Pal'tsev. Elements of control of voluntary movements. *Biofizika* 12:135–141, 1967.
9. Bendall, M. J., E. J. Bassey, and M. B. Pearson. Factors affecting walking speed of elderly people. *Age Aging* 18:327–332, 1989.
10. Berger, W., Dietz, V. and J. Quintern. Corrective reactions to stumbling in man: neuronal co-ordination of bilateral leg muscle activity during gait. *J. Physiol. (Lond.)* 357:109–125, 1984.
11. Binder, M. D., and L. M. Mendell (eds). *The Segmental Motor System.* New York: Oxford, 1990.
12. Black, S. E., B. E. Maki, and G. R. Fernie. Aging, imbalance, and falls. J. A. Sharpe and H. O. Barber, (eds). *The Vestibulo-Ocular Reflex and Vertigo.* New York: Raven Press, 1993, pp. 317–335.
13. Booth F. W., S. H. Weeden, and B. S. Tseng. Effect of aging on human skeletal muscle and motor function. *Med. Sci. Sports Exerc.* 26:556–560, 1994.
14. Brocklehurst, J. C., D. Robertson, and P. James-Groom. Clinical correlates of sway in old age-sensory modalities. *Age Aging* 11:1–10, 1982.
15. Brooks, S. V., and J. A. Faulkner. Contractile properties of skeletal muscles from young, adult, and aged mice. *J. Physiol. (Lond.)* 404:71–82, 1988.
16. Brooks, S. V., and J. A. Faulkner. Maximum and sustained power of extensor digitorum longus muscles from young, adult, and old mice. *J. Gerontol.* 46:B28–B33, 1991.
17. Brooks, S. V., and J. A. Faulkner. Skeletal muscle weakness in old age: underlying mechanisms. *Med. Sci. Sports. Exerc.* 26:432–439, 1994.
18. Brown, A. B., N. McCartney, and D. G. Sale. Positive adaptations to weight-lifting training in the elderly. *J. Appl. Physiol.* 69:1725–1733, 1990.
19. Brown, M. C. Sprouting of motor nerves in adult muscles: a recapitulation of ontogeny. *Trends Neurosci.* 7:10–14, 1984.
20. Brown, W. F. A method for estimating the number of motor units in thenar muscles and the changes in motor unit count with ageing. *J. Neurol. Neurosurg. Psychiat.* 35:845–852, 1972.
21. Brown, W. F. Functional compensation of human motor units in health and disease. *J. Neurol. Sci.* 20:199–209, 1973.
22. Bruce, S. A., D. Newton, and R. C. Woledge. Effect of age on voluntary force and cross-sectional area of human adductor pollicis muscle. *Q. J. Exp. Physiol.* 74:359–362, 1989.
23. Caligiuri, M. P., J. B. Lohr, and D. V. Jeste. Instrumental evidence that age increases motor instability in neuroleptic-treated patients. *J. Gerontol.* 46:197–200, 1991.
24. Campbell, M. J., A. J. McComas, and F. Petito. Physiological changes in ageing muscles. *J. Neurol. Neurosurg. Psychiat.* 36:174–182, 1973.
25. Carlson, B. M., and J. A. Faulkner. Reinnervation of long-term denervated rat muscle freely grafted into an innervated limb. *Exp. Neurol.* 102:50–56, 1988.
26. Carolan, B., and E. Cafarelli. Adaptations in coactivation after isometric resistance training. *J. Appl. Physiol.* 73:911–917, 1992.
27. Cartee, G. D. Aging skeletal muscle: response to exercise. J. O. Holloszy (ed.). *Exercise and Sport Sciences Reviews, Vol. 22.* Baltimore: Williams & Wilkins, 1994, pp. 91–120.
28. Charette, S. L., L. McEnvoy, G. Pyka, et al. Muscle hypertrophy response to resistance training in older women. *J. Appl. Physiol.* 70:1912–1916, 1991.
29. Chen, H. C. Stepping over obstacles: biomechanical analyses of the effects of age and attention. Ph.D. Dissertation. Department of Mechanical Engineering, Ann Arbor, University of Michigan, 1993.
30. Christ, C. B., R. A. Boileau, M. H. Slaughter, R. J. Stillman, J. A. Cameron, and B. H. Massey. Maximal voluntary isometric force production characteristics of six muscle groups in women aged 25 to 74 years. *Am. J. Human Biol.* 4:537–545, 1992.
31. Christakos, C. Analysis of synchrony (correlations) in neurol populations by means of unit-to-aggregate coherence computations. *Neuroscience* 58:43–57, 1994.

32. Christakos, C. A study of the muscle force waveform using a population stochastic model of skeletal muscle. *Biol. Cybern.* 44:91–106, 1982.
33. Chun, S. P., J. A. Ashton-Miller, N. B. Alexander, and A. B. Schultz. Impending fall response biomechanics in young and old adults. *J. Biomech.* in press.
34. Clarkson, P. M. The effect of age and activity level on simple and choice fractionated response time. *Eur. J. Appl. Physiol.* 40:17–25, 1978.
35. Cole, K. J. Grasp force control in older adults. *J. Motor Behav.* 23:251–258, 1991.
36. Cole, K. J., and C. L. Beck. The stability of precision grip force in older adults. *J. Motor Behav.* 26:171–177, 1994.
37. Comaish, S., and E. Bottoms. The skin and friction: deviations from Amonton's laws and the effects of hydration and lubrication. *Br. J. Dermatol.* 8:37–43, 1971.
38. Cordo, P. J. and L. M. Nashner. Properties of postural adjustments associated with rapid arm movements. *J. Neurophysiol.* 47:287–302, 1982.
39. Crosbie, W. J., M. A. Nimmo, M. A. Banks, M. G. Brownlee, and F. Meldrum. Standing balance responses in two populations of elderly women: a pilot study. *Arch. Phys. Med. Rehabil.* 70:751–754, 1989.
40. Cupido, C. M., A. L. Hicks, and J. Martin. Neuromuscular fatigue during repetitive stimulation in elderly and young adults. *Eur. J. Appl. Physiol.* 65:567–572, 1992.
41. Davey, N. J., P. H. Ellaway, J. R. Baker, and C. L. Friedland. Rhythmicity associated with a high degree of short-term synchrony of motor unit discharge in man. *Exp. Physiol.* 78:649–661, 1993.
42. Davies, C. T. M., D. O. Thomas, and M. J. White. Mechanical properties of young and elderly human muscle. *Acta. Med. Scand. Suppl.* 117:219–226, 1986.
43. de Haan, A., M. A. N. Lodder, and A. J. Sargeant. Age-related effects of fatigue and recovery from fatigue in rat medial gastrocnemius muscle. *Q. J. Exp. Physiol.* 74:715–726, 1989.
44. de Koning, P., G. Wieneke, D. van der Most Van Spijk, A. C. van Huffelen, W. H. Gispen, and F. G. I. Jennekens. Estimation of the number of motor units based on macro-EMG. *J. Neurol. Neurosurg. Psychiat.* 51:403–411, 1988.
45. Diez, V., J. Quintern, and W. Berger. Stumbling reactions in man: release of a ballistic movement pattern. *Brain Res.* 362:355–357. 1986.
46. Dietz, V., J. Quintern, and M. Sillem. Stumbling reactions in man: significance of proprioceptive and preprogrammed mechanisms. *J. Physiol. (Lond.)* 386:149–163, 1987.
47. Dietz, V., M. Faist, and E. Pierrot-Deseilligny. Amplitude modulation of the quadriceps H-reflex in the human during the early stance phase of gait. *Exp. Brain. Res.* 79:221–224, 1990.
48. Dietz, V., M. Trippel, and G. A. Horstmann: Significance of proprioceptive and vestibulospinal reflexes in the control of stance and gait. A. E. Patla, (ed). *Adaptability of Human Gait* New York: North-Holland, 1991, pp. 37–52.
49. Do, M. C., Y. Breniere, and P. A. Brenguire. A biomechanical study of balance recovery during the fall forward. *J. Biomech.* 15:933–939. 1982.
50. Doherty, T. J., A. A. Vandervoort, and W. F. Brown. Effects of ageing on the motor unit: a brief review. *Can. J. Appl. Physiol.* 18:331–358, 1993.
51. Duncan, P. W., D. K. Weiner, J. Chandler, and S. Studenski. Functional reach: a new clinical measure of balance. *J. Gerontol.* 45:M192–197, 1990.
52. Duncan, P. W., S. Studenski, J. Chandler, and B. Prescott. Functional reach: predictive validity in a sample of elderly male veterans. *J. Gerontol.* 47:M93–98, 1992.
53. Duthrie, E. H. Falls. *Geriatr. Med.* 73:1321–1336, 1989.
54. Duysens, J., M. Trippel, G. A. Horstmann, and V. Deitz. Gating and reversal of reflexes in ankle muscles during human walking. *Exp. Brain. Res.* 82:351–358, 1990.
55. Einsiedel, L. J., and A. R. Luff. Effect of partial denervation on motor units in the ageing rat medial gastrocnemius. *J. Neurol. Sci.* 112:178–184, 1992.
56. Enoka, R. M. Muscle strength and its development: new perspectives. *Sports Med.* 6:146–168, 1988.

57. Enoka, R. M., A. J. Fuglevand, and P. M. Barreto. Age does not impair the voluntary ability to maximally activate muscle. *J. Biomech.* 26:293, 1993.
58. Enoka, R. M., and D. G. Stuart. Neurobiology of muscle fatigue. *J. Appl. Physiol.* 72:1631–1648, 1992.
59. Eriksson, E., T. Haggmark, K.-H. Kiessling, and J. Karlsson. Effect of electrical stimulation on human skeletal muscle. *Int. J. Sports Med.* 2:18–22, 1981.
60. Fagg, G. E., S. W. Scheff, and C. W. Cotman. Axonal sprouting at the neuromuscular junction of adult and aged rats. *Exp. Neurol.* 74:847–854, 1981.
61. Fernie, G. R., C. I. Gryfe, P. J. Holliday, and A. Llewellyn. The relationship of postural sway in standing to the incidence of falls in geriatric subjects. *Age Aging* 11:11–16, 1982.
62. Feuerbach, J. W., and M. D. Grabiner. Invariant relative foot position during recovery from an impending forward fall. *Proceedings of the 18th Annual Meeting of the American Society of Biomechanics*, Columbus, OH, October, 1994.
63. Fiatarone, M. A., E. C. Marks, N. D. Ryan, C. N. Meredith, L. A. Lipsitz, and W. J. Evans. High-intensity strength training in nonagenarians. *J.A.M.A.* 263:3029–3034, 1990.
64. Fitts, R. H. Cellular mechanisms of muscle fatigue. *Physiol. Rev.* 74:49–94, 1994.
65. Frolkis, V. Syndromes of aging. *Gerontology* 38:80–86, 1992.
66. Frontera, W. R., V. A. Hughes, K. J. Lutz, and W. J. Evans. A cross-sectional study of muscle strength and mass in 45- to 78-yr-old men and women. *J. Appl. Physiol.* 71:644–650, 1991.
67. Frontera, W. R., C. N. Meredith, K. P. O'Reilly, H. G. Knuttgen, and W. J. Evans. Strength conditioning in older men: skeletal muscle hypertrophy and improved function. *J. Appl. Physiol.* 64:1038–1044, 1988.
68. Fuglevand, A. J., K. M. Zackowski, K. A. Huey, and R. M. Enoka. Impairment of neuromuscular propagation during human fatiguing contractions at submaximal forces. *J. Physiol. (Lond.)* 460:549–572, 1993.
69. Gabell, A., M. A. Simons, and U. S. L. Nayak. Falls in the healthy elderly: predisposing causes. *Ergonomics* 28:965–975, 1985.
70. Galganski, M. E., A. J. Fuglevand, and R. M. Enoka. Reduced control of motor output in a human hand muscle of elderly subjects during submaximal contractions. *J. Neurophysiol.* 69:2108–2115, 1993.
71. Gardner, E. Decrease in human neurones with age. *Anat. Rec.* 77:529–536, 1940.
72. Garland, S. J., R. M. Enoka, L. P. Serrano, and G. A. Robinson. Behavior of motor units in human biceps brachii during a submaximal fatiguing contraction. *J. Appl. Physiol.* 76:2411–2419, 1994.
73. Garrett, M., and R. G. Luckwill. Role of reflex responses of knee musculature during the swing phase of walking in man. *Eur. J. Appl. Physiol.* 52:36–41, 1983.
74. Gehlsen, G. M., and M. H. Whaley. Falls in the elderly. II. Balance, strength, and flexibility. *Arch. Phys. Med. Rehabil.* 71:739–741, 1990.
75. Ghori, G. M. U., and R. G. Luckwill. Pattern of reflex responses in lower limb muscles to a resistance in walking man. *Eur. J. Appl. Physiol.* 58:852–857, 1989.
76. Gilsing, M., C. VandenBosch, S. G. Lee, J. A. Ashton-Miller, N. B. Alexander and A. B. Schultz. Effects of age on the reliability of detecting ankle inversion and eversion, *Age Aging*, in press.
77. Glendinning, D. S., E. B. Montgomery, and R. M. Enoka. Recruitment of motor units in antagonist muscles in Parkinson's disease. *Soc. Neurosci. Abstr.* 20:1779, 1994.
78. Gordon, T., J. F. Yang, K. Ayer, R. B. Stein, and N. Tyreman. Recovery potential of a muscle after partial denervation: a comparison between rats and humans. *Brain Res. Bull.* 30:477–482, 1993.
79. Gottsdanker, R. Age and simple reaction time. *J. Gerontol.* 37:342–348, 1982.
80. Grabiner, M. D., and D. W. Jahnigen. Modeling recovery from stumbles: variable selection and classification efficacy. *J. Am. Geriatr. Soc.* 40:910–913, 1992.
81. Grabiner, M.D., T. J. Koh, T. M. Lundin, and D. W. Jahnigen. Kinematics of recovery from a stumble. *J. Gerontol.* 48:M97–M102, 1993.

82 Grabiner, M. D., T. M. Lundin, and J. W. Feuerbach. Converting Chattecx Balance System vertical reaction forces to center of pressure excursion. *Phys. Ther.* 73:316–319, 1993.

83. Grabiner, M. D., J. W. Feuerbach, and D. W. Jahnigen. Control of the trunk during the initial phase of recovery following a trip. *J. Biomech.* in press.

84. Greig, C. A., J. Botella, and A. Young. The quadriceps strength of healthy elderly people remeasured after eight years. *Muscle Nerve* 16:6–10, 1993.

85. Gutmann, E., and V. Hanzlikova. Motor units in old age. *Nature* 209:921–922, 1966.

86. Hagberg, J. M., D. R. Seals, J. E. Yerg, et al. Metabolic responses to exercise in young and older athletes and sedentary men. *J. Appl. Physiol.* 65:900–908, 1988.

87. Häkkinen, K., M. Alèn, and P. V. Komi. Changes in isometric force- and relaxation-time electromyographic and muscle fiber characteristics of human skeletal muscle during strength training and detraining. *Acta Physiol. Scand.* 125:573–585, 1985.

88. Häkkinen, K., and A. Pakarinen. Muscle strength and serum testosterone, cortisol and SHBG concentrations in middle-aged and elderly men and women. *Acta Physiol. Scand.* 148:199–207, 1993.

89. Halliday, A. M., and J. W. T. Redfearn. An analysis of the frequencies of finger tremor in healthy subjects. *J. Physiol. (Lond.)* 134:600–611, 1956.

90. Heitmann, D. K., M. R. Gossman, S. A. Shaddeau, and J. R. Jackson. Balance performance and step width in noninstitutionalized, elderly female fallers and nonfallers. *Phys. Ther.* 69:923–931, 1989.

91. Hicks, A., C. M. Cupido, J. Martin, and J. Dent. Muscle excitation in elderly adults: the effects of training. *Muscle Nerve* 15:87–93, 1992.

92. Horak, F. B., and L. M. Nashner. Central programming of postural movements: Adaptation to altered support surface configurations. *J. Neurophysiol.* 55:1369–1381, 1986.

93. Horak, F. B., C. L. Shupert, and A. Mirka. Components of postural dyscontrol in the elderly: a review. *Neurobiol. Aging* 10:727–738, 1989.

94. Hu, M.-H. and Woollacott, M. H. Multisensory training of standing balance in older adults. I. Postural stability and one-leg stance balance. *J. Gerontol.* 49:M52–M61, 1994.

95. Imms, F. J., and O. G. Edholm. Studies of gait and mobility in the elderly. *Age Aging* 10:147–156, 1981.

96. Inglin, B., and M. H. Woollacott. Age-related changes in anticipatory postural adjustments associated with arm movements. *J. Gerontol.* 43:M105–113, 1988.

97. Ishihara, A., and H. Araki. Effects of age on the number and histochemical properties of muscle fibers and motoneurons in the rat extensor digitorum longus muscle. *Mech. Age. Dev.* 45:213–221, 1988.

98. Jacob, J. M., and N. Robbins. Age differences in morphology of reinnervation of partially denervated mouse muscle. *J. Neurosci.* 10:1530–1540, 1990.

99. Jacob, J. M., and N. Robbins. Differential effects of age on neuromuscular transmission in partially denervated mouse muscle. *J. Neurosci.* 10:1522–1529, 1990.

100. Jebsen, R. H., N. Taylor, R. B. Treischmann, M. J. Trotter, and L. A. Howard. An objective and standardized test of hand function. *Arch. Phys. Med. Rehabil.* 50:311–319, 1969.

101. Johansson, R. S., and K. J. Cole. Sensory-motor coordination during grasping and manipulative actions. *Curr. Opin. Neurobiol.* 2:815–823, 1992.

102. Jones, D. A., O. M. Rutherford, and D. F. Parker. Physiological changes in skeletal muscle as a result of strength training. *Q. J. Exp. Physiol.* 74:233–256, 1989.

103. Joseph, J. A. (ed). Central determinants of age-related declines in motor function. *Ann. N. Y. Acad. Sci.* 515:1–430, 1988.

104. Joyner, M. J. Physiological limiting factors and distance running: influence of gender and age on record performances. J. O. Holloszy (ed). *Exercise and Sport Sciences Reviews* Vol. 21. Baltimore: Williams & Wilkins, 1993, pp. 103–133.

105. Kamen, G., and C. J. De Luca. Unusual motor unit firing behavior in older adults. *Brain Res.* 482:136–140, 1989.

106. Kanda, K., and K. Hashizume. Changes in properties of the medial gastrocnemius motor units in aging rats. *J. Neurophysiol.* 61:737–746, 1989.

107. Kaplan, F. S., J. E. Nixon, M. Reitz, L. Rindfleish, and J. Tucker. Age-related changes in proprioception and sensation of joint position. *Acta Orthop. Scand.* 56:71–74, 1985.

108. Kawamura, Y., H. Okazaki, P. C. O'Brien, and P. J. Dyck. Lumbar motoneurons of man. I: Numbers and diameter histograms of alpha and gamma axons and ventral roots. *J. Neuropathol. Exp. Neurol.* 36:853–860, 1977.

109. Keen, D. A., G. H. Yue, and R. M. Enoka. Training-related enhancement in the control of motor output in elderly humans. *J. Appl. Physiol,* 77, 1994 in press.

110. Kelly, S. S. The effect of age on neuromuscular transmission. *J Physiol. (Lond.)* 274:51–62, 1978.

111. Klitgaard, H., M. Mantoni, S. Schiaffino, et al. Function, morphology and protein expression of ageing skeletal muscle: a cross-sectional study of elderly men with different training backgrounds. *Acta Physiol. Scand.* 140:41–54, 1990.

112. Kokmen, E., R. W. Bossmeyer, and S. J. Williams. Quantitative evaluation of joint motion sensation in an aging population. *J. Gerontol.* 33:62–67, 1978.

113. Krebs, D. E., D. Wong, D. Jevsevar, P. O'Riley, and W. A. Hodge. Trunk kinematics during locomotor activities. *Phys. Ther.* 72:505–514, 1992.

114. Laforest S., D. M. M. St.-Pierre, J. Cyr, and D. Guyton. Effects of age and regular exercise on muscle strength and endurance. *Eur. J. Appl. Physiol.* 60:104–111, 1990.

115. Laidlaw, R. W., and M. A. Hamilton. A study of thresholds in apperception of passive movement among normal control subjects. *Bull. Neurol. Inst.* 6:268–273, 1937.

116. Larsson, L., G. Grimby, and J. Karlsson. Histochemical and biochemical changes in human muscle with age in sedentary males, age 22–65 years. *Acta Physiol. Scand.* 103:31–39, 1978.

117. Larsson, L., G. Grimby, and J. Karlsson. Muscle strength and speed of movement in relation to age and muscle morphology. *J. Appl. Physiol.* 46:451–456, 1979.

118. Laurent, M. Visual cues and processes involved in goal-directed locomotion. A. E. Patla (ed). *Adaptability of Human Gait.* New York: North-Holland, 1991, pp. 99–123.

119. Lee, S.-G. Theoretical and experimental biomechanical analyses of the effects of age and peripheral neuropathy on unipedal stance. Ph.D. Dissertation, Department of Mechanical Engineering, Ann Arbor University of Michigan, 1993.

120. Lee, W. A., T. S. Buchanan, and M. W. Rogers. Effects of arm acceleration and behavioral conditions on the organization of postural adjustments during arm flexion. *Exp. Brain. Res.* 66:257–270, 1987.

121. Lee, W. A., C. F. Michaels, and Y.-C. Pai. The organization of torque and EMG activity during bilateral handle pulls by standing humans. *Exp. Brain Res.* 82:304–314, 1990.

122. Lennmarken, C., T. Bergman, J. Larsson, and L.-E. Larsson. Skeletal muscle function in man: force, relaxation rate, endurance and contraction time-dependence on sex and age. *Clin. Physiol.* 5:243–255, 1985.

123. Lexell, J., and D. Y. Downham. The occurrence of fibre type and grouping in healthy human muscle: a quantitative study of cross-sections of whole vastus lateralis from men between 15 and 83 years. *Acta Neuropathol.* 81:377–381, 1991.

124. Lexell, J., C. C. Taylor, and M. Sjostrom. What is the cause of the aging atrophy? *J. Neurol. Sci.* 84:275–294, 1988.

125. Light, K. E., and W. W. Spirduso. Effects of adult aging on the movement complexity factor of response programming. *J. Gerontol.* 45:107–109, 1990.

126. Lichtenstein, M. J., S. L. Shields, R. G. Shiavi, and C. Burger. Clinical determinants of biomechanics platform measures of balance in aged women. *J. Am. Geriatr. Soc.* 36:996–1002, 1988.

127. Lichtenstein, M. J., M. C. Burger, S. L. Shields, and R. G. Shiavi. Comparison of biomechanics platform measures of balance and videotaped measures of gait with a clinical mobility scale in elderly women. *J. Gerontol.* 45:M49–54, 1990.

128. Lipsitz, L. A., P. V. Jonsson, M. M. Kelley, and J. S. Koestner. Causes and correlates of recurrent falls in ambulatory frail elderly. *J. Gerontol.* 46:M114–122, 1991.

129. Llewellyn, M., J. F. Yang, and A. Prochazka. Human H-reflexes are smaller in difficult beam walking than in normal treadmill walking. *Exp. Brain Res.* 83:22–28, 1990.

130. Luchies, C. W., A. B. Schultz, J. A. Ashton-Miller, and W. Alexander. Effects of age on the stepping response to impending falls. *Proc. ASME Biomech. Symp.* 120:315–318, 1991.

131. Luchies, C. W., N. B. Alexander, A. B. Schultz, and J. A. Ashton-Miller. Stepping responses of young and old adults to postural disturbances. I: Kinematics. *J. Am. Geriatr. Soc.*, in press.

132. Luchies, C. W., N. B. Alexander, A. B. Schultz, and J. A. Ashton-Miller. Stepping responses of young and old adults to postural disturbances. I. Dynamics. *J. Biomech.*, in press.

133. Lundin, T. M., M. D. Grabiner, and D. W. Jahnigen. Functional reserve influences the motor strategy of rising from a chair in elderly subjects. *J. Biomech*, in press.

134. MacKinnon, C. D., and D. A. Winter. Control of whole body balance in the frontal plane during human walking. *J. Biomech.* 26:633–644, 1993.

135. Maki, B. E. Biomechanical approach to quantifying anticipatory postural adjustments in the elderly. *Med. Biol. Eng. Comput.* 31:355–362, 1993.

136. Manchester, D., M. Woollacott, N. Zederbauer-Hylton, and O. Marin. Visual, vestibular, and somatosensory contributions to balance control in the older adult. *J. Gerontol.* 44:M118–127, 1989.

137. Man'kovskii, N. B., A. Y. Mints, A. Y., and V. P. Lysenyuk. Regulation of the preparatory period for complex voluntary movement in old and extreme old age. *Hum. Physiol. (Moscow)* 6:46–50, 1980.

138. Marsden, C. D., J. C. Meadows, G. W. Lange, and R. S. Watson. Variations in human physiological tremor, with particular reference to changes with age. *Electroencephalogr. Clin. Neurophysiol.* 27:169–178, 1969.

139. Marshall, J. The effect of ageing upon physiological tremor. *J. Neurol. Neurosurg. Psychiat.* 24:14–17, 1961.

140. Marshall, J., and E. G. Walsh. Physiological tremor. *J. Neurol. Neurosurg. Psychiat.* 19:260–267, 1956.

141. Mathias, S., U. S. L. Nayak, and B. Isaacs. Balance in the elderly patient: the "Get up and go" test. *Arch. Phys. Med. Rehabil.* 67:387–389, 1986.

142. Merletti, R., L. R. Lo Conte, C. Cisari, and M. V. Actis. Age-related changes in surface myoelectric signals. *Scand. J. Rehabil. Med.* 24:25–36, 1992.

143. Metter, E. J., D. Walega, E. L. Metter, et al. How comparable are healthy 60- and 80-year old men? *J. Gerontol.* 47:M73–M78, 1992.

144. Miller, R. G., D. Giannini, H. S. Milner-Brown, et al. Effects of fatiguing exercise on high-energy phosphates, force, and EMG: evidence for three phases of recovery. *Muscle Nerve* 10:810–821, 1987.

145. Milner-Brown, H. S., R. B. Stein, and R. G. Lee. Synchronization of human motor units: possible roles of exercise and supraspinal reflexes. *Electroencephalogr. Clin. Neurophysiol.* 38:245–254, 1975.

146. Milner-Brown, H. S., R. B. Stein, and R. Yemm. The contractile properties of human motor units during voluntary isometric contractions. *J. Physiol. (Lond.)* 228:285–306, 1973.

147. Mittal, K. R., and F. H. Logmani. Age-related reduction in the 8th cervical ventral nerve root myelinated fiber diameters and numbers in man. *J. Gerontol.* 42:8–10, 1987.

148. Moberg, E. Criticism and study of methods for examining sensibility in the hand. *Neurology* 12:8–19, 1962.

149. Moore, G. P., D. H. Perkel, and J. P. Segundo. Statistical analysis and functional interpretation of neuronal spike data. *Annu. Rev. Physiol.* 28:493–522, 1966.

150. Morgan, M., J. G. Phillips, J. L. Bradshaw, J. B. Mattingly, R. Iansek, and J. A. Bradshaw. Age-related slowness: Simply strategic? *J. Gerontol.* 49:M133–139, 1994.

151. Morse, J. M., S. J. Tylko, and H. A. Dixon. Characteristics of the fall-prone patient. *Gerontologist* 27:516–522, 1987.
152. Nako, M., Y. Ionue, and H. Murakami. Aging process of leg muscle endurance in males and females. *Eur. J. Appl. Physiol.* 59:209–214, 1989.
153. Narici, M. V., M. Bordini, and P. Ceretelli. Effect of aging on human adductor pollicis muscle function. *J. Appl. Physiol.* 71:1277–1281, 1991.
154. Narici, M. V., G. S. Roi, L. Landoni, A. E. Minetti, and P. Cerretelli. Changes in force, cross-sectional area and neural activation during strength training and detraining of the human quadriceps. *Eur. J. Appl. Physiol.* 59:310–319, 1989.
155. Nashner, L. M., Adapting reflexes controlling the human posture. *Exp. Brain. Res.* 26:59–72, 1976.
156. Nashner, L. M. Balance adjustments of humans perturbed while walking. *J. Neurophysiol.* 44:650–664, 1980.
157. Nashner, L. M., M. Woollacott, and G. Tuma. Organization of rapid responses to postural and locomotor-like perturbations of standing man. *Exp. Brain. Res.* 36:463–476, 1979.
158. Nelson, R. M., G. L. Soderberg, and N. L. Urbscheit. Alteration of motor-unit discharge characteristics in aged humans. *Phys. Ther.* 64:29–39, 1984.
159. Nevitt, M. C., S. R. Cummings, S. Kidd, and D. Black. Risk factors for recurrent nonsyncopal falls: a prospective study. *J. A. M. A.* 261:2663–2668, 1989.
160. Newell, K. M., and L. G. Carlton. On the relationship between peak force and variability in isometric tasks. *J. Motor Behav.* 17:230–241, 1985.
161. Nordstrom, M. A., A. J. Fuglevand, and R. M. Enoka. Estimating the strength of common input to human motoneurons from the cross-correlogram. *J. Physiol. (Lond.)* 453:547–574, 1992.
162. Nordstrom, M. A., and T. S. Miles. Instability of motor unit firing rates during prolonged contractions in human masseter. *Brain Res.* 549:268–274, 1991.
163. Oertel, G. Changes in human skeletal muscles due to aging. *Acta Neuropathol.* 69:309–313.
164. Overend, T. J., D. A. Cunningham, D. H. Paterson, and M. S. Lefcoe. Thigh composition in young and elderly men determined by computed tomography. *Clin. Physiol.* 12: 629–640, 1992.
165. Overstall, P. W., A. N. Exton-Smith, F. J. Imms, and A. L. Johnson. Falls in the elderly related to postural imbalance. *Br. Med. J.* 1:261–264, 1977.
166. Parkkola, R., U. Kujala, and U. Rytökoski. Response of the trunk muscles to training assessed by magnetic resonance imaging and muscle strength. *Eur. J. Appl. Physiol.* 65:383–387, 1992.
167. Patla, A. E. Visual control of human locomotion. A. E. Patla (ed). *Adaptability of Human Gait.* New York: North-Holland, 1991, pp. 55–97.
168. Paulus, W. M., A. Straube, and T. H. Brandt. Visual stabilization of posture: Physiological stimulus characteristics and clinical aspects. *Brain* 107:1143–1163, 1984.
169. Phelan, J. P. Genetic variability and rodent models of human aging. *Exp. Gerontol.* 7:147–159, 1992.
170. Phillips, C. G. *Movements of the Hand.* Liverpool: Liverpool University Press, 1986.
171. Phillips, S. K., S. A. Bruce, and R. C. Woledge. In mice, the muscle weakness due to age is absent during stretching. *J. Physiol. (Lond.)* 437:63–70, 1991.
172. Phillips, S. K., S. A. Bruce, D. Newton, and R. C. Woledge. The weakness of old age is not due to failure of muscle activation. *J. Gerontol.* 47:M45–M49, 1992.
173. Phillips, S. K., K. M. Rook, N. C. Siddle, S. A. Bruce, and R. C. Woledge. Muscle weakness in women occurs at an earlier age than in men, but strength is preserved by hormone treatment. *Clin. Sci.* 84:95–98, 1993.
174. Posiadlo, D., and S. Richardson. The timed "up and go": a test of basic functional mobility for frail elderly persons. *J. Am Geriatr. Soc.* 39:142–148, 1991.
175. Poulin, M. J., A. A. Vandervoort, D. H. Paterson, J. F. Kramer, and D. A. Cunningham. Eccentric and concentric torques of knee and elbow extension in young and older men. *Can. J. Appl. Sport Sci.* 17:3–7, 1992.

176. Pyka, G., E. Lindenberger, S. Charette, and R. Marcus. Muscle strength and fiber adaptations to a year-long resistance training program in elderly men and women. *J. Gerontol.* 49:M22–M27, 1994.

177. Pyykko, I., P. Jantti, and H. Aalto. Postural control in the oldest old. *Adv. Otorhinolaryngol.* 41:146–151, 1988.

178. Rafuse, V. F., T. Gordon, and R. Orozco. Proportional enlargement of motor units after partial denervation of cat triceps surae muscles. *J. Neurophysiol.* 68:1261–1276, 1992.

179. Robbins, A. S., L. Z. Rubenstein, K. R. Josephson, B. L. Schulman, D. Osterweil, and G. Fine. Predictors of falls among elderly people. *Arch. Phys. Med. Rehabil.* 149:1628–1633, 1989.

180. Rogers, M. A., and W. J. Evans. Changes in skeletal muscle with aging: Effects of exercise training. J. O. Holloszy (ed.). *Exercise and Sport Sciences Reviews, Vol. 21.* Baltimore: Williams & Wilkins, 1993, pp. 65–102.

181. Rogers, M. W., C. G. Kukulka, and G. L. Soderberg. Age-related changes in postural responses preceding rapid self-paced and reaction time arm movements. *J. Gerontol.* 47:M159–165, 1992.

182. Roman, W. J., J. Fleckenstein, J. Stray-Gundersen, S. F. Alway, R. Peshock, and W. J. Gonyea. Adaptations in the elbow flexors of elderly males after heavy-resistance training. *J. Appl. Physiol.* 74:750–754, 1993.

183. Rosenhall, U. Degenerative changes in the aging human vestibular geriatric neuroepithelia. *Acta Otolaryngol.* 76:208–220, 1973.

184. Rowe, J. W. Clinical research on aging: strategies and directions. *N. Engl. J. Med.* 297:1332–1336, 1977.

185. Rutherford, O. M., and D. A. Jones. The role of learning and coordination in strength training. *Eur. J. Appl. Physiol.* 55:100–105, 1986.

186. Sale, D. G. Neural adaptation to resistance training. *Med. Sci. Sports Exerc.* 20:S135–S145, 1988.

187. Sargeant, A. J., and D. Kernell (eds). *Neuromuscular Fatigue.* Amsterdam: North Holland, 1993.

188. Schultz, A. B., N. B. Alexander, and J. A. Ashton-Miller. Biomechanical analyses of rising from a chair. *J. Biomech.* 25:1383–1391, 1992.

189. Sears, T. A., and D. Stagg. Short-term synchronization of intercostal motoneurone activity. *J. Physiol. (Lond.)* 263:357–381, 1976.

190. Sekuler, R., and L. P. Hutman. Spatial vision and aging. I. *J. Gerontol.* 35:692–699, 1980.

191. Sheldon, J. H. The effect of age on the control of sway. *Gerontol. Clin.* 5:129–138, 1963.

192. Sherwood, D. E., and R. A. Schmidt. The relationship between force and force variability in minimal and near maximal static and dynamic contractions. *J. Motor Behav.* 12:75–89, 1980.

193. Spiegel, K., J. Stratton, J. R. Burke, D. S. Glendinning, and R. M. Enoka. Influence of age on the assessment of motor unit activation threshold in a human hand muscle. *Soc. Neurosci. Abstr.* 20:386, 1994.

194. Stålberg, E., O. Borges, M. Ericsson, et al. The quadriceps femoris muscle in 20-70-year-old subjects: relationships between knee extension torque, electrophysiological parameters, and muscle fiber characteristics. *Muscle Nerve* 12:382–389, 1989.

195. Stålberg, E., and P. R. W. Fawcett. Macro EMG in healthy subjects of different ages. *J. Neurol. Neurosurg. Psychiat.* 45:870–878, 1982.

196. Staron, R. S., D. L. Karpaondo, W. J. Kraemer, et al. Skeletal muscle adaptations during early phase of heavy-resistance training in men and women. *J. Appl. Physiol.* 76:1247–1255, 1994.

197. Stein, R. B. Reflex modulation during locomotion: functional significance. A. E. Patla (Ed). *Adaptability of Human Gait.* New York: North-Holland, 1991, pp. 21–36.

198. Stelmach, G. E., J. Phillips, R. P. DiFabio, and N. Teasdale. Age, functional postural reflexes, and voluntary sway. *J. Gerontolol.* 44:B100–106, 1989.

199. Stelmach, G. E., L. Populin, and F. Muller. Postural muscle onset and voluntary movements in the elderly. *Neurosci. Lett.* 117:188–193, 1990.
200. Stelmach, G. E., N. Teasdale, J. Phillips, and C. J. Worringham. Force production characteristics in Parkinson's disease. *Exp. Brain Res.* 76:165–172, 1989.
201. Stelmach, G. E., and C. J. Worringham. Sensorimotor deficits related to postural stability. *Clin. Geriatric Med.* 1:679–694, 1985.
202. Sutton, G. G., and K. Sykes. The variation in hand tremor with force in healthy subjects. *J. Physiol. (Lond.)* 191:699–711, 1967.
203. Taylor, J. A., and S. C. Kandarian. Advantage normalizing force production to myofibrillar protein in skeletal muscle cross-sectional area. *J. Appl. Physiol.* 76:974–978, 1994.
204. Tesch, P. A., G. A. Dudley, M. R. Duvoisin, B. M. Hather, and R. T. Harris. Force and EMG signal patterns during repeated bouts of concentric or eccentric muscle actions. *Acta Physiol. Scand.* 138:263–271, 1990.
205. Tinetti, M. E., Speechley, M., and S. F. Ginter. Risk factors for falls among elderly persons living in the community. *N. Eng. J. Med.* 319:1701–1707, 1988.
206. Tinetti, M. E., and M. Speechley. Prevention of falls among the elderly. *N. Eng. J. Med.* 320:1055–1059, 1989.
207. Tinetti M. E., T. F. Williams, and R. Mayewski. Fall risk index for elderly patients based upon number of chronic disabilities. *Am. J. Med.* 80:429–434, 1986.
208. Tomlinson, B. E., and D. Irving. Total numbers of limb motor neurons in the human lumbosacral cord throughout life. *J. Neurol. Sci.* 34:213–219, 1977.
209. Tötösy De Zepetnek, J. E., H. V. Zung, S. Erdebil, and T. Gordon. Innervation ratio is an important determinant of force in normal and reinnervated rat tibialis anterior muscles. *J. Neurophysiol.* 67:1385–1403, 1992.
210. Vallbo, Å. B., and J. Wessberg. Organization of motor output in slow finger movements in man. *J. Physiol (Lond.)* 469:673–691, 1993.
211. VanDenBosch, C., Gilsing, M., Richardson, J. K., Ashton-Miller, J. A. Effect of peripheral neuropathy on thresholds for detecting ankle inversion and eversion and their relation with nerve conduction parameters, *J. Am. Geriatr. Soc.*, in press.
212. Vandervoort, A. A., J. F. Kramer, and E. R. Wharram. Eccentric knee strength of elderly females. *J. Gerontol.* 45:B125–B128, 1990.
213. Vandervoort, A. A., and A. J. McComas. Contractile changes in opposing muscles of the human ankle joint with aging. *J. Appl. Physiol.* 61:361–367, 1986.
214. Videla, D. G., and J. A. Ashton-Miller. A simple method for measuring ankle isometric strength and endurance in the sagittal and frontal planes utilizing unipedal stance. *J. Biomech.*, in press.
215. Westing, S. H., A. G. Cresswell, and A. Thorstensson. Muscle activation during maximal voluntary eccentric and concentric knee extension. *Eur. J. Appl. Physiol.* 62:104–108, 1991.
216. Whipple, R. H., L. I. Wolfson, and P. M. Amerman. The relationship of knee and ankle weakness to falls in nursing home residents: an isokinetic study. *J. Am. Geriatr. Soc.* 35:13–20, 1987.
217. Winter, D. A., A. E. Patla, J. S. Frank, J. S. and S. E. Walt. Biomechanical walking pattern changes in the fit and elderly. *Phys. Ther.* 70:340–347, 1990.
218. Wolfson, L., R. Whipple, P. Amerman, and J. Tobin. Gait assessment in the elderly: a gait abnormality rating scale and its relation to falls. *J. Gerontol.* 45:M12–M19, 1990.
219. Woollacott, M., A. T. Shumway-Cook, and L. M. Nashner. Postural reflexes and aging. J. A. Mortimer (ed). *The Aging Motor System* New York: Praeger, 1982, pp. 98–119.
220. Woollacott, M., A. T. Shumway-Cook, and L. M. Nashner. Aging and posture control: changes in sensory organization and muscular coordination. *Int. J. Aging Hum. Dev.* 23:97–114, 1986.
221. Woollacott, M. H., and D. L. Manchester. Anticipatory postural adjustments in older adults: are changes in response characteristics due to changes in strategy? *J. Gerontol.* 48:M64–M70, 1993.

222. Wolle, S., C. Thornton, R. Jozefowicz, and M. Statt. Myofibrillar protein synthesis in young and old men. *Am. J. Physiol.* 27:E693–E698, 1993.
223. Yack, H. J. and R. C. Berger. Dynamic stability in the elderly: identifying a possible measure. *J. Gerontol.* 48:M225–M230, 1993.
224. Yarasheski, K. E., J. J. Zachwieja, and D. M. Bier. Acute effects of resistance exercise on muscle protein synthesis rate in young and elderly men and women. *Am. J. Physiol.* 28:E210–E214, 1993.
225. Young, A., M. Stokes, and M. Crowe. Size and strength of the quadriceps muscles of old and young women. *Eur. J. Clin. Invest.* 14:282–287, 1984.
226. Young, A., M. Stokes, and M. Crowe. The size and strength of the quadriceps muscles of old and young men. *Clin. Physiol.* 5:145–154, 1985.
227. Young, A., M. Stokes, J. M. Round, and R. H. T. Edwards. The effect of high-resistance training on the strength and cross-sectional area of the human quadriceps. *Eur. J. Clin. Invest.* 13:411–417, 1983.
228. Yue, G. H., A. J. Fuglevand, M. A. Nordstrom, and R. M. Enoka. Limitations of the surface-EMG technique for estimating motor unit synchronization. *Biol. Cybern.*, in press.
229. Yue, G. H., D. A. Keen, and R. M. Enoka. The voluntary strength of a human hand muscle cannot be predicted by its size. *Proceedings of the 18th Annual Meeting of the American Society of Biomechanics.* Columbus, OH, October 13–15, 1994.
230. Zhang, X., J. A. Ashton-Miller, A. B. Schultz, and N. B. Alexander. A biomechanical study of the effects of age on recovery from impending lateral falls. *Proceedings of the 16th Annual Meeting of the American Society of Biomechanics,* Iowa City, IA, October 21–23, 1992.

4
Influence of Exercise on Human Sleep

PATRICK J. O'CONNOR, Ph.D.
SHAWN D. YOUNGSTEDT, M.A.

The sleep of a labouring man is sweet.

———Ecclesiastes

This chapter reviews the body of scientific literature concerning the influence of exercise on human sleep. After introducing several key concepts and providing a rationale as to why this area of research deserves attention, the paper summarizes current knowledge and provides examples of the paradigms that have been used to gain insight into relationships between exercise and sleep.

KEY CONCEPTS

Basic sleep concepts are introduced in this section. A complete overview of sleep, or the related topics of sleepiness and circadian rhythms, is precluded by space limitations. Several comprehensive sources are available to the interested reader [90, 112, 119, 120, 160].

Sleep Basics
Adult humans, unlike most animals, usually sleep in a single continuous bout. The sleep state is typified by a daily occurrence that results in behavioral disengagement from, as well as a decreased sensory responsiveness to, the environment and in characteristic electroencephalographic (EEG), electro-oculographic (EOG), and electromyographic (EMG) patterns. Polysomnography is the term used to describe the simultaneous and continuous measurement of EEG, EOG, EMG, and other physiological parameters, such as body temperature or nasal air flow, during sleep.

Sleep contains two distinct states that alternate cyclically throughout the night: nonrapid eye movement (NREM) sleep and rapid eye movement (REM) sleep. NREM-REM cycles are thought to be the basic organizational unit of mammalian sleep, and they first appeared in evolutionary history in association with endothermy [187]. NREM sleep is characterized by physiological quiescence in which there is a gradual slowing of the frequency and an increase in the amplitude in the EEG. NREM sleep has been divided into four arbitrary stages (Stages 1, 2, 3, and 4) that are roughly indicative of the depth of sleep. Stage 4 is the deepest sleep, the stage during which whole-body oxygen consumption is lowest [26] and awakening a person is most difficult [39]. Standard EEG, EOG, and EMG criteria established by a consensus of experts more than 25 yr ago are used to determine sleep stage visually [138]; however, increasing attention is being paid to the use of computer-assisted scoring and powerful statistical techniques, such as spectral analysis, to quantify sleep physiology more accurately and meaningfully [53, 55].

In contrast to the quiescence of NREM sleep, portions of the central and peripheral nervous systems become highly active during REM sleep. The central nervous system changes include increases in neuronal firing rates [151], blood flow [105], metabolic rate [32], and temperature [131]. Peripheral changes include an increase in the sympathetic nerve traffic to the skeletal muscle vascular bed [150]. Muscle tone of the head and neck are lost during REM sleep [86], and thermoregulation is severely inhibited [66]. REM sleep is measured in the sleep laboratory by low voltage, fast activity of the EEG, phasic bursts of eye movements, and the loss of EMG activity in the muscles of the chin.

Although there is an incomplete database concerning what makes up normal adult sleep, certain generalizations can be made [39]. Most adults obtain between 7 and 8 hr of sleep per night, achieve sleep onset in less than 20 min, and have a sleep efficiency, defined as the total amount of time spent sleeping while in bed, that is greater than 90%. Sleep is initiated through NREM Stage 1. About 75% of a usual night's sleep is NREM (~5% Stage 1, ~50% Stage 2, and ~20% Slow-wave sleep, defined as Stages 3 and 4 combined) and approximately 25% is REM. The first NREM period, which lasts approximately 65–85 min, usually contains the greatest amount of a night's slow wave sleep (SWS) and is followed by a brief REM period of ~1–5 min. Typically, there are four to six NREM-REM cycles during sleep that alternate with a period of about 90 min. Most SWS occurs during the first three NREM cycles, whereas REM sleep predominates during the final third of the night.

In recent years, it has become apparent that the adequacy of sleep at night cannot be understood fully without considering daytime functioning, especially sleepiness. Although postprandial states, a warm room, or a boring book chapter can be associated with sleepiness during the day, excessive daytime sleepiness is primarily a symptom of inadequate sleep at night [112]. Sleepiness can be measured subjectively or objectively. Subjective assessments of sleepiness include standardized scales of the sleepiness-alertness construct such as the Stanford Sleepiness Scale [76], the Activation-Deactivation Check List [155], and Visual Analogue Scales of alertness [111]. The Multiple Sleep Latency Test (MSLT) is the most prominent objective measure of sleepiness [41]. The Multiple Sleep Latency Test involves the assessment of the spontaneous EEG, EOG, and chin EMG for 20 min under standardized conditions a minimum of four separate times. These tests are repeated every 2 hr, starting 1.5–3 hr after the subject wakes up. Subjects are placed in a dark, quiet, distraction-free bedroom and instructed to close their eyes and try to fall asleep. Under these conditions, it takes normal adults an average of 10–20 min to exhibit Stage 1 sleep, whereas sleep-deprived subjects or people with sleep abnormalities often fall asleep in less than 5 min [38].

Sleep Regulation
Research showing that the amount of SWS decreases as sleep progresses each night [39], that naps taken later in the day have greater amounts of SWS than those taken earlier in the day [52, 100], that sleep deprivation results in a dramatic increase in SWS during the recovery night, and that this increase in recovery-night SWS is a function of the duration of prior wakefulness [23, 177] has led Borbély and colleagues to postulate that slow wave activity is a homeostatically regulated process [22]. Other aspects of sleep, such as its duration and the presence of REM, are strongly dependent on the circadian system [46]. Consequently, there is an emerging consensus that sleep is regulated by both homeostatic and circadian mechanisms. The brain site responsible for generating circadian rhythms is localized within the suprachiasmatic nucleus [106]. In contrast, homeostatic sleep regulation is not localized to a small brain region and its neurobiology is less well understood. For example, slow wave activity measured during sleep is believed to be the result of synchronized events in millions of coupled neurons in the thalamus and the cerebral cortex [152]. Additional complexity in homeostatic sleep regulation is implied by animal research that has identified several endogenous substances (e.g., cytokines such as interleukin-1) that promote slow wave activity during sleep. The role of these substances in human sleep homeostasis, however, is not yet clear [24]. Several models have been proposed to explain how circadian and homeostatic mechanisms interact to regulate human sleep [1, 21, 22, 157]; these models offer important conceptual frameworks for exploring the regulation and function of sleep.

Circadian Basics
Circadian rhythms are regularly occurring oscillations that have a period (i.e., recur at a frequency) of about (*circa*) one 24-hr day (*dian*). A circadian rhythm can be described by its amplitude and phase. The term "amplitude" refers to the difference between the maximum (or minimum) and the mean value of an oscillating rhythm. The term "phase" refers to a particular state of a rhythm, for example, the location of a rhythm's peak or trough.

Several important discoveries about sleep have resulted from studying circadian aspects of sleep. For example, Czeisler and colleagues [46] studied polysomnographically recorded sleep from human subjects living for extended periods in an environment free of external time cues (e.g., clocks, sunlight) and showed that both the duration of a sleep bout and its organization (i.e., the amount of REM sleep) depended not on the length of prior wakefulness, but rather, on the circadian phase of the core body temperature rhythm at sleep onset. This observation, and a myriad of others, serves to underscore the importance of viewing the sleep-wake cycle as a circadian rhythm [176].

Circadian rhythms are produced endogenously by a pacemaker—a localizable, functional entity capable of self-sustained oscillations [120]. The suprachiasmatic nucleus of the hypothalamus is a circadian pacemaker in the mammalian brain [106]. Under conditions in which there is an absence of external time cues, circadian rhythms "free run"; that is, they are endogenously expressed without any modulation by environmental factors such as sunlight. The free-running period of the human sleep-wake cycle is about 25, not 24, hr [180]. This means that endogenous rhythms must be resynchronized (or entrained) daily to maintain a 24-hr schedule. Light is an important synchronizer of the human circadian pacemaker [47]; however, behaviors, such as the strict scheduling of meal or bed times, also have the ability to entrain the pacemaker [7, 180].

The effect of an entraining agent on the circadian pacemaker is critically dependent upon the timing of the stimulus. Studies examining such timing typically reference the presentation of a stimulus to an identifiable state of the circadian system such as the peak or trough of a particular rhythm. For example, exposing a human subject to a single 3-hr pulse of bright light centered 2 hr before the time of their body core temperature minimum (i.e., about 2 hr before usual wake time) significantly delays the subsequent circadian phase by about 2 hr; however, the same bright light exposure presented 4 hr later results in an advance of the circadian phase of about 2 hr [109]. In addition, at certain times during the 24-hr day, the circadian system is completely insensitive to bright light exposure. Thus, a key property of the circadian system is that its sensitivity to entraining agents changes throughout the 24-hr day. The relationship between the timing of exposures to a stimulus and the resultant phase shifts make up the phase response characteristics; these responses are frequently plotted as a phase response curve. The strength of a stimulus also can influence the magnitude of the phase shift. For instance, larger phase shifts have been reported with exposure to light of an intensity of 9000 lux compared with 5000 lux [109].

Experiments with rodents have shown the existence of a phase response curve to physical activity or one of its concomitants [59, 110, 124, 165, 169]. Recent work also suggests that a single bout of exercise can induce phase delays in the human circadian system [168]. Full elucidation of a phase response curve to physical activity in humans and a determination of the mechanism(s) underlying such effects are likely to provide a significant advance toward a fuller understanding of the influence of exercise on human sleep.

WHY STUDY THE SLEEP CONSEQUENCES OF EXERCISE?

Scientific scrutiny of the sleep consequences of exercise is warranted for both theoretical and practical reasons. Exercise can be an effective tool for testing theories about sleep. For example, exercise studies have helped to undermine the theory that the primary purpose of sleep is to recover from "wear and tear" caused by daytime activity [72, 78, 79].

In addition to shedding light on theories about sleep function, exercise may have a useful role in the prevention and treatment of sleep problems. Insomnia, a common sleep disorder, is a major public health problem. For example, in a study of 7954 community respondents living in five U.S. cities, the 6-mo prevalence of insomnia, defined by the investigators as 2 wk or more of trouble falling asleep, staying asleep, or waking up too early, was reported to be 10.2% [63]. Although both popular [166] and clinical [186] opinion holds that exercise promotes sleep onset, to the best of our knowledge there is only one published abstract concerning the influence of exercise on the sleep of insomniacs [16].

Despite the large scope of sleep problems—an estimated 40 million Americans suffer from chronic disorders of sleep and wakefulness and 20–30 million more are plagued by intermittent sleep disturbances [126]—the negative health consequences of inappropriate sleep are not widely appreciated. Some of the major public health concerns related to sleep include the following:

All-Cause Mortality
Sleep duration is associated with all-cause mortality. Hammond [69], in a study of 1,064,004 men and women, found that those aged 45 yr or older who reported sleeping more than 10 hr or fewer than 5 hr per night had an elevated mortality risk. Those who reported sleeping about 7 hr per night had the lowest death rate. Subsequent work has confirmed links between too little or too much sleep duration and increased mortality [27, 89, 184].

Cardiovascular Disease
The risk of acute coronary events is higher in the morning hours just after awakening from sleep [125, 182]. This observation suggests that the physiological consequences of sleep "set the stage" for the occurrence of adverse cardiac events in the morning. For example, REM sleep both dominates the last third of the sleep period and is characterized by profound increases in sympathetic nerve activity [150]. Somers et al. [150] have hypothesized that the sympathetic changes during REM sleep could initiate platelet aggregation, plaque, rupture, or coronary vasospasm, and thereby act as a trigger for cardiac events that appear clinically only after awakening. If this hypothesis is correct, then the reduction in the long-term risk for a heart attack associated with regular exercise may be, in part, due to influences of chronic exercise on sleep physiology. Resting sympathetic nerve activity is

reduced after endurance training [67]; however, the influence of exercise training on sympathetic nerve activity during REM sleep, to the best of our knowledge, has not yet been examined.

Mental Illness

Sleep disturbances are strongly related to mental illness. In a large study (N = 7954) conducted by the National Institutes of Mental Health [63], 40% of the respondents with insomnia also had a psychiatric disorder such as anxiety, depression, or substance abuse, whereas those who had no sleep complaints had a significantly lower rate of psychiatric disorder (16.4%). In addition, a meta-analysis of 177 studies that examined sleep polysomnographically in 7151 psychiatric patients reported that most psychiatric conditions were associated with a significant reduction in sleep efficiency as well as total sleep time; these reductions were accounted for by a decrease in NREM sleep [12]. Of the various psychiatric conditions studied, the sleep of patients with affective disorders (e.g., anxiety, depression) differed most frequently and significantly from that of normal control subjects [12]. Because acute and chronic exercise consistently have been associated with affective benefits [122, 129], it is plausible that mental health gains associated with exercise also may improve sleep. Alternatively, it is possible that improvements in affect associated with exercise may be mediated, in part, by the influence of exercise on sleep. To the best of our knowledge, the influence of exercise on sleep in patients suffering from psychological distress, including anxiety and depressive disorders, has not yet been investigated.

Excessive Daytime Sleepiness

Excessive daytime sleepiness has been estimated to be a problem for 4–5% of the general population [15, 94], and increased attention is being paid to the adverse consequences of daytime sleepiness. For example, excessive sleepiness in children is associated with learning disabilities [127], and adults with excessive daytime sleepiness exhibit a high rate of automobile accidents [95]. Only a few studies have addressed the possible role of exercise in minimizing excessive daytime sleepiness and the findings are inconclusive. Some studies show no positive effects of exercise [6], whereas others suggest that exercise may be useful in minimizing daytime sleepiness either by promoting nocturnal sleep or enhancing daytime alertness [173].

Consequences of Shift Work and Jet Lag

Poor sleep is a hazard for air travelers who fly across multiple time zones [130] and for night-shift workers [139]. Both these groups have frequent, nonspecific complaints such as malaise, fatigue, and difficulty concentrating that could be the result of sleep problems. Several studies have reported a high rate of gastrointestinal and cardiovascular disease in shift workers [87, 88]. Because it has been estimated that 48 million passengers return from international flights annually [167] and that approximately 50 million people in the United States are engaged in some form of shift work [113], the potential adverse health consequences of air travel and shift work are extensive. Perhaps an even greater public health risk stems from the loss of behavioral efficiency that can occur when circadian and environmental synchrony is disrupted because of air travel or shift work. For instance, major industrial accidents, including the Bhopal, Chernobyl, *Exxon Valdez*, and Three Miles Island disasters, have been attributed to the negative effects of working in the middle of the night [119]. There is a small amount of incomplete, yet tantalizing, evidence suggesting that physical fitness can explain some of the variance in tolerance to shift work [70], and that moderate physical training reduces work-dependent fatigue [71].

Sleep-Disordered Breathing
Sleep-disordered breathing, as evidenced by snoring, has been associated with an increased risk for hypertension, strokes, and myocardial infarctions [48, 141]. Moreover, the scope of sleep-disordered breathing problems is large. For instance, the prevalence of polysomnographically documented sleep-disordered breathing, defined as an average of 5 or more episodes of apnea and/or hypopnea per hour of sleep, was 9% for women and 24% for men in a sample of 602 employed, middle-aged women and men [185]. Surgery or the use of a nasal mask that delivers continuous positive pressure to the upper airway can be effective treatments for sleep-disordered breathing. However, some patients are unacceptable candidates for surgery and others find sleeping with a mask strapped to their face unacceptable; consequently, other treatments have been used. Exercise has been suggested as a possible treatment or adjunct in some obstructive sleep apnea cases [156]. In theory, weight loss associated with an exercise program could reduce "the soft tissue flabbiness and bulkiness that compromise the upper airway in the collapsible portion, where snoring and obstructive sleep breathing occurs (between the epiglottis and the nasopharynx)" [61]. To the best of our knowledge, no published studies have examined the influence of exercise training on patients with sleep-disordered breathing.

In summary, despite the enormity of sleep-related health problems and the potential for exercise to impact upon these concerns, the topic of sleep has been largely ignored by exercise scientists. For example, no information about the influence of exercise on sleep is given in 10 widely used exercise physiology textbooks [8, 28, 51, 64, 93, 103, 128, 137, 148, 183]. In addition, the topic has received scant attention in edited volumes that aspire to provide a summary of the scientific aspects of physical activity, fitness, and health [25]. Specialists in the area of exercise psychology also have largely disregarded this area of research [142, 149]. Equally unfortunate is that many sleep researchers with an interest in pursuing questions related to exercise have not collaborated with colleagues possessing expertise in exercise science; in many instances this has reduced the inter-pretability of findings obtained.

PARADIGMS FOR UNDERSTANDING THE EFFECTS OF EXERCISE ON SLEEP

This section provides selected examples of research strategies that have been used to better understand the influence of exercise on sleep. We have purposefully chosen this approach as a way to highlight both the strengths and limitations of different paradigms, and to complement other reviews of this literature [56, 77, 91, 143, 158, 162] (S. D. Youngstedt, P. J. O'Connor, and R. K. Dishman, unpublished data).

Epidemiology
Epidemiology is concerned with "quantifying the rate of health-related states or events that occur within the population being studied" and "iden-tifying potential causative factors that may be associated with disease or a health-related event" [42] Many epidemiological studies have documented significant associations between physical activity and a variety of health con-cerns including coronary heart disease [17], cancers [65, 69], diabetes [99], and mental depression [129]. Physical activity epidemiologists have acknowledged the potential influence of physical activity on sleep as it re-lates to overall well-being [43]; however, few epidemiological investigations have examined relationships between physical activity and sleep.

A large survey conducted in Finland illustrates an epidemiological ap-proach to exploring relationships between exercise and sleep [72, 166, 173]. A random sample of 1600 women and men (aged 36–50 yr) living in Tampere, Finland, were asked about the perceived effects of exercise on sleep. Complete data were obtained from 1190 subjects. In response to an open-ended question that asked the respondents: "Please state, in their or-der of importance, three practices, habits, or actions which you have ob-served to best promote or improve your falling asleep immediately or your perceived quality of sleep," 33% of the men and 30% of the women indi-cated that exercise was the most important sleep-promoting factor [166]. Exercise was among the top three sleep-promoting factors mentioned for 44% of both the female and male respondents.

Figure 4.1 illustrates the relationship observed between self-reported ex-ercise frequency and excessive daytime tiredness [173]. Sedentary people reported a higher rate of excessive daytime tiredness compared with regu-larly active respondents. These findings are consistent with cross-sectional comparisons showing that groups of physically fit athletes report more vigor and less fatigue compared with less fit subjects [121]. Moreover, the study by Vuori and colleagues [173] found that 43% of those subjects who in-creased their exercise over the previous 3 mo (n = 81) reported improved

FIGURE 4.1

The percentage of subjects reporting exercise of a frequency of 0, 1, and 2 or more days per week who also reported excessive daytime tiredness. Adapted from Vuori et al. [173].

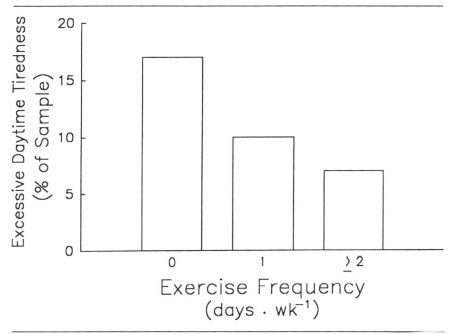

subjective sleep, whereas only 1% reported worsened sleep. In addition, 30% of those subjects who decreased their exercise over the previous 3 mo (n = 73) reported worsened sleep, whereas only 4% reported improved sleep. A smaller questionnaire study (N = 51) found that daily activity level was unrelated to daytime tiredness; however, the same study found that physically fit subjects went to bed later, fell asleep more rapidly, spent less total time asleep, and awoke feeling less tired than did people who were reported to be less physically fit [136].

The small amount of available epidemiological evidence suggests that exercise is perceived as helpful in promoting sleep. In addition, regular physical activity of a moderate intensity may be useful in improving sleep and thereby reducing daytime sleepiness. An equally plausible interpretation of the data, however, is that those who sleep better are less tired during the day and therefore are more willing to engage in regular exercise. Thus, the causal direction of these correlational data remains to be established.

There are methodological advantages and disadvantages in using epidemiological approaches [42]. One especially useful advantage is the feasibility of obtaining sleep reports on hundreds of thousands of respondents from various populations [69]. One limitation of epidemiological studies is that relationships between exercise and sleep may be spurious, driven by a strong relationship between exercise and another factor known to influence sleep, such as general health status. In addition, epidemiological investigations rely on subjective assessments of both physical activity and sleep; unfortunately, these measures often lack documented reliability and validity. For example, dissociations between subjective perceptions and objective measures of sleep can call into question the validity of subjective reports [40, 44]. This limitation is overcome by approaches that measure sleep directly.

Cross-Sectional Comparisons
A frequent research design used to examine relationships between exercise and sleep has been to compare the sleep of groups that differ in their physical activity histories or their degree of physical fitness [68, 114, 115, 117, 132–134, 136, 159, 161, 163, 164, 174, 175]. An Australian psychologist, John Trinder, and his associates have conducted a series of investigations of this type; one will be reviewed here [163].

Four groups of 10 men were recruited based on both their history of participation in competitive physical activities and their estimated $\dot{V}O_2$max. Studied were an "aerobic" group, characterized by a mean ($\pm$SD) $\dot{V}O_2$max of 68 ($\pm$11) ml·kg·min^{-1} and a history of running 45 ($\pm$19) miles·wk^{-1}; a "mixed" group, characterized by a $\dot{V}O_2$max of 55 ($\pm$18) ml·kg·min^{-1} and a history of training 4 days·wk^{-1}; in the sports of Australian-rules football, hockey, basketball, sprint-running or sprint-swimming; a "power" group, characterized by a $\dot{V}O_2$max of 46 ($\pm$6) ml·kg·min^{-1} and a history of lifting weights 12 ($\pm$3) hr·wk^{-1}; and a control group, characterized by a $\dot{V}O_2$max of 37.1 ($\pm$6) ml·kg·min^{-1} and a history of nonparticipation in sports. Sleep onset, defined as the first 30-s epoch of sleep Stage 2, occurred more quickly in the aerobic group compared with the power group (17 vs. 33 min), whereas the mean sleep latencies for the control and mixed groups were 25 and 26 min, respectively. The endurance-trained athletes also exhibited a greater amount of SWS compared with the power athletes, and these findings are illustrated in Figure 4.2.

The results of this study by Trinder et al. suggest that the type of physical training in which an athlete participates can influence both sleep-onset latency and the amount of SWS. One strength of a cross-sectional design is that groups with particular characteristics can be obtained with relative ease. However, when subjects are not randomly assigned to training conditions, the likelihood of group differences emerging on a variety of nuisance factors with potential to influence sleep is increased (e.g., diet, drug use, medical conditions, sleep history, etc.). Accordingly, conclusive evidence regarding the influence of exercise on sleep will never be generated from solely cross-sectional investigations. Biases inherent in cross-sectional studies often can be avoided using a randomized, longitudinal design.

FIGURE 4.2

Average (± SE) minutes of SWS for 10 inactive control subjects and three groups of 10 men with a history of training in either running (Aerobic), weight lifting (Power), or sports that combine endurance and power regimens (Mixed). Adapted from Trinder et al. [163].

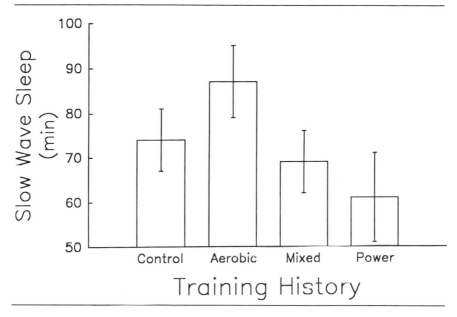

Longitudinal Investigations

Several longitudinal studies have been reported concerning the influence of exercise training on sleep [57, 62, 107, 147, 170, 171, 172]. A recent study by Vitiello and colleagues with elderly subjects, a population with frequent sleep problems that has infrequently been studied with regard to exercise and sleep [13, 60, 153], will be summarized for illustrative purposes [172]. It will be useful to review briefly a few of the most important age-related changes in sleep; readers with an interest in this topic are referred to an excellent review by Bliwise [18]. The literature suggests that sleep efficiency is reduced in the elderly, and this is due in large part to an increased number of nocturnal awakenings [19]. In addition, sleep-related breathing disorders and periodic limb movements during sleep are common in the elderly, and could contribute to an increased number of nocturnal awakenings or a change in sleep architecture [4, 5]. The primary changes in sleep architecture associated with aging are an increase in Stage 1 sleep and a decrease in SWS that is due to a decreased amplitude of the EEG [18]. In addition, the amplitude of the circadian endogenous body core temperature rhythm is decreased by 40% and its circadian phase occurs nearly

2 hr earlier in older compared with younger subjects [45]. It has been suggested that these changes in the output of the circadian pacemaker associated with aging may underlie complaints of sleep disturbances in the elderly [45]. To summarize, age-related changes in both homeostatic and circadian aspects of sleep have been documented.

Healthy but sedentary elders (mean age of 66 yr) with normal sleep patterns were randomly assigned to participate in 6 mo of thrice-weekly aerobic exercise or stretching and flexibility training [172]. Thirty (12 women and 18 men) completed aerobic training and 21 (9 women and 13 men) completed a stretching and flexibility program. $\dot{V}O_2$max was increased by 13% in the aerobic training group, but was unchanged for the stretching and flexibility group. Subjects slept in the laboratory on three nights (i.e., one adaptation and two recording nights) both before and after the 6-mo experimental conditions. Immediately after the last night of sleep in the laboratory subjects were monitored for approximately 32 additional hr to document their circadian rhythms.

Self-reported sleep quality was found to improve for both the aerobic exercise and the stretching and flexibility groups [171]. The SWS data are plotted in Figure 4.3. Note the small amount of SWS in both elderly groups compared with data from younger subjects shown in Figure 4.2. A statistically significant increase in SWS was reported for only the exercise group [172]. However, we calculated the effect size (post-test minus pretest values divided by the pooled standard deviation) for the change in SWS, and found the effect size to be 0.35 for the aerobic training group and 0.26 for the stretching and flexibility group. Thus, although statistical significance was reported for only the aerobic training group, the direction and the magnitude of the changes in SWS are similar for the two groups. A clearcut increase in the amplitude and delay in the phase of the body core temperature rhythm was observed for only the aerobic training group [170], suggesting that exercise training may enhance the strength of the circadian pacemaker and thereby result in improved sleep [45].

The results of the few studies that have examined the influence of exercise training on sleep have been mixed. Accordingly, strong conclusions about chronic exercise on sleep are presently not warranted. Because randomized, prospective studies that include appropriate control groups have obvious strengths from a design perspective, additional studies similar to that described in this section are needed if the influence of chronic exercise on sleep is to be better understood.

Acute Exercise Experiments
Most investigations concerning exercise and sleep have been aimed at documenting the influence of a single bout of exercise on various aspects of sleep [2, 10, 11, 13, 14, 29–31, 33–35, 49, 58, 60, 73–75, 81–85, 92, 102, 115, 116, 118, 132, 144–146, 159, 174). In an attempt to draw objective conclu-

FIGURE 4.3

Average (± SE) minutes of SWS in elderly subjects before and after 6-mo programs of either aerobic training or stretching and flexibility training. Adapted from Vitiello et al. [172].

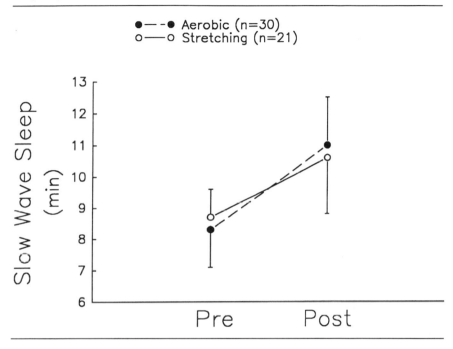

sions from this literature, we conducted a meta-analysis of the available acute exercise studies (S. D. Youngstedt, P. J. O'Connor, and R. K. Dishman, unpublished data). Acute exercise was found to be associated with a significant increase in total sleep time (mean effect size of 0.31 S D) as well as increases in both Stage 2 (mean effect size of 0.21) and SWS (mean effect of 0.18) when compared with control conditions. The magnitude of these effects is small from a clinical perspective. That is, the effects for total sleep time and SWS correspond to a mean nightly increase of 10.0 and 3.4 min, respectively. Larger effects were found for REM sleep variables. Acute exercise was associated with a delay in REM onset latency that averaged 12.3 min (mean effect size of 0.47) and a reduction in the total amount of REM sleep by 6.6 min (mean effect size of -0.39). These quantitative findings about REM sleep are inconsistent with a comprehensive and critical review of the exercise and sleep literature through 1980, conducted by sleep researcher James Horne, in which it was concluded that "the major sleep findings with human studies appear to be related to SWS and its components" [77].

A host of methodological considerations are especially important in attempting to evaluate the large number of studies that have been conducted concerning the influence of a single bout of exercise on sleep. Although Horne previously identified several important methodological issues [77], we wish to emphasize several major concerns. The activity history and fitness level of research participants frequently have been assessed inadequately or simply ignored. These factors are important because it is possible that exercise promotes sleep in physically fit or active persons [77], but is an arousing stressor for unfit and inactive persons. The sleep history of test subjects frequently has not been well documented in studies of exercise and sleep; however, it appears that this area of research has been limited almost exclusively to good sleepers. Thus, the small magnitude of the effects of acute exercise on sleep may be primarily because of the use of subjects who simply have little room for sleep improvement. Another major concern is the failure to control a myriad of factors to which subjects are exposed during the day that can and do influence sleep. These factors include the use of medications, dietary constituents such as caffeine, concern over job or other important responsibilities, exposure to sunlight, and even a warm bath or shower. Failure to control these nuisance variables adequately make it difficult conclusively to attribute effects observed to acute exercise per se.

Only a few studies have been aimed at testing hypotheses about how exercise might influence sleep. Horne concluded in his review that a high rate of energy expenditure during acute exercise has a greater effect on SWS than the total amount of energy expended. He also noted studies conducted in Russia which showed that a hot bath increased SWS in much the same way as exercise [97, 98]. On the basis of these observations, Horne speculated that exercise effects on SWS may be linked to exercise-induced increases in core body temperature. Horne's subsequent studies related to this hypothesis have had a significant impact on how the effects of exercise on SWS have been viewed, and consequently, they will be reviewed here.

Horne and Staff studied eight physically trained adults with an average ($\pm$SD) age and estimated $\dot{V}O_2$max of 25.4 ($\pm$4.4) yr and 62.0 ($\pm$7.6) ml·kg·min^{-1}, respectively [84]. After two adaptation nights, used to eliminate artifacts associated with sleeping in a novel laboratory environment [3], subjects completed three conditions within a 2-wk period: high- and low-intensity exercise and passive heating. The high-intensity exercise consisted of two 40-min bouts of level treadmill running at 80% of estimated $\dot{V}O_2$max with a 30-min rest period between the two bouts. The low-intensity exercise condition was designed as a control, matching the total energy expended in the high-intensity condition. This condition involved two 80-min treadmill runs at 40% of estimated $\dot{V}O_2$max with a 15-min rest period between the two bouts. Passive heating served as a second control; it was designed to produce the same core body temperature changes as those that occurred in response to high-intensity exercise. This condition consisted of subjects sitting in a tank of warm (42°C) water for two 40-min periods; these periods were separated by 30 min outside the tank at room temperature.

The findings for SWS are summarized in Figure 4.4. High-intensity exercise and the passive heating condition resulted in a significant increase in SWS compared with both baseline and the low-intensity exercise condition. Low-intensity exercise did not influence SWS, but did result in a significantly reduced mean (±SD) sleep latency (17.6 ± 14.1 vs. 34.5 ± 23.0 min) when compared with baseline sleep values. These findings discount the notion that SWS is increased simply as a by-product of increased total energy expenditure and support the idea that a large increase in core body temperature may be required to cause an increase in SWS after an acute bout of exercise.

Subsequent work by Horne and Moore explored this temperature hypothesis more directly [81]. Six physically fit ($\dot{V}O_2$max > 55 ml·kg·min^{-1}) women performed two conditions of high-intensity exercise (75% $\dot{V}O_2$max), similar to those used previously and described above [84]. In one

FIGURE 4.4

Average (± SE) minutes of SWS in eight physically trained adults on nights after low-intensity (40% estimated $\dot{V}O_2$max) and high-intensity (80% estimated $\dot{V}O_2$max) exercise bouts as well as baseline and a warm water (Heating) exposure condition during which the change in rectal temperature mimicked the pattern and magnitude observed during the high-intensity exercise condition. Adapted from Horne and Staff [83].

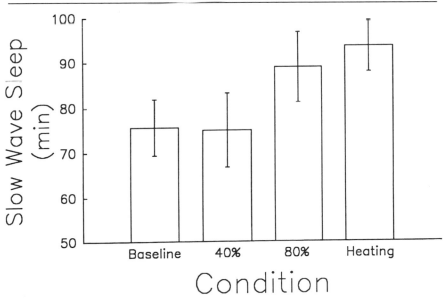

FIGURE 4.5

Average (± SE) minutes of SWS in six physically fit women on nights after high-intensity (75% estimated V̇O₂max) exercise during which core body temperature was manipulated by wearing extra clothing (HOT) or by dampening running clothes and increasing convective heat loss with electric fans (COOL). Adapted from Horne and Moore [81].

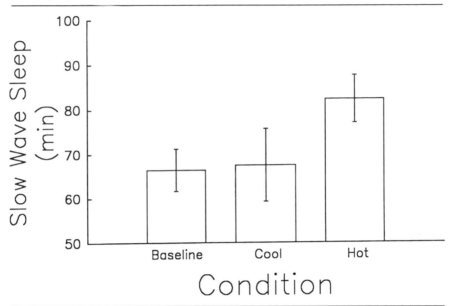

condition (HOT), subjects ran wearing a full tracksuit; in a second condition (COOL), running was performed while wearing only dampened shorts and a vest, and during exposure to a stream of air supplied by several electric fans. Body core temperature was successfully manipulated in the two conditions; the average (±SD) increase in rectal temperature was 2.3 (±0.7°C) in the HOT condition, but only 1.0 (±0.4°C) in the COOL condition. The main finding of this investigation is illustrated in Figure 4.5. Exercise in the HOT condition resulted in a significant increase in SWS compared with baseline; however, exercise of the same duration and intensity in which the increase in core body temperature was blunted by 1.3°C was not followed by an increase in SWS. These findings give more compelling credence to the idea that a large increase in core body temperature during exercise is a key element for observing subsequent increases in SWS.

Beyond playing a major role in hypotheses about how exercise effects sleep, the studies by Horne [80, 83] also have supported neuroanatomical, biochemical, and thermoregulatory evidence suggesting that SWS is a homeostatic feedback process that serves to lower brain temperature [104].

This brain-cooling–SWS hypothesis has been challenged by studies showing that increased amounts of SWS are not observed when core body temperature is elevated either artificially, such as after bright light exposure [36], or naturally, such as during prolonged (late-morning) sleep periods that are accompanied by a circadian-driven increase in core body temperature [54]. These arguments ignore an important nuance in the brain-cooling–SWS hypothesis; that is, the interaction between temperature and sleep is posited to result not from temperature per se, but from the activation of hypothalamic heat-loss mechanisms (i.e., sweating, shunting of blood flow to the skin) interacting with SWS mechanisms [104]. Because temperature elevations associated with both bright light exposure and the rising phase of the circadian temperature rhythm are associated with suppression of heat-loss mechanisms, these situations may not test the brain-cooling–SWS hypothesis adequately [9]. Thus, it remains tenable that vigorous exercise may be influencing SWS by acting indirectly on thermoregulation. Future work aimed at understanding relationships between exercise, thermoregulation, brain metabolism [80], and SWS has the potential to advance our understanding in this area.

Experiments with Rigorous Control over the Environment
A number of environmental factors, such as strictly controlled bed and meal times and exposure to light, are capable of influencing sleep and the circadian system in humans [7, 47]. Consequently, experiments that exert rigorous control over the environment are especially potent for understanding the effects of exercise *per se* on sleep.

THE CONSTANT ROUTINE TECHNIQUE. Because direct assessment of suprachiasmatic nucleus function (ie., the circadian pacemaker) is not possible with humans, information about the pacemaker is obtained by measuring markers that are strongly linked to the circadian pacemaker. Commonly used variables include urinary volume, cortisol, melatonin, subjective alertness ratings, and core body temperature. Assessment of circadian variation in these measures can be masked by a variety of factors including eating, ambient temperature, exercise, or exposure to sunlight. Accordingly, investigators have used the constant routine technique to expose endogenous circadian rhythms by minimizing and standardizing the masking effects of behavioral, environmental and social stimuli. The constant routine involves approximately 40 hr of continuous wakefulness while resting in bed in a room in which lighting, nourishment, posture, and interactions with research technicians are standardized [47].

The constant routine technique was used by Piercy and Lack to study the influence of morning versus evening exercise on the circadian pacemaker [135]. Six physically fit men who ran 8–12 km within 35–55 min at least five times per week were investigated. In one experimental condition, the subjects began their runs between 0600 and 0800 hr for 3 consecutive wk. In a second 3-wk condition, the exercise bouts were completed between 1700 and 1900 hr. After both conditions, core body temperature and urine formation were assessed during a constant routine. The 3-wk evening exercise period was associated with nearly a 2-hr phase delay in the circadian rhythm of both body core temperature and urinary output compared with the morning exercise condition. Because the exercise bouts were completed outdoors, these findings are only suggestive that appropriately timed, regular exercise may reset the human circadian pacemaker because the possible effects of exercise were potentially confounded by the effects of exposure to sunlight. Other field studies involving exercise that have used the constant routine technique are also limited by this confound [108].

Recent work by Van Reeth and colleagues [168] has yielded findings that are not confounded by exposure to sunlight. This study did not examine sleep per se; however, because certain aspects of sleep are controlled by the circadian system, the findings have implications for understanding exercise and sleep interactions. Seventeen young men completed two constant routines, one without the presentation of a stimulus (i.e., the control) and a second that incorporated a 3-hr exercise stimulus. The exercise involved five 36-min cycles, each consisting of 15 min of arm exercise and 15 min of leg exercise, followed by 6 min of rest. In addition, the exercise intensity alternated between moderate (60% $\dot{V}O_2$max) and low (40% $\dot{V}O_2$max) intensity during the 3-hr exercise period. The exercise bouts were performed at various times during the late night and early morning based on research with rodents showing that the largest phase shifts result when physical activity is timed to during periods in which the animals exhibit little activity [124]. Thus, for six subjects, the midpoint of exercise preceded the core body temperature minimum by 3–5 hr, for eight subjects the midpoint of exercise occurred within 2 hr of the core body temperature minimum, and for three subjects the midpoint of exercise occurred 3–4 hr after the core body temperature minimum. Fifteen of the 17 exercise bouts resulted in a delay in the phase of the circadian rhythms of both plasma melatonin and thyroid-stimulating hormone concentrations (measured at 20-min intervals throughout the constant routines), and the mean phase delay was statistically different from the control trials. The largest delays (mean of ~96 min, n = 6) were found when the exercise was timed 3–5 hr before the core temperature minimum; the smallest delays were found when exercise was performed 3–4 hr after the core temperature minimum (mean of ~30 min, n = 3). These findings show that appropriately timed exercise can produce large phase delays in the human circadian pacemaker that are equivalent to those seen after a 3-hr exposure to bright light of 5000 lux [109]. These findings imply that the influence of exercise on circadian-dependent aspects of sleep (i.e., sleep duration, REM periods) are likely to be critically influenced by the timing of the exercise. The finding that exercise can phase-delay the circadian pacemaker is consistent with the meta-analytically derived observation of a significant delay in REM latency after acute exercise (S.D. Youngstedt, P. J. O'Connor, and R. K. Dishman, unpublished data). These observations suggest that exercise may be similar to bright light in that it may be useful as a treatment for health problems related to asynchrony between environmental timing cues and the circadian system such as occur with seasonal affective disorder or jet lag [154].

BED REST STUDIES. One potentially useful strategy for understanding the influence of exercise on sleep is to determine the sleep consequences of complete physical inactivity. Campbell confined well-rested, healthy young adults to bed for 60 continuous hours in a sound-attenuated, temperature-controlled room isolated from daylight and other time-of-day cues [37]. Exogenous stimuli were minimized because the subjects were prevented from usual activities including exercise, reading, writing, watching television, or listening to music. Subjects were instructed to lie as quietly as possible, but could change position in bed, could go to the bathroom (in the room) at their convenience, and could sit up during meals that were served at irregular intervals during periods of wakefulness. Under these conditions, sleep and wakefulness patterns were clearly disrupted. The major changes were that the typical monophasic, prolonged sleep period (~8 hr) was replaced by short fragmented sleep bouts (~3 hr) that occurred throughout the 24-hr day. These findings suggest that behavior, including physical activity, may play a role in the consolidation of sleep into a single period.

Exercise has been incorporated into at least one bed rest study. Ryback and Lewis tested eight subjects during a 1-wk baseline period and during 5 wk of continuous supine bed rest either with (n = 4) or without (n = 4) a daily bout of total body ergometry that resulted in the expenditure of 600 kcal [140]. The duration, intensity, and timing of the exercise were not reported. Unlike the previous study by Campbell [37], subjects were prevented from napping during the day; this promoted monophasic sleep and prevents us from making a meaningful comparison between the two studies. No statistically significant influence of exercise on SWS was observed in the study by Ryback and Lewis [140]. Nevertheless, the potential influence of exercise on sleep parameters during extended periods of restriction to bed cannot be ruled out entirely because exercise effects are likely to be sensitive to both the timing of exercise and its intensity, two variables not manipulated in the investigation by Ryback and Lewis [140].

SLEEP DEPRIVATION STUDIES. Randy Gardner set the world record for continuous wakefulness in 1965 by refraining from sleep for 11 days, 12 min. Dr. William Dement, a pioneer in the field of sleep research, monitored Mr. Gardner during this event and summarized the experience by writing that, "The crucial factor in surmounting the effects of prolonged sleep loss is probably physical fitness. There is almost no degree of sleepiness that cannot be overcome if the subject engages in vigorous exercise. As the vigil wears on, almost continuous muscular activity is necessary to forestall overwhelming sleepiness" [50, p.12]. This case study highlights the paradoxical nature of the influence of exercise on sleep. Sleep onset is, of course, prevented *during* vigorous exercise, but after vigorous exercise certain aspects of sleep may be enhanced.

The mechanism(s) by which sleep is prevented during exercise and the time course of postexercise alterations in alertness have scarcely been studied. Clinical sleep specialists commonly recommend that vigorous late-night exercise should be avoided under the assumption that exercise inhibits sleep for several hours postexercise. There is, however, little research evidence to support this practice and a number of sleep deprivation studies have failed to find postexercise effects on sleepiness. For example, Angus and colleagues studied 12 healthy young men who were deprived of sleep for 60 hr on two occasions [6]. In one condition, subjects rested and in another the subjects completed 60 min of treadmill walking at 28% of $\dot{V}O_2$max every third hour. Self-reports of mood and sleepiness as well as a battery of cognitive tasks were completed at some point during the hour after the exercise or rest. Sleepiness, mood, and cognitive performance did not differ between the two conditions throughout the 60-hr sleep deprivation period. These findings show that after low-intensity exercise, sleepiness is not prevented or reduced during prolonged sleep deprivation. Other studies also have found no influence of exercise on recovery sleep after periods of sleep deprivation [123, 178]. However, in these and related studies [20, 96] several important methodological concerns have not been addressed fully. For example, little is known about (a) whether exercise influences objective measures of sleepiness, (b) possible relationships between the characteristics of exercise stimuli (e.g., intensity, duration, timing, amount of muscle mass activated) and subsequent sleepiness, and (c) whether exercise influences sleepiness during the immediate postexercise period (i.e., the first 20 min of recovery).

Sleep deprivation protocols have been employed widely to study sleep, and they are especially useful in identifying homeostatic aspects of sleep because the need for sleep is experimentally manipulated. Interpretation of sleep deprivation studies, however, needs to be tempered with an appreciation for the methodological limitations inherent in the design. Two principal concerns are that subjects cannot be blinded to the sleep deprivation condition, and that those who volunteer to participate in sleep deprivation studies may do so, in part, because they are more able to cope with sleep deprivation. These and other issues are addressed more fully in an excellent chapter that appeared previously in *Exercise and Sport Sciences Reviews* on the related topic of exercise performance and physiology after sleep loss [101].

CHRONIC TEMPORAL ISOLATION STUDIES. Physical activity was introduced in human circadian rhythm research as a control for reduced activity inherent in chronic temporal isolation experiments [179, 181]. The circadian rhythm changes in these experiments, namely the observed lengthening of the circadian sleep-wake period, were hypothesized to be partly due to lower energy outputs that "decrease the cues for sleep" accumulated during the day [179]. Webb and Agnew tested this hypothesis by isolating 14 young, healthy male subjects for 10–14 days in a 12 ft × 12 ft room that was specially constructed to eliminate all external time cues [179]. Four nights of baseline sleep records were obtained before the experiment. Brain electrocortical activity was monitored continuously for the presence of sleep during the experimental days, and the electrodes were channeled into a 20-ft umbilical cord that allowed for freedom of movement. Subjects were instructed to eat, sleep, and use their time as they wanted while living in the isolation room. Half the subjects were given no access to exercise equipment, but the other seven subjects were instructed to complete eight separate bouts of cycle ergometry as soon as possible after getting out of bed. The exercise regimen was designed to be equivalent to a hard day's work, and involved eight cycling bouts at approximately 100 watts for a distance of 4 km at a speed of 20 km/hr. Exercise did not influence either the period or the overall amount of sleep; however, greater variability in the distribution of sleep was observed for the exercise group.

Wever also studied male subjects (n = 9) who lived in an isolation unit for about 4 wk [181]. On half the days, no exercise was performed and on the other days, subjects were asked to pedal on a cycle ergometer seven separate times throughout the course of the day for about 20 min each time at a workload of 100 watts. It was concluded that the influence of the exercise on the period of free-running circadian rhythms of either sleep and activity or core body temperature was negligible. However, the lack of a group effect might be attributed to the low intensity of the exercise or to the repeated bouts of exercise that were performed throughout the day. Given that most entraining agents can induce both phase advances and phase delays, depending on the timing of the stimulus, it is likely that any activity-induced phase delays would have been neutralized by equivalent phase advances and visa versa. A stronger test of the potential effects of exercise on sleep in a time-free environment could be made by systematically manipulating and carefully controlling the exercise stimulus; this includes taking into consideration physical activity history and emphasizing factors such as the timing, the relative exercise intensity, its duration, and the amount of muscle mass employed during the exercise bout.

SUMMARY

Several research paradigms have been used to examine the influence of exercise on sleep. Epidemiological studies show that exercise is perceived as helpful in promoting sleep and suggest that regular physical activity may be useful in improving sleep quality and reducing daytime sleepiness. Additional epidemiological inquiry is clearly warranted based on the available evidence.

Acute exercise experiments that have measured sleep physiology directly from subjects who either performed, or refrained from, daytime exercise indicate that exercise is associated with a small, but reliable increase in Stage 2 and slow wave sleep. The mechanism(s) that underlie exercise-associated increases in SWS is unknown. However, there is evidence that links elevations in daytime core body temperature to increases in SWS.

Acute exercise experiments were found to be associated with a reduction in REM sleep and a delay in REM onset latency that were larger in magnitude than the effects observed for Stage 2 and SWS. These REM sleep observations highlight the need for continued study of the consequences of exercise on both circadian and homeostatic aspects of sleep. The delay in REM onset latency observed in the naturalistic acute exercise studies was consistent with the results of experiments in which environmental factors were more rigorously controlled and showed that physical exercise, or a concomitant, can induce a phase delay in markers of the human circadian pacemaker. It is worth pointing out that the most sophisticated and rigorous experiments from a standpoint of understanding sleep, such as those involving constant routines, bed rest, and temporal isolation, have for the most part used exercise in a crude manner. Because exercise is a stressor with diverse psychophysiological consequences that depends in part upon the interaction of multiple factors (e.g., the setting; degree of environmental heat stress; the activity history and fitness of the subject; the duration, intensity, and timing of the exercise bout; body position, etc.), understanding the influence of exercise on sleep will be stymied until carefully designed sleep studies also use exercise in an equally sophisticated and systematic way.

Exercise is widely believed to have large effects on sleep. However, the scientific evidence does not strongly support this common belief. This incongruity may well be explained in part by considering the paradigms that have been used to study exercise and sleep. The majority of research that has been conducted to date on this topic either has cross-sectionally compared groups possessing different levels of physical fitness or has examined the effects of acute exercise on the sleep of good sleepers. Accordingly, it is not yet possible to draw scientifically defensible summary statements about the influence of exercise on sleep, especially given the complexity of sleep, the variety of factors that can impinge upon sleep-wake cycles, the homogeneous samples that have been studied, and given that relatively few methodologically rigorous exercise studies have been conducted. Nevertheless, there is adequate evidence to warrant paying increased research attention to explicating the potential relationships between exercise and sleep, especially in light of the enormous toll that sleep problems take on the health of the public. If exercise were eventually proven to be useful in treating the myriad of health problems associated with inadequate sleep, it would have several advantages over current methods used to treat sleep problems, including low cost, easy availability, and few adverse side effects. Future research is needed to determine whether exercise benefits the sleep of people with sleep problems.

REFERENCES

1. Achermann, P., D. J. Dijk, D. P. Brunner, and A. A. Borbély. A model of human sleep homeostasis based on EEG slow-wave activity: quantitative comparison of data and simulations. *Brain Res. Bull.* 31:97–113, 1993.
2. Adamson, L., W. M., Hunter, O. O. Ogunremi, I. Oswald, and I. W. Percy-Robb. Growth hormone increase during sleep after daytime exercise. *J. Endocrinol.* 62:473–478, 1974.
3. Agnew H. W., W. B. Webb, and R. L. Williams. The first night effect: an EEG study of sleep. *Psychophysiol.* 2:263–266, 1966.
4. Ancoli-Israel, S., D. F. Kripke, M. R. Klauber, W. J. Mason, R. Fell, and O. Kaplan. Periodic limb movements in sleep in community dwelling elderly. *Sleep* 14:496–500, 1991.
5. Ancoli-Israel, S., D. F. Kripke, M. R. Klauber, W. J. Mason, R. Fell, and O. Kaplan. Sleep disordered breathing in community dwelling elderly. *Sleep* 14:486–495, 1991.
6. Angus R. G., R. J. Heslegrave, and W. S. Myles. Effects of prolonged sleep deprivation, with and without chronic physical exercise, on mood and performance. *Psychophysiol.* 22:276–282, 1985.
7. Aschoff, J., M. Fatranska, H. Giedke, P. Doerr, D. Stamm, and H. Wisser. Human circadian rhythms in continuous darkness: entrainment by social cues. *Science* 171:213–215, 1971.
8. Åstrand, P-O., and K. Rodahl. *Textbook of Work Physiology, 3rd ed.* New York: McGraw-Hill, 1986.
9. Badia, P., B. Myers, M. Boecker, J. Culpepper, and J. R. Harsh. Bright light effects on body temperature, alertness, EEG and behavior. *Physiol. Behav.* 50:583–588, 1991.
10. Baekland, F. Exercise deprivation, sleep and psychological reactions. *Arch. Gen. Psychiatry* 22:365–369, 1970.
11. Baekland, F., and R. Lasky. Exercise and sleep in college athletes. *Percept. Mot. Skills* 22:1203–1207, 1966.
12. Benca, R. M., W. H. Obermeyer, R. A. Thisted, and J. C. Gillin. Sleep and psychiatric disorders: a meta-analysis. *Arch. Gen. Psychiatry* 49:651–668, 1992.
13. Bevier, W. C., D. L. Bliwise, N. G. Bliwise, D. E. Bunnell, and S. M. Horvath. Sleep patterns of older adults and the effects of exercise. *J. Clin. Exp. Gerontol.* 14:1–15, 1992.
14. Bevier, W. C., D. E. Bunnell, and S. M. Horvath. Cardiovascular function during sleep of active older adults and the effects of exercise. *Exp. Gerontol.* 22:329–337, 1987.
15. Bixler, E. D., A. Kales, C. R. Soldatos, et al. Prevalence of sleep disorders in the Los Angeles metropolitan area. *Am. J. Psychiatry* 136:1257–1262, 1979.
16. Black, J., C. Guilleminault, and A. Clark. Non-drug trials in psycho-physiological insomnia. *Sleep Res.* 23:233, 1994.
17. Blair, S. N. Physical activity, fitness, and coronary heart disease. C. Bouchard, R. J. Shephard, and T. Stephens (ed). *Physical Activity, Fitness and Health.* Champaign, IL: Human Kinetics Publishers, 1994, pp. 579–590.
18. Bliwise, D. L. Sleep in normal aging and dementia. *Sleep* 16:40–81, 1993.
19. Bliwise, D. L., A. C. King, and W. L. Haskell. Prevalence of self-reported poor sleep in a healthy population aged 50–65. *Soc. Sci. Med.* 49–55, 1992.
20. Bonnet, M. H. Sleep, performance and mood after the energy-expenditure equivalent of 40 hours of sleep deprivation. *Psychophysiol.* 17:56–63, 1980.

21. Borbély, A. A. A two process model of sleep regulation. *Hum. Neurobiol.* 1:195–204, 1982.
22. Borbély, A. A. Sleep homeostasis and models of sleep regulation. M. H. Kryger, T. Roth, and W. C. Dement (eds). *Principles and Practice of Sleep Medicine, 2nd ed.* Philadelphia: W. B. Saunders, 1994, pp. 309–320.
23. Borbély, A. A., F. Baumann, D. Brandeis, et al. Sleep-deprivation: effect on sleep stages and EEG power density in man. *Electroencephalogr. Clin. Neurophysiol.* 51:483–493, 1981.
24. Borbély, A. A., and I. Tobler. Endogenous sleep-promoting substances and sleep regulation. *Physiol. Rev.* 69:605–670, 1989.
25. Bouchard, C., R. J. Shephard, and T. Stephens. *Physical Activity, Fitness and Health.* Champaign, IL: Human Kinetics Publishers, 1994.
26. Brebbia, R. D., and K. Z. Altshuler. Oxygen consumption rate and electroencephalographic state of sleep. *Science* 150:1621–1623, 1965.
27. Brock, B. M., D. P. Haefner, and D. S. Noble. Alameda county redux: replication in Michigan. *Prev. Med.* 17:483–495, 1988.
28. Brooks, G. A., and T. D. Fahey. *Exercise Physiology: Human Bioenergetics and Its Applications.* New York: John Wiley & Sons, 1984.
29. Browman C. P. Sleep following sustained exercise. *Psychophysiol.* 17:577–579, 1980.
30. Browman, C. P., and R. D. Cartwright. The influence of evening activity and psychological state on dream life. *J. Psychiat. Treat. Eval.* 4:307–311, 1982.
31. Browman, C. P., and D. I. Tepas. The effects of pre-sleep activity on all-night sleep. *Psychophysiol.* 13:536–540, 1976.
32. Buchsbaum, M. S., J. C. Gillin, J. Wu, et al. Regional cerebral glucose metabolic rate in human sleep assessed by positron emission tomography. *Life Sci.* 45:1349–1356, 1989.
33. Buguet, A., B. Roussel, R. Angus, B. Sabiston, and M. Radomski. Human sleep and adrenal individual reactions to exercise. *Electroencephalogr. Clin. Neurophysiol.* 49:515–523, 1980.
34. Bunnell, D. E., Bevier, and S. M. Horvath. Effects of exhaustive exercise on the sleep of men and women. *Psychophysiol.* 20:50–57, 1983.
35. Bunnell, D. E., W. Bevier, and S. M. Horvath. Nocturnal sleep, cardiovascular function, and adrenal activity following maximum capacity exercise. *Electroencephologr. Clin. Neurophysiol.* 56:186–189, 1983.
36. Cajochen, C. H., D. J. Dijk, and A. A. Borbély. Dynamics of EEG slow wave activity and core body temperature in human sleep after exposure to bright light. *Sleep* 15:337–343, 1992.
37. Campbell, S. S. Duration and placement of sleep in a "disentrained" environment. *Psychophysiol.* 21:106–113, 1984.
38. Carskadon, M. A. Measuring daytime sleepiness. M. H. Kryger, T. Roth, and W. C. Dement (ed). *Principles and Practice of Sleep Medicine, 2nd ed.* Philadelphia: W. B. Saunders, 1994, pp. 961–966.
39. Carskadon, M. A., and W. C. Dement. Normal human sleep: an overview. M. H. Kryger, T. Roth, and W. C. Dement (eds). *Principles and Practice of Sleep Medicine, 2nd ed.* Philadelphia: W. B. Saunders, 1994, pp. 16–25.
40. Carskadon, M. A., W. C. Dement, M. M. Mitler, C. Guilleminault, V. P. Zarcone, and R. Spiegel. Self-reports versus sleep laboratory findings in 122 drug-free subjects with complaints of chronic insomnia. *Am. J. Psychiatry* 133:1382–1388, 1976.
41. Carskadon, M. A., W. C. Dement, M. M. Mitler et al. Guidelines for the multiple sleep latency test (MSLT): a standard measure of sleepiness. *Sleep* 9:519–524, 1986.
42. Caspersen, C. J. Physical activity epidemiology: concepts, methods, and applications to exercise science. K. B. Pandolf (ed). *Exercise and Sport Sciences Reviews.* Baltimore: Williams & Wilkins, 1989, pp. 423–474.
43. Caspersen, C. J., K. E. Powell, and R. K. Merritt. Measurement of health status and well-being. C. Bouchard, R. J. Shephard, and T. Stephens (eds). *Physical Activity, Fitness and Health.* Champaign, IL: Human Kinetics Publishers, 1994, pp. 180–202.
44. Clodore, M., J. Foret, and O. Benoit. Diurnal variation in subjective and objective mea-

sures of sleepiness: the effects of sleep reduction and circadian type. *Chronobiol. Int.* 3:255–263, 1986.

45. Czeisler, C. A., M. Dumont, J. F. Duffy, et al. Association of sleep-wake habits in older people with changes in output of circadian pacemaker. *Lancet* 340:933–936, 1992.

46. Czeisler, C. A., E. D. Weitzman, M.C. Moore-Ede, et al. Human sleep: its duration and organization depend on its circadian phase. *Science* 210:1264–1267, 1980.

47. Czeisler, C. A., R. E. Kronauer, J. S. Allan, et al. Bright light induction of strong (Type 0) resetting of the human circadian pacemaker. *Science* 244:1328–1333, 1989.

48. D'Alessandro, R., C. Magelli, G. Gamberini, et al. Snoring every night as a risk factor for myocardial infarction: a case control study. *Br. Med. J.* 300:1557–1558, 1990.

49. Davies, B. C. M. Shapiro, A. Daggett, J. A. Gatt, and P. Jakeman. Physiological changes and sleep responses during and following a world record continuous walking record. *Br. J. Sports Med.* 18:173–180, 1984.

50. Dement, W. C. *Some Must Watch While Some Must Sleep.* San Francisco: W. H. Freeman and Company, 1972.

51. deVries, H. A., and T. J. Housh. *Physiology of Exercise, 5th ed.* Madison, WI: WCB Brown & Benchmark, 1994.

52. Dijk, D. J., D. G. M. Beersma, and S. Daan. EEG power density during nap sleep: reflections of an hourglass measuring the duration of prior wakefulness. *J. Biol. Rhythms* 2:207–219, 1987.

53. Dijk, D. J., D. P. Brunner, and A. A. Borbély. Time course of EEG power density during long sleep in humans. *Am. J. Physiol.* 258:R650–661, 1990.

54. Dijk, D., C. Cajochen, I. Tobler, and A. A. Borbély. Sleep extension in humans: sleep stages, EEG power spectra and body temperature. *Sleep* 14:294–306, 1991.

55. Dijk, D. J., B. Hayes, and C. A. Czeisler. Analysis of spindle activity by transient pattern recognition software and power spectral analysis. *Sleep Res.* 22:426, 1993.

56. Dishman, R. K. Mental Health. V. Seefeldt (eds). *Physical Activity & Well-Being.* Washington, D.C.: Hemisphere Publishing, 1986, pp. 303–341.

57. Driver, H. S., A. F. Meintjes, G. G. Rodgers, and C. M. Shapiro. Submaximal exercise effects on sleep patterns in young women before and after an aerobic training programme. *Acta Physiol. Scand. Suppl.* (574) 133:8–13, 1988.

58. Driver, H. S., G. G. Rodgers, D. Mitchell, et al. Prolonged endurance exercise and sleep disruption. *Med. Sci. Sports Exerc.* 26:903–907, 1994.

59. Edgar, D. M., and W. C. Dement. Regularly scheduled voluntary exercise synchronizes the mouse circadian clock. *Am. J. Physiol.* 261:R928–R933, 1991.

60. Edinger, J. D., M. C. Morey, R. J. Sullivan, et al. Aerobic fitness, acute exercise and sleep in older men. *Sleep* 16:351–359, 1993.

61. Fairbanks, D. N. F. Nonsurgical treatment of snoring and obstructive sleep apnea. *Arch. Otolaryngol. Head Neck Surg.* 100:633–635, 1989.

62. Felicetta, J. V., S. Kapen, and J. R. Sowers. Does fitness in the elderly promote sleep? *Sci. Med. Res.* 1:101–109, 1989.

63. Ford, D. E., and D. B. Kamerow. Epidemiologic study of sleep disturbances and psychiatric disorders. *J. A. M. A.* 262:1479–1484, 1989.

64. Fox, E., R. Bowers, and M. Foss. *The Physiological Basis for Exercise and Sport, 5th ed.* Madison, WI: WCB Brown & Benchmark, 1993.

65. Gerhardsson, M., S. E. Norrell, H. Kirviranta, N. L. Pedersen, and A. Ahlbam. Sedentary jobs and colon cancer. *Am. J. Epidemiol.* 123:775–780, 1986.

66. Glotzbach, S. F., and H. C. Heller. Temperature regulation. M. H. Kryger, T. Roth, and W. C. Dement (eds). *Principles and Practice of Sleep Medicine, 2nd Ed.* Philadelphia: W. B. Saunders, 1994, pp. 260–275.

67. Grassi, G. G. Seraville, D. A. Calhoun, and G. Mancia. Physical training and baroreceptor control of sympathetic nerve activity in humans. *Hypertension* 23:294–301, 1994.

68. Griffin, S. J., and J. Trinder. Physical fitness, exercise and human sleep. *Psychophysiol.* 15:447–450, 1978.
69. Hammond, E. C. Some preliminary findings on physical complaints from a prospective study of 1,064,004 men and women. *Am. J. Public Health* 54:11–23, 1964.
70. Härmä, M., J. Ilmarinen, and P. Knauth. Physical fitness and other individual factors relating to the shiftwork tolerance of women. *Chronobiol. Int.* 5:417–424, 1988.
71. Härmä, M., J. Ilmarinen, P. Knauth, J. Rutenfranz, and O. Hänninen. Physical training intervention in female shift workers: I. The effects of intervention on fitness, fatigue, sleep and psychosomatic symptoms. *Ergonomics* 31:39–50, 1988.
72. Hasan, J., H. Urponen, I. Vuori, and M. Partinen. Exercise habits and sleep in a middle-aged Finnish population. *Acta Physiol. Scand Suppl.* (574) 133:33–35, 1988.
73. Hauri, P. J. Effects of evening activity on early night sleep. *Psychophysiol.* 4:267–277, 1968.
74. Hauri, P. J. The influence of evening activity on the onset of sleep. *Psychophysiol.* 5:426–430, 1969.
75. Hauri, P. J. Evening activity, sleep mentation and subjective sleep quality. *J. Abnormal Psychol.* 76:270–275, 1970.
76. Hoddes, E., V. Zarcone, H. Smythe, R. Phillips, and W. C. Dement. Quantification of sleepiness: a new approach. *Psychophysiol.* 10:431–436, 1973.
77. Horne, J. A. The effects of exercise upon sleep: a critical review. *Biol. Psychol.* 12:241–290, 1981.
78. Horne, J. A. Human sleep and tissue restitution: some qualifications and doubts. *Clin. Sci.* 65:569–678, 1983.
79. Horne, J. A. *Why We Sleep: The Functions of Sleep in Humans and Other Mammals.* New York: Oxford University Press, 1988.
80. Horne, J. A. Human slow wave sleep: a review and appraisal of recent findings, with implications for sleep functions, and psychiatric illness. *Experientia* 48:941–954, 1992.
81. Horne, J. A., and V. J. Moore. Sleep EEG effects of exercise with and without additional body cooling. *Electroencephalogr. Clin. Neurophysiol.* 60:33–38, 1985.
82. Horne, J. A., and J. M. Porter. Exercise and human sleep. *Nature* 256:573–575, 1975.
83. Horne, J. A., and J. M. Porter. Time of day effects with standardized exercise upon subsequent sleep. *Electroencephalogr. Clin Neurophysiol.* 40:178–181, 1976.
84. Horne, J. A., and L. H. E. Staff. Exercise and sleep: body-heating effects. *Sleep* 6:36–46, 1983.
85. Iguchi, Y., T. Kobayashi, and T. Yamamoto. Slow wave sleep due to daytime activities and individual differences. *Jpn. J. Psychiatry Neurol.* 42:165–166, 1988.
86. Jacobson, A., A. Kales, D. Lehmann, and F. S. Hoedemaker. Muscle tonus in human subjects during sleep and dreaming. *Exp. Neurol.* 10:418–424, 1964.
87. Knutsson, A., T. Akerstedt, B. G., Jonsson, and K. Orth-Gomer. Increased risk of ischaemic heart disease in shift workers. *Lancet* 2:89–91, 1986.
88. Koller, M., M. Kundi, and R. Cervinka. Field studies of shift work at an Austrian oil refinery. I. Health and psychosocial well-being of workers who drop out of shift work. *Ergonomics* 10:835–847, 1978.
89. Kripke, D. F., R. N. Simons, L. Garfinkel, and E. C. Hammond. Short and long sleep and sleeping pills: is increased mortality associated? *Arch. Gen. Psychiatry* 36:103–116, 1979.
90. Kryger, M. H., T. Roth, and W. C. Dement (eds). *Principles and Practice of Sleep Medicine, 2nd ed.* Philadelphia: W. B. Saunders, 1994.
91. Kubitz, K. A., D. M. Landers, S. J. Petruzzello, W. Salazar, and M. Han. The effects of acute and chronic exercise on sleep: a meta-analytic review. *Sports Med.*, in press.
92. Kupfer, D. J., D. E. Sewitch, L. E. Epstein, C. Bulik, C. R. McGowen, and R. J. Robertson. Exercise and subsequent sleep in male runners: failure to support the slow wave sleep-mood-exercise hypothesis. *Neuropsychobiology* 14:5–12, 1985.
93. Lamb, D. R. *Physiology of Exercise, 2nd ed.* New York: MacMillan, 1984.

94. Lavie, P. Sleep habits and sleep disturbances in industrial workers in Israel: main findings and some characteristics of workers complaining of excessive daytime sleepiness. *Sleep* 4:147–158, 1981.

95. Leger, D. The cost of sleep-related accidents: a report for the national commission on sleep disorders research. *Sleep* 17:84–93, 1994.

96. Lubin, A., D. J. Hord, M. L. Tracy, and L. C. Johnson. Effects of exercise, bedrest and napping on performance decrement during 40 hours of sleep deprivation. *Psychophysiol.* 13:334–339, 1976.

97. Maloletnev, V. I., and M. G. Chachanaschvili. Changes in sleep structure in athletes after rapid weight reduction in steam bath [Russian]. *Bull. Acad. Sci. Georg. U. S. S. R.* 96:689–692, 1979.

98. Maloletnev, V. I., Z. A. Telia, and M. G. Chachanaschvili. Changes in the structure of night sleep in man after intensive muscular work [Russian]. *Sechnov. Physiol. J. U. S. S. R.* 63:11–20, 1977.

99. Manson, J. E., E. B. Rimm, M. J. Stampfer, et al. Physical activity and incidence of non-insulin-dependent diabetes mellitus in women. *Lancet* 338:774–778, 1991.

100. Maron, L., A. Rechtschaffen, and E. A. Wolpert. Sleep cycle during napping. *Arch. Gen. Psychiatry* 11:503–507, 1964.

101. Martin, B. J. Sleep deprivation and exercise. K. B. Pandolf (ed). *Exercise and Sport Sciences Reviews.* New York: MacMillan, 1986, pp. 213–229.

102. Matsumota, K., Y. Saito, M. Abe, and K. Furmi. The effects of daytime exercise on night sleep. *J. Hum. Ergol.* 13:137–145, 1988.

103. McArdle, W. D., F. I. Katch, and V. L. Katch. *Essentials of Exercise Physiology.* Philadelphia: Lea & Febiger, 1994.

104. McGinty, D., and R. Szymusiak. Keeping cool: a hypothesis about the mechanisms and functions of slow wave sleep. *Trends Neurosci.* 13:480–487, 1990.

105. Meyer, J. S., Y. Ishikawa, T. Hata, and I. Karacan. Cerebral blood flow in normal and abnormal sleep and dreaming. *Brain Cogn.* 6:266–294, 1987.

106. Meijer, J. H., and W. J. Reitveld. Organization and function of a central nervous system circadian oscillator: the suprahiasmatic nucleus. *Fed. Proc.* 42:2783–2789, 1989.

107. Meintjes A. F., H. S. Driver, and C. M. Shapiro. Improved physical fitness failed to alter the EEG patterns of sleep in young women. *Eur. J. Appl. Physiol.* 59:123–127, 1989.

108. Mermin, J. H., and C. A. Czeisler. Comparison of ambulatory temperature recordings at varying levels of physical exertion: average amplitude is unchanged by strenuous exercise. *Sleep Res.* 16:253, 1987.

109. Minors, D. S., J. M. Waterhouse, and A. Wirz-Justice. A human phase-response curve to light. *Neurosci. Lett.* 133:36–40, 1991.

110. Mistlberger, R. E. Scheduled daily exercise or feeding alters the phase of photic entrainment in Syrian hamsters. *Physiol. Behav.* 50:1257–1260, 1991.

111. Monk, T. H. A visual analogue scale technique to measure global vigor and affect. *Psychiatry Res.* 27:89–99, 1989.

112. Monk, T. H. *Sleep, Sleepiness and Performance.* New York: Wiley & Sons, 1991.

113. Monk, T. H. Shift work. M. H. Kryger, T. Roth, and W. C. Dement (eds). *Principles and Practice of Sleep Medicine, 2nd ed.* Philadelphia: W. B. Saunders, 1994, pp. 471–476.

114. Montgomery, I., J. Trinder, and S. Paxton. Energy expenditure and total sleep time: effect of physical exercise. *Sleep* 5:159–168, 1982.

115. Montgomery, I., J. Trinder, S. Paxton, and G. Fraser. Sleep disturbance following a marathon. *J. Sports Med.* 25:69–74, 1985.

116. Montgomery, I., J. Trinder, S. Paxton, and G. Fraser. Aerobic fitness and exercise: effects on the sleep of younger and older adults. *Aust. J. Psychol.* 39:259–272, 1987.

117. Montgomery, I., J. Trinder, S. Paxton, D. Harris, G. Fraser, and I. Corain. Physical exercise and sleep: the effects of the age and sex of the subjects and the type of exercise. *Acta Physiol. Scand. Suppl.* (574) 133:36–40, 1988.

118. Montmayeur, A., A. Buguet, H. Sollin, and J.-R. Lacour. Exercise and sleep in four African sportsmen living in the Sahel. *Int. J. Sports Med.* 15:42–45, 1994.
119. Moore-Ede, M. C. *The Twenty Four Hour Society.* Reading, MA: Addison-Wesley Publishing, 1993.
120. Moore-Ede, M. C., F. M. Sulzman, and C. A. Fuller. *The Clocks that Time Us.* Cambridge: Harvard University Press, 1982.
121. Morgan, W. P. Selected psychological factors limiting performance: a mental health model. D. H. Clarke and H. M. Eckert (eds). *Limits of Human Performance.* Champaign, IL: Human Kinetics Publishers, pp. 10–80, 1985.
122. Morgan, W. P. Physical activity, fitness, and depression. C. Bouchard, R. J. Shephard, and T. Stephens (eds). *Physical Activity, Fitness and Health.* Champaign, IL: Human Kinetics Publishers, 1994, pp. 851–867.
123. Moses, J. M., A. Lubin, P. Naitah, and L. C. Johnson. Exercise and sleep loss: effects on recovery sleep. *Psychophysiol.* 14:237–244, 1977.
124. Mrosovsky, N., S. G. Reebs, G. I. Honrado, and P. A. Salmon. Behavioral entrainment of circadian rhythms. *Experientia* 45:696–702, 1989.
125. Muller, J. E., P. H. Stone, Z. G. Turi, et al. Circadian variation in the frequency of onset of acute myocardial infarction. *N. Engl. J. Med* 313:1315–1322, 1985.
126. National Commission on Sleep Disorders Research: Wake Up America: A National Sleep Alert, Vol. 1, *Executive Summary and Executive Report, Report of the National Commission on Sleep Disorders Research.* Bethesda, MD: National Institutes of Health, 1993, pp. 1–76.
127. Navelet, Y., T. Anders, and C. Guilleminault. Narcolepsy in children. C. Guilleminault, W. C. Dement, and P. Passouant (eds). *Narcolepsy.* New York: Spectrum Publications, 1976, pp. 171–177.
128. Noble, B. J. *Physiology of Exercise and Sport.* St. Louis: Times Mirror/Mosby College Publishing, 1986.
129. O'Connor, P. J., L. E. Aenchbacher, and R. K. Dishman. Physical activity and depression in the elderly. *J. Aging Physical Activity* 1:34–58, 1993.
130. O'Connor, P. J., and W. P. Morgan, Athletic performance following rapid traversal of multiple time zones: a review. *Sports Med.* 10:20–30, 1990.
131. Parmeggiani, P.-L., G. Zamboni, E. Perez, and P. Lenzi. Hypothalamic temperature during desynchronized sleep. *Exp. Brain Res.* 54:315–320, 1984.
132. Paxton, S., I. Montgomery, J. Trinder, J. Newman, and A. Bowling. Sleep after exercise of variable intensity in fit and unfit subjects. *Aust. J. Psychol.* 34:289–296, 1982.
133. Paxton, S., J. Trinder, and I. Montgomery. Does aerobic fitness affect sleep? *Psychophysiol.* 20:320–324, 1983.
134. Paxton, S., J. Trinder, C. M. Shapiro, K. Adam, I. Oswald, and K. J. Graf. Effect of physical fitness and body composition on sleep and sleep-related hormone concentrations. *Sleep* 7:339–346, 1984.
135. Piercy, J., and L. Lack. Daily exercise can shift the endogenous circadian phase. *Sleep Res.* 17:393, 1988.
136. Porter, J. M., and J. A. Horne. Exercise and sleep behaviour: a questionnaire approach. *Ergonomics* 24:511–521, 1981.
137. Powers, S. K., and E. T. Howley (eds). *Exercise Physiology, 2nd ed.* Madison, WI: WCB Brown & Benchmark, 1994.
138. Rechtschaffen, A., and A. A. Kales. *A Manual of Standardized Terminology: Techniques and Scoring System for Sleep Stages of Human Subjects.* Los Angeles: UCLA Brain Information Service/Brain Research Institute, 1968.
139. Regestein, Q. R., and T. H. Monk. Is poor sleep of shift workers a disorder? *Am. J. Psychiatry* 148:1487–1493, 1991.
140. Ryback R. S., and O.F. Lewis. Effects of prolonged bed rest on EEG sleep patterns in young, healthy volunteers. *Electroencephalogr. Clin. Neurophysiol.* 31:399–395, 1971.

141. Schmidt-Nowara, W. W., D. B. Coultas, C. Wiggins, B. E. Skipper, and J. M. Samet. Snoring in a Hispanic-American population: risk factors and association with hypertension and other morbidity. *Arch. Intern. Med.* 150:597–601, 1990.

142. Seraganian, P. (ed.) *Exercise Psychology.* London: Wiley-Interscience, 1993, pp. 1–390.

143. Shapiro, C. M. Energy expenditure and restorative sleep. *Biol. Psychol.* 15:229–239, 1982.

144. Shapiro, C. M., R. Bortz, D. Mitchell, P. Bartel, and P. Jooste. Slow wave sleep: a recovery period after exercise. *Science.* 214:1253–1254, 1981.

145. Shapiro, C. M., R. D. Griesel, P. R. Bartel, and P. L. Jooste. Sleep patterns after graded exercise. *J. Appl. Physiol.* 39:187–190, 1975.

146. Shapiro, C. M. and G. J. Verchoor. Sleep patterns after a marathon. *S. Afr. J. Sci.* 75:415–416, 1979.

147. Shapiro, C. M., P. M. Warren, J. Trinder, et al. Fitness facilitates sleep. *Eur. J. Appl. Physiol.* 53:1–4, 1984.

148. Shephard, R. J. *Physiology and Biochemistry of Exercise.* New York: Praeger Publishing, 1982.

149. Singer, R. N., M. Murphey, and L. K. Tennant (eds). *Handbook of Research on Sport Psychology.* New York: MacMillan, 1993.

150. Somers, V. K., M. E. Dyken. A. L. Mark, and F. M. Abboud. Sympathetic-nerve activity during sleep in normal subjects. *N. Engl. J. Med.* 328:303–307, 1993.

151. Steriade, M., and J. A. Hobson. Neuronal activity during the sleep-waking cycle. *Prog. Neurobiol.* 6:155–376, 1976.

152. Steriade, M., D. A. McCormick, and T. J. Sejnowski. Thalamocortical oscillations in the sleeping and aroused brain. *Science* 262:679–685, 1993.

153. Stevenson J. S., and R. Topp. Effects of moderate and low intensity long-term exercise by older adults. *Res. Nurs. Health* 13:209–218, 1990.

154. Terman, M. Light treatment. M. H. Kryger, T. Roth, and W. C. Dement (eds). *Principles and Practice of Sleep Medicine, 2nd ed.* Philadelphia: W. B. Saunders, 1994, pp. 1012–1029.

155. Thayer, R. E. Factor analytic and reliability studies on the activation-deactivation adjective check list. *Psychol. Rep.* 42:747–756, 1978.

156. Thomas, E. E., J. B. Smith, and F. C. Hiller. Nutrition and exercise for weight control as a treatment for the obese with obstructive sleep apnea: patient education. *J. Polysomnographic Tech.* 12:11–16, 1991.

157. Tobler, I., P. Franken, L. Trachsel, and A. A. Borbély. Models of sleep regulation in mammals. *J. Sleep Res.* 1:125–127, 1992.

158. Torsvall, L. Sleep after exercise: a literature review. *J. Sports Med.* 21:218–224, 1981.

159. Torsvall, L., T. Akerstedt, and G. Lindbeck. Effects on sleep stages and EEG power density of different degrees of exercise in fit subjects. *Electroencephalogr. Clin. Neurophysiol.* 57:347–353, 1984.

160. Touitou, Y., and E. Haus. *Biological Rhythms in Clinical and Laboratory Medicine.* Berlin: Springer-Verlag, 1992.

161. Trinder, J., D. Bruck, S. Paxton, I. Montgomery, and A. Bowling. Physical fitness, exercise, age and human sleep. *Aust. J. Psychol.* 34:131–138, 1982.

162. Trinder, J., I. Montgomery, and S. Paxton. The effect of exercise on sleep: the negative view. *Acta Physiol. Scand. Suppl.* (574) 133:14–20, 1988.

163. Trinder, J., S. Paxton, I. Montgomery, and G. Fraser. Endurance as opposed to power training: their effect on sleep. *Psychophysiol.* 22:668–673, 1985.

164. Trinder, J., J. Stevenson, S. J. Paxton, and I. Montgomery. Physical fitness, exercise, and REM sleep cycle length. *Psychophysiol.* 19:89–93, 1982.

165. Turek, F. W. Effects of stimulated physical activity on the circadian pacemaker of vertebrates. *J. Biol. Rhythms* 4:135–147, 1989.

166. Urponen, H., I. Vuori, J. Hasan, and M. Partinen. Self-evaluations of factors promoting and disturbing sleep: an epidemiological survey in Finland. *Soc. Sci. Med.* 26:443–450, 1988.

167. U.S. Customs Bureau. *Statistical Abstract of the United States: 1990, 108th ed.* Washington, D.C., 1991.
168. Van Reeth, O., J. Sturis, M. M. Byrne, et al. Nocturnal exercise phase-delays the circadian rhythms of melatonin and thyrotropin secretion in normal men. *Am. J. Physiol. Endocrinol Metab.* 266:E964–E974, 1994.
169. Van Reeth, O., and F. W. Turek. Stimuated activity mediates phase shifts in the hamster circadian clock induced by dark pulses or benzodiazepines. *Nature* 339:49–51, 1989.
170. Vitiello, M. V., L. H. Larson, K. E. Moe, P. N. Prinz, and R. S. Schwartz. The circadian body temperature rhythm of healthy older men and women is enhanced with increased aerobic fitness. *Sleep Res.* 23:514, 1994.
171. Vitiello, M. V., P. N. Prinz, and R. S. Schwartz. The subjective sleep quality in healthy older men and women is enhanced by participation in two fitness training programs: a non-specific effect. *Sleep Res.,* in press.
172. Vitiello, M. V., P. N. Prinz, and R. S. Schwartz. Slow wave sleep but not overall sleep quality of healthy older men and women is improved by increased aerobic fitness. *Sleep Res.,* in press.
173. Vuori, J., H. Urponen, I. Hasan, and M. Partinen. Epidemiology of exercise effects on sleep. *Acta Physiol.* Scand. Suppl. (574) 133:3–7, 1988.
174. Walker, J. M., T. C. Floyd, G. Fein, C. Cavness, R. Lualhati, and I. Feinberg. Effects of exercise on sleep. *J. Appl. Physiol.* 44:945–951, 1978.
175. Walsh, B. T., J. Puig-Antich, R. Goetz, M. Gladis, H. Novacenko, and A. H. Glassman. Sleep and growth and hormone secretion in women athletes. *Electroencephalogr. Clin. Neurophysiol.* 57:528–531, 1984.
176. Webb, W. B. Sleep as a biological rhythm: a historical review. *Sleep* 17:188–194, 1994.
177. Webb, W. B., and H. W. Agnew. Stage 4 sleep: Influence of time course variables. *Science.* 174:1354–1356, 1971.
178. Webb, W. B., and H. W. Agnew. Effects on performance of high and low energy expenditure during sleep deprivation. *Percept. Mot. Skills* 37:511–514, 1973.
179. Webb, W. B., and H. W. Agnew. Sleep and waking in a time-free environment. *Aerospace Med.* 45:617–622, 1974.
180. Wever, R. A. *The Circadian System of Man.* New York: Springer-Verlag, 1979.
181. Wever, R. A. Influence of physical workload on freerunning circadian rhythms of man. *Pflügers Arch.* 381:119–126, 1979.
182. Willich, S. N., D. Levy, M. B. Rocco, G. H. Tofler, P. H. Stone, and J. E. Muller. Circadian variation in the incidence of sudden cardiac death in the Framingham Heart Study population. *Am. J. Cardiol.* 60:140–144, 1987.
183. Wilmore, J. H., and D. L. Costill. *Physiology of Sport and Exercise.* Champaign, IL: Human Kinetics Publishers, 1994.
184. Wingard, D. L., L.F. Berkman, and R. J. Brand. A multivariate analysis of health-related practices. *Am. J. Epidemiol.* 116:765–775, 1982.
185. Young, T., M. Palta, J. Dempsey, J. Skatrud, S. Webb, S. Weber, and S. Badr. The occurrence of sleep-disordered breathing among middle aged adults. *N. Engl. J. Med.* 328:1230–1235, 1993.
186. Zarcone, V. P. Sleep hygiene. M. H. Kryger, T. Roth, and W. C. Dement, W. C. (eds). *Principles and Practice of Sleep Medicine, 2nd ed.* Philadelphia: W. B. Saunders, 1994, pp. 542–546.
187. Zepelin, H. Mammalian sleep. M. H. Kryger, T. Roth, and W. C. Dement, W. C. (eds). *Principles and Practice of Sleep Medicine, 2nd ed.* Philadelphia: W. B. Saunders, 1994, pp. 69–80.

5
Exercise and Oxidative Stress: Role of the Cellular Antioxidant Systems

LI LI JI, Ph.D.

Oxygen free radical generation has been implicated to be a major cause for exercise-induced cell and tissue injury [50, 51, 89, 122]. It has been proposed that some of the oxygen intermediates, which are a byproduct of normal cell metabolism, can elicit a series of biochemical and physiological damage to organisms, and that these detrimental effects are indicative of an oxidative stress. To evaluate the efficacy of this free radical theory of tissue damage there are two underlying presumptions: (a) there is an increased production of free radicals and other reactive oxygen species (ROS) during physical exercise; and (b) the intrinsic antioxidant defense systems are not sufficient to protect the organisms against these toxic species.

There is now strong evidence that strenuous physical exercise is associated with an increased free radical generation primarily due to a dramatic increase in oxygen uptake both at the whole body and local tissue levels [4, 20, 50, 99]. Most of the oxygen consumed is utilized in the mitochondria for oxidative phosphorylation and is reduced to water. However, a small fraction of oxygen intermediates, i.e., O_2^-, H_2O_2, and $\cdot OH$, may be produced univalently and leak out of the electron transport chain [18, 19]. Several investigators have shown, using electron paramagnetic resonance spectroscopy, that free radical signals in biological tissues are indeed increased after acute exercise in vivo or in vitro, and that the increased free radical production coincides with oxidative tissue damage [20, 49, 70]. However, a direct linkage between free radical generation and the observed physiological and biochemical alterations has not been fully established.

The body is equipped with an efficient antioxidant defense system consisting of antioxidant vitamins, glutathione (GSH) and sulfhydryls, and antioxidant enzymes [81]. Each of these antioxidant systems plays a unique role but also complements each other functionally. In general, antioxidant vitamins (e.g., vitamin E and β-carotene) are involved in the direct trapping of free radicals and singlet oxygen [139]. GSH and other thiol sources play an important role in the maintenance of cellular oxidoreductive (redox) status [86]. Antioxidant enzymes, i.e., superoxide dismutase (SOD), catalase (CAT) and GSH peroxidase (GPX), catalyze the one-electron reduction of ROS [18]. Their functions are supported by a number of other enzymes involved in the supply of reducing powers (i.e., NADPH), such as glutathione

135

reductase (GR) and glucose-6-phosphate dehydrogenase (G6PDH). In addition, GSH-sulfur transferase (GST) is capable of conjugating GSH with a variety of xenobiotic compounds including organic and lipid peroxides [38]. Cellular levels of antioxidants are influenced by numerous physiological, pathological, and nutritional factors [39, 42, 81]. Recent evidence suggests that there might be interorgan transport of certain antioxidants during exercise-induced oxidative stress [52, 68]. According to the definition of oxidative stress, i.e., a shift of prooxidant/antioxidant balance in favor of the former [120], the efficiency of the cellular antioxidant defense system is of vital importance in determining the extent of oxidative stress and cell or tissue damage. The purpose of this article is to review the role and response of each of the antioxidant defense systems during acute and chronic exercise, and to discuss the factors that may impact on their regulation, such as nutritional deficiency and aging.

ANTIOXIDANT ENZYMES

Catalytic Mechanisms

SUPEROXIDE DISMUTASE. The primary defense in the cell offered by SOD is to dismutase O_2^- to H_2O_2.

$$2O_2^- + 2H^+ \rightarrow H_2O_2 + O_2$$

This reaction occurs naturally with a rather slow rate ($t_{1/2} = 7$ s) and is also pH dependent. With 0.35 μM SOD present, the rate of O_2^- dismutation is accelerated dramatically with a $t_{1/2} = 0.5$ ms regardless of pH [18]. Although O_2^- itself is not highly toxic, it can extract an electron from many biological compounds near its generation sites, such as the mitochondrial inner membrane, causing a free radical chain reaction [39]. Therefore, it is essential for the cell to keep the superoxide anion in check.

There are three types of SOD isozymes, depending on the cellular locations as well as the metal ion bound to its active site. CuZn SOD is found in the cytosolic compartment of eukaryotes. It is a dimer $M_r = 32,000$) and sensitive to cyanide inhibition [19]. Mn SOD is present in the mitochondrial matrix of eukaryotes and insensitive to cyanide. This distinction of cyanide sensitivity has been used to measure the activity of the two types of SOD in tissue extracts without separating the mitochondria and cytosol [45]. The distribution of SOD activity in the cell seems to vary from tissue to tissue. In rat liver, approximately two-thirds of SOD activity is in the cytosol and one-third is in the mitochondria [139]. In addition, bacteria contain a third type of SOD that requires Fe as a prosthetic group [19]. In mammals, the highest SOD activity is found in the liver, followed by kidney, brain, adrenal, and heart [39]. In the skeletal muscle, SOD activity is similar to that in the heart and, unlike some other antioxidant enzymes (see below), there is little difference among muscle fiber types [60] (Table 5.1).

Several characteristics of SOD kinetics are worth mentioning. First, unlike most enzymes, SOD lacks a Michaelis constant (K_m). Second, the enzyme is partially occupied by its substrate (O_2^-) and its catalytic activity increases with increasing O_2^- concentration within a wide range [19]. Furthermore, high levels of H_2O_2 has been shown to inhibit SOD in vitro [9]. Finally, because of the above-mentioned kinetic properties, assays of SOD are usually based on indirect methods, involving the inhibition of a reaction in which O_2^- is generated [32]. Therefore, it is difficult to compare maximal in vivo activity between studies using different assay methods.

CATALASE. The primary function of CAT is to decompose H_2O_2 to H_2O [18]. It shares this function with GPX, although the substrate specificity and affinity as well as the cellular location of the two antioxidant enzymes are different (see below).

$$2H_2O_2 \rightarrow 2H_2O + O_2$$

CAT is a tetramer with a relatively large molecular weight of ~240,000. Fe^{3+} is a required ligand to be bound to the enzyme's active site for its catalytic function. CAT resembles SOD in many kinetic properties such as the lack of an apparent K_m and V_{max}, and its activity increases enormously with an increase in H_2O_2. In the presence of H_2O_2, CAT is also capable of reducing a limited number of hydroperoxides (peroxidatic function), but not *t*-butyl hydroperoxide, to their respective aldehydes [18]. Azide and cyanide are both inhibitors of CAT. This inhibition is often used to parti-

TABLE 5.1
Antioxidant Enzyme Activity in Various Tissues

Tissues	SOD			GPX			CAT	GR	GST	G6 PDH
	CuZn	Mn	Total	Cyto	Mito	Total				
Liver	500	50	14400	550	430	85	670	40	940	8.0
Heart	65	21	2610	150	70	17	84	1.3	2.5	10.9
Soleus	ND	ND	1300	ND	ND	13	61	0.8	1.1	ND
DVL	21	8	1360	23	17	2	18	0.4	0.5	0.6
SVL	ND	ND	1400	ND	ND	0.9	15	0.3	0.2	ND
Erythrocytes	NA	NA	8.8	NA	NA	25	10	35	1.0	2.3

Units of enzyme activity in rat tissues: CuZn and Mn SOD, unit/mg protein; SOD total, unit/g wet wt; cytosolic and mitochondrial GPX, nmol/min·mg^{-1} protein; catalase, K × 10^{-2}/g wet wt; activity for other enzymes, μmol/min·g^{-1} wet wt; activity in human erythrocytes: units/g of hemoglobin. NA, not applicable; ND, not determined. Data from Ji et al. [54, 57, 60, 62].

tion CAT activity from GPX activity in enzyme assays of crude tissue extracts. CAT is widely distributed within the cell, and a high concentration is found in the peroxisomes [1]. However, mitochondria and other intracellular organelles also contain considerable CAT activity [80]. As shown in Table 5.1, the activity of CAT among mammalian tissues follows the order of SOD, with liver being the highest, and the skeletal muscle the lowest. Interfiber difference of muscle CAT activity, however, is much greater for CAT than for SOD.

Assays of CAT typically involve the addition of its substrate H_2O_2, and its removal is followed at 240 nm spectrophotometrically [1]. Caution should be paid to the reported catalytic activity because it is determined not only by the enzyme protein present in the assay medium but also by the concentration of H_2O_2 used. Without defining the conditions of the assay, the comparison of activities among studies is often meaningless.

GLUTATHIONE PEROXIDASE. GPX catalyzes the reduction of H_2O_2 and organic hydroperoxide to H_2O and alcohol, respectively, using GSH as the electron donor [31]

$$2GSH + H_2O_2 \rightarrow GSSG + 2\,H_2O$$

or

$$2GSH + ROOH \rightarrow GSSG + ROH$$

It should be clarified that GPX refers only to the selenium-dependent enzyme (EC 1.11.1.9). The often so-called selenium-independent GPX is actually a fraction of the GST (EC 2.5.1.18) activity, which also removes hydroperoxide [38]. The primary function of GST, however, is to conjugate GSH with a variety of xenobiotic substances, making them more water soluble, and hence easier to be metabolized [38]. Also, GST function is primarily limited to the hepatocytes. GPX is highly specific for its hydrogen donor GSH, but has low specificity for hydroperoxide, ranging from H_2O_2 to complex organic hydroperoxide, including long-chain fatty acid hydroperoxide and nucleotide-derived hydroperoxides [31]. This characteristic of GPX makes it a versatile hydroperoxide remover in the cell, thus playing an important role in inhibiting lipid peroxidation and preventing damage to DNA and RNA. It is also important to recognize that although GPX and CAT have an overlap of substrate H_2O_2, GPX (at least in mammals) has a much greater affinity for H_2O_2 at low concentrations ($K_m = 1$ μM) than CAT ($K_m = 1$ mM) [120]. GPX is susceptible to O_2^- and hydroperoxide in vitro because of the oxidation of the selenocysteine residue at the enzyme's active site [9]. Both SOD and GSH prevent the inactivation of GPX by removing O_2^- and reducing the sulfhydryls of the enzyme, respectively.

GPX is located in both the cytosol and mitochondrial matrix of the cell, with a distribution ratio of $\sim$2:1 [19]. This allows it to reach a number of cellular sources of hydroperoxide generation. The activity of GPX is high in the liver and erythrocytes; moderate in the brain, kidney, and heart; and low in the skeletal muscle (Table 5.1). However, the oxidative Type 1 muscle (soleus) possesses a GPX activity close to the level in the heart [59]. Selenium deficiency dramatically decreases tissue GPX activity in all body tissues in a dose-responsive fashion and this can be reversed by refeeding the animals with a diet containing an adequate amount of selenium [46]. There is evidence that mitochondria are more resistant to dietary selenium deficiency. When postneonatal rats were fed a low-selenium diet for 8 wk, cytosolic GPX activity in liver, heart, and muscle was decreased to 3–4% of control values, whereas mitochondrial GPX was maintained at 9, 20, and 24%, respectively [58, 61].

GLUTATHIONE REDUCTASE. Adequate function of GPX requires the regeneration of GSH from its oxidative product glutathione disulfide (GSSG). This is accomplished by the flavin-containing enzyme GR. NADPH is used as the reducing power of this reaction, which is coupled with G6PDH in erythrocytes and some other tissues [31]. When H_2O_2 concentration is increased in red cells, there is a tendency toward an elevated GSSG, which appears to impact on the regulation of the hexose monophosphate shunt. GSSG activates G6PDH directly; it decreases NADPH, which is normally inhibitory to G6PDH, and it elevates $NADP^+$, which is a substrate and allosteric activator of G6PDH [31]. In skeletal muscle, isocitrate dehydrogenase may play a more important role in supplying NADPH for GR than G6PDH [111]. Thus, although not classified as an antioxidant enzyme, GR has a subcellular distribution similar to that of GPX and is essential for normal antioxidant function.

OTHER ENZYMES OFFERING ANTIOXIDANT DEFENSE. In addition to the primary antioxidant enzymes mentioned above, the cell has a number of enzyme systems that function either to reduce the production of ROS or to facilitate the removal of ROS and their byproducts. Cytochrome *c* oxidase is the terminal enzyme in the mitochondrial respiratory chain, catalyzing the electron transfer from cytochrome a_3 to O_2. Chance et al. [18] pointed out the importance of this enzyme in preventing the release of O_2^- and H_2O_2 outside the respiratory chain by binding these ROS tightly with the enzyme. Recently, Yu [139] expanded the concept of antioxidant defenses to primary and secondary defenses. The former refers to the enzymes directly involved in scavenging ROS and chain-breaking antioxidant vitamins. The latter includes those enzymes participating in the degradation, removal, and repair of the damaged cell constituents. In this context, lipolitic enzymes, such as phospholipase A_2, play an important role in the removal of oxidized lipids, thus preventing extensive lipid peroxidation [139]. Degradation of oxidized protein is another important function the cell must accomplish to prevent accumulation of altered or damaged residues. There is considerable evidence that, under oxidative exposure, certain proteases are activated to preferentially degrade oxidized protein, including enzyme molecules [33, 96].

Response to Acute Exercise

SOD, CAT, GPX, and GR provide the first line of defense against the ROS generated during exercise; it is therefore expected that exercise may have a direct impact on these enzymes. Indeed, an acute bout of exercise has been shown to increase SOD activity in a number of biological tissues including heart [53], liver [3, 57, 58, 59], lung [110], blood platelets [12], and skeletal muscle [57, 75]. Because SOD can be activated by partial occupancy of the enzyme by O_2^- in vitro [19], it is proposed that the increased SOD activity may be an indication that O_2^- production is increased during exercise [53]. However, some skepticism still remains regarding the mechanism for SOD activation because O_2^- has a very short half-life [19, 31]. Furthermore, SOD activity has been reported in different units in the literature, making comparisons among various studies difficult.

An early study by Calderera et al [15] showed that CAT activity was increased significantly in rat heart, liver, and skeletal muscle after an acute bout of exercise. However, most of the reviewed literature revealed no significant alteration in CAT activity with acute exercise [89]. In our laboratory, CAT activity was found to increase significantly after both an acute bout of exhaustive exercise [55] and exercise at high intensity in the deep portion of vastus lateralis muscle (DVL) in rats [60]. However, the superficial vastus lateralis (SVL) and soleus muscle, as well as liver and heart, did not display significant changes in CAT activity with exercise. With a catalytic mechanism similar to SOD, one may expect CAT activity also to increase because of an increased H_2O_2 production during exercise. However, CAT is located primarily in the peroxisomes, whereas the main source of H_2O_2 is from the mitochondria under physiological conditions [19]. Mitochondrial and cytosolic GPX are probably more effective in competing for the H_2O_2 produced in these two cell compartments than CAT.

The effect of an acute bout of exercise on GPX activity in various tissues has not been reported consistently in the literature. Several previous studies showed no change in this enzyme in skeletal muscle after acute exercise [11, 57, 135], whereas others reported that GPX activity in muscle was elevated following intense exercise [55, 60, 108]. Furthermore, heart [108] and platelet [12] GPX activity has been shown to be elevated after exercise. There is no clear explanation for these discrepancies.

Although GR is not directly involved in removing ROS, it is responsible for supplying GSH to maintain GPX catalytic function and to maintain a reduced intracellular milieu during prolonged aerobic exercise. GR activity has been shown to increase in rat skeletal muscle after an acute bout of exercise along with an increased GPX activity [55, 60]. Also, erythrocyte GR activity was reported to be elevated after prolonged exercise in humans [28, 54, 95]. In addition, increased erythrocyte GST activity has been reported after prolonged exercise [28].

Overall, antioxidant enzymes may be activated selectively during an acute bout of strenuous exercise. This activation may reflect an increased production of ROS during exercise based on the kinetic properties of these enzymes. However, because of the different magnitudes of increase in oxygen consumption and the diverse intrinsic antioxidant enzyme activities, skeletal muscle may be subjected to a greater level of oxidative stress during exercise than liver and heart; therefore, greater changes in antioxidant enzymes are observed. There is no clear explanation for the increased enzyme activity during exercise, although several authors attribute it to an increased ROS production [53, 135]. Based on the current knowledge, mammalian tissues do not demonstrate a rapid up-regulation of gene expression of antioxidant enzymes in response to acute oxidative stress [42], although such a mechanism has been found in the prokaryotes [127]. Thus, increased binding of substrates (ROS) to enzymes causing allosteric or covalent modulation of the enzyme's catalytic activity remains the most viable explanation [53].

Adaptation to Chronic Training
Nature has made an almost perfect match between the antioxidant defense capacity of an organism and its living environment. Strict anaerobes have few, if any, antioxidant enzymes present in the body. Appearance of oxygen on the earth some 2 billion years ago provoked the development of the organism's antioxidant defense mechanism [39]. In mammals and birds, CAT activity in skeletal muscle was found to be greater in the wild species compared with the domestic counterparts [13]. Within the body, tissues that have a higher oxygen consumption rate, such as liver, heart, and brain, normally have higher antioxidant enzymes than those with lower oxygen consumption [51]. In skeletal muscle, a highly heterogeneous organ, antioxidant enzyme activity varies widely, depending on the metabolic characteristics of muscle types. For example, Type 1 muscle possesses greater activities of all antioxidant enzymes than Type 2a muscle and Type 2b muscle [60].

It has long been recognized that living organisms are also capable of inducing the antioxidant defense system by relatively rapid mechanisms to cope with oxidative stress. Both animals and certain plant species can induce SOD (only Mn SOD) upon increased exposure of oxygen, paraquat (a known producer of O_2^-), and x-irradiation [94]. Many bacteria can rapidly turn on genes coded for CAT and alkylhydroperoxidases and for SOD and G6PDH upon exposure to H_2O_2 and O_2^-, respectively [42]. Acute exposure of lung tissue to hypertensive oxygen (85%) has been shown to increase GSH content 5-fold within 24 hr [22]. Because an acute bout of strenuous physical exercise can cause a tremendous increase in oxygen consumption and oxidative stress to the body [20, 50, 89], and certain antioxidant systems seem to be activated in response to the exercise stress, it is expected that repeated exercise exposure will induce their cellular antioxidant systems to protect against the oxidative damage.

Over the last few decades, there is increasing evidence that chronic exercise training up-regulates antioxidant enzymes in those tissues actively involved in exercise, although some controversy still exists. Several reviews on this topic have been published previously [50, 53, 89]; therefore, only a brief summary will be provided in this chapter. In general, antioxidant enzymes in skeletal muscle show the most responsive training adaptation. SOD activity has been shown to increase significantly after training [45, 76, 104, 108], and there is evidence that Mn SOD is primarily responsible for the increase [45]. CAT activity has been shown by some authors [51, 108] to increase after training in skeletal muscle, but most studies report no change in muscle CAT with training [50, 89] and a few studies even reported a decrease [74, 76]. More consistent findings have been reported with respect to GPX adaptation to training, and with a few exceptions [11, 115] most studies show that there is an increase in GPX activity after training [58, 59, 74–76, 104]. Recently, a careful study was conducted by Powers et al. [104], who investigated the influences of exercise intensity, duration, and muscle fiber type on training response of antioxidant enzymes. They found that training increased SOD activity in Type 1 fiber only and SOD activity increased as a function of exercise duration rather than intensity. GPX activity was induced by training only in Type 2a fiber; again, only exercise duration was important in determining the level of training adaptation rather than exercise intensity. CAT was not altered by training in any muscle fiber type, regardless of exercise intensity and duration. It is noteworthy that as a striated muscle, diaphragm muscle also exhibits considerable training adaptation of antioxidant enzymes [105]. Interestingly, the level of up-regulation was found to be considerably greater in the costal versus crural diaphragm, possibly reflecting the different workload and metabolic rate between the two regions.

There is considerable controversy in the literature regarding myocardial antioxidant enzyme response to training. Higuchi et al. [45] reported that no alteration of myocardial antioxidant enzyme status occurred after training. This finding was consistent with the work of Ji et al. [62], in which rats consuming either a Se-adequate or Se-deficient diet revealed no significant change in heart antioxidant enzymes after 8 wk of endurance training. In contrast, Kanter et al. [63] showed that although virtually no change occurred in SOD, catalase, and GPX in the mouse heart after 9 wk of swim training, all three enzymes were increased significantly after 21 wk of training. Powers et al. [106] found that SOD activity was increased in the left ventricular tissues after training at various intensities and duration, whereas in the right ventricle only high-intensity exercise of a longer duration induced SOD. Thus, increased workload (and therefore oxygen consumption) seems to be a crucial factor in determining myocardial antioxidant enzyme response to training. Furthermore, because activities of catalase and GPX did not change at any intensity or duration in either left or right ventricle after training, the role of SOD in myocardial training adaptation was emphasized. Compared with other organs and tissues, myocardium has relatively low SOD activity, given its high oxidative potential and free radical generation (Table 5.1). Removal of O_2^- may thus be a rate-limiting step in the metabolism of ROS during high-intensity exercise. Recently, several authors reported that activities of antioxidant enzymes were decreased in the rat heart as a result of swim training [61, 65, 66]. These reductions may not necessarily reflect a down-regulation of antioxidant enzymes by training, but rather, were caused by an increased cardiac mass (hypertrophy), resulting in a decreased enzyme activity per unit of heart weight.

The physiological significance of a training induction of antioxidant enzymes is not totally clear at present. It is conceivable that an up-regulation of antioxidant enzymes offers a greater protection to the various tissues during exercise. Davies et al. [21] proposed that endurance training helps to reduce oxidative damage by increasing mitochondrial oxidative enzymes and consequently decreasing oxygen flux in each respiratory chain. Higuchi et al. [45], however, argued that the increase in mitochondrial Mn SOD with training is relatively small compared with increases in other mitochondrial enzymes and is therefore not likely to improve antioxidant protection significantly. Ji et al. [59] showed that trained rats had a lesser degree of mitochondrial sulfhydryl oxidation during acute exercise and that exercise-induced inactivation of muscle enzymes was less pronounced in the trained animals. These protective effects of training coincided with an enhanced antioxidant enzyme activity with training [58, 59]. In humans, a higher antioxidant enzyme activity was reported to correlate with $\dot{V}O_2$max, and trained athletes were shown to have greater SOD and CAT activities in skeletal muscle [51]. Mena et al. [88] reported that amateur and professional cyclists had higher erythrocyte SOD activity than the control subjects and the professionals cyclists had higher CAT and GPX activities than the control subjects and amateur cyclists. To establish a clear benefit of training, future studies should be directed to the investigation of muscle functional improvement as a result of antioxidant adaptation.

GLUTATHIONE AND THIOLS

Biochemical Properties and Cellular Distribution

GLUTATHIONE. GSH (γ-glutamylcysteinylglycine) is a major nonenzymatic antioxidant and the most abundant nonprotein thiol source in the cell. It has several important functions related to free radical metabolism [22, 86, 136]. GSH is a substrate for GPX, which removes H_2O_2 and lipid peroxide, as discussed in the previous section. By donating a pair of electrons to a hydroperoxide, 2GSH are oxidized to GSSG. The GSSG formed can be reduced back to GSH by NADPH, which is catalyzed by GR. This important step ensures that cells are kept in a reduced environment, which is essential for the function of many enzymes and cofactors. Recent evidence demonstrates that GSH is also an efficient scavenger of ·OH and singlet oxygen ($^1O_2$) [83, 139] (Fig. 5.1). In addition, GSH may be involved in the recycling of vitamin E radical and semidehydroascorbic (SDA) radicals [100]. Together, these reactions make GSH a "recyclable" and "master" antioxidant in the cell. However, when there is an excessive production of ROS that exceeds the recycling capacity of GR, GSSG levels will rise, resulting in a decreased GSH:GSSG ratio. Therefore, the GSH:GSSG ratio is a sensitive index of the cellular redox status [31]. To maintain the GSH:GSSG ratio and to alleviate oxidative stress, cells are capable of exporting GSSG

FIGURE 5.1.

Antioxidant function of GSH. GPX, glutathione peroxidase; GR, glutathione reductase; GST, glutathione sulfur-transferase; G6PDH, glucose-6-phosphate dehydrogenase; ICDH, isocitrate dehydrogenase; ROOH, hydroperoxide; ROH, aldehyde or H_2O; X, xenobiotics; GS·, glutathione radical; GSOO·, glutathione peroxyl radical.

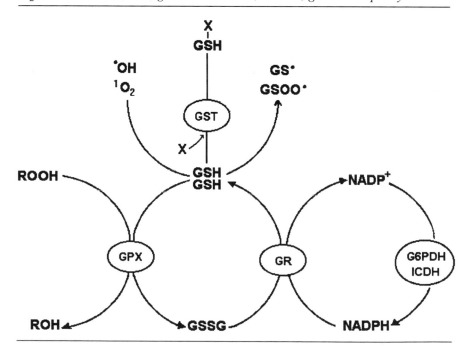

[86]. This important adaptive function has been demonstrated in the erythrocytes, liver, heart, and skeletal muscle [47, 86, 119, 125].

Most of the de novo synthesis of GSH occurs in the liver; therefore, the nonhepatic tissues import GSH from the circulation [22]. GSH is first cleaved into its constituent amino acids, glutamic acid, cysteine, and glycine by the membrane-bound enzyme γ-glutamyltranspeptidase (GGT) and transported into the cell. In a few steps, these amino acids are utilized for the resynthesis of GSH by γ-glutamylcysteine synthase (GCS) and GSH synthase (GS) [86]. Under physiological conditions, intracellular synthesis of GSH relies on the operation of the γ-glutamyl cycle [22]. GCS is considered the rate-limiting enzyme for GSH synthesis. There is evidence that some tissues, such as kidney, may take up intact GSH from the blood [86].

GSH concentration in the cell is in the millimolar range for most tissues. However, there is a great variability in GSH content in different tissues, depending on their function and oxidative capacity [39]. The eye lens has the highest GSH concentration ($\sim$10 mM) among all tissues, probably because of its essential role in protecting the lens from photoradiation. The concentration of GSH in the liver is about 5–7 mM, followed by kidney (3 mM) and heart (2 mM), whereas the muscle has about 1–2 mM, depending on fiber type [60]. GSH content is 2-fold higher in soleus than DVL and 5 fold higher than SVL [60, 76]. The concentration of GSH in the red blood cell is relatively high ($\sim$2 mM) compared with that of blood plasma (<0.05 mM). Within the cell, GSH seems to be particularly enriched in the cell membrane lipid bilayers [85].

DIHYDROLIPOATE AND OTHER THIOLS. In addition to GSH, dihydrolipoate (reduced form of α-lipoic acid) and other thiols (such as ubiquinol) have been recognized recently to have a "tocopherol-sparing effect" [83]. Their effect, however, may not be direct, but by means of the regeneration of ascorbate from the SDA radical, which is formed during the reduction of vitamin E radical [100]. It has been shown that addition of dihydrolipoate to a media that generates tocopheroxyl radicals can reduce electron paramagnetic resonance signals [100]. Cysteine, a precursor for GSH synthesis, is an important free thiol source in the cell, although its concentration is usually low. Another low molecular weight thiol, N-acetylcysteine, has been used to prevent ischemia-reperfusion damage in the heart [29] and recently has been shown to reduce an exercise-induced oxidative stress in humans [118].

Glutathione Status during Exercise
Tissue GSH status is largely regulated by GPX and GR-catalyzed reactions (Fig. 5.1) and in most tissues GPX activity usually far exceeds that of GR (Table 5.1). The GSH:GSSG ratio is therefore determined not only by hydroperoxide production, but also by the capacity of GR to reduce GSSG back to GSH and ultimately by the supply of reducing power NADPH [31]. Furthermore, extrahepatic tissues are capable of taking up GSH from the

circulation and supplement intracellular GSH by means of the γ-glutamyl cycle [22]. These factors should be kept in mind in studying the exercise response of the glutathione system.

Lew et al. [78] were the first to report that GSSG concentration was significantly increased in rat skeletal muscle, liver, and plasma after an acute bout of exhaustive exercise in rodents. GSH content was slightly decreased in the liver and muscle, whereas it was increased in the plasma. The total glutathione levels (GSH+GSSG) in the blood were significantly elevated after exercise. In a later study [107], the authors showed that during an acute bout of exhaustive exercise in rats, running time correlated significantly (r = −0.79) with the GSH content in the liver and that depletion of hepatic GSH under these conditions was approximately 20%.

Because of its important antioxidant function, GSH and the related enzymes in the γ-glutamyl cycle have drawn renewed interest among exercise physiologists in recent years. Available data indicate that GSH content and redox status undergo dynamic changes during exercise, and a complicated picture regarding GSH homeostasis has started to emerge. Sen et al. [117] showed that GSH content was decreased in skeletal muscle and liver of rats after an acute bout of exhaustive exercise. Along with the decreased GSH was a down-regulation of GGT activity in the muscle. Durarte et al [25] reported a marked decline of muscle GSH immediately after 1 hr of treadmill exercise and 48 hr postexercise in mice. Allopurinol, an endothelial xanthine oxidase inhibitor, was found to be effective in protecting the muscle from exercise-induced GSH loss. In skeletal muscle, GSSG concentration has been found to be elevated after an acute bout of prolonged exercise, indicating ROS production exceeding the redox capacity of GR [60]. The level of GSSG increase depends on exercise intensity as well as muscle fiber type. In DVL muscle, GSSG was found to increase by 40% after 1 hr of exercise at ~75% $\dot{V}O_2$max. Soleus showed only a modest increase in GSSG and no change was found in SVL. As much as a 60% increase in GSSG was reported in DVL of rats running to exhaustion [55]. In contrast to Sen et al. [117] and Durarte et al. [25], Ji and Fu [55] showed that the large increase in muscle GSSG was accompanied by concomitant increases in GSH and total glutathione (GSH+GSSG) in exercised rats. As a result, there is little change in the GSH:GSSG ratio in the various muscle fibers after an acute bout of exercise, and only a modest decrease in GSH:GSSG ratio at exhaustion. This unique response of the GSH system in skeletal muscle was previously displayed by Pyke et al. [107], indicating that muscle has some mechanism to maintain its glutathione redox status during exercise. In the liver, a decreased GSH content after exercise has been reported in several rodent studies [77, 78, 117], whereas GSSG was found to be either unchanged [55] or decreased [77]. This GSSG response was explained by a much higher hepatic GSH content and possible release of GSSG into the bile under oxidative stress [86].

There are few data regarding heart GSH response to acute exercise. In one study, Packer et al. [102] found no significant difference in either total glutathione (GSH+GSSG) or GSSG in the heart between rested and exhaustively exercised guinea pigs. Recently, however, we investigated GSH status in the myocardium of mice swimming to exhaustion [77]. GSH content decreased from 0.9 μmol/g wet wt at rest to 0.7 μmol/g wet wt after exercise (P<0.05), whereas GSSG concentration was also significantly reduced. Thus, although myocardial GSH+GSSG was reduced by ~20% at the end of the swimming lasting 3.5 hr, the GSH:GSSG ratio was maintained relatively constant.

Several investigators have shown that prolonged exercise can cause a disturbance to blood GSH status in both animals and humans [26, 28, 35, 116, 118, 134]. However, the results were inconsistent and often confusing. Gohil et al. [35] showed in human subjects that blood GSH levels were significantly decreased, whereas GSSG levels were increased in a reciprocal fashion during 90 min of exercise. However, short-term maximal exercise did not alter blood GSH status. Duthie et al. [26], evaluating antioxidant function in human erythrocytes in response to a half-marathon, found a ~50% reduction of GSH immediately after the race but no change in GSSG. GPX and G6PDH activities were also found unaltered prerace and postrace. In contrast, Evelo et al. [28] showed that GSH levels in human blood were unchanged after a 15-km race and significantly elevated after a half-marathon. Marin et al. [82] and Kretzschmar et al. [69] reported no change in plasma GSH or GSSG after maximal bicycle exercise. These findings seem to agree with Gohil et al. [35] regarding the GSH response to maximal exercise. However, Sen et al. [118] recently showed that blood concentration of GSSG, but not GSH, was significantly elevated after an acute bout of treadmill exercise at both maximal and submaximal intensities. Furthermore, Sahlin et al. [114] showed that total GSH in the blood and plasma were significantly increased during bicycle exercise at progressively increased workloads. Ji et al. [54] also reported an increased blood GSH and total glutathione concentration during a prolonged exercise bout lasting several hours. These discrepancies may reflect the levels of severity of the exercise protocols used as well as the training status of the subjects in the various studies. It should be kept in mind that blood GSH has two separate pools, i.e., erythrocyte (~2 mM) and plasma (0.05 mM). To obtain meaningful results, the two GSH sources should be separated immediately after exercise. Caution also has to be exercised to prevent rapid oxidation of GSH to GSSG.

Interorgan transport of GSH has been proposed to occur during prolonged strenuous exercise [54, 68, 78]. However, there are two conflicting scenarios regarding the role of liver and skeletal muscle in the maintenance of GSH homeostasis. First, Lew et al. [78] and Ji et al. [55] hypothesized that liver exports GSH under the hormonal influence, such as glucagon and vasopressin, which are known to increase during prolonged exercise. Circulating GSH may be taken up by skeletal muscle under exercise-induced oxidative stress. In support of this hypothesis, blood GSH content was shown to be elevated without changing GSSG concentration during prolonged bicycle exercise at 75% $\dot{V}O_2$max. Furthermore, when the subjects were supplied with a carbohydrate drink during exercise, the elevated GSH response to exercise was abolished [54]. Presumably, carbohydrate ingestion inhibited glucagon response, which under normal conditions stimulates the liver to release GSH to the blood circulation [79]. There is an increase in GSH in oxidative types of skeletal muscle during exercise [55, 60]. Because de novo synthesis of GSH is small in the muscle, there must be an increased uptake of GSH, either directly or indirectly, from the circulation. In contrast to the first hypothesis, Kretzschmar et al. [68] proposed that skeletal muscle exports GSH into, instead of importing GSH from, the plasma during prolonged exercise to cope with the oxidative stress in the whole body. This hypothesis was supported by the notion that muscle and liver both have low GGT activity, and by their finding that plasma GSH levels were sustained 6 hr after surgery in hepectomized rats. Given the large volume of muscle mass, this hypothesis seems attractive. However, the mechanism to export GSH from muscle cells has not been postulated and the signals stimulating muscle GSH efflux remain to be identified. To clarify the role of skeletal muscle in GSH homeostasis during prolonged exercise, two crucial pieces of information are required: (a) there is an activation of membrane transport of GSH, by either an increased GGT activity or a decreased K_m for GSH, or both, during acute exercise; and (b) that the elevated GSH in muscle cells comes from liver. So far there are few data to substantiate these scenarios.

In addition to GSH homeostasis, an acute bout of exercise has been shown to decrease mitochondrial protein thiols in skeletal muscle, which correlates with the activity of some key mitochondrial enzymes, such as citrate synthase and malate dehydrogenase [59]. Dithiothreitol, a disulfide-reducing agent, was found effective to reverse such enzyme inactivation occurring during exercise. This exercise-induced down-regulation recently has been reported in muscle phosphofructokinase [75], although the role of thiol-disulfide status in this alteration was not defined. It is interesting to note that oxidatively injured cardiac muscle was shown to restore its contractile function after being treated with dithiothreitol [27]. These studies have raised the possibility that strenuous exercise may cause a general disturbance of cellular thiol-disulfide status because of increased ROS production and that additional reducing power may be required to cope with the increased oxidative stress.

Effect of Training on the Glutathione System
Chronic exercise training at high intensity and long duration has been shown to increase GSH content in liver, lung, and leg muscles of beagle dogs [68, 117]. The data indicate that muscle is capable of adapting to chronic

oxidative stress by increasing its uptake of extramuscular GSH. This scenario is consistent with two related findings: (a) along with an increased GSH, activities of enzymes in the γ-glutamyl cycle, such as GGT, GCS, and GS, were also significantly elevated in the trained dog muscles [82]; and (b) GSH content was increased in rat hind limb muscle after an acute bout of exercise [55, 60, 107]. To clarify whether the increased GSH was attributed to an increased cysteine uptake (the rate-limiting amino acid for GSH synthesis) during training, we have recently conducted a study wherein rats were fed a nutritionally well-defined, purified diet. Trained and untrained rats were pair-fed to ensure that dietary intake of cysteine was equal between the two experimental groups. After 10 wk of training consisting of 2 hr/day treadmill running at 25 m/min, 10% grade, trained rats displayed a 28% increase in GSH content without changing the GSH:GSSG ratio in the DVL muscle compared with the untrained counterparts (unpublished data). This study suggests that training may stimulate an enhanced synthesis of GSH in working muscle against the exercise-induced oxidative stress without increasing dietary cysteine intake. Whether this training adaptation in muscle GSH was at the expense of GSH in other organs is unknown at present.

The effect of training on GSH content seems to vary between muscle fiber types and among different tissues. Sen et al. [117] reported no alteration of GSH content in red gastrocnemius, mixed vastus lateralis, and longissimus dorsi of rats after 10 wk of training. Leeuwenburgh et al. [76] recently found that, whereas GSH levels were unaltered in rat DVL muscle, soleus muscle decreased GSH content as well as the GSH:GSSG ratio and GGT activity after 8 wk of training. The reason for these discrepancies is not clear. It may be related to the rate of GSH utilization versus the capacity of GSH synthesis within each fiber type. In addition to skeletal muscle, myocardial GSH was reported to be elevated after swim training in the rat, and this increase was hypothesized to provide a greater protection against ischemia-reperfusion injury [61, 65]. However, treadmill training has not been proven to be effective in raising myocardial GSH content or GGT activity [30, 117]. Erythrocyte GSH content has been shown to increase significantly, along with an increased GR activity, after 20 wk of physical training in previously sedentary men [28]. Robertson et al. [113] reported that blood GSH concentration increased with training distance in long-distance runners during a training season. Also, plasma GSH levels appear to be higher in long distance runners versus untrained control subjects [69].

ANTIOXIDANT VITAMINS

It is generally accepted that vitamins E, C, and β-carotene play an important role in protecting the cells from free radical damage during heavy exercise. The readers are referred to a more detailed review of antioxidant vitamins and exercise in this volume [64] and to several previous reviews on this topic [37, 101]. The following is a brief summary of the biological functions and exercise response of the various antioxidant vitamins.

Biological Function

VITAMIN E. Vitamin E (α-tocopherol) is the most important fat-soluble chain-breaking antioxidant in the body. Although it is incorporated into virtually all cell membrane bilayers, a major portion of tissue vitamin E is concentrated in the inner mitochondrial membrane, where the respiratory electron transport system is located [36]. However, vitamin E concentration in the cell membrane is rather small, about one in several thousand molecules of phospholipid [100]. Vitamin E content is relatively constant (60–70 nmol/g) across several major body tissues such as liver, heart, lung, and adipose tissue, but is most abundant in brown adipose tissue [34]. Skeletal muscle, however, has only 20–30 nmol/g vitamin E, depending on the fiber type. These differences in vitamin E levels probably reflect the differences of mitochondrial content as well as the oxidative potential among the various tissues [36]. Despite the relatively low content, vitamin E concentration in tissue is very stable and difficult to deplete acutely. This is because after vitamin E quenches an electron from a free radical species and is converted to a vitamin E radical, it can be reduced back to vitamin E by ascorbate (vitamin C) and/or GSH, either enzymatically or nonenzymatically [100] (Fig. 5.2). Vitamin E deficiency has been consistently linked to lipid peroxidation [20, 23]. There is some evidence that animals fed a low vitamin

FIGURE 5.2.
Synergistic function of antioxidant vitamins and thiols. R·, free radicals; VE, vitamin E; VE·, vitamin E radical; ASC, ascorbate, SDA·, semidehydroascorbate; α-LA, α-lipoic acid; OH-LA, dihydrolipoate.

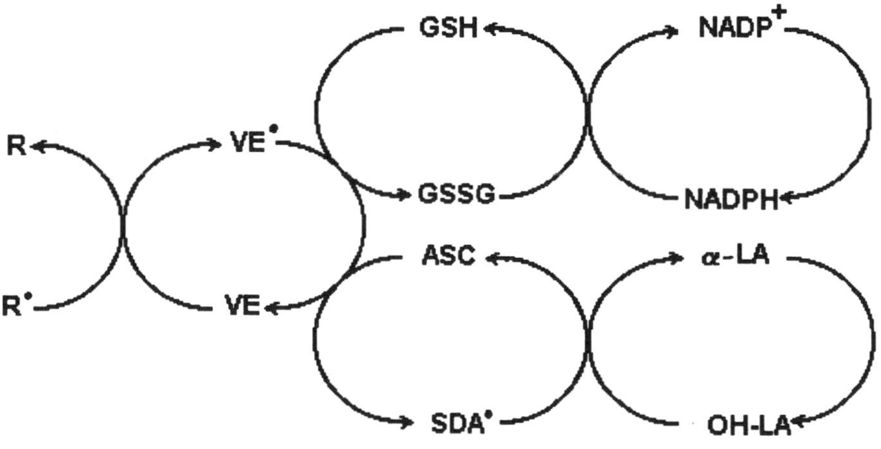

E diet suffer from loss of cell membrane fluidity, reduction of mitochondrial respiratory coupling, skeletal muscle damage, and increased incidence of cardiomyopathy [20, 24, 48].

VITAMIN C. Vitamin C (ascorbate) is a water-soluble vitamin present in the cytosolic compartment of the cell and the extracellular fluid [83]. Its antioxidant function is closely related to that of vitamin E. The spatial arrangement of the two vitamins is such that vitamin C has direct access to the vitamin E radicals generated in the cell membrane phase [39]. After donating an electron to the vitamin E radical, ascorbate is oxidized to an SDA radical, a less reactive compound. The latter can either be recycled by dihydrolipoate (Fig. 5.2), or go through a disproportionation reaction to form dehydroascorbate. In the presence of GSH, the enzyme dehydroascorbate reductase catalyzes the regeneration of ascorbate. In animals, SDA radicals can also be converted directly to ascorbate by the enzyme SDA reductase, using NADH as the reducing power. It should be pointed out that high concentration of ascorbate (~ 1 mM) may act as a prooxidant in the presence of transition metal ions such as Fe^{3+} and Cu^{2+} [39, 139].

β-CAROTENE. β-Carotene, a major carotenoid precursor of vitamin A, has recently received broad attention as an antioxidant [14]. Although its best defined antioxidant function is to quench singlet oxygen (not a free radical), it may also be involved in other free radical reactions [81, 83]. β-Carotene has an inhibitory effect on lipid peroxidation initiated by oxygen- or carbon-centered free radicals [139].

In addition to vitamins E, C, and β-carotene, several low-molecular-weight biological compounds also exhibit antioxidant function. These are uric acid, glucose, billirubin [139], and ubiquinol [100]. Uric acid recently has been found to be a potent antioxidant both intracellularly and extracellularly [6]. Its function may be related to preserving plasma ascorbate by chelating transition metal ions such as iron and copper.

Effect of Acute and Chronic Exercise
Tissue vitamin E depletion as a result of acute physical exertion has been reported in the literature. Kumar et al. [70] reported that an acute bout of exercise in rats caused an increase in free radical production and a decrease in serum and heart vitamin E concentration, and that vitamin E supplementation corrected these effects. An acute bout of exercise has been reported to decrease muscle vitamin E levels in rats fed a normal diet with adequate vitamin E [10]. This finding seems to support the previous notion by Packer [99] that vitamin E consumption was increased during prolonged aerobic exercise, resulting in a net deficiency of vitamin E in endurance-trained animals. However, conflicting reports emerged as Tiidus et al. [129] showed that vitamin E content was not affected by an acute bout of exercise in rats at either vitamin E adequate or depleted state. Because both studies used female rats and exercise intensity appeared similar between the two

studies, the possibility was raised that the younger animals (5–6 wk old) used in the former study might not provide sufficient sex hormone (estradiol) to serve an antioxidant function compared with the more mature rats used in the later study.

Exercise-induced alteration of plasma vitamin E levels also has been reported; however, there is a lack of consistency. Pincemail et al. [103] showed an increase in plasma and erythrocyte vitamin E concentration during exercise in humans. It was hypothesized that exercise might mobilize vitamin E from other tissues to blood plasma and that skeletal muscle might utilize circulating vitamin E to protect against oxidative damage. Lang et al. [73], while reporting no significant change in vitamin E content in liver, muscle, and brown adipose tissues, found a decrease in plasma vitamin E concentration after exhaustive exercise in rats. In studying plasma antioxidant response to a half-marathon running, Duthie et al. [26] found no change in vitamin E concentration; instead, they found that vitamin C concentration was significantly elevated immediately after exercise. An increased vitamin C output from the adrenal gland in response to cortisol release was proposed to be the cause.

Except for a few species, antioxidant vitamins (vitamins E, C, and β-carotene) cannot be synthesized by most mammals. Therefore, endurance training theoretically can reduce tissue levels of these vital compounds that are actively consumed during exercise, unless they are supplemented in the diet. Vitamin E concentration has been shown to decrease in a number of tissues, such as skeletal muscle and liver, in rats undergoing endurance training [2, 99]. More dramatic changes were observed when tissue vitamin E levels were expressed per unit of mitochondrial ubiquinone content [34]. The reduction of vitamin E concentration in the inner mitochondrial membrane can render the mitochondria more susceptible to free radical damage. Available data show that vitamin E content in the heart undergoes only a marginal decrease after a chronic treadmill training program as compared with the decreases in the skeletal muscle [34, 129]. Swim training was found to decrease vitamin E content in the endosubmyocardial sections of the left ventricle in rats, but in the episubmyocardium and right ventricle, the differences were not significant [65]. The differences in the training response of vitamin E between heart and other tissues may be explained in part by a higher vitamin E content in the former ($\sim$70 nmol/g), next only to brown adipose tissue.

EXERCISE AND NUTRITIONAL ANTIOXIDANT DEFICIENCY

The vital role of many antioxidants during exercise has been studied under nutritionally deficient conditions, and there is an abundance of literature dealing with the effects of various nutritional deficiencies on cellular antioxidant response to acute and chronic exercise. It is important to note that deficiency of most antioxidant nutrients is rare in sedentary experimental animals fed a commercial diet or in sedentary humans consuming a balanced diet. Most of the studies to be mentioned were designed to elucidate the mechanisms of antioxidant protection against exercise-induced oxidative stress in laboratory animals. Nevertheless, people involved in routine severe exercise can be predisposed to antioxidant deficiency if an adequate dietary intake of certain nutrients is not secured, making them more vulnerable to oxidative tissue damage [99].

Selenium Deficiency
Although Se itself is not an antioxidant, its essential role in GPX makes it an indispensible micronutrient for normal cell functions [31]. Se deficiency causes a variety of biochemical and physiological alterations in the body, which are well reviewed in the literature [46, 67, 121, 124]. However, its role in protecting exercise-induced oxidative injury has not been studied extensively. Lang et al. [73] showed that rats fed a Se-deficient diet significantly decreased muscle and liver GPX (-80%), but increased total GSH in liver, muscle, and plasma. Se-deficient rats had higher muscle cytochrome *c* oxidase activity and ubiquinone content compared with rats receiving adequate Se in the diet. Furthermore, Se deficiency had no significant effect on endurance capacity in rats and did not enhance exercise-induced decline of vitamin E or elevation of GSSG in the plasma. It was concluded that residual GPX was sufficient to prevent an exercise-induced oxidative stress in Se-deficient animals. Ji et al. [58] studied dietary Se deficiency, endurance training, and an acute bout of exercise on antioxidant systems in rats. It was found that although Se deficiency decreased GPX activity in the cytosol of liver and skeletal muscle to ~4% of control levels, GPX in the mitochondria of these tissues was maintained at higher levels (10–20%). Furthermore, training up-regulated Se-independent GPX (a fraction of GST) in muscle of Se-depleted rats, possibly as a partial compensation for the reduced GPX activity. However, Se deficiency increased lipid peroxidation in the liver and muscle mitochondria after an acute bout of exercise and abolished training adaptation of some enzymes involved in the muscle intermediary metabolism.

Although the role of Se in overall heart function has been well recognized [67], Se deficiency seems to be well tolerated by both sedentary and physically stressed experimental animals, especially if adequate vitamin E is present in the diet [112]. Ji et al. [62] showed that rats fed a Se-deficient diet (<0.01 ppm) and trained for 8 wk did not display abnormal profiles in the heart in terms of lipid peroxidation and metabolic enzyme activities, although their heart mitochondrial and cytosolic GPX were reduced to 20 and 4%, respectively, compared with their Se-adequate counterparts. However, it has been reported that when animals suffered from Se and vitamin

E double deficiencies, the oxidative damage observed was more severe than with deficiency of either antioxidant alone [97].

Vitamin E and Vitamin C Deficiencies

Vitamin E deficiency has been well documented to increase the susceptibility of skeletal muscle to exercise-induced oxidative injury [20, 36, 37, 109]. Davies et al. [20] found that vitamin E deficiency enhanced muscle and liver free radical generation in both rested and exhaustively exercised rats. Lipid peroxidation was increased and the mitochondrial respiratory control index was decreased by both vitamin E deficiency and exhaustive exercise. Activity of several mitochondrial enzymes involved in substrate oxidation was reported to be reduced by vitamin E deficiency, particularly after exercise to exhaustion [36]. Vitamin E-deficient rats also showed a greater degree of lysosomal membrane fragility and loss of sarcoplasmic and endoplasmic reticulum integrity [109]. In addition, endurance performance also has been reported to decrease in rats fed vitamin E-deficient diets [20]. Vitamin E deficiency also has been linked to muscle fiber damage, as measured by enzyme efflux in an in vitro preparation [48]. Amelink et al. [5] reported an increased creatine kinase leakage and ultrastructural damage in skeletal muscle of rats fed a vitamin E-deficient diet and run for 2 hr on a treadmill. Furthermore, it was found that male rats exhibited a greater degree of muscle damage than the female rats under the same conditions. The authors hypothesized that circulating estradiol might serve as an antioxidant to compensate for the impaired vitamin E function during exercise. Studies of exercising diaphragm muscle have generated similar results. It has been shown that vitamin E deficiency can enhance lipid peroxidation, activate the GSH-GSSG redox cycle, and cause early fatigue during resistance breathing [8].

There are insufficient data to conclude whether normal physiological functions of the heart are impaired by vitamin E deficiency, even though rats fed a vitamin E-deficient diet consistently showed reduced vitamin E levels in the myocardium [36, 128]. Gohil et al. [36] reported that the myocardia of rats fed a vitamin E-deficient diet displayed normal mitochondrial respiratory function using several electron donors, except for 2-oxoglutarate. They further demonstrated that an acute bout of exhaustive exercise had no significant effect on myocardial oxidative capacity in either vitamin E-deficient or control rats. However, Tiidus et al. [130] recently showed that rats maintained with a vitamin E-free AIN-76 diet for 8 and 16 wk had increased lipid peroxidation in the heart compared with rats with adequate vitamin E. An acute bout of exercise did not cause a significant increase in the thiobarbituric acid-reactant substance thiobarbituric in rats fed the vitamin E-deficient diet for 8 wk, but resulted in more than a 2-fold increase in acid-reactant substance in rats fed the same diet for 16 wk and also involved in a training program.

There are few data dealing with the effect of vitamin C deficiency on exercise-induced tissue oxidative damage. By reducing dietary vitamin C content to 10% of the normal values (0.2 g/kg), Packer et al. [102] demonstrated that vitamin C-deficient animals had markedly increased plasma total glutathione in response to exhaustive exercise compared with controls. Myocardial capacity to oxidize pyruvate, 2-oxoglutarate, and succinate was reduced and endurance time was also significantly shortened by dietary vitamin C deficiency [98, 99]. Interestingly, a group of guinea pigs supplemented with twice the normal amount of vitamin C in the diet also exhibited similar metabolic defects in the heart and early fatigue during prolonged exercise. Other tissues such as liver and skeletal muscle were not as susceptible as the heart.

Glutathione Deficiency
GSH deficiency is associated with a spectrum of physiological and biochemical disorders [87]. Although there has been active research on GSH regulation during exercise over the years, as discussed in the previous sections, little is known about the consequence of GSH deficiency on exercise-induced oxidative stress in various tissues. Recently, we have investigated the effect of GSH deficiency on tissue glutathione status, exercise capacity, and antioxidant systems in male Swiss-Webster mice [77]. GSH was depleted by injecting the mice with buthionine sulfoximine, a specific inhibitor of GCS (the rate-limiting enzyme for GSH synthesis). GSH-depleted and control mice were either subjected to an acute bout of swimming to exhaustion or rested before being killed. Buthionine sulfoximine treatment depleted the GSH content in liver, kidney, heart, and muscle to 23, 15, 10, and 7% of the normal values, respectively. After swimming to exhaustion, GSH content in the control mice was decreased as a function of time in all tissues studied except quadriceps muscle, which showed a slight increase. In the GSH-depleted mice, exercise further suppressed GSH levels in all tissues and increased lipid peroxidation in the liver and muscle. In the GSH-adequate mice, swimming to exhaustion decreased both GSH and GSSG by ~20% (P<0.05) without altering the GSH:GSSG ratio. GSH depletion was found to increase significantly the activity of SOD in the heart and kidney and GPX activity in the liver, kidney, and muscle. Furthermore, GR and GST activities were elevated with GSH depletion in the liver and kidney. Despite these disturbances of antioxidant systems, endurance performance was similar between the GSH-depleted and control mice (207 ± 30 vs. 198± 26 min).

Although not classified as an antioxidant, riboflavin (vitamin B_2) is an important nutrient serving as a prosthetic group for GR, thereby maintaining tissue GSH-GSSG redox status [31]. It is well known that riboflavin deficiency can cause impairment of work performance [131, 132]. Chronic physical exercise has been shown to increase riboflavin requirement in both young and old women [138]. Recently, Soares et al. [123] reported that an acute bout of exercise caused a deterioration of riboflavin status (measured by the GR activation coefficient, defined as the GR activity without added riboflavin as a fraction of GR activity with added riboflavin) in marginally riboflavin-deficient men. Thus, riboflavin deficiency potentially can jeopardize GSH recycling and affect tissue susceptibility to oxidative stress.

ANTIOXIDANTS, EXERCISE, AND AGING

Aging has been proposed to be caused by the accumulative action of the deleterious oxygen free radicals throughout the life span [41]. It is well known that aging influences both free radical production and cellular antioxidant defense systems in various organs and tissues. [For detailed reviews in this area, see refs. 7, 89, 90, and 139.] However, each tissue seems to undergo different changes during aging; therefore, there is a need to discuss the tissue-specific response of antioxidants to aging and exercise. Skeletal muscle and heart will be highlighted because of their well-defined function during exercise.

Skeletal Muscle

Aging is associated with a decline of cellular antioxidant defenses in most biological tissues [16, 84]. However, despite a general decline of physiological and biochemical function with age [17], senescent skeletal muscle appears to have an enhanced antioxidant enzyme system [55, 72, 80, 133]. Lammi-Keefe et al. [72] were among the first to observe that, contrary to the aging response of most tissues, several skeletal muscles showed an increased SOD activity with aging. Ji et al. [57] showed that activities of all major antioxidant enzymes, such as SOD, CAT, and GPX, were significantly higher in muscle of old versus young rats. In addition, the activity of GST, GR, and G6PDH were also increased with age [57]. Leeuwenburgh et al. [76] reported a similar increase in antioxidant enzyme activity with aging in both DVL and soleus muscles in rats. However, this age-related increase in antioxidant enzymes did not seem to prevent lipid oxidation in senescent muscles [57, 76, 126]. Luhtala et al. [80] recently discovered that elevation of muscle antioxidant enzymes during aging was markedly affected by dietary restriction in Fischer 344 rats. The progressive increases in CAT and GPX activities from 11 to 34 mo of age were prevented by a 30% reduction of food intake, whereas an age-related increase in Mn SOD was also attenuated in hind limb muscles. It has been proposed by Meydani and Evans [89] that even though antioxidant enzyme activities increase with age, these enzymes may become less efficient in protecting the muscle from oxidative damage. There is evidence that an acute bout of eccentric exercise may cause more severe oxidative injury to muscles in aged mice [140] and men [89] than their young counterparts.

An acute bout of exercise did not cause a different antioxidant response in old versus young rats [57, 75]. Endurance training, however, has been shown to increase some antioxidant enzyme activities in the senescent muscle [40, 56]. Ji et al. [56] showed a training induction of muscle GPX in 27-mo-old Fischer 344 rats, but SOD and CAT activities remained unchanged with training. Hammeren et al. [40] also reported a training adaptation of GPX in various muscle fibers in old Fischer 344 rats. Leeuwenburgh et al. [76] found that 10 wk of endurance training increased GPX and SOD in DVL of the young rats, but had little effect on antioxidant enzyme activity in either DVL or soleus in the old rats. There are two potential problems associated with training studies of antioxidant enzymes in senescent muscle: (a) the oxidative stress imposed on old animals might be limited by their exercise ability and (b) the training threshold of senescent muscles might be raised because of an age-related increase in the antioxidant enzymes activity. Therefore, it is difficult to conclude whether training is more or less effective to induce antioxidant enzymes in senescent skeletal muscle.

Aging is associated with a decline of cellular thiol reserve in most tissues [84]. GSH content has been found to be lower in liver, kidney, heart, and erythrocytes in aged mice, with no significant alteration in GSSG [43, 93]. However, skeletal muscle seems to be spared this effect. In a recent study, Leeuwenburgh et al. [76] showed that aging caused no significant alteration of GSH content or GSH:GSSG ratio in rat DVL muscle, whereas in soleus there was a 37% increase in GSH content in old rats, and the GSH:GSSG ratio was also increased with aging. Endurance training did not seem to affect muscle GSH content and redox status in aged rats [76]. As for antioxidant vitamins, the limited data show that aging does not provoke any significant change in α-tocopherol levels in rat skeletal muscle [126]. So far, there is no clear evidence that training can protect the senescent muscle from lipid peroxidation caused either by an acute bout of exercise [75, 76] or by an in vitro oxidative challenge [126].

Heart

Aging is associated with an increased mitochondrial free radical generation and overall oxidative stress in the heart [91]. However, there is no clear consensus as to whether aging results in an increase or decrease of myocardial antioxidant capacity. Myocardial SOD and GPX activities have been found to decrease or remain unchanged, whereas CAT activity is increased with aging. [See ref. 84 for a detailed review.] Hazelton and Lang [44] showed that GPX activity was significantly decreased, whereas GR activity was unchanged with age in the mouse heart. Cand and Verdetti [16] found no alteration in SOD and GPX activities but an increase in CAT activity in the myocardium of old rats. Ji et al. [53] studied myocardial antioxidant enzyme response to aging in various cell compartments and showed that activities of the cytosolic fractions of SOD (CuZn) and GPX decreased, whereas mitochondrial Mn SOD and GPX increased with age. These findings were in agreement with an early report by Nohl and Hegner [92]. The diverse responses of antioxidant enzymes probably reflect the age-related increase in free radical production in certain cell compartments in the heart, such as mitochondria and peroxisomes, and a cellular adaptation to the increased oxidative stress. However, the observed antioxidant enzyme adaptation did not appear to prevent mitochondrial and tissue lipid peroxidation in the senescent heart [53, 90, 92]. GSH content in the heart appears to decrease with age in rodents, as does vitamin C levels [43, 84]. Interestingly, vitamin E concentration seems to increase in a number of tissues, including the heart, in senescence [137]. So far, there is little evidence that the observed oxidative changes are directly related to the functional deterioration in aged heart such as excitation-contraction coupling, sarcoplasmic reticulum function, protein synthesis, and ATP generation [71].

The effect of exercise on antioxidant systems has not been found different between aged versus young animals. One reason may be the age limitation of exercise ability, such that aged animals are subjected to a reduced oxidative stress. In a previous study, we found no significant alteration in most myocardial antioxidant enzymes after 1 hr of treadmill running in either young or aged rats, except CuZn SOD, which showed an increase [53]. Recently, we have investigated the effect of 10 wk of exercise training on heart antioxidant function in aged rats [30]. Although aging per se increased GPX, GR, and SOD activities, there was no significant alteration in any antioxidant enzyme with training in young or old rats.

CONCLUSION

The production of reactive oxygen species is a normal process in the life of aerobic organisms. Under physiological conditions, these deleterious species are removed effectively by the cellular antioxidant systems, including antioxidant vitamins, GSH and sulfhydryls, and antioxidant enzymes. However, existing data show that antioxidant defenses are not perfect and the antioxidant reserve capacity in most tissues is rather marginal. Therefore, an increased production of ROS, or a weakening of the antioxidant systems, or both, can subject the organisms to oxidative stress and tissue damage (Fig. 5.3).

Heavy physical exercise is associated with a remarkable increase in oxygen consumption, and hence, a challenge to the antioxidant systems. Antioxidant enzymes provide the first line of defense by reducing O_2^- and H_2O_2

FIGURE 5.3.

Hypothetical scenario of antioxidant response and adaptation during exercise. Solid lines indicate direct influence; dotted lines indicate possible moduration.

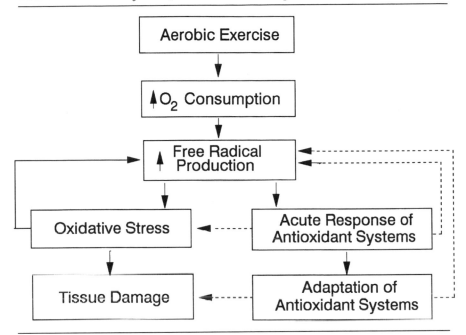

to relatively harmless species. Free radical species that escape the antioxidant enzymes are quenched by the chain-breaking antioxidant vitamin E, and incidentally formed OH are scavenged by vitamin E and GSH. Vitamin C, dihydrolipoate, and GSH serve to maintain vitamin E in the reduced state. Thus, each antioxidant plays a unique role in protecting the tissues from exercise-induced oxidative damage. Deficiency of an antioxidant nutrient can severely hamper the corresponding antioxidant system during exercise.

An acute bout of exercise of sufficient intensity has been shown to activate antioxidant enzymes and the GSH-GSSG redox cycle. This activation can be viewed as a defensive mechanism of the cell in face of an increased oxidative challenge. However, exhaustive exercise may cause a transient reduction of tissue vitamin E content and change glutathione redox status. Disturbance of the antioxidant homeostasis may exacerbate the exercise-induced oxidative stress and tissue damage, and has been linked to some fundamental cell dysfunction, such as energy production and excitation-contractile coupling, but so far such evidence is still circumstantial. Chronic exercise training seems to have dual effects: it induces antioxidant enzymes and perhaps stimulates GSH synthesis, thus theoretically facilitating the removal of various ROS produced during acute oxidative stress (Fig. 5.3). However, training appears to increase the consumption of vitamin E and therefore reduces its tissue concentration, if dietary intake remains unchanged. Therefore, the supplementation of certain antioxidant nutrients seems to be justified in physically actively people.

REFERENCES

1. Aebi, H. Catalase. *Methods Enzymol.* 105:121–126, 1984.
2. Aikawa, K. M., A. T. Quintanilha, B. O. deLumen, G. A. Brooks, and L. Packer. Exercise endurance training alters vitamin E tissue levels and red blood cell hemolysis in rodents. *Biosci. Rep.* 4:253–257, 1984.
3. Alessio, H. M., and A. H. Goldfarb. Lipid peroxidation and scavenge enzymes during exercise: adaptive response to training. *J. Appl. Physiol.* 64:1333–1336, 1988.
4. Allesio, H. M. Exercise-induced oxidative stress. *Med. Sci. Sports Exerc.* 25:218–224, 1993.
5. Amelink, G. J., W. A. A. v. d. Wal, J. H. J. Wokke, B. S. van Asbeck, and P. R. Bar. Exercise-induced muscle damage in the rat: the effect of vitamin E deficiency. *Pflugers Arch.* 419: 304–309, 1991.
6. Ames, B. N., R. Cathcart, E. Schwiers, and P. Hochstein. Uric acid provides an antioxidant defense in humans against oxidant and radical-caused aging and cancer: a hypothesis. *Proc. Natl. Acad. Sci. U.S.A.* 78:6858–6862, 1981.
7. Ames, B. N., M. K. Shigenaga, and T. M. Hagen. Oxidant, antioxidants, and degenerative diseases of aging. *Proc. Natl. Acad. Sci. U. S. A.* 90:7915–7922, 1993.
8. Anzueto A, F. H. Andrade, L. C. Maxwell, et al. Diaphragmetic function after resistive breathing in vitamin E-deficient rats. *J. Appl. Physiol.* 74:267–271, 1993.
9. Blum, J., and I. Fridovich. Inactivation of glutathione peroxidase by superoxide radical. *Arch. Biochem. Biophys.* 240:500–508, 1985.
10. Bowles, D. K., C. E. Torgan, J. P. Kehrer, J. L. Ivy, and J. W. Starnes. Effects of acute, submaximal exercise on skeletal muscle vitamin E. *Free Rad. Res. Commun.* 14:139–143, 1991.
11. Brady, P. S., L. J. Brady, and D. E. Ullrey. Selenium, vitamin E and the response to swimming stress in rats. *J. Nutr.* 109:1103–1109, 1979.
12. Buczynski, A., J. Kedziora, W. Tkaczewski, B. and Wachowicz. Effect of submaximal physical exercise on antioxidative protection of human blood platelets. *Int. J. Sports Med.* 12:52–54, 1991.
13. Burge, W. E., and A. J. Neil. Comparison of the amount of catalase in the muscle of large and of small animals. *Am. J. Physiol.* 43:433–437, 1916–1917.
14. Burton, G. W. and K. V. Ingold. Beta carotene: an unusual type of lipid antioxidant. *Science* 224:569–573, 1984.
15. Calderera, C. M., C. Guarnierri, and F. Lazzari. Catalase and peroxidase activity in cardiac muscle. *Bull. Italian Exp. Biol. Soc.* 49:72–77, 1973.
16. Cand, F., and J. Verdetti. Superoxide dismutase, glutathione peroxidase, catalase, and lipid peroxidation in the major organs of the aging rats. *Free Rad. Biol. Med.* 7:59–63, 1989.
17. Cartee, G. Aging skeletal muscle: response to exercise. J. O. Hollozsy (ed.) *Exercise and Sports Sciences Reviews.* Baltimore: Williams & Wilkins, 1993, pp. 91–120.
18. Chance, B., C. Saronio, and J. S. Leigh, Jr. Functional intermediates in the reaction of membrane bound cytochrome oxidase with oxygen. *J. Biol. Chem.* 250:9226–9237, 1975.
19. Chance, B. H. Sies, and A. Boveris. Hydroperoxide metabolism in mammalian organs. *Physiol. Rev.* 59:527–605, 1979.
20. Davies, K. J. A., A. T. Quantanilla, G. A. Brooks, and L. Packer. Free radicals and tissue damage produced by exercise. *Biochem. Biophys. Res. Commun.* 107:1198–1205, 1982.

21. Davies, K. J. A., L. Packer, and G. A. Brooks. Biochemical adaptation of mitochondria, muscle and whole animal respiration to endurance training. *Arch. Biochem. Biophys.* 209:539–554, 1981.

22. Deneke, S. M., and B. L. Fanburg. Regulation of cellular glutathione. *Am. J. Physiol.* 257:L163–L173, 1989.

23. Dillard, C. J., R. E. Litov, W. M. Savin, E. E. Mumelin, and A. L. Tappel. Effect of exercise, vitamin E, and ozone on pulmonary function and lipid peroxidation. *J. Appl. Physiol.* 45:927–932, 1978.

24. Diplock, A. T. Antioxidant nutrients and disease prevention: an overview. *Am. J. Clin Nutr.* 53:189S–193S, 1991.

25. Durarte, J. A. R., H. J. Appell, F. Carvalho, M. Bastos, and J. M. Soares. Endothelium-derived oxidative stress may contribute to exercise-induced muscle damage. *Int. J. Sports Med.* 14:440–443, 1993.

26. Duthie, G. G., J. D. Robertson, R. J. Maughan, and P. C. Morrice. Blood antioxidant status and erythrocyte lipid peroxidation following distance running. *Arch. Biochem. Biophys.* 282:78–83, 1990.

27. Eley, D. W., B. Korecky, and H. Fliss. Dithiothreitol restores contractile function to oxidant-injured cardiac muscle. *Am. J. Physiol.* 257:H1321–H1325, 1989.

28. Evelo, C. T. A., N. G. Palmen, Y. Artur, and G. M. E. Janssen. Changes in blood glutathione concentrations, and in erythrocyte glutathione reductase and glutathione S-transferase activity after running training and after participation in contests. *Eur. J. Appl. Physiol.* 64:354–358, 1992.

29. Ferrari, R., C. Ceconi, S. Curello, et al. Oxygen free radicals and myocardial damage: protective role of thiol-containing agents. *Am. J. Med.* 91:95S–105S, 1991.

30. Fiebig, R., C. Leeuwenburgh, and L. L. Ji. The effects of aging and training on myocardial antioxidant systems and lipid peroxidation. *Med. Sci. Sports Exerc.* 26:S133, 1994.

31. Flohe, L. Glutathione peroxidase brought into focus. W. Pryor (ed.) *Free Radical in Biology and Medicine, Vol. 5.* New York: Academic Press, 1982, pp. 223–253.

32. Fridovich, I. Quantitation of superoxide dismutase. R. A. Greenwald (ed). *Handbook of Methods for Oxygen Free Radical Research.* Boca Raton, FL: CRC Press, 1985, pp. 211–215.

33. Fucci, L., C. M. Liver, M. J. Coon, and E. R. Stadtman. Inactivation of key metabolic enzymes by mixed-function oxidation reaction: possible implication in protein turnover and ageing. *Proc. Natl. Acad. Sci. U. S. A.* 80:1521–1525, 1983.

34. Gohil, K., L. Rothfuss, J. Lang, and L. Packer. Effect of exercise training on tissue vitamin E and ubiquinone content. *J. Appl. Physiol.* 63:1638–1641, 1987.

35. Gohil, K., C. Viguie, W. C. Stanley, G. A. Brooks, and L. Packer. Blood glutathione oxidation during human exercise. *J. Appl. Physiol.* 64:115–119, 1988.

36. Gohil, K., L. Packer, B. deLumen, G. A. Brooks, and S. E. Terblanche. Vitamin E deficiency and vitamin C supplementation: exercise and mitochondrial oxidation. *J. Appl. Physiol.* 60:1986–1991, 1986.

37. Goldfarb, A. H. Antioxidants: role of supplementation to prevent exercise-induced oxidative stress. *Med. Sci. Sports. Exerc.* 25 232–236, 1993.

38. Habig, W. H., M. J. Pabst, and W. B. Jakoby. Glutathione S-transferases. *J. Biol. Chem.* 249:7130–7139, 1974.

39. Halliwell, B., and J. M. C. Gutteridge. *Free Radicals in Biology and Medicine.* Oxford: Clarendon Press, 1989.

40. Hammeren, J., S. Powers, J. Lawler, D. Criswell, D. Lowenthal, and M. Pollock. Exercise training-induced alterations in skeletal muscle oxidative and antioxidant enzyme activity in senescent rats. *Int. J. Sports Med.* 13:412–416, 1993.

41. Harman, D. Aging: a theory based on free radical and radiation chemistry. *J. Gerontol.* 11:298–300, 1956.

42. Harris, E. D. Regulation of antioxidant enzymes. *FASEB J.* 6:2675–2683, 1992.

43. Hazelton, G. A., and C. A. Lang. Glutathione content in the aging mouse. *Biochem J.* 188:25–30, 1980.
44. Hazelton, G. A., and C. A. Lang. Glutathione peroxide and reductase activity in the aging mouse. *Mech. Aging Dev.* 29:71–81, 1985.
45. Higuchi, M., L-J. Cartier, M. Chen, and J. O. Holloszy. Superoxide dismutase and catalase in skeletal muscle: adaptive response to exercise. *J. Gerontol.* 40:281–286, 1985.
46. Hill, K. E., R. F. Burk, and J. M. Lane. Effect of selenium depletion and repletion on plasma glutathione and glutathione-dependent enzymes in the rat. *J. Nutr.* 117:99–104, 1987.
47. Ishikawa, T., and H. Sies. Cardiac transport of glutathione disulfide and S-conjugate. *J. Biol. Chem.* 259:3838–3843, 1984.
48. Jackson, M. J., D. A. Jones, and R. H. T. Edwards. Vitamin E and skeletal muscle. R. Porter and J. Whelan (eds.) *Biology of Vitamin E.* London: Pitman Books, 1983, pp. 224–239.
49. Jackson, M. L., R. H. T. Edwards, and M. C. R. Symons. Electron spin resonance studies of intact mammalian skeletal muscle. *Biochim. Biophys. Acta* 847:185–190, 1985.
50. Jenkins, R. R. Free radical chemistry: relationship to exercise. *Sports Med.* 5:156–170, 1988.
51. Jenkins, R. R. Exercise, oxidative stress and antioxidant: a review. *Int. J. Sports Nutr.* 3:356–375, 1993.
52. Jenkins, R. R., R. Friedland, and H. Howald. The relationship of oxygen uptake to superoxide dismutase and catalase activity in human muscle. *Int. J. Sports Med.* 95:11–14, 1984.
53. Ji, L. L. Antioxidant enzyme response to exercise and aging. *Med. Sci. Sports Exerc.* 25:225–231, 1993.
54. Ji, L. L., A. Katz, R. G. Fu, M. Parchert, and M. Spencer. Alteration of blood glutathione status during exercise: the effect of carbohydrate supplementation. *J. Appl. Physiol.* 74:788–792, 1993.
55. Ji, L. L., and R. G. Fu. Responses of glutathione system and antioxidant enzymes to exhaustive exercise and hydroperoxide. *J. Appl. Physiol.* 72:549–554, 1992.
56. Ji, L. L., E. Wu, and D. P. Thomas. Effect of exercise training on antioxidant and metabolic functions in senescent rat skeletal muscle. *Gerontology* 37:317–325, 1991.
57. Ji, L. L., D. Dillon, and E. Wu. Alteration of antioxidant enzymes with aging in rat skeletal muscle and liver. *Am. J. Physiol.* 258:R918–R923, 1990.
58. Ji, L. L., F. W. Stratman, and H. A. Lardy. Antioxidant enzyme systems in rat liver and skeletal muscle. *Arch. Biochem. Biophys.* 263:150–160, 1988.
59. Ji, L. L., F. W. Stratman, and H. A. Lardy. Enzymatic down regulation with exercise in rat skeletal muscle. *Arch. Biochem. Biophys.* 263:137–149, 1988.
60. Ji, L. L., R. G. Fu, and E. W. Mitchell. Glutathione and antioxidant enzymes in skeletal muscle: effects of fiber type and exercise intensity. *J. Appl. Physiol.* 73:1854–1859, 1992.
61. Ji, L. L., R. G. Fu, E. Mitchell, M. Griffiths, T. G. Waldrop, and H. M. Swartz. Cardiac hypertrophy alters myocardial response to ischemia and reperfusion in vivo. *Acta Physiol. Scand.* 151:279–290, 1994.
62. Ji, L. L., F. W. Stratman, and H. A. Lardy. The impact of selenium deficiency on myocardial antioxidant enzyme systems and related biochemical properties. *J. Am. Coll. Nutr.* 11:79–86, 1992.
63. Kanter, M. M., R. L. Hamlin, D. V. Unverferth, H. W. Davies, and A. J. Merola. Effect of exercise training on antioxidant enzymes and cardiotoxicity of doxorubicin. *J. Appl. Physiol.* 59:1298–1303, 1985.
64. Kanter, M. M. Free radical and exercise: effect of antioxidant nutritional supplementation. J. O. Holloszy (ed.) *Exercise and Sports Sciences Review.* Baltimore: Williams & Wilkins, 1995.
65. Kihlstrom, M. Protection effect of endurance training against reoxygenation-induced injuries in rat heart. *J. Appl. Physiol.* 68:1672–1678, 1990.
66. Kihlstrom, M, J. Ojala, and S. Salminen. Decreased level of cardiac antioxidants in endurance-trained rats. *Acta Physiol. Scand.* 135:549–554, 1989.

67. Konz, K. H., M. Haap, K. E. Hill, R. F. Burk, and R. A. Walsh. Diastolic dysfunction of perfused rat hearts induced by hydrogen peroxide. Protective effect of selenium. *J. Mol. Cell. Cardiol.* 21:789–795, 1989.

68. Kretzschmar, M., and D. Muller. Aging, training and exercise: a review of effects of plasma glutathione and lipid peroxidation. *Sports Med.* 15:196–209, 1993.

69. Kretzschmar, M., U. Pfeifer, G. Machnik, and W. Klinger. Influence of age, training and acute physical exercise on plasma glutathione and lipid peroxidation in man. *Intr. J. Sports Med.* 12:218–222, 1991.

70. Kumar, C. T., V. K. Reddy, M. Plasad, K. Thyagaraju, and P. Reddanna. Dietary supplementation of vitamin E protects heart tissue from exercise-induced oxidant stress. *Mol. Cell. Biochem.* 111:109–115, 1992.

71. Lakatta, E. G. Cardiac muscle changes in senescence. *Annu. Rev. Physiol.* 49:519–531, 1987.

72. Lammi-Keefe, C. J., P. B. Swan, and P. V. J. Hegarty. Copper-zinc and manganese superoxide dismutase activities in cardiac and skeletal muscles during aging in male rats. *Gerontology* 30:153–158, 1984.

73. Lang, J. K., K. Gohil, L. Packer, and R. F. Burk. Selenium deficiency, endurance exercise capacity, and antioxidant status in rats. *J. Appl. Physiol.* 63:2532–2535, 1987.

74. Laughlin M. H., T, Simpson, W. L. Sexton, O. R. Brown, J. K. Smith and R. J. Korthuis. Skeletal muscle oxidative capacity, antioxidant enzymes, and exercise training. *J. Appl. Physiol.* 68:2337–2343, 1990.

75. Lawler, J. M., S. K. Powers, T. Visser, H. Van Dijk, M. J. Korthuis, and L. L. Ji. Acute exercise and skeletal muscle antioxidant and metabolic enzymes: effect of fiber type and age. *Am. J. Physiol.* 265:R1344–R1350, 1993.

76. Leeuwenburgh, C., R. Fiebig, R. Chandwaney, and L. L. Ji. Aging and exercise training in skeletal muscle: Response of glutathione and antioxidant enzyme systems. *Am. J. Physiol.* 267:R439–R445, 1994.

77. Leeuwenburgh, C., R. Fiebig, R., and L. L. Ji. Glutathione regulation during prolonged exercise in glutathione adequate and depleted mice. *Med. Sci. Sports. Exerc.* 26:S133, 1994.

78. Lew, H., S. Pyke, and A. Quintanilha. Change in the glutathione status of plasma, liver and muscle following exhaustive exercise in rats. *FEBS Lett.* 185:262–266, 1985.

79. Lu, S. C., C. Garcia-Ruiz, J. Kuhlenkamp, M. Ookhtens, M. Salas-Prato, and N. Kaplowitz. Hormonal regulation of glutathione efflux. *J. Biol. Chem.* 265:16088–16095, 1990.

80. Luhtala, T., E. B. Roecher, T. Pugh, R. J. Feuers, and R. Weindruch. Dietary restriction opposes age-related increases in rat skeletal muscle antioxidant enzyme activities. *J. Gerontol.* 1994, in press.

81. Machlin, L. J., and A. Bendich. Free radical tissue damage: protective role of antioxidant nutrients. *FASEB J* 1:441–445, 1987.

82. Marin, E., O. Hanninen, D. Muller, and W. Klinger. Influence of acute physical exercise on glutathione and lipid peroxide in blood of rat and man. *Acta Physiol. Hung.* 76:71–76, 1990.

83. Mascio, P. D., M. E. Murphy, and H. Sies. Antioxidant defense systems: the role of carotenoids, tocopherols, and thiols. *Am. J. Clin. Nutr.* 53:194S–200S, 1991.

84. Matsuo, M. Age-related alterations in antioxidant defense. Yu, B. P. (ed.). *Free Radical in Aging.* Boca Raton, FL: CRC Press, 1993, pp. 143–181.

85. Mbemba, F., A. Houbion, M. Raes, and J. Remacle. Subcellular localization and modification with ageing of glutathione, glutathione peroxidase and glutathione reductase activities in human fibroblasts. *Biochim. Biophys. Acta* 838:211–220, 1985.

86. Meister, A., and M. E. Anderson. Glutathione. *Annu. Rev. Biochem.* 52:711–760, 1983.

87. Meister, A. Glutathione deficiency produced by inhibition of its synthesis, and its reversal; applications in research and therapy. *Pharmacol. Ther.* 51:155–194, 1991.

88. Mena, P., M. Maynar, J. M. Gutierrez, J. Maynar, J. Timon, and J. E. Campillo. Erythrocyte free radical scavenger enzymes in bicycle professional racers. Adaptation to training. *Int. J. Sports Med.* 12:563–566, 1991.

89. Meydani, M., and W. J. Evans. Free radicals, exercise, and aging. B. P. Yu (ed). *Free Radical in Aging.* Boca Raton, FL: CRC Press, 1993, pp. 183–204

90. Nohl, H. Involvement of free radicals in aging: a consequence or cause of senescence. *Br. Med. Bull.* 49:653–667, 1993.

91. Nohl, H. D. Oxygen free radical release in mitochondria: influence of age. J. E., Johnson, R. Walford, D. Harmon, and J. Miquel (eds). *Free Radicals, Aging, and Degenerative Diseases.* New York: Alan R. Liss, Inc., 1986, pp. 77–98.

92. Nohl, H., and D. Hegner. Response of mitochondrial superoxide dismutase, catalase, and glutathione peroxidase activities to aging. *Mech. Aging Dev.* 11:145–151, 1978.

93. Oberley, L. W., and T. D. Oberley. Free radicals, cancer, and aging. J. E. Johnson, R. Walford, D. Harmon, and J. Miquel (eds). *Free Radicals, Aging, and Degenerative Diseases.* New York: Alan R. Liss, Inc., 1986, pp. 77–98.

94. Oberley, L. W., D. K. St. Clair, A. P. Autor, and T. D. Oberley. Increase in manganese superoxide dismutase activity in the mouse heart after X-irradiation. *Arch. Biochem. Biophys.* 254:69–80, 1987.

95. Ohno, H., S. Gasa, Y. Habara, A. Kuroshima, Y. Sato, N. Miyazawa, and N. Taniguchi. Effects of exercise stress and cold stress on glutathione and gamma-glutamyltransferase in rat liver. *Biochem. Biophys. Acta* 1033:19–22, 1990.

96. Oliver, C. N., B. Ahn, E. J. Moerman, S. Goldstein, and E. R. Stadtman. Age-related changes in oxidized proteins. *J. Biol. Chem.* 262:5488–5491, 1987.

97. Oster, O., M. Mahm, H. Oelert, W. Prellwitz. Concentrations of some trace elements (Se, Zn, Cu, Fe, Mg, K) in blood and heart tissue of patients with coronary heart disease. *Clin. Chem.* 35:851–856, 1989.

98. Packer, L. Vitamin E, physical exercise and tissue damage in animals. *Med. Biol.* 62:105–109, 1984.

99. Packer, L. Oxygen radicals and antioxidants in endurance training. G. Benzi, L. Packer, and N. Siliprandi (eds). *Biochemical Aspects of Physical Exercise.* New York: Elsevier Science Publishers, 1986, pp. 73–92.

100. Packer L. Synergy between α-lipoic acid and vitamin E. E. Cadenas and L. Packer (eds). *Biological Oxidants and Antioxidants: New Developments in Research and Health Effects.* Hippokrates: Verlag, 1994, in press.

101. Packer L. Protective role of vitamin E in biological systems. *Am. J. Clin. Nutr.* 53:1050S–1055S, 1991.

102. Packer, L., K. Gohil, B. DeLumen, and S. E. Terblanche. A comparative study on the effects of ascorbic acid deficiency and supplementation on endurance and mitochondrial oxidative capacities in various tissues of the guinea pig. *Comp. Biochem. Physiol.* 83B:235–240, 1986.

103. Pincemail, J., D. C. G. Camus, F. Pirnay, R. Bouchez, L. Massaux, and R. Goutier. Tocopherol mobilization during intensive exercise. *Eur. J. Appl. Physiol.* 57:189–191, 1988.

104. Powers, S. K., D. Criswell, J. Lawler, et al. Influence of exercise intensity and fiber type on antioxidant enzyme activity in skeletal muscle. *Am. J. Physiol. (Regul. Int. Comp. Physiol.)* 266:R375–R380, 1994.

105. Powers, S. K., D. Criswell, J. Lawler, D. Martin, L. L. Ji, and G. Dudley. Training-induced oxidative and antioxidant enzyme activity in the diaphragm: influence of exercise intensity and duration. *Respir. Physiol.* 95:226–237, 1994.

106. Powers, S. K., D. Criswell, J. Lawler, D. Martin, F. K. Lieu, L. L. Ji, and R. A. Herb. Rigorous exercise training increases superoxide dismutase activity in ventricular myocardium. *Am. J. Physiol.* 265:H2094–H2098, 1993.

107. Pyke, S., H. Lew, and A. Quintanilha. Severe depletion in liver glutathione during physical exercise. *Biochem. Biophys. Res. Commun.* 139:926–931, 1986.

108. Quintanilha, A. T. The effect of physical exercise and/or vitamin E on tissue oxidative metabolism. *Biochem. Soc. Trans.* 12:403–404, 1984.

109. Quintanilha, A. T., L. Packer, J. M. S. Davies, T. Racanelli, and K. J. A. Davies. Membrane

effects of vitamin E deficiency: bioenergetics and surface charge density studies of skeletal muscle and liver mitochondria. *Ann. N. Y. Acad. Sci.* 399:32–47, 1982.

110. Reddy, V. K., C. T. Kumar, M. Prasad, and P. Reddanna. Exercise-induced oxidant stress in the lung tissue: role of dietary supplementation of vitamin E and selenium. *Biochem. Int.* 26:863–871, 1992.

111. Reed, D. Regulation of reductive processes by glutathione. *Biochem. Pharmacol.* 35:7–13, 1986.

112. Rinstad, J., P. M. Tande, G. Norheim, and H. Refsum. Selenium deficiency and cardiac electrophysiological and mechanical function in the rat. *Pharmacol. Toxicol.* 63:189–192, 1988.

113. Robertson, J. D., R. J. Maughan, G. G. Duthie, and P. C. Morrice. Increased blood antioxidant systems of runners in response to training. *Clin. Sci.* 80:611–618, 1991.

114. Sahlin, K., K. Ekborg, and S. Cizinsky. Changes in plasma hypoxanthine and free radical markers during exercise in man. *Acta Physiol. Scand.* 142:275–281, 1991.

115. Salminen, A., and V. Vihko. Endurance training reduces the susceptibility of mouse skeletal muscle to lipid peroxidation in vitro. *Acta Physiol. Scand.* 117:109–113, 1983.

116. Sastre, J., M. Asensi, E. Gasco, et al. Exhaustive physical exercise causes oxidation of glutathione status in blood: prevention by antioxidant administration. *Am. J. Physiol.* 263:R992–R995, 1992.

117. Sen, C. K., E. Marin, M. Kretzschmar, and O. Hanninen. Skeletal muscle and liver glutathione homeostasis in response to training, exercise and immobilization. *J. Appl. Physiol.* 73:1265–1272, 1992.

118. Sen, C. K., T. Rankinen, S. Vaisanen, and R. Rauramaa. Oxidative stress following human exercise: effect of N-acetylcysteine supplementation. *J. Appl. Physiol.* 76:2570–2577, 1994.

119. Sen, C. K., P. Rahkila and O. Hanninen. Glutathione metabolism in skeletal muscle derived cells of the L6 line. *Acta Physiol. Scand.* 148:21–26, 1993.

120. Sies, H. (ed). *Oxidative Stress.* London: Academic Press, 1985.

121. Simmons, T. W., I. S. Jamall, and R. A. Lockshin. The effect of selenium deficiency on peroxidative injury in the house fly, *Musca domestica. FEBS Lett.* 218:251–254, 1987.

122. Sjodin, B., Y. Hellsten, and F. S. Apple. Biochemical mechanisms for oxygen free radical formation during exercise. *Sports Med.* 10:236–254, 1990.

123. Soares, M. J., K. Satyanarayana, M. S. Bamji, C. M. Jacom, Y. V. Ramana, and S. S. Rao. The effect of exercise on the riboflavin status of adult men. *Br. J. Nutr.* 69:541–551, 1993.

124. Spallholz, J., J. L. Martin, and H. E. Ganther. *Selenium in Biology and Medicine.* Westport, CT: AVI Press, 1981.

125. Srivastava, S. K., and E. Beutler. The transport of oxized glutathione from human erythrocytes. *J. Biol. Chem.* 244:9–16, 1969.

126. Starnes, J. W., G. Cantu, R. P. Farrar, and J. P. Kehrer. Skeletal muscle lipid peroxidation in exercise and food-restricted rats during aging. *J. Appl. Physiol.* 67:69–75, 1989.

127. Storz, G., L. A. Tartaglia, and B. N. Ames. Transcriptional regulator of oxidative stress-inducible genes: direct activation by oxidation. *Science* 248:189–194, 1990.

128. Tiidus, P. M., and M. E. Houston. Vitamin E status does not affect the responses to exercise training and acute exercise in female rats. *J. Nutr.* 123:834–840, 1993.

129. Tiidus, P. M., W. A. Behrens, R. Madere, and M. E. Houston. Muscle vitamin E levels following acute submaximal exercise in female rats. *Acta Physiol. Scand.* 147:249–250, 1993.

130. Tiidus, P. M., W. A. Behrens, R. Madere, J. J. Kim, and M. E. Houston. Effects of vitamin E status and exercise training on tissue lipid peroxidation based on two methods of assessment. *Nutr. Res.* 13:219–224, 1993.

131. van Dokkum, W., and E. J. van der Beek. Vitamins and physical performance *Voeding* 46:50–56, 1985.

132. van der Beek, E. J., W. van Dokkum, and J. Schrijver. Thiamin, riboflavin, and vitamins B-6 and C: impact of combined restricted intake on functional performance in man. *Am. J. Clin. Nutr.* 48:1451–1462, 1988.

133. Vertechy, M., M. B. Cooper, O. Chirardi, and M. T. Ramacci. Antioxidant enzyme activities in heart and skeletal muscle of rats of different ages. *Exp. Gerontol.* 24:211–218, 1989.
134. Viguie, C. A., B. Frei, M. K. Shigenaga, B. Ames, L. Packer, and G. A. Brooks. Antioxidant status and indexes of oxidative stress during consecutive days of exercise. *J. Appl. Physiol.* 75:566–572, 1993.
135. Vihko, V., A. Salminen, and J. Rantamaki. Oxidative lysosomal capacity in skeletal muscle of mice after endurance training. *Acta Physiol. Scand.* 104:74–79, 1978.
136. Vina, J. *Glutathione: Metabolism and Physiological Function.* J. Vina (ed). Boca Raton, FL: CRC Press, 1993.
137. Weglicki, W. B., Z. Luna, and P. P. Nair. Sex and tissue specific differences in concentrations of ∝-tocopherol in mature and senescent rats. *Nature* 221:185, 1969.
138. Winter, L. R. T., J. S. Yoon, H. J. Kalkwarf, et al. Riboflavin requirements and exercise adaptation in older women. *Am. J. Clin. Nutr.* 56:526–532, 1992.
139. Yu, B. P. Cellular defenses against damage from reactive oxygen species. *Physiol Rev.* 74:139–162, 1994.
140. Zerba, E., T. E. Komorowski, and J. A. Faulkner. Free radical injury to skeletal muscle of young, adult and old mice. *Am. J. Physiol.* 258:C429–C435, 1990.

6
Functional Morphology and Motor Control of Series-Fibered Muscles

JOHN A. TROTTER, Ph.D.
FRANCES J. R. RICHMOND, Ph.D.
PETER P. PURSLOW, Ph.D.

Muscles occur in a diversity of forms. These forms do not exist merely to give a pleasing shape to the body, as was once suggested by Aristotle [46]. It is now well established that adaptations in neuromuscular architecture confer useful functional specializations. Previous reviews of muscle physiology in this and other sources have discussed in great detail the physiological consequences of pinnate fiber arrangements [47, 48, 101] and intramuscular compartmentalization [104, 137, 152], and have drawn attention to the important roles of aponeuroses and tendons for the storage of energy and redirection of force [e.g., 3, 48]. Often ignored in these discussions are the seemingly simpler, straplike or sheetlike muscles with parallel fibers. This lack of attention presumably stems from implicit or even explicitly stated assumptions that fibers composing straplike muscles run the whole length of their fascicles no matter how long the muscle is [3]. The physiological properties of such muscles are therefore often modeled as if they were scaled-up versions of a single muscle fiber. However, a history of observations has shown this assumption to be false. Strap muscles are often composed of relatively short, serially arranged muscle fibers with interdigitated ends. This structure clearly has a number of implications for muscle function and dysfunction. The occurrence in a wide range of species and a basic description of the architecture of series-fibered muscles have been reviewed recently by Gaunt and Gans [51] and Trotter [151]. This review will concentrate on the functional implications of the series-fibered muscle architecture. We will explore the ways such muscles must work to generate useful forces and will speculate how certain pathologies may affect their performance.

ANALYSES OF FIBER ARCHITECTURE

Studies on Human Muscles

In the introduction to a recent textbook on muscle, Hoyle [64] noted that scientists have a penchant for "losing knowledge about muscle." The history of architectural studies on parallel-fibered muscles seems to support his

167

contention. On numerous occasions over the past century or more, anatomists have studied the internal structure of parallel-fibered muscles by softening the connective tissues of such muscles and then dissecting their constituent fascicles, one fiber at a time. A favorite preparation for such work has been human sartorius, which, at a length of 50–60 cm, is considered to have the longest span of any parallel-fibered muscle in the human body. In the earliest studies, Froriep [45] and Felix [42] noted the presence of fibers that tapered and ended intrafascicularly. The longest fibers dissected by Felix were approximately 12 cm. Since that time, the presence of relatively short, serially arranged fibers has been confirmed by additional investigators, but inconsistencies can be noted in the reported lengths of single fibers. Lockhardt and Brandt [83] dissected single fibers up to 34 cm long, the longest of which had broken ends, indicating that its length was underestimated. In contrast, the intact fibers reported by others [8, 58, 127] tended to be shorter, with most fibers ranging between 5 and 18 cm long. Some of the variability seen in the reported numbers might be expected because of the technical difficulties associated with the dissections in sartorius. A single muscle fiber 15 cm long is generally no more than 50 μm in diameter, yielding an aspect ratio (length/diameter) of 3000! These long, delicate fibers are often further weakened by the pretreatments necessary to break down intramuscular connective tissues. Thus, it would not be surprising to find that most reported data are skewed by a sampling bias toward shorter fibers. Nevertheless, all of these investigators agree that fibers with intrafascicular terminations are a characteristic of human sartorius.

Do other human muscles have short, in-series fiber arrangements or is sartorius a special case? The only other long human muscle to be microdissected systematically is gracilis, where a similar architecture of relatively short, intrafascicularly terminating fibers has been observed [127]. A number of human muscles in the back, neck, and limbs also have long spans and parallel fiber fascicles, but many of these muscles remain to be studied. It is clear, however, that serial fiber arrangements are not present in all skeletal muscles. Microdissections in a variety of relatively short muscles such as those of the hand or larynx have shown that their constituent fibers run from the aponeurosis of origin to that of insertion [26, 40, 127]. Some of the longer muscles, such as semitendinosus and rectus abdominis, are crossed by bands of connective tissue that serve as points of insertion for fibers [30]. In these muscles, sets of muscle fibers can be arranged in series by attaching to the inscriptions rather than by terminating intrafascicularly. (However, even within a compartment of fibers bounded by inscriptions, intrafascicularly terminating fibers can be found [30].)

What remains unclear is the arrangement of fibers in muscles lacking tendinous inscriptions whose fascicles have lengths of between about 10 and 40 cm. The detailed reports of von Schwarzacher [127] suggest that muscles in this category, such as pectoralis minor, biceps brachii, and trapezius, are composed of fibers that run the entire distance between the muscle origin and insertion. However, more recent observations in at least one of these muscles, biceps brachii, may be inconsistent with this simple view. Most skeletal muscle fibers have a single point of innervation (motor-end-plate) at approximately the middle of their lengths. Using acetylcholinesterase staining, both Christensen [23] and Aquilonius [5] showed that biceps brachii had two end-plate bands, suggesting the presence of short fibers running only part of the muscle length. The presence of more than one end-plate zone was also demonstrated electrophysiologically by McComas and his colleagues [96]. Unfortunately, no microdissections have been performed since in this muscle to confirm the conclusions of von Schwarzacher [127] that all of its fibers run from tendon to tendon. In obliquus externus, another long muscle containing parallel fiber fascicles, Bardeen [7] found no fibers that ran the entire length of the "muscle-bundle" from which they were taken. Thus, in-series arrangements of fibers may be more common than generally has been assumed, but more information will be necessary if we are to understand the occurrence of serial fiber arrangements in human muscles.

Microdissections of Animal Muscles
Further insight into the occurrence of in-series fiber architectures can be obtained from animal studies, in which a broader range of muscles can be examined more conveniently. In 1916, Huber [65] demonstrated convincingly that many long muscles in avian and mammalian species were composed of fibers that were shorter than the fascicles in which they were found. These fibers seldom ran for more than 1–3 cm before tapering and ending intrafascicularly. In the cat, a similar pattern of in-series fiber architecture has since been identified in several long limb muscles (Fig. 6.1), including gracilis [27], biceps femoris [22], tenuissimus [2, 18, 28, 84], sartorius [28, 79, 84], and semitendinosus [84]. In all of these parallel-fibered muscles, single muscle fibers were usually 2–3 cm long. In a muscle such as feline sartorius, fibers were found to run about one-fifth to one-third of the length of the 10-cm fascicles in which they were found. This ratio is interesting because it is similar to the ratio of fiber lengths to fascicle lengths reported in the human sartorius [58]. Thus, the feline muscle looks in some ways like a shrunken version of its counterpart in man. The shrinkage is, however, in one axis only. Feline and human muscle fibers have similar cross-sectional areas [58, 132]. Thus, the aspect ratios of feline muscle fibers are lower than those in man. Because aspect ratios are lower, microdissections of animal muscles are technically less difficult, although still very tedious and time consuming.

From the published data on feline hindlimb muscles, it is tempting to conclude that fiber length may be specified by some as-yet unrecognized rule. In-series fiber organization might therefore be expected in muscles whose fascicle lengths exceed the limit on fiber length specified for a given

FIGURE 6.1.

Microscopic appearance of a tapered muscle fiber from feline rhomboideus muscle. Thicker muscle-fiber shafts can be identified in the same field. Bar = 100 μm.

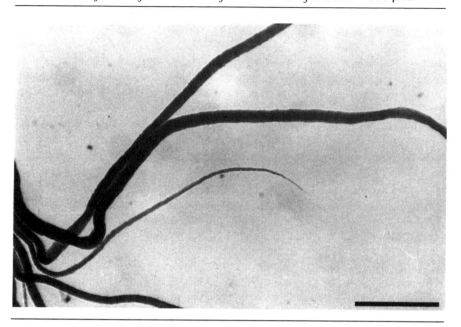

species. However, some recent architectural studies on short and long muscles in the cat may argue against such a simple view. For example, the fascicle lengths in the pinnate soleus muscle, which contains only continuous fibers, are 4 cm, and are thus longer than the typical lengths of single muscle fibers in series-fibered hindlimb muscles [136]. On the other hand, in the feline diaphragm and a variety of neck muscles, fascicle lengths are shorter than 4 cm, but still contain many fibers with intrafascicular terminations. In the neck muscles, biventer cervicis and splenius, for example, fibers with intrafascicular terminations appear to have somewhat shorter lengths (1–2 cm) than those dissected in hindlimb muscles (2–3 cm) [117, 119, 129].

Do the lengths of fibers with intrafascicular terminations scale simply with the relative size of the species, as comparisons between human and feline sartorius muscles might imply? The weight of the current evidence suggests that the answer is "no." However, relatively few quantitative studies have been conducted in other mammalian species, especially large species, and some of these results require confirmation. In the rat, fiber lengths seem similar to those reported in feline muscles. For example, intrafascicularly terminating fibers from the gracilis and rectus abdominis muscles, are reported to measure 1.5–3.0 cm long [60, 61, 153]. Electrophysiological recordings from muscle fibers in semitendinosus and biceps femoris also suggest that most fibers have a similar range of lengths [87]. However, von Schwarzacher [126] reported that fibers with intrafascicular terminations were longer, from 4 to 8 cm, in rodent gracilis. Fibers with intrafascicular terminations also have been reported to have relatively short lengths in some mammalian species at the other end of the size continuum. For example, microdissections in limb muscles in the goat have revealed the presence of many 2-cm fibers and electrophysiological recordings suggested that fibers longer than 6 cm are rare, even though the fascicle lengths in the goat muscles are much longer than those in the cat or rat [49]. Fibers ranging between 2 and 3 cm are also typical in shoulder muscles of the horse [123]. However, rather longer fibers (about 5 cm) have been dissected from the sternomandibularis of the cow [111].

Muscles with in-series fibers are not found only in mammalian taxa. Fibers with tapering ends have been reported in turtles [20], frogs [28, 93], and birds [50, 150]. Avian muscles contain particularly short fibers with tapered ends (0.4–2.6 cm) [50].

From the careful fiber-length studies done so far, a curious inconsistency seems to emerge. Muscle fibers in humans (and possibly other primates) seem to be significantly longer than those in other species. Why this difference should be present is not at all clear, but it suggests that the relatively shorter lengths of fibers in the other animals do not occur because of some limiting mechanical or electrical property of individual fibers, as has been previously suggested [84, 85]. Indeed, the observation that specific muscles have their own characteristic patterns of relative fiber lengths raises the question whether this aspect of muscle structure is associated with some specific functional advantages, although what these advantages might be remains an open question.

INNERVATION OF MUSCLES WITH IN-SERIES FIBERS

Muscles containing short, in-series fibers have different patterns of innervation than those in which fibers run from tendon to tendon. Motor nerves must course proximally and distally to innervate fibers at different levels between the muscle origin and insertion. Thus muscles with serially arranged fibers can generally be recognized following reaction for acetylcholinesterase activity by the presence of two or more motor-end-plate bands crossing the muscle at different proximodistal levels. In the longest muscles, fascicles may be crossed by multiple bands in a ladderlike pattern (illustrated, for example, in refs. 1, 27, 49, 52, 84, 127, and 150). The end-plate bands seldom appear to cross the whole width of the muscle in a contiguous line, as is generally observed in muscles with short fascicles. Instead, adjacent sets of fascicles often have bands that are out of register, although the spacings between the bands are similar from one column to the next. The multiple motor-end-plate bands are present at birth in human infants and in other animals [1, 23, 50, 53]. Their spacings in the small neonatal muscles are appropriately scaled down. As the fascicles grow longer, the end-plate bands become more widely spaced.

The patterns of nerve branching in muscles with serially arranged fibers can be quite complex. In the cat, where most experimental work has been carried out, perhaps the most specialized patterns are found in the neck and trunk. The long muscles in the neck, for example, are supplied by a number of separate nerve bundles that arise from different spinal segments and enter the muscle at different rostrocaudal levels (Fig. 6.2) [117, 118, 119]. The motor axons in these nerve bundles supply muscle fibers in territories close to the site of nerve entry. As a consequence, the fibers comprising a single motor unit are confined both rostrocaudally and mediolaterally within a small subvolume of the muscle. The splenius muscle has a particularly interesting organization that exemplifies the range of innervation patterns that can exist in neck muscles (Fig. 6.2B). It is innervated by sets of motor axons from four cervical segments; each set supplies muscle fibers at different rostrocaudal levels. In the lateral regions of splenius, tendinous inscriptions separate the motor territories supplied by each segmental nerve (Fig. 6.3). Between these inscriptions, muscle-fiber fascicles are short (usually less than 2–3 cm), and fibers with intrafascicular terminations are rare. In medial regions, however, no inscriptions are present; fibers supplied from one segment have tapering ends that interdigitate with the ends of fibers innervated by adjacent spinal segments [117].

Long limb muscles can also be supplied by motoneurons from more than one spinal segment, but these axons become grouped to form a single muscle-nerve bundle. Thus, cursory inspection might suggest that the nerve supply to the long limb muscles is simpler than that to axial muscles. However, closer analysis of the nerve supply to at least one long muscle, the feline sartorius, has shown some interesting complexities. Sartorius in the cat is a long, sheetlike muscle that originates from the iliac crest and runs to a wide insertion. The anterior part of the muscle inserts onto the patellar ligament, whereas more medial fascicles attach progressively along the tibial plateau (Fig. 6.4). This distributed insertion is paralleled by a specialized pattern of nerve branching in which single nerve branches from the parent bundle supply different strips of muscle fibers lying in parallel to one another [84]. Stimulation of branches serving the anterior part of sartorius leads to a mechanical action that tends to flex the hip but extend the knee. However, stimulation of strips in medial sartorius flexes both the hip and the knee. The capacity to control these motor units separately is reflected in the differing patterns of recruitment recorded in the two muscle parts during natural behaviors such as locomotion. When the alert cat walks, the anterior part of sartorius is active at different times than is the medial part of the same muscle [62, 109].

FIGURE 6.2.

Innervation of feline splenius muscle. The top line drawing shows the distribution of muscle nerve branches with respect to anatomical features on the ventral surface of the muscle. The schematic below shows the distribution of depleted muscle fibers following prolonged stimulation of C3 nerve bundles. Dense hatching represents an area composed almost exclusively of depleted fibers; light hatching shows regions containing a mixture of depleted and nondepleted profiles. Modified from ref. 117.

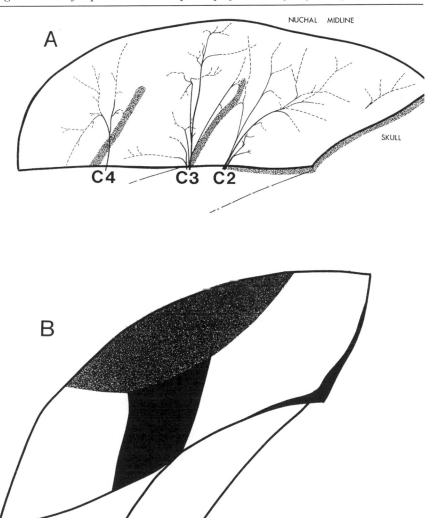

FIGURE 6.3.

Arrangement of short, serially arranged fibers in the splenius muscle. The lower panel shows the lengths and proximodistal positions of individual fibers dissected from the corresponding regions marked in the line drawing above. Note in B that an inscription divides the fascicles into two in-series regions.

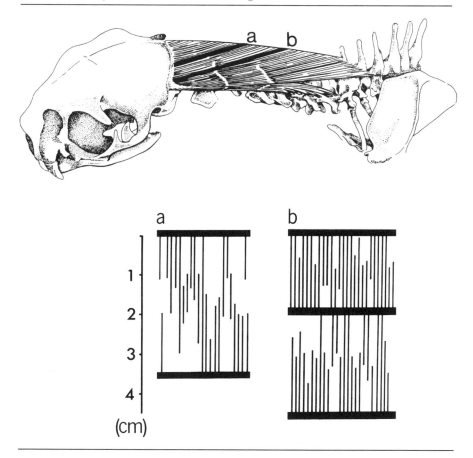

What was not expected from the behavioral observations of in-parallel compartmentalization was an additional nonuniformity in motor-unit distribution. This nonuniformity occurs in the in-series organization of motor units in anterior sartorius. The main nerve bundle that approaches anterior sartorius divides in a relatively predictable way: two main nerve branches course in opposite directions to enter the proximal and distal parts of the muscle, whereas a third (smaller) branch often enters the muscle centrally. Stimulation of a proximal or distal branch causes contractions that are stronger at one muscle end. When the stimulation is continued and the innervated motor units are glycogen-depleted, depleted fibers are found to be distributed

FIGURE 6.4.

Distribution of fibers belonging to a single motor unit in the anterior head of feline sartorius. A, schematized line drawing of the muscle to show its anatomical relationships with the skeleton. B, distribution of fibers depleted after intracellular stimulation of a single motoneuron, shown as dots on spaced muscle cross-sections. Note that more depleted profiles are present in proximal than distal cross-sections. Modified from ref. 132.

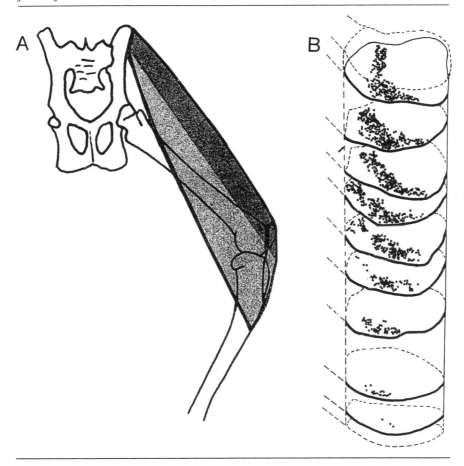

more densely at one end of the muscle than the other [141]. Further evidence that the proximal and distal motor-unit populations are largely separate has been provided by neuroanatomical studies in which the proximal and distal nerve branches were exposed to different retrograde tracers [54]. Relatively few motoneurons were double-labeled by this approach. Interestingly, the motoneurons labeled from proximal and distal nerve branches were intermixed in a common territory within the sartorius motor nucleus.

More definitive examinations of single motor units in feline sartorius have recently been conducted by impaling and stimulating single sartorius motoneurons using intracellular electrodes [132]. In anterior sartorius, the glycogen-depleted fibers belonging to the stimulated motor unit were scattered among nondepleted fibers belonging to other motor units (Fig. 6.5). They were confined within only a part of a muscle cross-section and were also distributed asymmetrically along the proximodistal axis (Fig. 6.4). In most of these motor units, a few fibers were found at the end opposite to that with the largest concentration of fibers. However, at least one case was observed in which the territory of the motor unit did not extend from one end of the muscle to the other. A few motor units were also depleted in medial sartorius, but fibers in these motor units were distributed more uniformly from the origin to insertion. In either part of sartorius, the number of fibers lying in parallel to one another at any one cross-sectional level was only a fraction of the total number of muscle fibers contained in the motor unit.

If some of the fibers in a motor unit are in series rather than in parallel, there are important consequences for the capacity of the motor unit to develop force. This is because the total force that can be developed by a motor unit is related to the sum of forces generated by fibers (or, more basically, myofilaments) lying in parallel, not in series, to one another. Thus, as previously argued by Edgerton and his colleagues [37], the forces developed by single motor units in sartorius might be predicted to be smaller than those in a muscle with continuous fibers such as soleus, even though motor units in the two different muscles contain similar numbers of fibers. This problem is illustrated in Figure 6.6, which attempts to show how force development will depend upon the way in which muscle fibers of a single motor unit are distributed. If all of the fibers were arranged in parallel (e.g., Fig. 6.6A) the motor unit would retain maximum force-generating capacity but might encounter problems in transferring those forces through the remaining muscle in which it had no fibers. Balanced force production would then seem to depend upon the synchronous activation of motor units at different proximodistal levels. In muscles such as biventer cervicis and splenius, where in-series compartments of motor units are seen, electromyogram records from different compartments have indeed shown well-matched patterns of activity [120]. Alternatively, muscle fibers comprising a single motor unit might be distributed in serial arrays from the muscle origin to insertion (Fig. 6.6, B and C). This arrangement would ensure relatively even levels of force production along the proximodistal axis of the muscle but would reduce the effective functional cross-sectional area of the single motor unit. In anterior sartorius, an intermediate pattern, like that illustrated in Figure 6.6C, is observed.

It is not yet clear whether motor units with primarily proximal or distal territories in anterior sartorius are used differently during normal behaviors or reflexes. As early as 1910, Sherrington [131] made the provocative observation that flexion reflexes in decerebrate cats caused the *proximal* but not the *distal* part of anterior sartorius to contract. Crossed-extension

FIGURE 6.5.

Sizes and distribution of depleted muscle fibers in feline sartorius. Top, transverse sections at different proximodistal levels, approximately 5 mm apart, to show the same depleted fibers marked by arrows. Both of these profiles have become smaller in the lower photomicrograph. Bottom, histogram to show the cross-sectional areas of muscle fibers intersected by a single transverse section through sartorius; the column marked by an asterisk presumably represents profiles of tapering fiber ends like those in the photomicrograph above. Modified from ref. 132.

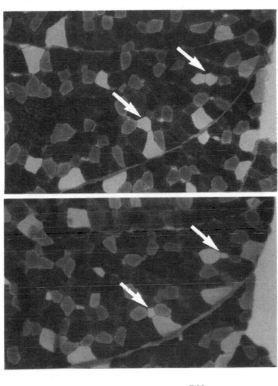

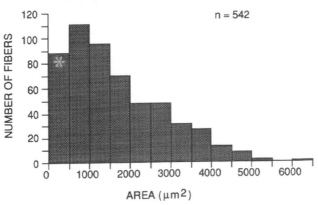

FIGURE 6.6.

Diagrammatic representation of possible arrangements of fibers composing a single motor unit in a long, straplike muscle. In A, all fibers lie in parallel at one level (e.g., biventer cervicis, splenius, semitendinosus). In this situation, muscle fibers have their largest cross-sectional area at one level, but face the problem of transmitting those forces through the motor units in series with them. In B, fibers are distributed evenly along the long axis of the muscle. This arrangement may avoid gross heterogeneities of force production at different cross-sectional levels, but may reduce the force-developing capacity of the motor unit because fewer fibers are functionally in parallel at any one level. No muscles have been identified in which depleted fibers all tie tightly apposed to one another as illustrated here for simplicity, but in medial sartorius, fibers in a single motor unit seem to be distributed quite evenly in a narrow column (see ref. 132). In C, most fibers are concentrated at one level of the muscle and the number of fibers diminishes progressively with distance from the level of maximum density (e.g., anterior sartorius). This arrangement combines the functional consequences of the more extreme arrangements in A and B.

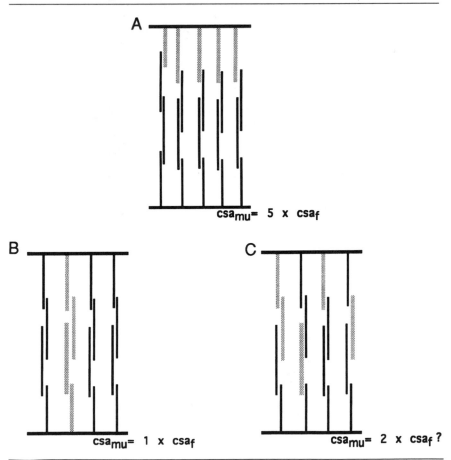

reflexes produced an opposite pattern of contraction in the distal but not the proximal part of anterior sartorius. In contrast, EMG recordings made from different proximodistal levels of anterior sartorius in chronically instrumented, alert animals showed no clear evidence for nonuniform motor-unit activation during flexion reflexes elicited by electrical stimulation of the sensory fibers in saphenous or sural nerves [108]. However, EMG methods are not ideal for demonstrating anything but the most robust differences in the recruitment of motor units at the two muscle ends. Even if motor units at one end were recruited much more strongly than those at the other end, EMG signals might still be detected at all proximodistal levels.

It is difficult to understand whether the nonuniform distribution of motor units at different proximodistal levels of muscles such as the feline anterior sartorius and splenius has some functional advantage related, for example, to the recruitment of different combinations of motor units or whether it is simply an adaptively neutral aspect of intramuscular design that must be accommodated by appropriate neural programming. Some insight into the mechanical problems inherent in an in-series fiber arrangement can be gained by stimulating one of the two or more muscle nerve branches entering the muscle at different proximodistal levels in isolation and comparing the resulting contractions with those produced by stimulating all branches concurrently, an approach taken in studies of canine semimembranosus [88] and feline anterior sartorius [128]. When only one nerve branch was stimulated, one muscle end shortened at the expense of the other even though the muscle was held isometrically. Furthermore, the forces produced by the contracting motor units were found to be relatively low, as might be expected of shortening rather than isometrically held fibers [128]. The apparent force length curve was shifted to the right; it was only at long lengths that the weakly activated region at one muscle end was stretched to a sufficiently high level of passive force that it resisted further stretching by the opposite, strongly contracting end.

Experiments such as those conducted by Scott et al. [128] are unlikely to reflect a physiological pattern of activation. In the normal animal, motor units are generally recruited according to a size principle in which the smallest, slowest motor units are activated first [57]. If the whole population of motoneurons supplying anterior sartorius were to be activated as a single pool, fibers at all proximodistal levels (which have a relatively even fiber-type composition [F. J. R. Richmond, unpublished observations]) should be activated in a relatively uniform manner. An interesting question that yet must be explored experimentally is whether the compliance of the muscle is greater at low levels of motor-unit activation—when large numbers of passive fibers must be interspersed between relatively small numbers of active ones—than at high levels, when most fibers are active. The presence of such a compliance would seem to make it more difficult for the few active motor units to transmit their forces effectively along the muscle length. However, slow, oxidative fibers (which are the only fibers thought to be recruited at the lowest levels of motorneuron activation) have a specialized pattern of distribution that might enhance their abilities to transfer forces to active neighbors. These fibers are confined to central locations in muscle fascicles, forming a core that is surrounded by fast fiber subtypes. When a slow-oxidative motor unit has been stimulated until its glycogen is depleted, it is not uncommon to see more than one depleted profile in the core of each fascicle. Thus, even if only a few motor units were recruited at different proximodistal levels, these contracting fibers might be distributed in a way that would optimize force transmission between active fibers by reducing the distance between them occupied by inactive fibers. Additionally, it is argued below that, on theoretical grounds, the compliance contributed by passive cellular and extracellular components could be too small to have any functional significance.

In-series muscles function quite effectively under normal conditions, but there are situations in which this architecture may pose special problems. The most obvious of these situations is that which presents when the muscle has been paralyzed by spinal-cord damage and reanimation can only be achieved by electrically stimulating the muscle clinically. In muscles with short fascicles and a single end-plate band, stimuli can be delivered to a single proximodistal level without fear that nonuniform contractions will occur along the muscle length. However, in a series-fibered muscle, recent experiments suggest that stimulation at a single level may activate fibers unevenly. In this situation strong contractions may occur at only one level of the muscle (T. Cameron, unpublished observations). The strongly active fibers presumably will stretch the more weakly activated fibers in series with them, in a way comparable with that described by Scott et al. [128]. To develop effective clinical therapies, it will be critical to identify those muscles in which reanimation can be achieved only by stimulating at more than one intramuscular site.

Markee and Lowenbach [88] also identified an additional concern when long in-series muscles are traumatized or subjected to surgical manipulation. They stated that "a new concept must be adopted of the functional significance of the branches of the nerve supplying a given muscle. Interruption of a branch may diminish the effective work produced by contraction of a muscle because that part of the length of the muscle may stretch . . . This new concept . . . suggests the necessity of meticulously avoiding, in surgical procedures, interference with even the minor branches of motor nerve supply."

FORCE TRANSMISSION IN MUSCLES WITH IN-SERIES FIBERS

The growing numbers of studies that document the presence of in-series fiber arrangements are at odds with the common view that skeletal muscle fibers act as parallel independent force-generating elements embedded in a frictionless matrix [47]. Such an organization is clearly not present in muscles containing discontinuous fibers because in-series muscle fibers are not attached to their own stiff tendinous strands that span the distance between the fiber ends and the distant tendon [147, 150]. Therefore they cannot function exclusively in parallel. In some muscles the in-series fibers are mechanically coupled through myomyous junctions [9, 16, 43, 61, 95, 139, 145, 155]. In most instances, however, the muscle fibers lack such junctions, and are instead embedded in a continuous network of endomysium, to which they must transmit tension. Furthermore, a number of studies have shown that the fibers that compose a motor unit usually are not adjacent to one another [13, 14, 79, 102, 132]. Therefore, the tension applied to the tendons of a muscle in which a single motor unit contracts must be transmitted not only through the endomysium, but also through passive fibers [147, 149, 150, 151], some of which are in parallel and some of which are in series with the active fibers. The concept that arises from these developing facts is that an in-series skeletal muscle is functionally a composite material in which active and passive fibers and the connective tissue that binds them together all contribute to its mechanical output.

Two important consequences derive from this model. First, the development of intramuscular shear forces must be a necessary condition for the transmission of force. Second, the intramuscular distribution and regional concentration of these shear forces must be affected by the amount and characteristics of the connective tissue matrix (i.e., the endomysium and the perimysium) by which the fibers and fascicles are surrounded and by the shear properties of both active and passive muscle fibers. However, relatively little research has been directed at understanding the role of intramuscular connective tissue in force transmission, and no studies have been done on the shear properties of muscle fibers. The remainder of this review will consider the interactions between muscle fibers and connective tissue in the muscle-connective tissue composite.

Functional Consequences of Fiber Morphology

Because all skeletal muscles consist of long muscle fibers embedded in a connective tissue matrix, they can be treated as members of the class of load-bearing materials known as fiber-reinforced composites [66, 71, 106]. This class of materials can be divided into two broad subclasses on the basis of the length of the fibers relative to the length of the structure. In continuous-fibered composites the fibers are as long as the structure, whereas in discontinuous-fibered composites they are shorter, sometimes much shorter, than the structure (Fig. 6.7). The tensile properties of continuous-fibered composites conform to the "Rule of Mixtures," which expresses the concept that the fibrous and nonfibrous phases are functionally in parallel and therefore act independently of one another. According to this rule the

FIGURE 6.7.

Schematic drawing of a continuous (A) and discontinuous (B) fibered composite strained by a tensile load (σ_c). See text for explanation.

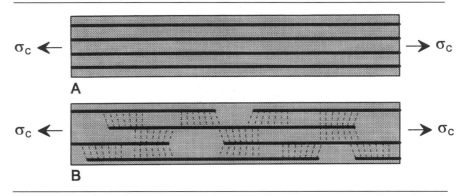

elastic modulus (E) of the composite (c) is the summed elastic moduli of the fibers (f) and the interfiber matrix (m), proportional to the volume fraction (V) of each. In algebraic notation:

$$E_c = E_f V_f + E_m V_m \qquad (1)$$

where $V_f + V_m = 1$.

The elastic (Young's) modulus is, for linearly elastic materials, the proportionality constant that relates stress (σ) to strain (ϵ), i.e., $E = \sigma/\epsilon$, and is therefore an expression of the stiffness of the material. The isometric tension (or stress) of vertebrate muscles contracting at their optimum lengths is, on average, about 300 kPa [25]. The strain within single contracting frog muscle fibers associated with this stress is about 1.3% [68]. Thus we can calculate that for single muscle fibers contracting isometrically near their optimum lengths, $E_f = 23$ MPa.

Collagen constitutes on the order of 5% of the dry mass of muscle [4, 10] and, we can assume, contributes a similar fraction to the muscle volume. Thus, even though the endomysial matrix has a negligible tensile modulus at the optimum length of the muscle, as is discussed below, the tensile properties of the composite muscle would be reduced by no greater amount than the volume fraction of the matrix. Because of difficulties associated with obtaining accurate cross-sectional areas of muscles or muscle fibers, stress estimates for skeletal muscles generally do not achieve an accuracy of ±5%. The small volume fraction of the connective tissue matrix together with the lack of accuracy of stress determinations on whole muscles have led to the concept that the mechanical contributions of the connective tissues to the active stiffness of a skeletal muscle are negligible. This view has found support in the numerous observations that the only regions of most muscle fibers in which the specific morphology has any mechanical significance are the ends, where muscle fibers form specialized muscle-tendon junctions (MTJs) with the tendon [144, 151] or with other muscle fibers through myomyous junctions [9, 16, 43, 61, 95, 139, 145, 155]. But the apparent morphological suitability of the MTJ to transmit stress between muscle and connective tissue, together with the absence of any such specialized junctions along the lateral surfaces of most muscle fibers, should not be interpreted to mean that stress transfer occurs only at the MTF or at myomyous junctions. Even in continuous-fibered muscles there is good evidence, some of which is discussed below, for lateral mechanical coupling between muscle fibers and endomysium [19, 29, 35].

In contrast to continuous-fiber composites, those with discontinuous fibers possess fibrous and nonfibrous phases that are functionally in series, rather than in parallel, and therefore do not function independently of each other. This situation is shown diagramatically in Figure 6.7, in which the interfiber matrix is seen to transfer stress between fibers through shearing interactions. Because the fibers and the matrix are functionally in series, the rule of mixtures has to be modified by the incorporation of additional terms, including those that express the size, spacing, and packing geometry of the fibers as well as the shear modulus of the matrix (G_m). Several slightly different expressions have been derived for cylindrical fibers of circular cross-section, all of which have the general properties expressed in the following equation [66]:

$$\sigma_c = \{E_f V_f (1-[(\tanh(\beta 1/2)/(\beta 1/2)] + E_m V_m\}\epsilon_c \qquad (2)$$

where the value of β depends on the ratio of the shear modulus of the matrix, G_m, to the tensile modulus of the fiber, E_f (i.e., G_m/E_f), and on the specific packing geometry and spacing of the fibers. As 1 becomes large, the expression $\tanh(\beta 1/2)/(\beta 1/2)$ approaches 0 and the composite modulus approaches that of continuous fibered composites, i.e., the equation for discontinuous fibered composites reduces to the Rule of Mixtures. Because the value of $\tanh(\beta 1/2)/(\beta 1/2)$ also decreases toward 0 as the values of G_m and s (the fiber aspect ratio) increase, similarly stiff composites can result from having fibers of high aspect ratio in a low modulus matrix or vice versa.

As in all discontinuous-fiber composite materials, the aspect ratio of the fiber and the shape of the fiber end play crucial roles in the distribution of stress and strain in the composite formed from muscle and connective tissue. Figure 6.8 represents an idealized composite consisting of a single muscle fiber in an amorphous matrix, the modulus of which is significantly

FIGURE 6.8.

Schematic drawing of the strain pattern in the matrix of a single-fiber composite in which the fiber is a circular cylinder, unloaded (A) and loaded in tension (B). Tensile stress is indicated by σ_c. The interfacial shear stress (τ_i) and fiber tensile stress (σ_f) are shown in C and D, respectively.

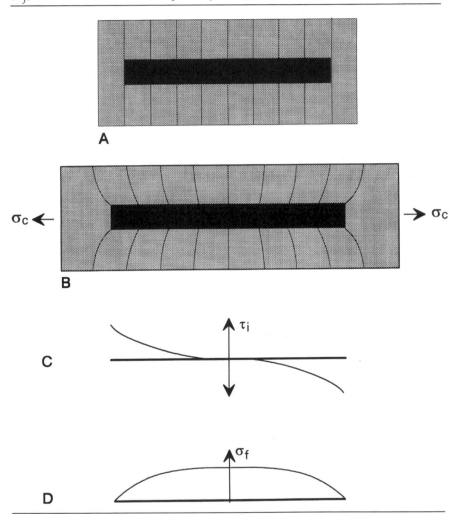

lower than that of the fiber. When the composite is loaded in tension there are stress and strain in the composite as a whole (σ_c and ϵ_c), as well as in the fibers and the matrix. The strain pattern in the matrix is indicated by the skew of the vertical lines in Figure 6.8, A and B. The end of the fiber is assumed to have no special adherence to the matrix. The composite tensile stress (σ_c) includes the tensile stress in the fiber (σ_f) and the matrix (σ_m)

and also produces an interfacial shear stress between the fiber and the matrix (τ_i). As shown in Figure 6.8, the load is transferred between the matrix and the fiber nonuniformly. The interfacial shear stress is maximal at the fiber ends and declines toward the middle of the fiber. On the other hand, the tensile stress within the fiber is maximal in the center of the fiber and declines toward the fiber ends. There are two significant consequences of these physical properties of composites. First, toward the ends of the fiber, its tensile strength is unused because the internal tensile stress drops as the interfacial shear stress increases, and so there is more material in the cross-section than necessary. This is obviously an inefficient use of the fiber end. Second, the interfacial shear stress near the fiber ends is significantly greater than elsewhere. If the matrix has uniform shear properties, the strain near the fiber end is thus greater than elsewhere. These nonuniformities are undesirable because they create stress concentrations within the composite, and it is well understood that stress concentrations lead to the failure of materials [74, 106].

It can be appreciated from Figure 6.8 that the transfer of stress between the fiber and the matrix occurs over a finite length of the fiber, the "transfer length." Fiber composite theory has established that fibers of a given radius must be as long as or longer than a critical transfer length (l_c) for the tensile stress in the fiber to reach its breaking stress. The critical length is directly proportional to the tensile strength of the fiber (σ_{fu}) and to its radius (r_f), and inversely proportional to the yield strength of the matrix (τ_{my}):

$$l_c = r\sigma_{fu}/\tau_{my} \tag{3}$$

Therefore, in terms of fiber diameter, the critical aspect ratio for the fiber ($s_c = l_c/d_d$) is given by the expression:

$$s_c = \sigma_{fu}/2\tau_{my} \tag{4}$$

The ultimate strength of an active muscle fiber during stretch is about 1.8 times the isometric stress of about 300 kPa, or about 540 kPa [97]. Thus, if a fiber 50 μm in diameter were only 1.25 cm long, its aspect ratio ($1/d$) would be 250. It could conceivably carry its maximum tensile load in a matrix with a yield strength of only 1 kPa. A yield strength of 1 kPa is very low; it approaches that of strong gelatin. The interesting and significant inference from this is that a muscle composed of discontinuous fibers that lack specific myomyous junctions can be macromechanically indistinguishable from a continuous-fibered muscle despite the fact that the micromechanics are distinctly different. This follows from the high aspect ratios of skeletal muscle fibers. It is also not unreasonable to suppose that the shear strength of passive muscle fibers could easily approach this value, which could be an important supposition because passive fibers also have to transmit shearing loads in series-fibered muscles [150].

The preceding discussion of the stress distribution along a cylindrical fiber naturally leads to a consideration of the possibility of modifying the stress distribution by altering the fiber shape. If that part of the muscle fiber associated with stress transfer had a conical shape, both the interfacial shear stress and the internal tensile stress of the fiber would remain constant [21, 150]. Figure 6.9 diagramatically illustrates the uniform shear and tensile stresses achieved by conical ends. The magnitude of the average surface stress in a conical end can be calculated by resolving the tensile stress in the fiber (σ_f) into its two orthogonally related components, one normal to the tapered surface (σ_t) and one parallel to it (τ_i), as illustrated in Figure 6.10A, in which

$$\sigma_t = \sigma_f \sin^2 \varphi \qquad (5)$$

and

$$\tau_i = \sigma_f \sin \phi \cos \varphi \qquad (6)$$

where φ is the taper angle. Because the cosine of small angles is close to unity, the shear stress along the tapered surfaces is approximately proportional to $\sin\varphi$.

Only a few estimates have been made of the average taper angle of muscle fibers. In a serial-section study of slow and fast fibers from cat tibialis anterior muscles, Eldred et al. [39] estimated the average taper angle to be 0.61° for fast and 0.45° for slow fibers. Callister et al. [20] studied the isolated fibers from the head retractor muscle of a turtle, which varied in length between 4 and 60 mm and had tapering ends between 1 and 26 mm long. They did not estimate taper angles, but average taper angles can be estimated from the data in their Figure 6.2. The maximum taper angle for the most bluntly ended fiber they studied was about 1.3° over the last 0.1 mm of the fiber, and about 0.8° over the last 1 mm of the fiber. Most of the fibers had smaller taper angles. Trotter [147] estimated from diameter measurements on scanning electron micrographs that the taper angle of isolated cat biceps femoris muscles was about 0.72°. From unpublished serial section data on quail pectoralis fibers, Trotter et al. estimated the average taper angle to be about 0.38°. From these data (ignoring the extreme taper angle value of 1.3°) and from Equation 6 it can be estimated that the average shear stress along the fiber surface is about 0.67% to 1.25% of the tensile stress within the fiber. If the maximal tensile stress is taken to be 540 kPa, then the average shear stress is apt to be between 3.6 and 6.8 kPa. These values are in the same order of magnitude as that calculated above for the yield strength of the matrix given a fiber aspect ratio of 250. Furthermore, the stress-reduction factor (membrane amplification factor) for tapered ends

FIGURE 6.9.
Schematic drawing of the strain pattern in the matrix of a single-fiber composite in which the fiber has conical ends, unloaded (A) and loaded in tension (B). Tensile stress is indicated by σ_c. The interfacial shear stress (τ_i) and fiber tensile stress (σ_f) are shown in C and D, respectively.

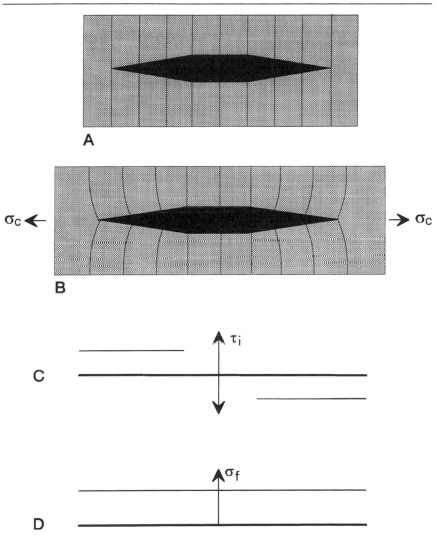

($1/\sin\varphi$) is on the order of 100. This value exceeds that calculated for MTJs by a factor of about 5 to 10 [144, 151].

Eldred et al. [39] found that the absolute length of the tapered region of singly tapered cat tibialis anterior fibers was fairly constant (11–12 mm) re-

FIGURE 6.10.

A, the interfacial shear stress and perpendicular tensile stress at the surface of a cone-ended fiber under a tensile load. B, the surface load distribution in a paraboloidal end of a fiber under tension. The areas of the rings and the circle at the tip of the fiber are equal and proportional to the load that is transmitted across each surface segment, whereas the areas of the surface segments decrease toward the fiber tip.

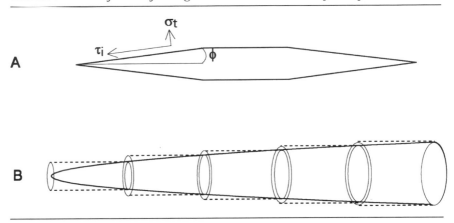

gardless of the length (18.9–58 mm) or contraction speed of the fibers. Callister et al. [20] found that the average percent taper length in the fibers they studied was 40.6 ± 16.2%. In both of these studies the fibers were predominately tapered at only one end. Trotter found that the doubly tapered fibers from the quail pectoralis muscle tapered over essentially 100% of their length, but no fibers in that study were more than 10 mm long (J. A. Trotter, unpublished data). The hypothesis emerges from these data that the end morphology of tapered fibers is quantitatively determined by their mechanical function [151]. Muscle fibers might have a way of sensing interfacial strain and of adjusting their morphology to maintain it within predetermined limits.

This brings us to a consideration of the actual shapes of tapered fiber ends. Eldred et al. [39] noted that in the tapered regions of cat fibers the cross-sectional area decreased nearly as a linear function of distance. A generally similar result has been obtained by serial section analysis of quail pectoralis fibers (J. A. Trotter et al., unpublished observations) on a much more limited data set. In contrast, Callister et al. [20] found that their data could be fitted to a "saturating function." Based on their regression analyses, Eldred et al. modeled the fiber ends as paraboloids rather than cones. Trotter found the data fit an ellipsoidal model slightly better than a paraboloidal one (J. A. Trotter, unpublished data). Although the available data do not really justify a strict geometric description of the tapered ends, it seems clear that diameter is a roughly curvilinear function of distance from the tapered end. Eldred et al. have discussed the consequence that, as the end is approached, increasingly greater stress is applied to the interface. This is because the quantity of force transmitted across the surface of a segment of unit length is proportional to the difference in cross-sectional area at the start and end of the segment. This is shown in Figure 6.10B. In a paraboloid, the same quantity of force is transmitted across all segments of equal length because the cross-sectional area changes as a linear function of length. On the other hand, the surface area of equal length segments decreases as the end is approached. As a consequence, the shear stress (force/area) increases.

This result appears to be paradoxical: the tapering of the fiber end is a geometric mechanism to eliminate stress concentrations, whereas the paraboloidal shape of the cat fibers studied by Eldred et al. [39] creates a mild stress concentration. It should be pointed out, however, that the notion that the fiber shape produces stress concentrations at the fiber ends results from the assumption that the actual end of the fiber is a paraboloid, whereas the light-microscopic data only justify concluding that the end region is approximately paraboloidal, ellipsoidal, or conical. Scanning and transmission electron micrographs of fiber ends, such as are seen in Figure 6.11, have shown that, at an ultrastructural level of resolution, their morphology may be locally variable. Corrugations and fingerlike projections are seen near the ends of some fibers, and shape analysis of electron micrographs has shown a tendency for the ends of tapered fibers to have increased surface area by an increased deviation from circularity [148]. It should also be emphasized that the tapered ends of muscle fibers are very finely attenuated, with average taper angles generally less than 1°. Given this morphology, it is quite doubtful that there would be a highly significant difference between cones, paraboloids, ellipsoids, or irregular shapes. Carrara and McGarry [21], for example, showed that for engineering fibers conical ends eliminated stress concentrations but that ellipsoidal ends worked essentially just as well. The actual distribution of shear stresses at the surfaces of the fiber ends will be better estimated by finite element analysis based on detailed fiber morphology. Preliminary finite element studies of the curvilinear processes of an MTJ have found that the shape of the processes essentially eliminates nonuniformities in the three-dimensional shear stresses [92]. Similar studies of the tapered ends of muscle fibers are underway [24].

In summary, it can be said that the characteristic tapering of fiber ends is apt to reduce significantly stress inequalities in the fiber and at the fiber-matrix interface, and to increase significantly the overall efficiency of force transmission in series-fibered muscles. It seems likely that the specific shape of individual ends may be produced by a dynamic response of individual fibers to the local mechanical environment. Muscle tissue may be viewed in this light as an example of a biological "smart material."

FIGURE 6.11.

A, the tapered end of a quail latissimus dorsi fiber as seen in the scanning electron microscope (from ref. 151). Note the irregular shape of the fiber end (arrowhead) *and the lateral processes, one of which is indicated by the arrow. Bar = 10 μm. B, transmission electron micrograph of the tapered end of a feline anterior latissimus dorsi fiber. Note the collagen fibrils in cross-section* (straight arrow) *and in oblique/longitudinal section* (wavy arrow). *Note also the lamina densa of the basement membrane* (arrowhead). *Bar = 0.25 μm.*

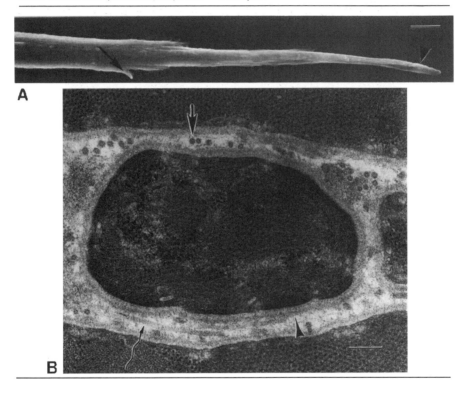

The Cross-Sectional Shapes of Skeletal Muscle Fibers

The formalisms of composite mechanics provide a useful approach but they are only approximately applicable to in-series fibered muscles because, among other considerations, muscle fibers do not have a geometrically regular cross-sectional shape. Rather, they assume irregular shapes that permit the surfaces of neighboring fibers to conform closely to each other, as can be appreciated by looking at any cross-section of any skeletal muscle. This close packing of irregularly shaped fibers decreases the distance between the fibers, greatly reduces the volume fraction of the matrix, and also allows the distance between fiber surfaces to remain more or less constant, which cannot be achieved even by very close packing of rigid circular cylinders.

The question naturally arises: What forces produce the specific cross-sectional shapes of muscle fibers? A plausible answer is that the adhesive forces between adjacent fibers are greater than the radial and longitudinal (internal) forces that would act to resist changes in cross-sectional shape. According to this view, fibers that might, if they were alone, have circular cross-sections, assume in a tissue the shapes dictated by the ratio of surface to internal forces. This principle of close packing is well known [140]. Were the fibers all of equal diameter, and the internal forces negligible, they would be hexagonally arrayed. Because muscle fibers differ in diameter and their internal forces are not negligible, their packing is not hexagonal but pleomorphic, and the surfaces of adjacent fibers are complementary.

A second aspect of the cross-sectional shape of individual fibers has to do with interfacial surface area because the fiber surface constitutes the interface across which force is transmitted. In most mechanical arguments about muscle it is usually assumed that the volume of the muscle and of individual fibers within it remains constant at all sarcomere lengths. Accepting these assumptions for the moment, it also follows that the volume of the connective tissue, neural, and vascular components also remain constant. In an individual fiber that undergoes length excursions of $\pm 20\%$ from the normal rest length while retaining a constant volume, either the cross-sectional shape or the surface area of the fiber has to change. This is shown in Figure 6.12, where the change in length (L) of a constant-volume, constant-cross-sectional-shape fiber between $0.8L_0$ and $1.2L_0$ produces a change in surface area of $\pm \sim 10\%$. In other words, about 10% new surface has to be added to the fiber as its length increases from L_0 to $1.2L_0$, whereas about 10% of the surface has to be removed as the fiber shortens from L_0 to $0.8L_0$. As the fiber length (L) changes, the cross-sectional area is required to change proportionately to maintain a constant volume (L $\times$ CSA = [constant] volume). The fiber perimeter for each muscle length varies as the square root of the cross-sectional area at that length. This follows from the assumption of a constant cross-sectional shape for the fiber. The relative surface area is then the product of perimeter and length (SA = PL). It is seen that the relative surface area increases as the fiber lengthens and decreases as it shortens. Within a physiological range of fiber lengths the surface area could change by more than $\pm 10\%$ from the value at L_0. Although several mechanisms, including transient caveolae and circumferential ruffling ("festoons") have been proposed that might allow the surface membrane (plasmalemma) to increase and decrease in apparent area with fiber length, none can realistically explain the concomitant changes that would also be required in the endomysial surface area.

However, if we eliminate the assumption that muscle fibers contract with a constant cross-sectional shape and assume instead that the shape can change to maintain a constant surface area, then the change in shape can be quantified by calculating the factor by which the constant-shape perime-

FIGURE 6.12.

The relative changes in cross-sectional area (CSA), perimeter (P), and surface area (SA) in a muscle fiber that maintains a constant volume and cross-sectional shape as it changes length.

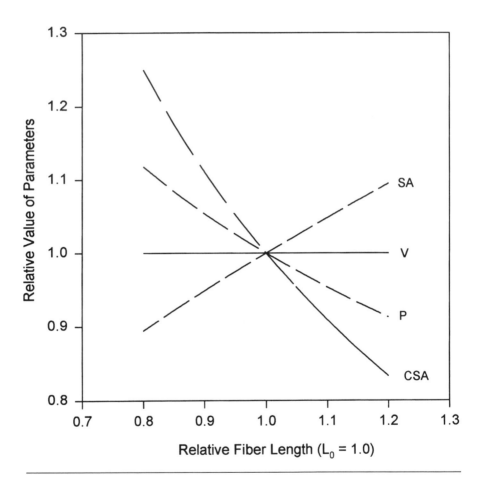

CONSTANT VOLUME AND SHAPE

ter value has to be multiplied to maintain a constant surface area (PL). This "form factor" (FF) was shown previously [150] to be the square root of the ratio of the fiber lengths, for any shaped fiber. That is, $FF = (L_0/L)^{0.5}$. Hence, under the constant surface area assumption, FF varies in exactly the same way that P varies in the constant shape case. Thus, the line marked P in Figure 6.12 for the constant-shape model is equivalent to the value of FF required to maintain a constant SA in the alternative, constant surface area model.

It should be noted here that, if the volume of the endomysium also remains constant, the constant fiber shape model requires that the distance between muscle fibers should increase as muscles shorten and decrease as they lengthen. Quantitatively it can be shown that the change in interfiber distance is the same as the change in perimeter. This is shown graphically in Figure 6.13.

Accordingly, it is possible to maintain constant both volume and surface area if the cross-sectional shape of the fiber changes systematically with fiber length. Figure 6.13, which shows this effect graphically for the simple case of rectangles, represents in Panel B a section through four fibers at muscle length L_0. Panels A and C represent a section through the same region after the muscle has shorted to 0.8 L_0 while maintaining constant shaped fibers (A) or constant fiber surface area (C). The smallest perimeter of a rectangle occurs when the sides are equal (i.e., in a square). Any deviation from squareness increases the relative length of the perimeter. Thus the rectangles in Panels A and C have the same area but those in Panel C have a 20% longer perimeter. Furthermore, in Panel C the distance between muscle fibers remains constant, whereas in Panel A it increases.

Two important questions then are: Do muscle fibers change cross-sectional shape as they change length; and is the surface area kept constant? A single study of the relationship of fiber shape to sarcomere length in cat muscles showed that the shape of the fibers changed in a way that was both qualitatively and quantitatively consistent with the maintenance of constant surface area [148]. The shape of the fibers was represented as the deviation from circularity and was quantitatively expressed as the ratio of true fiber perimeter to the perimeter of a circle with the same cross-sectional area.

FIGURE 6.13.
Schematic drawing of the changes in size and spacing (A) or size and shape (C) that occur when four adjacent muscle fibers (B) shorten by 20% while maintaining a constant shape (A) or surface area (C). See text for details.

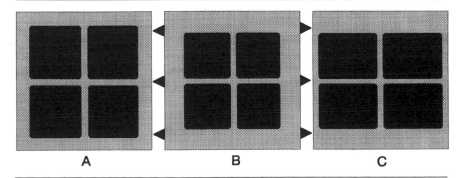

A   B   C

This ratio is mathematically identical to the form factor (FF) that was defined above. Hence the FF values calculated from measurements could be compared with the values predicted by the model. The experimentally obtained exponent was 0.29. It thus had the correct sense and was on the order of the predicted value of 0.5. But the change in shape in this single study was quantitatively somewhat smaller than predicted, which could be because the constant volume assumption is invalid, as has been suggested [100, 146].

From the above study it seemed that the shape of the fiber was, within the physiological range of sarcomere lengths, a dynamic function of the fiber length. The major contribution to the change in shape was a large-scale change in overall form rather than a change in the smaller-scale surface roughness (fine surface complexity). As mentioned above, every micrograph of skeletal muscle made has shown fibers of a variety of shapes closely matched to maintain a small endomysial space. It has also been the experience of anyone observing serial sections of muscle over long distances (millimeters) that an individual fiber changes shape dramatically such that the same fiber usually cannot be identified in sections 1 mm or so apart. There have also been observations of changing cross-sectional area along a single nontapered fiber [11, 38]. The picture that emerges from these studies is of dynamic changes in fiber shape (and perhaps fiber volume) acting so as to maintain a more or less constant surface area, which would maintain in turn a constant thickness of endomysium and so possibly conserve the geometry of the stress-transfer mechanism at the fiber surface.

The alterations in shape that occur as muscle fibers change length, as well as the inconstant shape along the length of a single muscle fiber, are consistent with the notion stated above that the adhesion forces holding fiber surfaces together are greater than internal forces that would act to resist changes in cross-sectional shape. The close packing of complementarily shaped fibers, the change in fiber shape with muscle length, and the inconstant shape along individual muscle fibers may thus be morphological manifestations of relatively strong interfibrous adhesion and relatively weak intrafibrous resistance. This line of thought emphasizes the mechanical connections between the surfaces of adjacent muscle fibers, where the adhesive is, of course, the endomysium.

THE ENDOMYSIUM

The argument that force transmission in series-fibered muscles is by shear linkage by means of the endomysium concentrates attention on the structure and mechanical properties of this connective tissue. Previous reviews detailing the structure and, especially, the biochemical composition of the endomysium are given by Mayne and Sanderson [94] and by Purslow and

Duance [110], who also review other possible roles of intramuscular connective tissue in phenomena such as muscle development. Variations in the composition and structure of intramuscular connective tissue due to increased mechanical demands on the muscle during exercise training, or decreased demands due to immobilization, show a linkage between endomysial collagen synthesis and muscle activity [72, 73, 75, 76]. This also supports the argument that this connective tissue is involved in the functional activity of muscle, because adaptive changes in the muscle in response to increased activity also include adaptive changes in this component. In briefly reviewing our knowledge of the endomysium here, it is important to emphasize those structures that provide linkages through the thickness of the endomysium; however, there is scant information in this regard because, to date, translaminar linkages have not been well considered. Reports in the literature on either the morphology or biochemical composition of endomysium have not made any explicit distinction between the endomysium of continuous or series-fibered muscle. It is possible that the structure of endomysia in these two muscle architectures may be fundamentally different, because of possible differences in their functional role in each case. On the other hand, there may not appear to be obvious differences in structure (and therefore properties) of the endomysium in continuous and series-fibered muscles. The possibility then exists that endomysium in continuously fibered muscle is similarly constructed so as to be able to link adjacent muscle fibers mechanically and enable load sharing between them, as suggested by the experimental results of Street [135] and of Buchthal and Knappies [19]. This would appear to be a promising subject for future investigation. Where possible we shall specifically cite examples of the structure of endomysium from muscle that has been shown to be series-fibered.

General Structure

Figure 6.14A is an electron micrograph of the extracellular matrix separating two adjacent muscle cells in a series fibered muscle, the feline biceps femoris. The whole membrane covering a muscle fiber historically has been termed the sarcolemma, and originally was described as a uniform, featureless structure [17]. Subsequent light and electron microscope studies have shown the whole structure to be composed of (a) the plasmalemma of the muscle cell itself, which is approximately 9 nm thick [124]; (b) the basement membrane, or basal lamina, which is about 50 nm thick [92, 124]; and (c) the outer reticular layer, which Mauro and Adams [92] describe as a "braided weave" of collagen fibrils. In frog sartorius muscle [124] this layer is 0.2–1 μm thick. In the series-fibered feline biceps femoris muscle it appears to be on the order of 1 μm thick [150]. The overall arrangement is shown diagrammatically in Figure 6.14B. Mauro and Adams [92] also identify a thin layer of fine fibrils external to the reticular layer, but this is not

FIGURE 6.14.

A, transmission electron micrograph of a longitudinally sectioned feline biceps femoris muscle prepared as described in ref. 147. Note the collagen fibrils sectioned at different angles (arrows) and the lamina densa (wavy arrow). Bar = 1 μm. B, a schematic explanation of A.

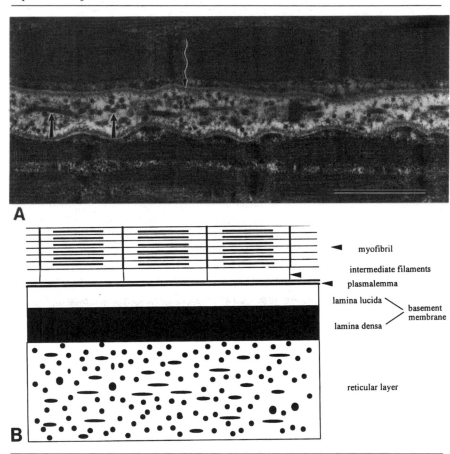

apparent in electron micrographs of sections through the endomysium such as that shown in Figure 6.14A.

The historical term "sarcolemma" is still often used to describe the whole extracellular structure shown in Figure 14 [124], but confusingly can be used to refer to just the plasma membrane of the muscle cell plus the basement membrane [12, 122]. Purslow and Duance [110] adopted the convention of referring to the whole of the structure outside the plasmalemma (i.e., the basement membrane plus the reticular layer) as the endomysium, and we will follow that convention here. From studies on the properties of isolated muscle fibers from a variety of muscle sources, but usually from frog muscles [86, 99, 107, 143], it is apparent that muscle fibers can be separated from each other with a physiologically intact endomysium surrounding each one. This indicates that the reticular layer may be divided through its thickness in such dissection procedures, leaving an intact plasmalemma, basement membrane, and some fraction of the reticular layer surrounding the isolated fiber. The ability to isolate single fibers with "intact" endomysium surrounding them has given rise to the concept that the endomysium is a sheath that surrounds each muscle fiber [17, 121]. However, it now seems more reasonable to view the endomysium as a continuous structure that separates two adjacent muscle cells [111, 138, 150], but one which may be cleaved through its thickness when one fiber is peeled off another.

The Basement Membrane
The basement membrane or basal lamina is composed of a dense layer (the laminal densa) and a less dense layer (lamina rara or lamina lucida). The lamina rara is equivalent to the 20-nm "gap zone" reported by Schmalbruch [124] as separating the muscle cell plasma membrane from the lamina densa. The basement membrane has a number of components. Principal among these is type IV collagen, which is specifically located within the basement membrane of the endomysium [55, 133]. Type IV collagen is thought to form the major structural backbone of basement membrane [94]. Kühn et al. [77] have proposed that it aggregates into tetrameric units which are linked together in open "chicken wire" planar meshworks. Other open planar meshworks based on hexagonal structures have been proposed by Yurchenco et al. [154]. Both Kühn et al. and Yurchenco et al. propose schemes of the molecular packing of type IV collagen parallel to the plane of the membrane, although one of the models of Yurchenco et al. does have small parts of the molecules lying through the thickness of the membrane.

Considering the basement membrane structure from the point of view of providing mechanical shear linkage between the plasmalemma and the reticular layer, transbasement membrane linkages are obviously of interest. These may be provided by crosslinks between overlying planar assemblies of type IV collagen, or by glycoproteins and proteoglycans. Laminin is a large glycoprotein found in all basement membranes and has been localized in skeletal muscle basement membranes [55, 133]. It is distributed throughout the lamina densa and lamina rara. Yurchenco et al. [154] postulate that it is important in providing cell-basement membrane interactions because of its ability to bind to type IV collagen, proteoglycan, and cell surface receptors, as well as to aggregate with itself. Similarly, fibronectin, another large glycoprotein, is present in the basement membrane, extending between the plasma membrane and the reticular layer [55]. Both of these glycoproteins have RGD sequences in their structure, a motif known to interact with cell surface receptors (integrins). The proteoglycan heparan sulfate is a predominant proteoglycan in basement membrane [56] that binds to both type IV collagen and to laminin [154]. Discrete filamentous structures (junctional filaments) that bridge the lamina rara of basement membrane in the myotendinous junctions of skeletal muscle are thought to have a functional role in force transmission [78, 144, 151]. They are also observed in intrafascicularly terminating muscle fibers, where they are enriched at membrane sites associated with subsarcolemmal densities [130, 147]. It is interesting to note that the lamina rara is thicker in the endomysia of fibers directly adjacent to the endomysium (fascia) surrounding the gastrocnemius and soleus muscles of the rat [70]. These endomysia also contain invaginations similar to those of the myotendinous junction, and the inference is that these myoepimysial or myofascial junctions may also have a role in force transmission [70].

Transmission of contractile force from the myofibrils through the plasmalemma and into the basement membrane also requires strong lateral intracellular linkages. Thornell and Price [142] envisage the intermediate filament lattice fulfilling this role, and review the evidence for this. Briefly, transverse intermediate filaments, principally composed of the protein desmin, are found to connect between Z-discs of adjacent myofibrils and form a continuous link out to the plasmalemma, where they are anchored to the sarcolemma by regular structures termed costomeres, which contain vinculin, spectrin, ankyrin, talin, and g-actin. Interactions with the extracellular matrix via transmembrane proteins of the integrin superfamily seem to occur preferentially here. This scheme provides a reasonable explanation of how contractile force could be transmitted through to the extracellular matrix by regular structures occurring at least once per sarcomere in most muscles. In some muscles, extra links at the level of the M line are envisaged. Tight linkages between extracellular and intracellular structures of this nature at specific points along the myofibril would leave the plasmalemma free between these attachments to form the invaginated foldings into calveoli on either side of the Z-disc, as reported by Dulhunty and Franzini-Armstrong [35].

The Reticular Layer
The reticular layer or reticular lamina forms the bulk of the material between adjacent muscle cells, as is evident in Figure 6.14A. The fibrillar collagen types I, III, and V and the microfibrillar collagen type VI are found in the endomysium [6, 33, 59, 82]. The ratio between types I and III is approximately 0.45:0.55 in a number of bovine muscles [80, 81]. Although there is little variation in the endomysial collagen content and type I:III ratio between these muscles, there are some suggestions that muscle with a higher collagen content overall may have proportionately less type III [110]. The precise roles of the different molecular types of collagen are unknown. Structurally, the collagen in the reticular layer is organized in fibrils in a

somewhat disorganized or distributed planar network described as a weave by Mauro and Adams [92] and Rowe [121], and as a feltwork by Trotter and Purslow [150]. Figure 6.15 shows the arrangement of the collagen fibrils in the reticular layer of a known series-fibered muscle, bovine sternomandibularis [111]. The pseudorandom orientation of the collagen fibrils with respect to the longitudinal axis of the muscle fibers is easily seen. A high proportion of the fibrils are curvilinear. The general appearance of this quasirandom feltwork is in agreement with that shown by feline biceps femoris, another series-fibered muscle [150]. The question arises as to whether the structure of this, the major element of the endomysium, is fundamentally different in continuous as opposed to series-fibered muscles. A brief survey of the available evidence from electron micrographs in the literature indicates that the reticular layers in all vertebrate skeletal muscles have a similar morphology [15, 116, 121, 124]. Schmalbruch [124] showed micrographs of endomysial networks from frog sartorius muscle with a degree of randomness in fibril orientation similar to Figure 6.15, but described

FIGURE 6.15.
Scanning electron micrograph of bovine sternomandibularis endomysium, prepared as described in ref. 111 by removal of muscle fibers and basement membrane. Note in this oblique view that the collagen fibrils of the reticular layer compose a disorganized or quasirandom feltwork. Bar = 6 μm.

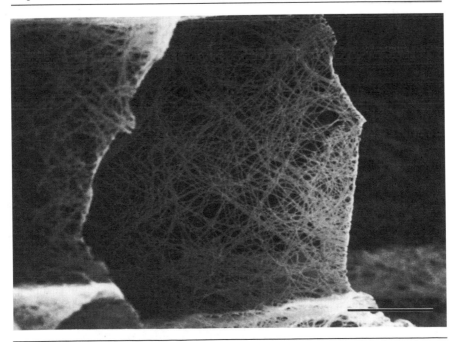

this as a helical arrangement. Borg and Caulfield [15] described a similar reticular morphology in the endomysium of six muscles in the rat (diaphragm, adductor major, gastrocnemius, pectoralis, biceps, and psoas major). Similarly, Rowe [121] did not find any qualitative differences in the organization of endomysium on surveying the morphology of intramuscular connective tissue in a variety of muscles (psoas major, biceps brachii, longissimus dorsi, semitendinosus, semimembranosus, anterior tibialis, and adductor magnus) from a variety of species (rat, rabbit, sheep, and cattle), describing them all as dense feltworks of collagen fibrils. Although some of these muscles are known to be series-fibered [151], it is not clear whether others are definitely continuously fibered.

The orientation of collagen fibrils in the reticular layer alters as the muscle fibers change length, becoming more circumferentally aligned as the muscle shortens and more aligned with the muscle fiber axis as the muscle lengthens. This has been reported qualitatively by a number of authors [121, 124, 125, 138, 150]. Trotter and Purslow [150] proposed a mathematical model to explain this reorientation quantitatively, based on an inference from earlier work [148] that the surface area of a muscle fiber may remain constant while the fiber changes length. This is in addition to the normal assumption that muscle contracts isovolumetrically. As demonstrated above and in Figures 6.12 and 6.13, the consequence of fibers maintaining both volume and surface area constant as they change length would be that the shape of their cross-section altered with length, and would be expected to become more circular at long sarcomere lengths. This change in shape is seen in the series-fibered feline biceps femoris muscle [148]. Trotter and Purslow [150] also used this model (the isoareal model) to explain on a quantitative basis why the majority of collagen fibrils in the reticular layer would be curvilinear at most muscle fiber lengths.

A quantitative analysis of the change in morphology of the reticular network with changing muscle length has been performed by Purslow and Trotter [111]. They studied the distribution of collagen fibril orientations in the endomysial reticular layer of a series-fibered muscle, bovine sternomandibularis, over a wide range of muscle lengths. The distribution of collagen orientations was very broad at all muscle lengths (i.e., many fibrils were found at all angles), reflecting the disorganized nature of the network. At muscle rest length the collagen fibril network was not completely random, but had a slight preference for fibrils to be more circumferentally oriented. The orientation distribution showed a progressive skewing toward the circumferential direction as the muscle was shortened, and conversely a shift toward a longitudinal bias as the muscle was lengthened. From each distribution of orientations, a number-weighted mean orientation could be calculated, and this is shown in Figure 6.16. This figure shows that the mean orientation changes progressively with sarcomere length, and this reorientation is compared with the predicted behavior of two models of such a net-

FIGURE 6.16.

Endomysial collagen fibril orientation as a function of sarcomere length in the series-fibered bovine sternomandibularis muscle (from ref. 111). Data points are the numerically weighted means of orientation distributions obtained by image analysis (open squares) or manual analysis (closed squares) or scanning electron micrographs of the reticular layer. The two lines shown are the predicted relationships between orientation and sarcomere length for the isoareal (open circles) and the constant shape (open triangles) models, as explained in the text.

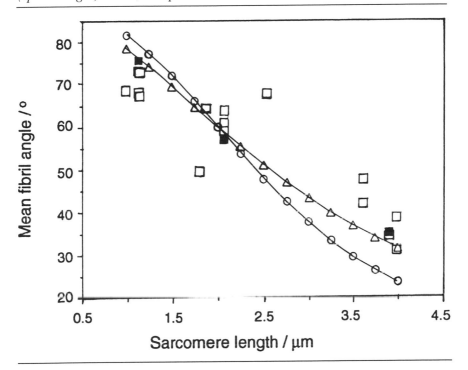

work. The first of these models, the isoareal model from Trotter and Purslow [150] based on the assumption of constant muscle fiber surface area and volume, predicts that the orientation of any one collagen fibril (e.g., one lying at an angle θ_0) changes to a new angle θ_1 when the muscle fiber is extended from length L_0 to L_1 according to the following relationship: $\tan \theta_1 = \tan \theta_0 \, \lambda^2$, where $\lambda = L_1/L_0$. The other model relationship shown is based on the assumption that the cross-sectional shape of the fiber remains constant, but that the area changes so that the fiber remains at constant volume (e.g., a cylindrical fiber with a circular cross-section on lengthening remains a cylinder, but the radius of the circular cross-section diminishes so that the volume of the whole remains constant). This constant shape model predicts reorientation according to the different relationship:

$\tan \theta_1 = \tan \theta_0 \lambda^{3/2}$. Both models show the same trend in mean orientation with muscle length as seen in the data, but the constant-shape model fits the observed rate of change of mean collagen fibril orientation more closely. Although it remains to rule definitively between these two models describing the behavior of the reticular network, it is clear from these results that substantial reorientation of the network does occur when the muscle changes length.

Mechanical Properties of the Endomysium

Experimental studies of the mechanical properties of endomysia have principally measured their tensile contribution to the passive elasticity of single muscle fibers. Compared with mammalian muscle it appears to be relatively easier to separate individual muscle fibers with intact endomysium from frog muscles, and so many single fiber experiments have been carried out on frog muscle (e.g., sartorius, semitendinosus). If the notable ease of separation in frog fibers is due to the lateral connections through the extracellular matrix being particularly weak in these muscles, then it is possible that they are not the best source of material for examining the normal workings of intramuscular connective tissue. The longitudinal length-tension relationship of endomysium has been measured by taking the difference between intact fiber properties and the properties of fibers after mechanical removal of the endomysium [86, 99, 107] or by length-tension studies of the endomysial tube produced when single intact fibers are pinched so that the myofibrillar material ruptures and retracts [91, 112, 114]. An alternative approach was used by Rapaport [113], who measured the tensile modulus of the endomysium by sucking a bleb on the surface of the fiber into a flat-mouthed pipette. The consensus of these studies is that the longitudinal tensile properties of the endomysium are nonlinear, the structure becoming progressively stiffer at higher extensions along the fiber direction. The longitudinal tensile stiffness of the endomysium near rest length is seen to be relatively low, and the tensile loads generated in the endomysium near rest length are only a small proportion of the total passive elastic response of the whole fiber on extension.

From their analysis of collagen fibril or orientation distributions at various muscle lengths, Purslow and Trotter [111] were able to model the change in longitudinal tensile stiffness of the endomysium due to collagen reorientation using fibrous composites theory. This modeling showed qualitative agreement with the experimental studies of endomysial stiffness, i.e., that the longitudinal tensile stiffness is low at rest length, and increases progressively with increasing muscle length. This result reiterates the conclusion that has previously appeared to argue against the involvement of the endomysium in force transmission, namely that because muscles (including series-fibered muscles) can produce high isometric tensions at or near rest length, the endomysium, with its low tensile stiffness at muscle rest length, must not function mechanically in series with muscle fibers, i.e., must not transmit force by longitudinal tension. However, in series-fibered muscles that lack myomyous junctions, it is only via the endomysium that intrafascicularly terminating fibers are connected to other fibers and thus eventually to the tendons. It therefore seems possible for series-fibered muscle to function only if the endomysium does indeed transmit contractile force between adjacent fibers.

A resolution of this apparent paradox has been proposed [111, 150, 151] that postulates that the mode of force transmission is not in tension, but in shear. Laterally adjacent fibers in a series-fibered muscle typically overlap each other for 60–75% of their length [151]. Forces produced in one fiber are thus most likely to be transmitted to the neighboring cell by shear through the thickness of the endomysial connective tissue which links them. Evidence for mechanically competent lateral linkages has previously been published by Street [135] and postulated by Buchthal and Knappeis [19]. It is axiomatic that tensile experiments on single fibers or on isolated endomysial tubes are inherently incapable of measuring any contributions of the endomysium to the shear linkages between fibers.

Purslow and Trotter [111] inferred from fibrous composites theory that the translaminar shear stiffness of the endomysial reticular layer is likely to be substantially independent of the orientation of collagen fibrils in the plane of the membrane. This inference implies that the translaminar shear stiffness will be independent of the reorientation caused by changes in muscle length. The rationale behind this is as follows. The reticular layer is in itself a composite of collagen fibrils in an amorphous matrix. In practice, the shear properties of the reticular layer will be dominated by the relatively compliant amorphous matrix, which will mask the effects of preferred collagen orientation. From a functional point of view, then, the reorientation of the collagen fibril network in the plane of the reticular layer can be seen as a mechanism that allows large extensions of the endomysium, to follow muscle fiber length changes. However, the translaminar shear stiffness of the reticular layer is likely to be nearly constant at all muscle lengths, which may be more suitable for efficient force transmission.

It is informative to estimate the axial compliance that shear strain in the endomysium would contribute to the overall compliance of an active series-fibered muscle. Say that the endomysial thickness between any two fiber surfaces is 2 μm and the shear stress applied during maximal loading (i.e., during an eccentric contaction) is, from the calculations made above, about 5 kPa. Say also that the shear modulus of the endomysium is 5 kPa, so that a 5-kPa load produces a shear strain of 1.0. Given the definition of shear strain as the displacement divided by the thickness of the sheared material, this is equivalent to a 2-μm longitudinal displacement of the two fiber surfaces. This is the longitudinal strain contributed by endomysial shear compliance regardless of the thickness of the muscle. Say finally that the muscle has, on average, 10 overlapping muscle fibers in series between its origin and its insertion. These 10 fibers will be connected by 9 adhesive overlaps. The total longitudinal compliance will then be 18 μm. If the muscle is, like the human sartorius, about 50 cm long, the muscle strain contributed by endomysial compliance will be 0.0036%! If we say for the sake of this argument that the shear modulus of passive muscle fibers is the same as that of the endomysium, that the average fiber diameter is 50 μm, and that 50% of the fibers are active throughout the length and breadth of the muscle, then passive muscle fibers will contribute a longitudinal strain of 50 μm each, or 450 μm total, equivalent in the 50-cm sartorius to a strain of 0.09%. The conclusion from these hypothetical (but not unrealistic) calculations is that the amount of strain contributed by compliance within the endomysium and within passive muscle fibers is too small to be significant in the overall mechanical performance of the muscle. This conclusion is consistent with the proposition (stated above) that the macromechanics of a discontinuous fibered composite can be indistinguishable from those of a continuous fibered composite despite the fact that the micromechanics are very different.

The shear linkage through the endomysium is clearly of prime importance in series-fibered muscle where the endomysium is the only obvious path through which an intrafascicularly terminating muscle fiber can transmit its contractile force. However, if endomysium from continuously fibered muscle is similar in structure and composition, then it will also be similar in properties. This raises the intriguing question of some role for lateral linkage between muscle fibers in continuously fibered muscle also. Lateral connectivity between muscle fibers (and between myofibrils within fibers) provides two obvious advantages: (a) the ability to sustain force output from a fiber that has been damaged at any point along its length; and (b) the ability to interrupt longitudinal continuity in the structure of fibers during growth and development, while still retaining the functional output from the whole contractile column. If force transmission in continuous fibers is only via the myotendinous junction at each end of the fiber, then interruption at any point along its length renders the whole fiber useless from a force production point of view. Lateral linkages between adjacent fibers would serve to transmit force produced in an interrupted fiber through its neighbors, so retaining the functional output of most of the damaged fiber. Reddy et al. [115] studied rabbit extensor digitorum longus muscle strained to the point where fibers ruptured near the myotendinous junction. They observed gross hypercontraction in the sarcomeres near to the point of fiber rupture due to disruption of the sarcolemma and influx of extracellular calcium. However, the length of sarcomeres further away progressively approached the normal length until, at a distance of 500 μm away from the rupture site, sarcomere length in the damaged fibers had become restored to the sarcomere length normal to this muscle. Good lateral linkage by shear between damaged fibers and their neighbors would enable the force produced by these "normal" sarcomeres to be usefully transmitted.

Evidence for Endomysial Force Transmission from Muscle Pathologies

Conventional explanations of force production and transmission within muscle do not invoke any argument of stresses in and across the endomysium. However, recent investigations of the structural causes of some muscle pathologies is focusing attention very much on the lateral connections between myofibrils and the cell membranes and provides evidence for the occurrence of stresses in and across the cell surface membranes in normally functioning muscle.

Misra et al. [98] show that muscle from a patient with adult-onset myotubular myopathy has an abnormal distribution of vimentin and desmin, so that the network of intermediate filaments laterally connecting myofibrils to the plasmalemma is poorly defined. The loss of muscle function associated with this condition indicates the importance of these intermediate filaments in providing lateral mechanical connections between myofibrils and the plasmalemma.

Duchenne muscular dystrophy is also a degeneative muscle disease in which normal muscle function is lost. There is an extensive proliferation of fibrotic connective tissue within affected muscle [34, 103]. The increasing collagen content and collagen crosslink content in dystrophic muscle has been observed to result in a large increase in the passive elastic response of a series-fibered muscle, the chicken pectoralis [41]. However, the disease is caused by a deficiency of a single gene product, dystrophin [63]. Dystrophin is absent in the *mdx* strain of mice, which acts as a model for Duchenne muscular dystrophy, except that none of the normal human muscle dysfunction is seen in any but the diaphragm muscle. Dystrophin is localized on the internal surface of the plasmalemma in dense circumferential rings at costomeres aligned with the Z-discs of adjacent myofibrils and also in finer longitundinal interconnections between costameres [31, 32, 89, 134]. Associated with dystrophin is a laminin-binding glycoprotein that may provide interactions between dystrophin and extracellular basement membrane across the plasmalemma [69, 105]; certainly dystrophin is tightly bound mechanically to the plasmalemma [134]. Duncan [36] suggests that a lack of dystrophin may change the permeability of stretch-activated cation channels in the plasmalemma. Franco and Lansman [44] ascribed the increased permeability of *mdx* muscle cell membranes to a change in the balance of activity between stretch-activated and stretch-inactivated ion channels. Conceivably this could result from an increased extensibility of cell membranes in the absence of dystrophin. They found no difference in the tensile strength of normal and *mdx* membranes, however. Hutter et al. [67] measured a significant decrease in the tensile strength of the surface membranes of flexor digitorum brevis muscle fibers from *mdx* mice, but believed that the decrease was too small for membrane rupture to be the cause of the osmotic fragility that accompanies Duchenne muscular dystrophy. In contrast, Petrof et al. [105] strongly suggest that dystrophin acts to reinforce mechanically the plasmalemma and protect it against forces produced in muscle contraction. In normal and *mdx* mouse muscles they showed a progressive incidence of cell membrane disruption with increased forces of active muscle contraction, and observed a higher incidence of cell membrane disruption in *mdx* muscle fibers than in normal fibers at any given muscle force. These findings are not necessarily contradictory to those of Franco and Lansman or Hutter et al.: increased membrane disruption could be the result of increased ion influx, in turn caused by an increased extensibility of dystrophin-deficient membrane. Petrof et al. [105] speculate that dystrophin could either spread contractile forces produced in the fiber over a broad membrane area by interactions with cytoskeletal elements or transmit these forces out into the basement membrane by means of the dystrophin-associated glycoprotein, so presumably enlisting the support of the extracellular matrix in sharing the forces involved. Whichever mechanism is involved, these two speculations both implicitly accept that significant shear forces are transmitted across the cell surface during normal muscle contraction.

CONCLUSION

The arrangement of discontinuous muscle fibers and intramuscular connective tissue into a composite structure appears to have been selected for by evolution because the presence of this architecture is widespread among vertebrates and is not simply a function of muscle length. Such a statement implies that there are specific functional advantages conferred by this structural configuration, but it is presently unclear what these advantages might be. Nevertheless, the scientific attention recently given to series-fibered muscles has revealed a number of morphological adaptations and has suggested specific mechanical functions for macromolecular assemblies both in the sarcoplasm and in the endomysium. The study of such muscles has only just begun, and some of the most interesting biomechanical and neuromotor questions remain to be answered. How are such muscles used in the control of limb movement and position? How are motor units distributed throughout the substance of such muscles, and does the nervous system recruit motor units in a manner that makes use of their distribution to achieve appropriate power outputs at different muscle lengths? Perhaps the next time this subject is reviewed in this publication it will be possible to provide some answers to questions such as these.

ACKNOWLEDGMENTS

The authors' research has been supported by grants from the National Institutes of Health (J.A.T.), the Agricultural and Food Research Council (AFRC) Biotechnology and Biological Sciences Research Council (BBSRC) of the United Kingdom (P.P.P.), and the Medical Research Council of Canada and

Canadian Networks of Centres of Excellence Program (F.J.R.R.). The suggestions of Drs. Keith Condon and G. E. Loeb were greatly appreciated. Thanks also to J. Creasy for assistance with some of the figures.

REFERENCES

1. Adams, D., and B. Mackay. The distribution of motor end-plates in mammalian muscles. *Bibl. Anat.* 2:153–154, 1961.
2. Adrian, D. E. The spread of activity in the tenuissimus muscle of the cat and in other complex muscles. *J. Physiol. (Lond.)* 60:301–315, 1925.
3. Alexander, R. M. *Animal Mechanics.* Oxford: Blackwell Scientific Publications, 1983, pp. 1–293.
4. Alnaqueeb, M. A., N. S. Al Said, and G. Goldspink. Connective tissue changes and physical properties of developing and ageing skeletal muscle. *J. Anat.* 139:677–689, 1984.
5. Aquilonius, S.-M., H. Askmark, P.-G. Gillberg, . Nandedkar, Y. Olsson, and E. Stålberg. Topographical localization of motor endplates in cryosections of whole human muscles. *Muscle Nerve* 7:287–293, 1984.
6. Bailey, A. J., and T. J. Sims. Meat tenderness: distribution of molecular species of collagen in bovine muscle. *J. Sci. Fed. Agric.* 28:565–570, 1977.
7. Bardeen, C. R. Variations in the internal architecture of the M. obliquus abdominis externus in certain animals. *Anat. Anz.* 23:241–249, 1903.
8. Barrett, B. The length and mode of termination of individual muscle fibers in the human sartorius and posterior femoral muscles. *Acta Anat.* 48:242–257, 1962.
9. Bartels, H. Myomuscular junctions in the gill-sac muscle of the atlantic hagfish, Myxine glutinosa: analogy with myotendinous junctions. *Cell Tissue Res.* 246:223–225, 1986.
10. Bendall, J. R. The elastin content of various muscles of beef. *J. Sci. Fd. Agric.* 18:553–558, 1967.
11. Blinks, J. R. Influence of osmotic strength on cross-section and volume of isolated single muscle fibers. *J. Physiol.* 177:42–57, 1965.
12. Bloom, W., and Fawcett, D. W. *A Textbook of Histology.* Philadelphia: W. B. Saunders, 1968.
13. Bodine, S. C., A. Garfinkel, R. R. Roy, and V. R. Edgerton. Spatial distribution of motor unit fibers in the cat soleus and tibialis anterior muscles: local interactions. *J. Neurosci.* 8:2142–2152, 1988.
14. Bodine-Fowler, S., A. Garfinkel, R. Roy, and V. R. Edgerton. Spatial distribution of muscle fibers within the territory of a motor unit. *Muscle Nerve* 13:1133–1145, 1990.
15. Borg, T. K., and J. B. Caulfield. Morphology of connective tissue in skeletal muscle. *Tiss. Cell* 12:197–207, 1980.
16. Bormioli, S. P., and S. Schiaffino. Myomuscular junctions in re-innervated rat skeletal muscle. *J. Anat.* 124:359–370, 1977.
17. Bowman, W. On the minute structure and movements of voluntary muscle. *Philos. Trans. R. Soc. Lond. (Biol.)* 130:457–501, 1840.
18. Boyd, L. A. The tenuissimus muscle of the cat. *J. Phyisol. (Lond.)* 133:35–36, 1956.
19. Buchthal, F., and G. G. Knappeis. Diffraction spectra and minute structure of cross-striated muscle fibre. *Scand. Arch. Physiol.* 83:281–307, 1940.
20. Callister, R. J., R. Callister, and E. H. Peterson. Design and control of the head retractor muscle in a turtle, pseudemys (trachemys) scripta. I. Architecture and histochemistry of single muscle fibers. *J. Comp. Neurol.* 325:405–421, 1992.
21. Carrara, A. S., and F. J. McGarry. Matrix and interface stresses in a discontinuous fiber composite model. *J. Comp. Material.* 2:222–243, 1968.
22. Chanaud, C. M., C. A. Pratt, and G. E. Loeb. Functionally complex muscles of the cat hindlimb. II. Mechanical and architectural heterogeneity in the biceps femoris. *Exp. Brain Res.* 85:257–270, 1991.

23. Christensen, E. Topography of terminal motor innervation in striated muscles from still-born infants. *Am. J. Phyusiol. Med.* 38:65–78, 1959.
24. Clift, S. E., A. Crighton, P. P. Purslow, and J. A. Trotter. Finite element modeling of the transfer of contractile force from short muscle fibres. *Proc. 2nd World Biomechanics Congress,* 1994, in press. 1:86a, 1994.
25. Close, R. I. Dynamic properties of mammalian skeletal muscles. *Physiol. Rev.* 52:129–197, 1972.
26. Cöers, C. Contribution à l'étude de la jonction neuro-musculaire. II. Topographie zonale de l'innervation motrice terminale dans les muscles striés. *Arch. Biol.* 64:495–505, 1953.
27. Cöers, C., and J. Durand. La répartition des appareils cholinestérasiques en cupule dans divers muscles striés. *Arch. Biol.* 68:209–215, 1957.
28. Cooper, S. The relation of active to inactive fibers in functional contraction of muscle. *J. Physiol. (Lond.)* 67:1–13, 1925.
29. Craig, S. W., and J. V. Pardo. Gamma actin, spectrin, and intermediate filament proteins colocalize with vinculin at costameres, myofibril to sarcolemma attachment sites. *Cell Motil* 3:449–462, 1983.
30. Cullen, T. S., and M. Brödel. Lesions of the rectus abdominis muscle simulating an acute intra-abdominal condition. I. Anatomy of the rectus muscle. *Bull. John Hopkins Hosp.* 61:295–316, 1937.
31. Dickson, G. A. Azad, G. E. Morris, H. Simon, M. Noursadeghi, and F. S. Walsh. Colocal-ization and molecular association of dystrophin with laminin at the surface of mouse and human myotubes. *J. Cell Sci.* 103:1223–1233, 1992.
32. Dmytrenko, G. M., D. W. Pumplin, and R. J. Bloch. Dystrophin in a membrane skeletal network: localization and comparison to other proteins. *J. Neurosci.* 13:547–558, 1993.
33. Duance, V. C., D. J. Restall, H. Beard, F. J. Bourne, and A. J. Bailey. The location of three collagen types in skeletal muscle. *FEBS Lett.* 79:248–252, 1977.
34. Duance, V. C., H. R. Stephens, M. Dunn, A. J. Bailey, and V. Dubowitz. A role for collagen in the pathogenesis of muscular dystrophy? *Nature* 284:470–472, 1980.
35. Dulhunty, A. F., and C. Franzini-Armstrong. The relative contributions of the folds and calveolae to the surface membrane of frog skeletal muscle fibres at different sarcomere lengths. *J. Physiol. (Lond.)* 250:513–539, 1975.
36. Duncan, C. J. Dystrophin and the integrity of the sarcolemma in Duchenne muscular dy-strophy. *Experientia* (Basel) 45:175–177, 1989.
37. Edgerton, V. R., R. R. Roy, and R. J. Gregor. Motor unit architecture and interfiber matrix in sensormotor partitioning. *Behav. Brain Sci.* 12:651–652, 1989.
38. Eldred, E., A. Garfinkle, E. S. Hsu, M. Ounjian, R. R. Roy, and V. R. Edgerton. The physi-ological cross-sectional area of motor units in the cat tibialis anterior. *Anat. Rec.* 235:381–389, 1993.
39. Eldred, E., M. Ounjian, R. R. Roy, and V. R. Edgerton. Tapering of the intrafascicular endings of muscle fibers and its implications to relay of force. *Anat. Rec.* 236:390–398, 1993.
40. Feinstein, B., B. Lindegård, E. Nyman, and G. Wohlfart. Morphologic studies of motor units in normal human muscles. *Acta Anat.* 23:127–142, 1955.
41. Feit, H., K. Masataka, and A. S. Mostafapour. The role of collagen crosslining in the in-creased stiffness of avian dystrophic muscle. *Muscle Nerve* 12:486–492, 1989.
42. Felix, W. Die länge der Muskelfaser bei dem Menschen und einigen Säugethieren. *Fest schrift, Albert von Kölliker,* Leipzig: Englemann, 1887, as cited by Huber, 1916.
43. Floyd, K. Junctions between muscle fibers in cat extraocular muscles. *Nature* 227:185–186, 1970.
44. Franco, A., and Lansman, J. B. Calcium entry through stretch-inactivated ion channels in *mdx* myotubes. *Nature* 344:670–673, 1990.
45. Froriep, A. Ueber das sarcolemm und die muskelkerne. *Arch. Anat. Phisiol. Anat. Abt.* 2:416–428, 1878.

46. Fulton, J. F. *Selected Readings in the History of Physiology.* Sprinfield, Ill: Charles C Thomas, 1966, pp. 201–207.
47. Gans, C. Fiber architecture and muscle function. *Exerc. Sport Sci. Rev.* 10:160–207, 1982.
48. Gans, C., and F. de Vree. Functional bases of fiber length and angulation in muscle. *J. Morphol.* 192:63–85, 1987.
49. Gans, C., G. E. Loeb, and F. de Vree. Architecture and consequent physiological properties of the semitendinosus muscle in domestic goats. *J. Morphol.* 199:287–297, 1989.
50. Gaunt, A. S., and C. Gans. Architecture of chicken muscles: short-fiber patterns and their ontogeny. *Proc. R. Soc. Lond. (Biol.)* 240:351–362, 1990.
51. Gaunt, A. S., and C. Gans. Serially arranged myofibers: an unappreciated variant in muscle architecture. *Experientia* (Basel) 48:864–868, 1992.
52. Gaunt, A. S., and C. Gans. Variations in the distribution of motor end-plates in avian pectoralis. *J. Morphol.* 215:65–88, 1993.
53. Gordon, D. C., C. G. M. Hammond, J. T. Fisher, and F. J. R. Richmond. Muscle-fiber architecture, innervation, and histochemistry in the diaphragm of the cat. *J. Morphol.* 201:131–143, 1989.
54. Gordon, D. C., G. E. Loeb, and F. J. R. Richmond. Distribution of motoneurons supplying cat sartorius and tensor fasciae latae, demonstrated by retrograde multiple-labelling methods. *J. Comp. Neurol.* 304:357–372, 1991.
55. Hantai, D., J. Gautron, J. Labat-Robert. Immunolocalization of fibronectin and other macromolecules of the intercellular matrix in the striated muscle fiber of the adult rat. *Collagen Relat. Res.* 3:381–391, 1983.
56. Hassell, J. R., P. G. Robey, H. J. Barrach, J. Wilczek, S. I. Rennard, and G. R. Martin. Isolation of heparin sulfate containing proteoglycan from basement membrane. *Proc. Natl. Acad. Sci. U. S. A.* 55:119–126, 1966.
57. Henneman, E., H. P. Clamann, J. D. Gillies, and R. D. Skinner. Rank order of motoneurons within a pool: law of combination. *J. Neurophysiol.* 34:1338–1349, 1974.
58. Heron, M. I., and F. J. R. Richmond. In-series fiber architecture in long human muscles. *J. Morphol.* 216:35–45, 1993.
59. Hessle, H., and E. Engvall. Type VI collagen. *J. Biol. Chem.* 259:3955–3961, 1984.
60. Hijikata, T., H. Wakisaka, and T. Yohro. Architectural design, fiber-type composition, and innervation of the rat rectus abdominis muscle. *Anat. Rec.* 234:500–512, 1992.
61. Hijikata, T., H. Wakisaka, and S. Nida. Functional combination of tapering profiles and overlapping arrangements in nonspanning skeletal muscle fibers terminating intrafascicularly. *Acta. Anat.* 236:602–610, 1993.
62. Hoffer, J. A., G. E. Loeb, N. Sugano, W. B. Marks, M. J. O'Donovan, and C. A. Pratt. Cat hindlimb motoneurons during locomotion. III. Functional segregation in sartorius. *J. Neurophsiol.* 57:554–562, 1987.
63. Hoffman, E. P., R. H. Fischbeck, R. H. Brown, et al. Characterization of dystrohin in muscle-biopsy specimens from patients with Duchenne's or Becker's muscular dystrophy. *N. Engl. J. Med.* 318:1363–1368, 1988.
64. Hoyle, G. *Muscles and Their Neural Control.* New York: John Wiley & Sons, 1983, pp. 1–16.
65. Huber, G. C. On the form and arrangement in fasciculi of striated voluntary muscle fibers. *Anat. Rec.* 11:149–168, 1916.
66. Hull, D. *An Introduction to Composite Materials.* New York: Cambridge University Press, 1981.
67. Hutter, O. F., F. L. Burton, and D. L. Bovell. Mechanical properties of normal and *mdx* mouse sarcolemma: bearing on function of dystrophin. *J. Musc. Res. Cell Motil.* 12:585–589, 1991.
68. Huxley, A. F., and R. M. Simmons. Mechanical properties of the cross-bridges of frog striated muscle. *J. Physiol. (Lond.)* 218:59P–60P, 1971.
69. Ibraghimov-Beskrovnaya, O., J. M. Ervasti, C. J. Leveille, C. A. Slaughter, S. W. Sernett, and K. P. Campbell. Primary structure of dystrophin-associated glycoproteins linking dystrophin to the extracellular matrix. *Nature* 355:696–702, 1992.

70. Järvinen, M., L. Jozsa, M. Kvist, M. Lehto, T. Vieno, J. Isola, and P. Kannus. Ultrastructure and collagen composition of the myo-fascial junction in rat calf muscles. *Acta Anat.* 145:216–219, 1992.

71. Jeronimidis, G., and J. F. V. Vincent. Composite materials. D. W. L. Hukins, (ed). *Connective Tissue Matrix.* Weinheim: Verlag Chemie, 1984, pp. 187–210.

72. Karpakka, J., K. Väänänen, S. Orava, and T. E. S. Takala. The effects of preimmobilization training and immobilization on collagen synthesis in rat skeletal muscle. *Int. J. Sports Med.* 11:484–488, 1990.

73. Karpakka, J., P. Virtanen, K. Väänänen, S. Orava, and T. E. S. Takala. Collagen synthesis in rat skeletal muscle during immobilization and remobilization. *J. Appl. Physiol.* 70:1774–1780, 1991.

74. Kinloch, A. J. *Adhesion and Adhesives.* London: Chapman and Hall, 1987.

75. Kovanen, V., H. Suominen, and L. Peltonen. Effects of aging and life-long physical training on collagen in slow and fast skeletal muscle in rats. *Cell Tissue Res.* 248:247–255, 1987.

76. Kovanen, V., and H. Suominen. Age- and training-related changes in the collagen metabolism of rat skeletal muscle. *Eur. J. Appl. Physiol.* 58:765–771, 1989.

77. Kühn, K., H. Weidemann, R. Timpl, et al. Macromolecular structure of basement membrane collagens. *FEBS Lett.* 125:123–128, 1981.

78. Law, D. J. Ultrastructural comparison of slack and stretched myotendinous junctions, based on a three-dimensional model of the connecting domain. *J. Musc. Res. Cell Motil.* 14:401–411, 1993.

79. Lev-Tov, A., C. A. Pratt, and R. E. Burke. The motor-unit population of the cat tenuissimus muscle. *J. Nuerophysiol.* 59:1128–1142, 1988.

80. Light, N. D., and A. E. Champion. Characterization of muscle epimysium, perimysium and endomysium collagens. *Biochem. J.* 219:1017–1026, 1984.

81. Light, N. D., A. E. Champion, C. A. Voyle, and A. J. Bailey. The role of epimysial, perimysial and endomysial collagen in determining the texture in six bovine muscles. *Meat Sci.* 13:137–149, 1985.

82. Linsenmeyer, T. F., A. Mentzer, M. H. Irwin, N. K. Waldrep, and R. Mayne. Avian type VI collagen. *Exp. Cell Res.* 165:518–529, 1986.

83. Lockhart, R. D., and W. Brandt. Length of striated muscle-fibres. *J. Anat.* 72:470, 1938.

84. Loeb, G. E., C. A. Pratt, C. M. Chanaud, and F. F. R. Richmond. Distribution and innervation of short interdigitated muscle fibers in parallel-fibered muscles of the cat hindlimb. *J. Morphol.* 191, 1–15, 1987.

85. Loeb, G. E., and F. J. R. Richmond. Architectural features of multiarticular muscles. *Hum. Mov. Sci.* in press.

86. Magid, A., and D. J. Law. Myofibrils bear most of the resting tension in frog skeletal muscle. *Science* 230:1280–1282, 1985.

87. Manzano, G., and A. J. McComas. Longitudinal structure and innervation of two mammalian hindlimb muscles. *Muscle Nerve* 11:1115–1122, 1988.

88. Markee, J. E., and H. Lowenbach. The relations between multiple innervation and "segmental" response of skeletal muscle of the dog. *J. Neurophsiol.* 8:409–420, 1945.

89. Masuda, T., N. Fujimaki, E. Ozawa, and H. Ishikawa. Confocal laser microscopy of dystrophin localization in guinea pig skeletal muscle fibers. *J. Cell Biol.* 119:543–548, 1992.

90. Mattheck, C., H. Huber, and P. Purslow. Assessment of shape optimisation of the myotendinous junction. *Animal and Related Cell Abstracts of the Annual Meeting, Soc. Exp. Biol.* 37, 1992.

91. Mauro, A., and O. Sten-Knudsen. The role of the sarcolemma in muscle physiology. *Acta Med. Scand.* 142 (suppl. 266):715–724, 1952.

92. Mauro, A., and W. R. Adams. The structure of the sarcolemma of the frog skeletal muscle fiber. *J. Biophys. Biochem. Cytol.* 10:177–183, 1961.

93. Mayeda, R. Ueber die kaleberverhaltnisse der quergestreiften muskelfasern. *Zeit. Biol.* 27:119–152, 1890.

94. Mayne, R., and R. D. Sanderson. The extracellular matrix of skeletal muscle. *Collagen Relat. Res.* 5:449–468, 1985.

95. Mayr, R., H. Gottschall, H. Gruber, and W. Neuhuber. Internal structure of cat extraocular muscle. *Anat. Embryol.* 148:25–34, 1975.

96. McComas, A. J., S. Kereshi, and G. Manzano. Multiple innervation of human muscle fibers. *J. Neurol. Sci.* 64:55–64, 1984.

97. McMahon, T. A. *Muscles, reflexes, and locomotion.* Princeton: Princeton University Press, 1984, pp. 3–21.

98. Misra, A. K., K. M. Nirmala, and S. K. Mishra. Abnormal distribution of desmin and vimentin in myofibers in adult onset myotubular myopathy. *Muscle Nerve* 15:1246–1252, 1992.

99. Natori, R. The role of myofibrils, sarcoplasma and sarcolemma in muscle contraction. *Jikei Med. J.* 1:18–28, 1954.

100. Neering, I. R., L. A. Queensberry, V. A. Morris, and S. R. Taylor. Nonuniform volume changes during muscle contraction. *Biophys. J.* 59:926–932, 1991.

101. Otten, E. Concepts and models of functional architecture in skeletal muscle. *Exerc. Sports Sci. Rev.* 16:89–137, 1988.

102. Ounjian, M., R. R. Roy, E. Eldred, et al. Physiological and developmental implications of motor unit anatomy. *J. Neurobiol.* 22:547–559, 1991.

103. Peltonen, L., R. Myllylä, U. Tolonen, and V. V. Myllylä. Changes in collagen metabolism in diseased muscle. II. Immunohistochemical studies. *Arch. Neurol.* 39:756–759, 1982.

104. Peters, S. E. Structure and function in vertebrate skeletal muscle. *Am. Zool.* 29:221–234, 1989.

105. Petrof, B. J., J. B. Shrager, H. H. Stedman, A. M. Kelly, and H. L. Sweeney. Dystrophin protects the sarcolemma from stresses developed during muscle contraction. *Proc. Natl. Acad. Sci. U. S. A.* 90:3710–3714, 1993.

106. Piggott, M. R. *Load-bearing fibre composites.* Oxford: Pergamon Press, 1980.

107. Podolsky, R. J. The maximum sarcomere length for contraction of isolated myofibrils. *J. Physiol. (Lond.)* 170:110–123, 1964.

108. Pratt, C. A., C. M. Chanaud, and G. E. Loeb. Functionally complex muscles of the cat hindlimb. IV. Intramuscular distribution of movement command signals and cutaneous reflexes in broad, bifunctional thigh muscles. *Exp. Brain Res.* 85:281–299, 1991.

109. Pratt, C. A., and G. E. Loeb. Functionally complex muscles of the cat hindlimb. I. Patterns of activation across sartorius. *Exp. Brain Res.* 85:243–256, 1991.

110. Purslow, P. P. and V. C. Duance. Structure and function of intramuscular connective tissue. Hukins, D. W. L. (ed). *Connective Tissue Matrix Part 2.* London: MacMillan Press, 1990, pp. 127–166.

111. Purslow, P. P., and J. A. Trotter. The morphology and mechanical properties of endomysium in series-fibred muscles; variations with muscle length. *J. Musc. Res. Cell Motil.* 15:299–304, 1994.

112. Ramsay, R. W., and S. F. Street. The isometric length-tension diagram of isolated skeletal muscle fibers of the frog. *J. Cell. Comp. Physiol.* 15:11–34, 1940.

113. Rapaport, S. I. Mechanical properties of the sarcolemma and myoplasm in frog muscle as a function of sarcomere length. *J. Gen. Physiol.* 59:559–585, 1972.

114. Rapaport, S. I. The anisotropic elastic properties of the sarcolemma of the frog semitendinosus muscle fiber. *Biophys. J.* 13:14–36, 1973.

115. Reddy, A. S., M. K. Reedy, A. V. Seaber, W. E. Garrett. Restriction of the injury response following an acute muscle strain. *Med. Sci. Sports Exerc.* 25:321–327, 1993.

116. Reed, R., and K. M. Rudall. Electron microscope studies of muscle structure. *Biophys. Biochim. Acta* 2:19–26, 1948.

117. Richmond, F. J. R., D. R. R. MacGillis, and D. A. Scott. Muscle-fiber compartmentalization in cat splenius muscles. *J. Neurophysiol.* 53:868–885, 1985.

118. Richmond, F. J. R., and V. C. Abrahams. Morphology and enzyme histochemistry of dorsal muscles of the cat neck. *J. Neurophysiol.* 38:1313–1321, 1975.
119. Richmond, F. J. R., and R. B. Armstrong. Fiber architecture and histochemistry in the cat neck muscle, biventer cervicis. *J. Neurophysiol.* 60:46–59, 1988.
120. Richmond, F. J. R., D. B. Thomson, and G. E. Loeb. Electromyographic studies of neck muscles in the intact cat. I. Patterns of recruitment underlying posture and movement during natural behaviors. *Exp. Brain Res.* 88:41–58, 1992.
121. Rowe, R. W. D. Morphology of perimysial and endomysial connective tissue in skeletal muscle. *Tissue Cell* 13:681–690, 1981.
122. Rowe, R. W. D. Electron microscopy of bovine muscle. I. The native state of post rigor sarcolemma and endomysium. *Meat Sci.* 26:271–279, 1989.
123. Ryan, J. M., M. A. Cobb, and J. W. Hermanson. Elbow extensor muscles of the horse: postural and dynamic implications. *Acta Anat.* 144:71–79, 1992.
124. Schmalbruch, H. The sarcolemma of morphology muscle fibres as demonstrated by a replica technique. *Cell Tissue Res.* 150:377–387, 1974.
125. Schmalbruch, H. *Skeletal Muscle.* Berlin: Springer-Verlag, 1985.
126. von Schwarzacher, H. G. Zur lage der motorischen endplatten in den skeletmuskeln. *Acta. Anat.* 30:758–774, 1957.
127. von Schwarzacher, H. G. Über die länge und anordnung der muskelfasern in menschlichen skelettmuskeln. *Acta Anat.* 37:217–231, 1959.
128. Scott, S. H., D. B. Thomson, F. J. R. Richmond, and G. E. Loeb. Neuromuscular organization of feline anterior sartorius. II. Intramuscular length changes and complex length-tension relationships during stimulation of individual nerve branches. *J. Morphol.* 213:171–183, 1992.
129. Selbie, W. S., D. B. Thomson, and F. J. R. Richmond. Suboccipital muscles in the cat neck: morphometry and histochemistry of the rectus capitis muscle complex. *J. Morphol.* 216:47–63, 1993.
130. Shear, C. R., and R. J. Bloch. Vinculin in subsarcolemmal densities in chicken skeletal muscle: localization and relationship to intracellular and extracellular structure. *J. Cell Biol.* 101:240–256, 1986.
131. Sherrington, C. S. Flexion-reflex of the limb, crossed extension-reflex and reflex stepping and standing. *J. Physiol. (Lond.)* 40:28–121, 1910.
132. Smits, E., P. K. Rose, T. Gordon, and F. J. R. Richmond. Organization of single motor units in feline sartorius. *J. Neurophysiol.* 72:1885–1896, 1994.
133. Stephens, H. R., M. Bendayan, and M. Silver. Immunocytochemical localization of collagen types and laminin in skeletal muscle with the protein-A gold technique. *Biol. Cell* 44:81–84, 1982.
134. Straub, V., R. E. Bittner, J. J. Léger, and T. Voit. Direct visualization of the dystrophin network on skeletal muscle fiber membrane. *J. Cell Biol.* 119:1183–1191, 1992.
135. Street, S. F. Lateral transmission of tension in frog myofibers: a myofibrillar network and transverse cytoskeletal connections are possible transmitters. *J. Cell. Physiol.* 114:346–364, 1983.
136. Stickland, N. C. The arrangements of muscle fibres and tendons in two muscles used for growth studies. *J. Anat.* 136:175–179, 1983.
137. Stuart, D. G., T. M. Hamm, and S. Vanden Noven. Partitioning of monosynaptic Ia EPSP connections with motorneurons according to neuromuscular topography: generality and functional implications. *Prog. Neurobiol.* 30:437–447, 1988.
138. Swatland, H. J. Morphology and development of endomysial connective tissue in porcine and bovine muscle. *J. Anim. Sci.* 41:78–86, 1975.
139. Teravainen, H. Localization of acetylcholinesterase activity in myotendinous and myomyous junctions of the striated skeletal muscles of the rat. *Experientia* (Basel) 25:524–525, 1969.
140. Thompson, D. W. *On Growth and Form.* London: Cambridge, 1961.

141. Thomson, D. B., S. H. Scott, nd F. J. R. Richmond. Neuromuscular organization of feline anterior sartorius. I. Asymmetric distribution of motor units. *J. Morphol.* 210:147–162, 1991.
142. Thornell, L. E. and M. G. Price. The cystoskeleton in muscle cells in relation to function. *Biochem. Soc. Trans.* 19:1116–1120, 1991.
143. Tidball, J. G. Energy stored and dissipated in skeletal muscle basement membranes during sinusoidal oscillations. *Biosphys. J.* 50:1127–1138, 1986.
144. Tidball, J. G. Myotendinous junction injury in relation to junction structure and molecular composition. *Exerc. Sports Sci. Rev.* 19:419–445, 1991.
145. Torigoe, K., and T. Nakamura. Fine structure of myomyous junctions in the mouse skeletal muscles. *Tissue Cell* 19:243–250, 1987.
146. Trombitas, K., P. Baatsen, J. Schreuder, and G. H. Pollack. Contraction-induced movements of water in single fibers of frog skeletal muscle. *Biophys. J.* 64:A28, 1993.
147. Trotter, J. A. Interfiber tension transmission in series-fibered muscles of the cat hindlimb. *J. Morphol.* 206:351–361, 1990.
148. Trotter, J. A. Dynamic shape of tapered skeletal muscle fibers. *J. Morphol.* 207:211–223, 1991.
149. Trotter, J. A., J. D. Salgado, R. Ozbaysal, and A. S. Gaunt. The composite structure of quail pectoralis muscle. *J. Morphol.* 212:27–35, 1992.
150. Trotter, J. A., and P. P. Purslow. Functional morphology of the endomysium in series fibered muscles. *J. Morphol.* 212:109–122, 1992.
151. Trotter, J. A. Functional morphology of force transmission in skeletal muscle. *Acta Anat.* 146:205–222, 1993.
152. Windhorst, U., T. M. Hamm, and D. G. Stuart. On the function of muscle and reflex partitioning. *Behav. Brain Sci.* 12:629–645, 1989.
153. Wines, M. W., and E. C. B. Hall-Craggs. Neuromuscular relationships in the muscle having segregated motor endplate zones. I. Anatomical and physiological considerations. *J. Comp. Neurol.* 249:147–151, 1986.
154. Yurchenco, P. D., E. C. Tsilibary, A. S. Charonis, and H. Furthmayr. Models for the self-assembly of basement membrane. *J. Histochem. Cytochem.* 34:93–102, 1986.
155. Zenker, W., D. Snobl, and R. Boetschi. Multifocal innervation and muscle length. *Anat. Embryol.* 182:273–283, 1990.

7
The Impact of Exercise on the Immune System: NK Cells, Interleukins 1 and 2, and Related Responses

ROY J. SHEPHARD, M.D. (LOND.), Ph.D.
SHAWN RHIND, M.Sc.
PANG N. SHEK, Ph.D.

The present review focuses upon two cytokines, interleukin-1 and interleukin-2 (IL-1 and IL-2), and their place in reactions involving natural killer (NK) cells and T and B lymphocytes. Many immunological responses to exercise persist for only 30–60 min postexercise and are thus of limited clinical significance. However, strenuous exercise can depress the NK/IL-2 system for 7 days or longer (Shek et al., manuscript in preparation, 1993), probably explaining much of the vulnerability to acute infection that is associated with high-level competition and chronic overtraining [16, 132, 134, 176]. Changes in levels of IL-1 also modify the rate of progression of atherosclerosis [171], with important implications for preventive cardiology.

IL-1, IL-2 AND THEIR RECEPTORS

Interleukin-1

IL-1 exists in two forms [31]: $IL-1_\alpha$ (typically cell-associated), and $IL-1_\beta$ (the soluble mediator). IL-1 is produced by various cell types, particularly antigen-presenting macrophages [188, 229]. It stimulates T-helper lymphocytes to produce IL-2 and to express IL-1 and IL-2 receptors, at the same time upgrading the production of major histocompatibility complex (MHC) class II proteins on antigen-exposed B cells. It is involved in exercise-related elevations of body temperature, inflammation, and prostaglandin secretion. The biological activity of IL-1 is inhibited by prostaglandin E_2 and by a specific receptor antagonist (IL-1 RA), both of which are produced by alveolar macrophages and by monocytes [95].

Interleukin-2

IL-2 affects both adjacent cells and the cells where it has been secreted. It thus serves as both a paracrine and an autocrine immunoregulator. Sources include activated T-helper cells, to a lesser extent NK cells [170, 222], and possibly in small quantities T-suppressor cells [57]. It stimulates thymocyte maturation [161], proliferation of T and B cells [122, 204], increase of IL-2 receptor expression on both T and B cells [197], release of other cytokines such as interferon [43, 183], and the proliferation and cytotoxicity of NK cells, lymphokine-activated killer cells, and monocytes [81, 101].

Lymphocyte proliferation can also be initiated by plant lectins and by antigens. Lectins nonspecifically activate 30–60% of peripheral blood mononuclear cells, whereas antigens act only on the 0.02–0.1% of peripheral blood mononuclear cells expressing receptors specific to that antigen. Activation induces the transcription of certain genes (particularly the IL-2 receptor gene). After stimulation with phytohemagglutinin (PHA), IL-2 mRNA is detectable at 4 hr, and peaks at 12–15 hr [183]. IL-2 receptor density is greatly increased 24–72 hr after T-cell activation [183], but by 6–14 days the receptor count has returned to resting values.

Cytokine Receptor Structure
The typical cytokine receptor is a glycoprotein. A terminal amino acid chain lies outside the cell membrane, a hydrophobic sector spans the membrane, and there is an intracellular domain that differs from one receptor to another [121].

The amino acid sequencing of the external part of the molecule places the B-cell antigen receptor, the α and β chains of the T-cell antigen receptor, and the type I IL-1 receptor in the immunoglobulin superfamily [8]. Each of these receptors has about 110 amino acid residues, including at least one pair of external cysteine residues, and an extensive antiparallel β sheet structure [34].

The IL-2 receptor comprises three noncovalently associated subunits. A 55-kD α chain can be detected by CD25 monoclonal antibodies [2]. It does not belong to any well-defined immunoglobulin family. A second (β) subunit [71] belongs to the hemopoietin superfamily; the external, ligand-binding domain of this receptor contains about 210 amino acid residues, including 4 terminal cysteine residues, and a Trp-Ser-X-Trp-Ser motif close to the membrane [28, 121]. Mikβ-1 and TU-27 monoclonal antibodies identify the β receptor chain [23]; Mikβ-1 reacts with a 70-kD molecule [206], whereas TU-27 reacts with a 75-kD molecule [192]. There is also a 64-kD (γ) chain, again a member of the hemopoietin superfamily [192], but unfortunately no convenient antibody has yet been developed for this subunit.

The α chain binds IL-2 on amino acids 33–56; the Michaelis constant (K_m) of 10^{-8} M implies that a free IL-2 concentration of 10^{-8} M will occupy a half of the binding sites [218]. The intracellular portion of the α receptor, only 13 amino acids, is insufficient for signal transduction [103], and there is no discernible biological response if binding occurs only at this site.

Amino acids 11–20 of the β chain have a stronger affinity for IL-2 ($K_m = 10^{-9}$ M) [218], and T cells that express both α and β receptors bind IL-2 even more strongly $K_m = 10^{-11}$ M) [166]. IL-2 binding can be blocked by antibodies to either α or β receptors, implying that the two receptors act jointly to form a high-affinity receptor complex; this permits IL-2 to transmit signals at very low concentrations. The β chain has a large (286-amino acid) intracytoplasmic domain; the serine-rich portion probably mediates the IL-2 signal [167, 194], binding a lymphocyte-specific phosphotyrosin sequence [37, 120]. Signal transmission seems independent of calcium-dependent phosphatidylinositol and protein kinase C pathways, and does not require cAMP or GMP as second messengers [201].

Some 35% of resting peripheral lymphocytes express the IL-2 α chain, and 10% the IL-2 β chain, both at levels of less than 500 copies per cell [83, 102, 232]; however, a subpopulation of large granular lymphocytes stain strongly for such receptors [139]. The α receptor is expressed by a significant proportion of T-helper (CD4+) cells, but not by T-suppressor (CD8+) cells [180]. The CD8+ cells express relatively high levels of β receptors, whereas the expression of this antigen is weak in CD4+ and B (CD19+) cells [143, 232]. Most NK cells express the β chain, but very few express the α chain [180]; substantial (1 nM) concentrations of IL-2 are thus required for their activation [205].

Stimulation of lymphocytes by PHA or pokeweed mitogen (PWM) induces a major (30–100-fold) up-regulation of α receptors (to >30,000 copies per cell), but little (3–4-fold) up-regulation of β receptors [6]. Induction of the α receptor alone does not make the lymphocytes responsive to IL-2; there must also be subtle quantitative or qualitative changes in the β receptor [233].

METHODS OF EVALUATION

General Considerations

Immune function may be investigated in terms of the counts of secreting or targeted cells, the rates of cell proliferation, the immunoglobulin content of body fluids, in vitro production of immunoglobulins, and more direct cytokine assay procedures.

Differential Blood Counts

The meaning of cell counts remains uncertain, given that 90–99% of all lymphocytes are normally found outside the circulating blood [228]. However, analysis has been facilitated greatly by the introduction of automated flow cytometers and fluorochrome-labeled monoclonal antibodies. Large numbers of cells can now be enumerated, and classification is more certain than was possible with earlier techniques such as microscopic morphology, adherence to specific surfaces, rosetting, and enzyme histochemistry. If several differing concentrations of monoclonal antibody are used, the surface density of the receptors can be determined [178]. Cell populations of particular interest are the pan T cell count (CD3+), T-helper/inducer cells (CD4+), T-suppressor cells (CD8+ CD3+), cytotoxic T cells (CD8+ CD3−), B cells (CD19+), and natural killer cells (CD16+, with a subpopulation carrying the CD56+ marker).

CD4+ Cells

CD4+ cells recognize and bind foreign antigens ingested by monocyte macrophages (CD14+ cells) and presented on the surface of the macrophages in the context of MHC class II molecules [220]. The macrophages then release IL-1 as a second signal to activate the CD4+ cells. Despite occasional contrary reports [109, 122], most authors believe that IL-2 cannot trigger the proliferation of either T cells [191] or B cells [14, 90] except in the presence of a second signal such as IL-1 or the mitogen concanavalin A; such responses are enhanced not only by other interleukins and interferons, but also by substances such as L-carnitine and acetylcholine [211] that apparently act by altering membrane structures.

Activated CD4+ cells produce IL-2 and express increasing numbers of IL-2 receptors. IL-2 also stimulates the CD4+ cells to secrete a third lymphokine (IL-3). This last substance sends a signal to cytotoxic (CD8+, CD3) T cells previously sensitized at the IL-2 β receptor; they then recognize the foreign surface constituents of abnormal or virus-transformed cells and initiate their destruction [230]. The response depends on the rate of recirculation of cells through the lymphatic and general circulation [231]. Subpopulations of slow, intermediate, and fast-moving cells can be distinguished by the use of selective antibodies. Motility is influenced by adhesion molecules and their receptors on the lymphocytes and the vascular endothelium, intracellular contraction proteins, the rate of lymphocyte metabolism, and levels of interleukin-8 [52, 209, 231].

The CD4+ cells interact with the B lymphocytes. Initially, there seems to be a low-affinity, nonspecific reaction between the CD4+ protein and a class II MHC protein on the CD19+ cells [84, 140], although dendritic cells may also play a role [119, 127]. Activation increases the affinity of a CD4+ surface protein (LFA-1) for a second protein on the surface of the B cells (ICAM-1). Adhesion and interaction between the two cell types is assured by up-regulation of other T-cell surface proteins (CD2+ and CD28+) [4, 86]. After 4–8 hr, the CD4+ cells synthesize an as-yet unidentified factor that initiates B-cell proliferation; the B cells then become responsive to IL-4 and IL-5 [77, 141], differentiating into plasma cells, with a resultant release of antibodies. Several subclasses of CD4+ cells are now distinguished. The classical T_{h1} cells produce IL-2 in response to antigens and use this cytokine as an autocrine factor to stimulate their own growth. The T_{h2} cells make and respond to IL-4; they can also respond to IL-2, but do not secrete it [125]. CD4+ cells are also differentiated in terms of the CD45RA marker; CD4+

CD45RA+ cells are selectively stimulated by concanavalin A, and induce CD8+ cells to suppress immunoglobulin production. In contrast, CD4+ CD45RA− cells respond to PHA and enhance immunoglobulin production [137].

CD8+ Cells

CD8+ cells provide a negative feedback that regulates the CD4+ cells. They also recognize foreign antigens in association with the MHC class I protein molecules found on abnormal and virus-infected target cells [10, 33]. Susceptibility to viral infections is increased if the ratio of CD4+ to CD8+ cells drops below 1.5 [12, 48].

NK Cells

The NK cells [85, 111, 144, 169] are found mainly in the spleen, liver, and lungs [72, 228]. They have a much higher surface density of LFA-1 than the CD4+ cells, with a correspondingly greater potential for modulation of their motility [52]. Most NK cells express CD16, but not the CD3 surface marker [68, 99]. Such cells recognize and destroy a wide range of tumor, abnormal, and virus-infected cells [199] without the intervention of MHC proteins [124]. The NK cells pass selectively to injured muscle, assisting in the repair process, but cannot migrate between blood and lymph nodes, as do the lymphocytes [228]. NK activity is increased by various soluble factors, including IL-1, IL-2, interferons, growth hormone, L-carnitine, and acetylcholine [13, 175, 191, 193, 211). Cytotoxic activity is not inhibited by antibodies that block the IL-2 α receptor, suggesting that IL-2 regulates cytolysis by means of the β chain [93, 146, 180]. Interferon may increase susceptibility to IL-2 either by altering receptor affinity or by inducing additional IL-2 receptors [75]. NK proliferation does not occur until a high IL-2 affinity is realized through the combined action of newly synthesized α and existing β chains. About 10% of NK cells are normally CD56 bright but CD16 negative. Such cells have an excess of free β chains [128], and respond to 10–100 times lower concentrations of IL-2 than do CD56 dim cells [61].

Factors Modifying Cell Counts and Activity

Extraneous factors that can modify peripheral blood counts and/or activity during exercise include (a) a decrease of blood volume; (b) an increase of cardiac output, a decrease of visceral blood flow, and possibly an alteration of surface adhesion molecules [52, 177, 231], leading to a demargination and/or a mobilization of cells sequestered in the lungs, liver [51], and spleen [5]; (c) an up-regulation of cytokine receptors [115]; (d) an activation of α- or β-adrenoreceptors [100, 110, 115, 212], reducing the attachment of leucocytes to the vascular endothelium for any given level of circulating catecholamines; (e) autonomic activity related to pain and/or emotional stress [11, 129, 173, 187]: a release of catecholamines and co-transmitters depresses the response to mitogens, but also decreases cell margination [24, 89, 92, 203]; (f) cortisol secretion that suppresses the function of CD4+ cells [45, 154, 162, 224], counters the action of IL-1 [32, 162], suppresses IL-2 receptor expression [45], and induces a release of granulocytes from bone marrow [27]; and (g) a migration of cells from the bloodstream into injured tissues [148].

There are also effects from dietary modification [7], nutrient deficiencies [20, 108, 130, 131, 152, 153], and circadian and seasonal rhythms [157, 196].

Cell Proliferation

The rate of lymphocyte proliferation can be estimated from incorporation of tritiated thymidine [82], assuming that DNA synthesis parallels cell proliferation [117]. Counts depend on many technical factors such as sample type and size, choice of scintillation mixture, container shape and size, counter efficiency, and impurities [189]. Cells are incubated with nonspecific lectins. PHA binds mainly to the CD3 complex; it is a potent mitogen for all T cells [225], but also has an indirect effect on B cells through increases of cytokine secretion. PWM is predominantly a B-cell mitogen, although it also causes some increase in CD8+ cell proliferation [227].

Analyses are based on either whole blood or washed peripheral mononuclear cells. The recovery of washed cells is incomplete, although with careful technique, the two data sets agree fairly closely [178]. A correction can be applied for overall losses, but the proportion of CD8+ cells is also somewhat lower in washed cells than in whole blood. Whole blood responses may be modified by soluble factors [172]. A further practical problem is to find an optimal dose of mitogen. Because of the difficulties, and the absence of a close linkage between intravascular cell numbers and immune function, differing inferences about the effects of exercise may be drawn from cell proliferation rates and CD4+/CD8+ cell ratios [210].

Cellular Activity

NK cytolytic activity is commonly assessed by the in vitro release of radioactive chromium [145] from human myeloid tumor cells (K-562) tested at several differing effector/target ratios [178]. Lytic activity can be expressed per unit volume of blood or per CD16+ cell [68, 99]. Discrepancies can arise relative to studies based on the CD56+ marker, particularly if there has been a differential migration of CD16+ cells out of the circulation.

The activity of B cells can be assessed from immunoglobulin levels in plasma, saliva, and mucosal secretions. Immunoglobulin concentrations are reduced both by very heavy exercise and by very heavy training [112, 113, 126, 202, 213, 226], but it is as yet unclear whether concentrations are reduced by more moderate aerobic activity [63, 113, 126, 213].

Interleukin Assay

Interleukin assay procedures must detect extremely low concentrations [200]. For example, resting serum levels of IL-2 are in the range of 0–250 pg/ml. After 36–72 hr of incubation with PHA, peripheral blood mononuclear cells still yield no more than 2500 pg/ml. Bioassays depend on the incorporation of tritiated thymidine into a leukemic T-cell line [1, 118]. There can be problems of both reproducibility and specificity [39] because responses are vulnerable to natural interleukin inhibitors [185] and the target cells must respond to IL-2, but not to other cytokines, such as IL-4 [76].

A radioimmunoassay (RIA) or an enzyme-linked inmmunosorbent assay compares experimental IL-2 concentrations [3] with standard international preparations of either natural IL-2 [54, 118] or recombinant IL-2 [30]. Unfortunately, there is not as yet world-wide agreement on methods of expressing concentrations (protein concentration, picograms per milliliter, or units capable of inducing 50% of maximal proliferation per milliliter). Immunoassays are quicker (4–6 hr vs. 2–4 days) and simpler than bioassays, but the antibodies that are used can react not only to active IL-2, but also to inactive precursors and partially cleaved forms of IL-2 [21, 56]. It is also difficult to incorporate radioisotope without modifying either antigenicity or binding capacity. The threshold of RIA (20–50 pg/ml) is thus marginal for low but biologically active concentrations of cytokine. Enzyme-linked immunosorbent assay reagents have a longer shelf life, and avoid problems arising in the handling of radioactive material, but have even less sensitivity than RIA [138]. A final option is to infer production of IL-2 from the transcription of the corresponding mRNA.

IL-2 receptor density can be determined by dual-parameter immunofluorescence flow cytometry, one axis indicating the percentage of cells of a given type, and the other axis the percentage carrying the receptor marker. Changes in cell responsiveness can also be examined in terms of proliferation rates after PHA or PWM stimulation. Soluble IL-2 receptor (released in a reaction of IL-2 with the α-receptor chain) can finally be assayed in plasma or in urine.

RESPONSES OF THE NK–IL SYSTEM TO ACUTE EXERCISE

Cell Counts and Exercise

Exercise-induced changes in cell counts are typically biphasic. Multipoint blood sampling is thus essential [69, 178]. Appropriate corrections must also be applied for any changes of blood volume. Many of the reported changes seem too transient to affect immune defenses significantly, and they may reflect little more than a redistribution of cells within the lymphatic system [207].

Reactions vary with the type and duration of exercise (short-term activity mobilizes sequestrated cells, but these escape to damaged tissues with prolonged or eccentric exercise), the relative intensity of effort [94], opportunity for recovery from previous exercise bouts, and associated psychological or environmental stresses (including habituation to the test laboratory) [164].

T Cells and B Cells

Absolute T cell numbers show large increases (up to 150%) during or immediately after vigorous exercise, whether submaximal [41, 44, 58, 104] or maximal [58, 67, 208]. However, the percentage of CD3+ cells is unchanged after all-out treadmill exercise [9] or 30 min of exercise at 80% of maximal oxygen intake [214], and the latter stress does not change CD19+ cell percentages [214]. Others have seen a decrease of CD3+ counts with 1 hr of exercise at 25, 50, or 75% of maximal oxygen intake [208], but no change in CD3+ or CD4+ counts after prolonged exercise such as marathon running [59, 123, 134].

Some authors find increments of CD19+ counts [41, 44]. Others [29, 144, 164, 207] report no change in CD19+ counts, but (perhaps because the CD4+/CD8+ ratio is decreased, unpublished data of Shek et al., 1993), plasma levels of immunoglobulin are reduced [67] and the cells show a reduced in vitro production of immunoglobulin [74] with 1–2 hr of submaximal exercise. Shinkai et al. [178] noted increases in CD3+, CD4+, and CD8+ cells and less marked increments of CD19+ counts when sedentary young men (maximal oxygen intake, $\dot{V}O_2max$ = 41.3 ml/[kg·min]) undertook 60 min of cycle ergometer exercise at 60% of $\dot{V}O_2max$. Shek et al. (unpublished data, 1993) observed a similar response when fit subjects ($\dot{V}O_2max$ = 66.5 ml/[kg·min]) undertook a 90–120-min bout of treadmill exercise at 65% of $\dot{V}O_2max$; CD3+ counts peaked at a 43% increase 30 min postexercise, but there were no significant changes in CD19+ counts.

The CD4+/CD8+ ratio has been suggested as influencing mitogen-induced cellular proliferation [78, 100]. However, the in vitro response to mitogens does not always agree with what might be inferred from CD4+/CD8+ ratios [214, 217]. The CD4+/CD8+ ratio commonly decreases because of a decrease of CD4+ count after a maximal test [9, 44], or longer periods of submaximal exercise: 15 min [73, 100], 30 min [214], 45 min [136], 60 min [164], and 120 min [147]. Hack et al. [67], Shinkai et al. [178] and Shek et al. (unpublished data, 1993) noted that the CD4+/CD8+ ratio decreased despite increases in both CD4+ and CD8+ counts: by 36% with 1 hr of exercise [178] and by 57% with 90–120 min (Shek et al., unpublished data, 1993); after exercise, both CD4+ and CD8+ counts became subnormal, but (perhaps in compensation for this) the CD4+/CD8+ ratio was increased (Shek et al., unpublished data, 1993).

In vitro determinations of cellular proliferation are based on culturing a fixed number of cells, and because exercise induces a lymphocytosis, there can be a decreased mitogen response per cell, despite an unchanged or even an enhanced proliferative response per unit volume of blood [168, 184]. Acute exercise generally suppresses cell proliferation, sometimes by as much as 50% [59, 73, 147, 207, 208], but changes last no more than 2 hr, even with vigorous exercise [49, 132, 137], and are thus unlikely to have a major effect on immune function [133, 214]. Sometimes the response to both mitogens and antigens is reduced for several hours [40, 114]. The effect is not modified by administering antibodies to IL-1, but is countered by antibodies to tumor necrosis factor-α; prostaglandin release may also modify the response by decreasing IL-2 release or blocking IL-2 receptors [208], although responsiveness cannot be restored by adding substantial quantities of exogenous IL-2 [163].

Strenuous exercise increases the sensitivity of T-cell β-adrenoreceptors (by 121% on CD4+ cells, and by 80% on CD8+ cells) [214]. The CD4+/CD8+ ratio may remain elevated for as long as 24 hr after exercise (Shek et al., unpublished data, 1993), apparently because of a cortisol-induced reduction in the number of CD8+ cells. Intercell differences in the number of β-adrenoceptors, and thus sensitivity to exercise-induced secretion of catecholamines, probably contribute to changes in subset counts during and after exercise. CD19+ cells have almost 3 times as many β-adrenoreceptors as T cells, and CD4+ cells also have 4 times as many receptors as CD8+ cells. The density of the receptors is modulated by habitual catecholamine and cortisol levels, and also by training [214].

The expression of CD3+, CD4+, CD8+, and CD19+ antigens decreases by 2–3% immediately after exercise [178]. As with the CD4+/CD8+ ratio [41, 91], this change probably reflects a mobilization of cells with a 10–20% weaker expression of marker antigens. However, humoral factors could also down-regulate expression of surface antigens [178].

Natural Killer Cell Numbers and Activity
Moderate exercise leads to early increases in the number, percentage and activity of NK cells [9, 29, 38, 41, 46, 51, 94, 98, 104, 112, 132, 159, 178, 195, 208, 223]. Nieman et al. [137] saw a 176% increase of count immediately after a 30-s all-out effort. Others had similar findings with 60 s of anaerobic exercise [62]. Shinkai et al. [178] found CD16+ numbers were almost doubled after 60 min of exercise, although there was no change in the density of surface receptors. Shek et al. (unpublished data, 1993) noted a 40–50% increase of NK counts when fit subjects performed similar exercise for 90–120 min. Pedersen [156] maintained that although the CD16+ CD56+ count was increased, the CD16− CD56+ count was unaffected by exercise. Furthermore, the magnitude of the CD16+ response seems to depend on the relative work rate and the extent of eccentric contractions [50].

The proportion of activated killer cells increases during and immediately after exercise. Edwards et al. [38] noted increased cytolysis after 5 min of staircase running, although cytolytic activity had normalized by 1 hr post-exercise. Hanson and Flaherty [70] found enhanced cytolysis both immediately and 24 hr after a 12.8-km run. Mackinnon et al. [113] found a 40% increase of NK activity 1 hr after exercise. Kotani et al. [98] commented that whereas the percentage of NK cells had normalized within 15 min of ceasing a 3-min bout of treadmill walking, cytotoxic activity remained elevated for at least 30 min. Naloxone inhibits the early increase of NK activity (although the NK count is unchanged); this could imply a mediator role for endogenous opioids [46], although the fact that responses are unaffected by epidural anesthesia [156] argues against this possibility. Passive heating to a core temperature of 39.5°C increases CD16+ counts [87, 88, 156]. Exercise-induced changes in the concentration of the interleukins and interferons may modify lytic activity in vivo. However, having due regard to the potential mobility of the NK cells [231], redistribution may also recruit into the bloodstream NK cells with a high IL-2 response capacity [105, 155, 173].

Increased NK activity may persist for 24 hr after moderate exercise [70]. However, exhausting exercise has a less favorable effect. Pedersen et al. [159] and Tvede et al. [208] argued that there was a prostaglandin-mediated down-regulation of cytolytic activity per NK cell after 1 or 2 hr of exercise at 75–80% of $\dot{V}O_2$max. The findings of Brahmi et al. [15] are typical: NK activity peaked immediately after cycle ergometer exercise to exhaustion, subsequently dropping to a subnormal nadir 120 min postexercise, and recovering over the next 20 hr. Berk et al. [9] reported a 31% decrease of NK cell activity 1.5 hr after a 3-hr marathon run; there was a 50% decrease in CD16+ cells (which persisted for 21 hr), but no change in the number of CD56+ cells. Because, in their view, the CD56+ cells were responsible for much of the NK activity, Nieman and Nehlsen-Cannarella [133] argued that the decrease in cytolysis reflected a temporary down-regulation of CD56+ cells. Shinkai et al. [178] noted that the CD16+ activity of unfit subjects moved in close parallel with CD16+ count, and it was only 50% of baseline 60 min after 1 hr of cycle ergometer exercise at 60% of $\dot{V}O_2$max. Changes in cell distribution [173] seem a more likely explanation than a down-regulation of NK activity, particularly because normal counts and activity were restored within 2 hr of ceasing exercise. Mackinnon et al. [113] also observed recovery of a depressed count within 2 hr and recovery was complete 6 hr after participation in a triathlon competition [179]. However, for reasons that have yet to be elucidated, Shek et al. (unpublished data, 1993) saw a more profound disturbance of NK function; they used a relatively long exercise bout (90–120 min at 60% of $\dot{V}O_2$max) and sampled blood for 7 days. At the end of this period, NK cell counts were still only 75% of baseline, and NK activity was only about 50% of baseline. Their observations obviously have major clinical implications; therefore it is important that their study be replicated and the reasons for the severe response be ascertained.

The rise of NK count during exercise is correlated with the increase in heart rate [50] and with endogenous [116] or infused [87] levels of epinephrine. It probably reflects a decrease of cell margination, but it is unclear whether the primary association is with increased cardiac output, catecholamine release, or changes in cell adherence factors. The NK cell has receptors for many neuroendocrine factors [11, 160]. NK activity is negatively correlated with the late, exercise-induced surge of serum cortisol levels [133], and cortisol has a negative effect on in vitro NK activity [53]. The decreased activity is also correlated with the increment of monocyte numbers; the release of prostaglandins from monocytes and neutrophils that have migrated into damaged muscle tissue may thus be involved, suggesting a potential for therapeutic administration of indomethacine [17, 159, 208].

Neutrophils
Moderate exercise increases the neutrophil count and "primes" the capacity of the neutrophils to produce peroxides and free radicals for several hours, thereby increasing their capacity to kill bacteria and viruses; however, intensive exercise suppresses neutrophil counts for 24 hours or longer [36, 74, 132, 208, 210].

Soluble Factors
When testing for exercise-induced changes of cytokine concentrations, due allowance must be made for exercise-induced decreases of plasma volume [182].

IL-1. Sprenger et al. [186] found no changes in plasma IL-1 β when well-trained runners had completed a 20-km road race; however, urinary clearance (and thus the presumed production of IL-1β) was augmented. Radioimmunoassay also showed increased plasma levels of IL-1 3–6 hr after exercise at 60% of $\dot{V}O_2$max [19]. Isolated mononuclear cells secrete more IL-1 after heavy exercise [18, 66, 104]. Microtraumata in the active muscles may be one trigger to IL-1 release; if so, this would explain why some forms of exercise do not increase IL-1 levels [156]. Passive heating has a suppressant effect on in vitro production of IL-1β but no IL-1α [88].

IL-2. The reported impact of exercise upon plasma levels and in vitro production of IL-2 differs from one laboratory to another. Lewicki et al. [104] exercised 11 trained cyclists for about 20 min to exhaustion. They noted that the in vitro IL-2 production of PHA-stimulated peripheral blood mononuclear cells was decreased by 30% 3 min after exercise, and by 40% 2 hr postexercise. Rhind et al. [163] also found a decreased in vitro production of IL-2 at the 60th min of heavy exercise, with an even larger decrement 2 hr postexercise. Likewise, Espersen et al. [41] noted a 50% decrease in plasma IL-2 levels "immediately" after 11 well-conditioned runners had completed a 5-km run; recovery occurred over the next 2 hr, and values were 50% greater than normal 24 hr postexercise. Tvede et al. [208] also found a decreased in vitro production during and for 2 hr after exercise at 75% of maximal oxygen intake. In contrast, Haahr et al. [66] found no change in either radioimmunoassay or bioassay estimates of in vitro IL-2 production when 10 subjects completed an hour of cycle ergometry at 75% of $\dot{V}O_2$max. Schectman et al. [174] reported that in vitro IL-2 production had increased by 40% immediately after 1 hr of cycle ergometer exercise at 60% of $\dot{V}O_2$max. Output was still 31% above normal 30 min postexercise. Passive heating increased IL-2 levels by a similar amount [87, 88, 174]; changes may thus be due to a combination of catecholamine and cortisol secretion plus a rising core temperature. In support of a thermal effect, Gmünder et al. [59] measured serum IL-2 on 3 women and 13 men after they had completed a 21-km run under snowy conditions (when any rise of core temperature was probably small); concentrations of IL-2 were normal immediately after the race, and remained so 2 days later. Concentrations of IL-2 seem unrelated to circulating lymphocyte counts postexercise. The cytokines may therefore be liberated extravascularly, through inflammation of the active muscles [41]. Plasma levels of IL-2 may also change if an increased proportion of the lymphocyte population are active and thus are binding circulating IL-2 [163]. Other factors that could modify IL-2 production [104] are an effect of exercise-induced glucocorticoid secretion upon the production of the endogenous leukotriene B_4 [26, 60] or the CD4+/CD8+ cell ratio [150].

IL-2 Receptors
Soluble IL-2 receptor concentrations reflect interactions between T cells and circulating IL-2. Dufaux and Order [35] found increased plasma concentrations for 2 days after a 150-min bout of running, and Northoff and Berg [142] noted a peak immediately after participation in a triathlon. Sprenger et al. [186] also saw an increased urinary excretion of soluble IL-2 receptor (IL-2R) after a 20-km run. Lewicki et al. [104] observed that 20 min of maximal exercise induced a 3-fold increase in the percentage of unstimulated cells expressing the IL-2 p55 (CD25+) receptor. Several authors [22, 49, 178] have confirmed an immediate increase in the percentage of CD25+ cells with exercise, although Shinkai et al. [178] noted a 40% decrease 1 hr postexercise. In contrast, after mitogen stimulation, the percentage of CD25+ cells is reduced by a brief (1-min) bout of anaerobic exercise [62, 104].

Rhind et al. [163] found a doubling in the percentage of lymphocytes expressing p70 and p75 receptors at 30 and 60 min of submaximal exercise; there was a 30% decrease in the percentage of cells expressing the p55 receptor, but when percentages were multiplied by the corresponding cell counts, the p55 receptors showed a marginal increase, and the p70–75 receptors a 200% increase over baseline. This dose of exercise also led to an increase in serum levels of soluble IL-2R [163]. All changes were reversed 30 min postexercise.

EFFECTS OF ENDURANCE TRAINING

Cross-sectional Comparisons

When comparing immune responses between endurance athletes and sedentary subjects, it is important to match the relative intensity of exercise for the two groups, and to allow adequate recovery from the stresses of competition, training, and heavy travel schedules.

The resting immune status of athletes is relatively normal [147], although phagocytic activity is sometimes poorer during heavy training. During moderate, controlled training, athletes tend to have low total lymphocyte, CD3+, CD4+, and NK cell counts, and low CD4+/CD8+ ratios [106]. Green et al. [64] observed that 10 of 20 marathon runners had lymphocyte counts of <1500 cells/mm^3; however, 5 of the 10 subjects with low counts had completed a long run in the previous 3 days.

Other studies of well-trained subjects have seen evidence of enhanced metabolic activity in the lymphocytes: an increased number of insulin receptors [96], an increase in mitogen-stimulated lymphocyte proliferation [97, 114], increased antibody-dependent cytotoxic and NK cell counts or activity [158, 163], and an increase in resting plasma IL-1-like activity [42, 155]. Both CD16+ and CD56+ counts are high in athletes [163]. The percentage of CD25+ cells is normal [163] or subnormal [62, 148, 151], but the 70–75-kD IL-2 receptor density is about twice that observed in sedentary people [163]. There are close correlations between $\dot{V}O_2$max and IL-2 β-chain expression: r=0.914 for Mikβ-1, P<0.001; r=0.890 for TU-27, P<0.005, but IL-2α receptor expression is unrelated to $\dot{V}O_2$max. The increase in p70–75 receptors reflects in part the high NK counts of the athletes because the IL-2β receptor is coexpressed with CD8 dim CD16+ and CD56+ cells [163].

There are no major differences in overall T-cell or subset responses to exercise between trained and untrained human subjects. In general, there is an increase in CD4+ cells, but a larger increase in CD8+ cells. Increases in the CD3+ count seen when well-trained persons undertake maximal exercise [104] may be matched by sedentary subjects when they undertake submaximal exercise [44, 94]. Whereas exercise invariably decreases the percentages of CD3+ and CD4+ cells, in trained athletes, exercise markedly increases CD8+ and NK counts [147].

Evans et al. [42] reported that exercise induced a larger increase of IL-1 activity in untrained than in trained people, but this observation must be interpreted cautiously because some of the trained subjects had undertaken vigorous exercise in the previous 48 hr.

MacNeil et al. [114] noted that exercise decreased mitogen-induced lymphocyte proliferation, this effect being greatest in subjects who were well trained. Others have found either no change [64, 112, 147] or even increased mitogen responsiveness [184] in well-trained people.

Longitudinal Training Studies
The training response depends on the intensity, frequency, and duration of exercise on the subject's initial condition. Moderate training is beneficial, but exhausting training depresses immune function [190]. In the rat and the mouse, moderate training increases the proliferative response to mitogens [79, 198], but heavy training decreases the mass of the thymus, and splenic lymphocytes become less responsive to mitogens [190]. Potential causes include an alteration in the relative proportions of T and B cells, and suppressant actions of CD8+ cells or of macrophage-secreted prostaglandin E_2.

MODERATE TRAINING. Light walking (5 days/wk, 40–50 min/day at 60% of the heart rate reserve, with no gain of aerobic power) decreased resting lymphocyte and T-cell counts in sedentary obese women, changes being greater at 6 than at 15 wk [132]. The CD4+/CD8+ cell ratio was unchanged. Soppi et al. [184], using the somewhat dated technique of rosette formation, reported decreased T-cell counts after 6 wk of training of naval conscripts. In contrast, Watson et al. [223], also using the rosetting method, claimed that the T-cell counts of sedentary young men were increased after 15 wk of training at 70–85% of $\dot{V}O_2$max; in their study, final blood samples were collected within 20 hr of the last training session. Völker et al. [219] noted a decrease in both resting lymphocyte counts and T-cell subsets when endurance runners reduced the intensity of their training program for 5 wk.

Shore et al. (unpublished data, 1993) had sedentary male subjects exercise for 30 min at 70% of $\dot{V}O_2$max 4 times a week for 12 wk. Twenty-four hours after the last training bout, the CD3+ count was decreased, and the CD19+ count was unchanged at rest, during, and after a standard exercise challenge (60 min of exercise at 60% of $\dot{V}O_2$max). Typically, training attenuates the early circulatory mobilization of lymphocytes that accompanies exhausting exercise in a sedentary person. T cells also account for a larger percentage of the total lymphocytes after training, but the CD4+/CD8+ ratio may be decreased. Possibly, the fit person must mobilize fewer lymphocytes to yield an adequate immune response [184].

In elite athletes, 5 mo of normal training had no effect upon resting lymphocyte counts or percentages, but acute maximal exercise again induced smaller increases in CD4+ counts than initially [44].

Moderate training does not change the rate of spontaneous blastogenesis [132]. Mitogen-induced lymphocyte proliferation is either unchanged [49] or increased [184, 223]. Adequate recovery from the final training session has an important influence on response; Hoffman-Goetz et al. [79] observed a decreased mitogen response immediately postexercise, but proliferation was increased when 72 hr of recovery were allowed. Shore et al. (unpublished data, 1993) also found that after 12 wk of training, sedentary male subjects had an increased response to both PWM and PHA, at rest, during an exercise challenge, and during a 2-hr recovery period. Others have found that moderate training attenuates the decrease of lymphocyte proliferation seen with a standard exercise challenge [79, 80, 184].

Moderate treadmill training increases NK cytolytic activity in animals [181], although very heavy training has a negative effect. Human studies are inconsistent. Nieman et al. [135] found a 57%increase of resting NK activity after 6 wk of moderate training, but Watson et al. [223] reported decreased NK activity when sedentary students had completed 15 weeks of training. Shore et al. (unpublished data, 1993) found no change of resting activity per NK cell over a 12 wk training period, but because of a rise in NK count, the cytotoxic activity per unit volume of blood was increased, this change being moderately correlated (r = 0.61) with gains in $\dot{V}O_2$max. Crist et al. [25] and Fiatarone et al. [47] both found that light training increased resting NK-cell activity in geriatric populations. Nieman et al. [135] had similar findings, although their study was marred by the use of program drop-outs as control subjects.

Rhind et al. [163] noted that 12 wk of moderate training reduced the exercise-induced decrease of in vitro IL-2 production in sedentary young men; moreover, the training regimen increased the expression of both IL-2Rα and IL-2Rβ, with a lesser exercise-induced increase in serum concentrations of soluble IL-2R.

HEAVY TRAINING. Heavy training has adverse effects even on international-class competitors. The total resting lymphocyte count may not change, but Surkina [190] saw a drop in resting T-cell counts and activity in Soviet athletes after 4 mo of intense competition. Liesen et al. [107] noted that a combination of psychological stress and intensive interval training led to a tremendous decrease of resting T-cell counts in the German Olympic Field Hockey team; the CD4+/CD8+ ratio for the team dropped as low as in AIDS patients. Likewise, Verde et al. [215, 216] saw decreases in the resting T-cell percentage and the CD4+/CD8+ ratio when distance runners deliberately undertook 3 wk of very heavy training. The T-cell percentage decreased further over the first 3 wk of the recovery period, but by this stage the CD4+/CD8+ ratio had risen above its initial level. In this study, very heavy training did not change the CD4+/CD8+ response to a standard 30-min submaximal exercise challenge [215].

Verde et al. [215] noted that 3 weeks of heavy training increased the mitogen response of peripheral blood mononuclear cells, but Fry et al. [49] observed no change after an intensive interval training program. Verde et al. [215] reported further that the immediate suppression of mitogen response of a standard exercise challenge was augmented by heavy training.

The resting NK count was decreased, possibly because of migration to injured tissues, or conversion to cytotoxic T cells [215]. The in vitro production of IL-2 by isolated splenocytes is suppressed by heavy training [149].

A shortage of glutamine seems one possible component of an adverse response to exercise [130, 131]. Macrophages depend upon glutamine for IL-1 synthesis [221], and the normal in vitro response of T and B cells to mitogens is also suppressed by low plasma glutamine levels [65]. Glutamine levels can be depressed for as long as 6 wk after exhausting training [152]. Swimmers training 18 hr/wk increase their CD4+/CD8+ ratio and plasma IgA levels in response to glutamine supplements; however, CD3+ counts and proliferation rates do not change.

CONCLUSIONS

Whereas moderate endurance exercise has a beneficial effect upon the interleukin/NK system, more intense and more stressful exercise causes an adverse response. The negative impact of a brief bout of exercise is short-lived, but in one study 90–120 min of exercise at 60% of maximal oxygen intake reduced NK counts and activity for at least 1 wk, with potential implications for resistance to viral infections. The likelihood of an adverse response depends on not only the duration but also the relative intensity of effort. Moderate training thus reduces the impact of a standard exercise challenge. In contrast, excessive training can give rise to cumulative disturbances of immune function. Given the importance of the immune system to many aspects of health, we must learn much more about how to optimize training and we need therapies that can alleviate adverse effects as athletes prepare for major competition.

ACKNOWLEDGMENT

This research was supported in part by a Ministry of Defence research contract to one of us (R. J. S.).

REFERENCES

1. Aarden, L. and M. Helle. Biological assay of interleukins. I. Lefkowitz and B. Pernis (eds). *Immunological Methods IV*. San Diego: Academic Press, 1990, pp. 165–174.
2. Abbas, A. K., A. H. Lichtman, and J. S. Pober. *Cellular and Molecular Immunology*. Philadelphia: W. B. Saunders, 1991.
3. Abraham, R. T., S. N. Ho, and D. J. McKean. Bioassay of interleukins. *J. Tissue Cult. Methodol.* 10:93–99, 1986.
4. Alberola-Ila, J., L. Places, O. de la Calle, et al. Stimulation through the TCR/CD3 complex upregulates the CD2 surface expression of human T lymphocytes. *J. Immunol.* 146: 1085–1092, 1991.

5. Allsop, P., A. M. Peters, R. N. Arnot, et al. Intrasplenic blood cell kinetics in man before and after brief maximal exercise. *Clin. Sci.* 83:47–54, 1992.

6. Audrain, M., F. Boeffard, J.-P. Soulillou, and Y. Jacques. Synergistic action of monoclonal antibodies directed at p55 and p75 chains of the IL-2 receptor. *J. Immunol.* 146:884–892, 1991.

7. Barone, J., J. R. Herbert, and M. M. Reddy, Dietary fat and natural killer cell activity. *Am. J. Clin. Nutr.* 50:861–867, 1989.

8. Beaman, K. D., W. C. Barker, and J. J. Marchalonis. *Antigen-specific T Cell Receptors and Factors.* Boca Raton, FL: CRC Publishing, 1987.

9. Berk, L. S., D. C. Nieman, W. S. Youngberg, et al. The effect of long endurance running on natural killer cells in marathoners. *Med. Sci. Sports Exerc.* 22:207–212, 1990.

10. Berke, G. The cytolytic T lymphocyte and its mode of action. *Immunol. Lett.* 20:169–178, 1989.

11. Blalock, J. E. A molecular basis for bidirectional communication between the immune and neuroendocrine systems. *Physiol. Rev.* 69:1–32, 1989.

12. Bloom, B. R., P. Salgame, and B. Diamond. Revisiting and revising suppressor T cells. *Immunol. Today* 13:131–136, 1992.

13. Bonavida, B., and S. C. Wright. Multistage model of natural killer cell mediated cytotoxicity involving NKCF as soluble cytotoxic mediators. *Adv. Cancer Res.* 49:169–187, 1987.

14. Boom, W. H., D. Llano, and A. K. Abbas. Heterogeniety of helper/inducer T lymphocytes. II. Effects of interleukin 4 and interleukin 2 producing T cell clones on resting B lymphocytes. *J. Exp. Med.* 167:1350–1363, 1988.

15. Brahmi, A., J. E. Thomas, M. Park, and I. R. G. Dowdeswell. The effect of acute exercise on natural killer-cell activity of trained and sedentary human subjects. *J. Clin. Immunol.* 5.921–928, 1985.

16. Brenner, I., P. N. Shek, and R. J. Shephard. Acute infections and exercise. *Sports Med.* 17:86–107, 1994.

17. Brunda, M. J., R. B. Herberman, and T. Holden. Inhibition of murine natural killer cell activity by prostaglandins. *J. Immunol.* 124:2682–2687, 1980.

18. Cannon, J. G., and M. J. Kluger. Endogenous pyrogen activity in human plasma after exercise. *Science* 220:617–619, 1983.

19. Cannon, J. G., W. J. Evans, V. A. Hughes, C. N. Meredith, and C. A. Dinarello. Physiological mechanisms contributing to increased interleukin-1 secretion. *J. Appl. Physiol.* 61:1869–1874, 1986.

20. Chandra, R. K. Effect of vitamin and trace-element supplementation on immune responses and infection in elderly subjects. *Lancet* 340:1124–1127, 1992.

21. Chard, T. An introduction to radioimmunoassay and related techniques. A. Fallon, R. F. G. Booth, and L. D. Bell (eds). *Laboratory Techniques in Biochemistry and Molecular Biology, 3rd Ed.* Amsterdam: Elsevier Publications, 1986, pp. 256–274.

22. Ciusani, E., L. Grazzi, A. Salmaggi, et al. Role of physical training on the immune function: preliminary data. *Int. J. Neurosci.* 51:249–252, 1990.

23. Cosman, D., S. D. Lyman, R. L. Idzerda, M. P. Beckmann, and C. J. March. A new cytokine receptor superfamily. *Trends Biochem. Sci.* 15:265–269, 1990.

24. Crary, B., S. L. Hauser, M. Borysenko, et al. Epinephrine-induced lymphocyte subsets in peripheral blood of humans. *J. Immunol.* 131:1178–1181, 1983.

25. Crist, D. M., L. T. Mackinnon, R. F. Thompson, H. A. Atterbom, and P. A. Egan. Physical exercise increases natural cellular mediated tumor cytotoxicity in elderly women. *Gerontology* 35:66–71, 1989.

26. Cupps, T. R., and A. S. Fauci. Corticosteroid-mediated immunoregulation in man. *Immunol. Rev.* 65:133–155, 1982.

27. Dale, D. C., A. S. Fauci, I. V. D. Guerry, and S. M. Wolff. Comparison of agents producing a neutrophilic leucocytosis in man: hydrocortisone, prednisone, endotoxin and citocholanone. *J. Clin. Invest.* 56:808–813, 1975.

28. D'Andrea, A. D., G. D. Fasman, and H. F. Lodish. Erythropoietin receptor and IL-2 receptor beta chain: A new receptor family. *Cell* 58:1023–1024, 1989.

29. Deuster, P. A., A. M. Curiale, M. L. Cowan, and F. D. Finkelman. Exercise-induced changes in populations of peripheral blood mononuclear cells. *Med. Sci. Sports Exerc.* 20:276–280, 1988.

30. Devos, R., G. Plaetinck, H. Cheroutre, et al. Molecular cloning of the human IL-2 cDNA and its expression in E Coli *Nucleic Acids Res.* 11:4307–4323, 1983.

31. diGiovine F. S., and G. W. Duff. Interleukin I: the first interleukin. *Immunol. Today* 11:13–20, 1990.

32. Dinarello, C. A., and J. W. Mier. Lymphokines. *N. Engl. J. Med.* 317:940–945, 1987.

33. Dorf, M. E., V. K. Kuchroo, and M. Collins. Suppressor T cells: some answers but more questions. *Immunol. Today* 13:241–243, 1992.

34. Dower, S. K., J. E. Sims, J. H. Stanton, et al. Molecular heterogeneity of interleukin-1 receptors. *Ann. N. Y. Acad. Sci.* 594:231–239, 1990.

35. Dufaux, B., and U. Order. Plasma elastase-alpha-1-antitrypsin, neopterin, tumor necrosis factor, and soluble interleukin-2 receptor after prolonged exercise. *Int. J. Sports Med.* 10:434–438, 1989.

36. Dugger, K. O., and J. N. Galgiani. Neutrophil killing of single micro-organisms as measured by a new method. *Diagn. Microbiol. Infect. Dis.* 12:199–203, 1989.

37. Eck, M. J., S. E. Shoelson, and S. C. Harrison. Recognition of a high-affinity phosphotyrosyl peptide by the Src homnology-2 domain of p56.[lck] *Nature* 362, 87–89, 1993.

38. Edwards, A. J., T. H. Bacon, C. A. Elms, R. Verardi, M. Felder and S. C. Knight. Changes in the populations of lymphoid cells in human peripheral blood following physical exercise. *Clin. Exp. Immunol.* 58:420–427, 1984.

39. Eskandari, M. K., and Remick, D. G. Quantitation of the biological activities of cytokines. S. L. Kunkel and D. G. Remick (eds). *Cytokins in Health and Disease.* New York: Marcel Dekker, 1992, pp. 1–14.

40. Eskola, J., O. Ruuskanen, E. Soppi, et al. Effect of sport stress on lymphocyte transformation and antibody formation. *Clin. Exp. Immunol.* 32:339–345, 1978.

41. Espersen, G. T., A. Elbaek, E. Ernst, et al. Effect of physical exercise on cytokines and lymphocyte populations in human peripheral blood. *Acta Pathol. Microbiol. Immunol. Scand.* 98:395–400, 1990.

42. Evans, W. J., C. N. Meredith, J. G. Cannon, et al. Metabolic changes following eccentric exercise in trained and untrained men. *J. Appl. Physiol.* 61:1864–1868, 1986.

43. Farrar, J. J., W. R. Benjamin, M. L. Hilfiker, M. Howard, W. L. Farrar, and J. Fuller-Farrar. The biochemistry, biology and the role of IL-2 in the induction of cytotoxic T cell and antibody-forming B cell responses. *Immunol. Rev.* 63:129–166, 1982.

44. Ferry, A., F. Picard, A. Duvallet, B. Weill, and M. Rieu. Changes in blood leucocyte populations induced by acute maximal and chronic submaximal exercise. *Eur. J. Appl. Physiol.* 59:435–442, 1990.

45. Ferry, A., P. Rieu, C. LePage, A. Elhabazi, F. Laziri, and M. Rieu. Effect of physical exhaustion and glucocorticoids (dexamethasone) on T cells of trained rats. *Eur. J. Appl. Physiol.* 66:455–460, 1993.

46. Fiatarone, M. A., J. E. Morley, E. T. Bloom. D. Benton, T. Makinodan, and G. F. Solomon. Endogenous opioids and the exercise-induced augmentation of natural killer cell activity. *J. Lab. Clin. Med.* 112:544–552, 1988.

47. Fiatarone, M. A., J. E. Morley, E. T. Bloom, D. Benton, G. F. Solomon, and T. Makinodan. The effect of exercise on natural killer cell activity in young and old subjects. *J. Gerontol.* 44:M37–M45, 1989.

48. Fitzgerald, L. Exercise and the immune system. *Immunol. Today* 9:337–339, 1988.

49. Fry, R. W., A. R. Morton, and D. Keast. Acute intensive interval training and T-lymphocyte function. *Med. Sci. Sports Exerc.* 24:339–34, 1992.

50. Gabriel, H., L. Schwarz, G. Steffens, and W. Kindermann. Immunoregulatory hormones, circulating leucocyte and lymphocyte subpopulations before and after endurance exercise of different intensities. *Int. J. Sports Med.* 13:359–366, 1992.
51. Gabriel, H., L. Schwarz, P. Born, and W. Kindermann. Differential mobilization of leucocyte and lymphocyte subpopulations into the circulation during endurance exercise. *Eur. J. Appl. Physiol.* 65:529–534, 1992.
52. Gabriel, H., B. Schmitt. A. Urhausen, and W. Kindermann. Adhäsionsmolekül LFA-1 auf der Zelloberfläche von Lymphozytensubpopulationen während und nach akuter körperlicher Belastung. *Dtsch. Z. Sportmed.* 44:436–444, 1993.
53. Gatti, G., R. Cavallo, M. L. Satori, et al. Inhibition by cortisol of human natural killer cell activity. *J. Steroid Biochem.* 26:49–58, 1987.
54. Gearing, A. J. H. and R. Thorpe. The international standard for human IL-2. Calibration by international collaborative study. *J. Immunol. Methods* 114:3–9, 1988.
55. Gearing, A. J. H., A. P. Johnstone, and R. Thorpe. Production and assay of interleukins. *J. Immunol. Methods* 83:1–27, 1985.
56. Gearing, A. J. H., J. E. Cartwright, and M. Wadhwa. (1991). Biological and immunological assays for cytokines. A. Thomson (ed). *The Cytokine Handbook.* London: Academic Press, 1991, pp. 339–350.
57. Gillis, S., and K. A. Smith. Long-term culture of tumor specific cytotoxic T cells. *Nature* 268:154–156, 1977.
58. Gimenez, M., T. Mohan-Kumar, J. C. Humbert, N. de Talance, and J. Buisine. Leukocyte, lymphocyte and platelet response to dynamic exercise. Duration or intensity effect? *Eur. J. Appl. Physiol.* 55:465–470, 1986.
59. Gmünder, F. K., G. Lorenzi, B. Bechler, et al. Effect of long-term physical exercise on lymphocyte reactivity: similarity to space flight reactions. *Aviat. Space Environ. Med.* 59:146–151, 1988.
60. Goodwin, J. S., D. Atluru, S. Sierakowski, and E. A. Lianos. Mechanism of action of glucocorticosteroids. *J. Clin. Invest.* 77:1244–1250, 1986.
61. Graham, H. M. H., R. M. Douglas, and P. Ryan. Stress and acute respiratory infection. *Am. J. Epidemiol.* 124:389–401, 1986.
62. Gray, A. B., Y. C. Smart, R. D. Telford, M. J. Weidmann, and T. K. Roberts. Anaerobic exercise causes transient changes in leukocyte subsets and IL-2R expression. *Med. Sci. Sports Exerc.* 24:1332–1338, 1992.
63. Green, R. G., and M. L. Green. Relaxation increases salivary immunoglobulin AI. *Psychol. Rep.* 61:623–629, 1987.
64. Green, R. L., S. S. Kaplan, B. S. Rabin, C. L. Stanitski, and U. Zdziarski. Immune function in marathon runners. *Ann. Allergy* 47:73–75, 1981.
65. Griffiths, M. and D. Keast. The effect of glutamine on murine splenic leukocyte responses to T- and B-cell mitogens. *Immunol. Cell Biol.* 68:405–408, 1990.
66. Haahr, P. M., B. K. Pedersen, A. Fomsgaard, et al. Effect of physical exercise on in vitro production of interleukin-1, interleukin-6, tumor necrosis factor-alpha, interleukin-2 and interferon-gamma. *Int. J. Sports Med.* 12:223–227, 1991.
67. Hack, V., M. Weiss, and H. Weicker. Lymphozytensubpopulationen und Belastung von hochausdauertrainierten Athleten während zweier Trainingsphasen. *Dtsch. Z. Sportmed.* 44:430–435, 1993.
68. Hannel I., F. Erkeller-Yuksel, P. Lydyard, V. Deneys, and M. DeBruyé. Developmental and maturational changes in human blood lymphocyte subpopulations. *Immunol. Today* 13:215–218, 1992.
69. Hansen, J-B., L. Wilsgard, and B. Osterud. Biphasic changes in leukocytes induced by strenuous exercise. *Eur. J. Appl. Physiol.* 62:157–161, 1991.
70. Hanson, P. G., and D. K. Flaherty. Immunological responses to training in conditioned runners. *Clin. Sci.* 60:225–228, 1981.

71. Hatakeyama, M., M. Tsudo, S. Minamoto, et al. Interleukin-2 receptor beta chain gene generation of three receptor forms by cloned human alpha and beta chain cDNAs. *Science* 244 (4904):551–556, 1989.

72. Heberman, R. B. Natural killer cells. *Annu. Rev. Med.* 37:347–352, 1986.

73. Hedfors, E., G. Holm, M. Ivansen, and J. Wahren. Physiological variation of blood lymphocyte reactivity: T cell subsets, immunoglobulin production and mixed lymphocyte reactivity. *Clin. Immunol. Immunopathol.* 27:9–14, 1983.

74. Heine, O., B. Dufaux, U. Prinz, and R. Rost. Auswirkungen einer korperlichen Belastung auf die Granulozyten. *Dtsch. Z. Sportmed.* 44:412–422, 1993.

75. Henney, D. S., K. Kuribayashi, D. E. Kern, and S. Gillis Interleukin-2 augments natural killer cell activity. *Nature* 291:335–338, 1981.

76. Ho, S., R. T Abraham, S. Gillis, and D. J. McKean. Differential bioassay of IL-2 and IL-4. *J. Immunol. Methods* 98:99–104, 1987.

77. Hodgkin, P. D., L. C. Yamashita, R. L. Coffman, and M. R. Kehry. Separation of methods mediating B cell proliferation and Ig production by using T cell membranes and lymphokines. *J. Immunol.* 145:2025–2034, 1990.

78. Hoffman-Goetz, L., R. Keir, R. Thorne, M. E. Houston, and C. Young. Chronic exercise stress in mice depresses splenic T lymphocyte mitogenesis in vitro. *Clin. Exp. Immunol.* 66:551–557, 1986.

79. Hoffman-Goetz, L., R. J. Thorne, J. A. R. Simpson, and Y. Arumugan. Exercise stress alters murine lymphocyte subset distribution in spleen, lymph nodes and thymus. *Clin. Exp. Immunol.* 76:307–310, 1989.

80. Hoffman-Goetz, L., R. J. Simpson, and M. E. Houston. Lymphocyte subset responses to repeated submaximal exercise in men. *J. Appl. Physiol.* 68:1069–1074, 1990.

81. Holter, W., C. K. Goldman, L. Casabo, D. L. Nelson, W. C. Greene, and T. A. Waldmann. Expression of functional IL-2 receptors by lipopolysaccharide and interferon-gamma stimulated human monocytes. *J. Immunol.* 138:2917–2922, 1987.

82. Isakov, N., and A. Altman. Lymphocyte activation and immune regulation. *Immunol. Today* 7:155–157, 1986.

83. Jackson, A. L., H. Matsumoto, M. Janszen, V. Maino, A. Blidy, and S. Shye. Expression of p55 IL-2 receptor (CD25) on normal T cells. *Clin. Immunol. Immunopathol.* 54:126–133, 1990.

84. Janeway, C. J., S. Carding, B. Jones, et al. CD4+ T cells: specificity and function. *Immunol. Rev.* 101:39–80, 1988.

85. Jondal, M. The human NK cell—a short overview and an hypothesis on NK recognition. *Clin. Exp. Immunol.* 70:255–262, 1987.

86. June, C. H., J. A. Ledbetter, P. S. Linsley, and C. B. Thompson. Role of the CD8 receptor in T cell activation. *Immunol. Today* 11:211–216, 1990.

87. Kappel, M., N. Tvede, H. Galbo, et al. Evidence that the effect of physical exercise on NK cell activity is mediated by epinehphrine. *J. Appl. Physiol.* 70:2530–2534, 1991.

88. Kappel, M., C. Stadeager, N. Tvede, H. Galbo, and B. K. Pedersen. Effects of in vivo hyperthermia on natural killer cell activity, *in vitro* proliferative responses and blood mononuclear cell populations. *Clin. Exp. Immunol.* 84:175–180, 1991.

89. Kappel, M., M. Diamant, M. B. Hansen, M. Klokker, and B. K. Pedersen. Effects of *in vitro* hyperthermia on the proliferative response of blood mononuclear cell subsets, and detection of interleukins 1 and 6, tumour necrosis factor-alpha and interferon-gamma. *Immunology* 73:304–308, 1991.

90. Karasuyama, H., A. Rolinck, and F. Melchers. Recombinant Interleukin 2 or 5 but not 3 or 4 induces maturation of resting mouse B lymphocytes and propagates proliferation of activated B cell blasts. *J. Exp. Med.* 167:1377–1390, 1988.

91. Keast, D., and A. R. Morton. Long-term exercise and immune function. R. R. Watson and M. Eisinger (eds). *Exercise and Disease.* Boca Raton, FL.: CRC Publishing, 1992, pp. 89–120.

92. Keast, D., K. Cameron, and A. R. Morton. Exercise and immune responses. *Sports Med.* 5:248–267, 1988.
93. Kehrl, J. H., M. Dukovich, G. Whalen, P. Katz, A. S. Fauci and W. C. Greene. Novel IL-2 receptor appears to mediate IL-2 induced activation of NK cells. *J. Clin. Invest.* 81:200–205, 1988.
94. Kendall, A., L. Hoffman-Goetz, M. Houston, B. MacNeiland, and Y. Arumugam. Exercise and blood lymphocyte subset responses: intensity, duration and subject fitness effects. *J. Appl. Physiol.* 69:251–260, 1990.
95. Kline, J. N., M. M. Monick, and G. W. Hunninghake. IL-1 receptor antagonist release is regulated differently in human alveolar macrophages than in monocytes. *J. Appl. Physiol.* 73:1686–1692, 1992.
96. Koivisto, V. A., V. R. Soman. P. Conrad, R. Hendler, E. Nadel, and P. Felig. Insulin binding to monocytes in trained athletes: changes in resting state after exercise. *J. Clin. Invest.* 64:1011–1015, 1979.
97. Kono, I., H. Kitao, M. Matsuda, S. Haga, H. Fukushima, and Y. Sato. Weight reduction in athletes may adversely affect the phagocytic function of monocytes. *Phys. Sportsmed.* 16:56–65, 1988.
98. Kotani, T., Y. Aratke, R. Ishiguro, et al. Influence of physical exercise on large granular lymphocytes. Leu-7 bearing mononuclear cells and natural killer cell activity in peripheral blood NK cell and NK activity after exercise. *Acta Haematol. Jpn.* 50:1210–1216, 1987.
99. Krensky, A. M., L. L. Lanier, and E. G. Engleman. Lymphocyte subsets and surface molecules in man. *Clin. Immunol. Rev.* 4:95–138, 1985.
100. Landmann, R. M. A., F. B. Muller, C. H. Perini, M. Wesp, P. Erne, and F. R. Buhler. Changes of immuno-regulatory cells induced by psychological and physical stress: relationship to catecholamines. *Clin. Exp. Immunol.* 58:127–135, 1984.
101. Lanier, L. L., C. J. Benike, J. H. Phillips, and E. G. Engleman. Recombinant IL 2 enhanced natural killer cell mediated cytotoxicity in human lymphocyte subpopulations expressing the Leu 7 and Leu 11 antigens. *J. Immunol.* 134:794–801, 1985.
102. Le Mauff B., H. Gascan, D. Olive, et al. Parameters of interaction of a novel monoclonal antibody with human IL-2 receptors. *Hum. Immunol.* 19:53–68, 1987.
103. Leonard, W. J., J. M. Deeper, G. R. Crabtree, R. J. Robb, T A. Waldmann and W. C. Greene. Molecular cloning and expression of cDNAs for human IL 2 receptor. *Nature* 311:626–631, 1984.
104. Lewicki, R., H. Tchorzewski, E. Majewska, Z. Nowak and Z. Baj. Effect of maximal physical exercise on T-lymphocyte subpopulations and on interleukin 1 (IL 1) and interleukin 2 (IL 2) production in vitro. *Int. J. Sports Med.* 9:114–117, 1988.
105. Liesen, H., and G. Uhlenbruck. Sports immunology. *Sports Sci. Rev.* 1:94–116, 1992.
106. Liesen, H., H. Reidel, U. Order, S. Mücke, and W. Widenmayer. Reference values of leucocytes and lymphocyte subsets during a controlled moderate training period. *Dtsch. Z. Sportmed.* 40:4–14, 1989.
107. Liesen, H., K. Kleiter, S. Mücke, U. Order, W. Widenmayer and H. Riedel. Leucocytes and lymphocyte subpopulations in players of the German field hockey team during the preparatory training period for the Olympic Games in 1988. *Dtsch. Z. Sportmed.* 40:41–52, 1989.
108. Liesen, H., M. Baum, M. Weiss, and J. Enneper. Die Bedeuting ausgesuchter Mineralien und Spurenelemente für die Veränderung immunologischer Parameter bei unterschiedlichen Trainingsbelastungen von Leistungssportlern. *Dtsch. Z. Sportmed.* 44:441–444, 1993.
109. Lifson, J., A. Raubitschek, C. Benike, et al. Purified IL-2 induces proliferation of fresh human lymphocytes in the emphasis of exogenous stimuli. *J. Biol. Resp. Modif.* 5:61–72, 1986.
110. Locke, S., L. Kraus, I. Kutz, S. Edbril, K. Phillips, and H. Benson. Altered natural killer cell activity during norepinephrine infusion in humans. N. H. Spector (ed). *Neuroim-*

munomodulation. Proceedings of First International Workshop on Neuroimmunomodulation. Bethesda: National Institutes of Health, 1984, p. 297.

111. Lotzova, E., and W. Ades. Natural killer cells: definition, heterogeneity, lytic mechanisms, functions and clinical application. *Nat. Immun. Cell Growth Regul.* 8:1–9, 1989.

112. Mackinnon, L. *Exercise and Immunology.* Champaign, IL: Human Kinetics Publishers, 1992.

113. Mackinnon, L. T., T. W. Chick, A. van Es, and T. B. Tomasi. The effect of exercise on secretory and natural immunity. *Adv. Exp. Med. Biol.* 216A:869–876, 1988.

114. MacNeil, B., L. Hoffman-Goetz, A. Kendall, M. Houston, and Y. Arumugam. Lymphocyte proliferation responses after exercise in men; fitness, intensity and duration effects. *J. Appl. Physiol.* 70:179–185, 1991.

115. Maisel, A. S., T. Harris, C. A. Rearden, and M. C. Michel. Beta-adrenergic receptors in lymphocyte subsets after exercise. *Circulation* 82:2003–2010, 1990.

116. Masuhara, M., K. Kami, K. Umebayasi, and N. Tasumi. Influences of exercise on leukocyte count and size. *J. Sports Med. Phys. Fitness* 27:285–290, 1987.

117. Maurer, H. R. Potential pitfalls of ^{3}H thymidine techniques to measure cell proliferation. *Cell Tissue Kinet.* 14:111–120, 1981.

118. Meager, A. *Cytokines.* Buckingham: Open University Press, 1990.

119. Metlay, J. P., E. Puré, and R. M. Steinman. Control of the immune response at the level of the antigen presenting cells: a comparison of the function of dendritic cells and B lymphocytes. *Adv. Immunol.* 47:45–116, 1989.

120. Michiel, D., G. G. Garcia, G. A. Evans, and W. Farrar. Regulation of the IL-2 receptor complex tyrosinase kinase activity *in vitro. Cytokine* 3:428–438, 1991.

121. Miyajima, A., T. Kitamura, N. Harada, T. Yokata, and K. Arai. Cytokine receptors and signal transduction. *Annu. Rev. Immunol.* 10:295–331, 1992.

122. Mookerjee, B. K., and J. L. Pauly. Mitogenic effect of IL-2 on unstimulated human T cells: an editorial review. *J. Clin. Lab. Anal.* 4:138–149, 1990.

123. Moorthy, A. V., and W. Zimmerman. Human leucocyte response to an endurance race. *Eur. J. Appl. Physiol.* 38:271–276, 1978.

124. Moretta, L., E. Ciccone, A. Moretta, P. Hoglund, C. Ohlen, and K. Karre. Allorecognition by NK cells: nonself or no self? *Immunol. Today* 13:300–306, 1992.

125. Mosmann, T. R., and R. L. Coffman. Heterogeneity of cytokine secretion patterns and functions of T helper cells. *Adv. Immunol.* 46:111–147, 1989.

126. Müns, G., H. Liesen, H. Riedel, and K.-C. Bergmann. Influence of long distance running on IgA in nasal secretion and saliva. *Dtsch. Z. Sportmed.* 40:63–65, 1989.

127. Myers, C. D. Role of B cell antigen processing and presentation in the humoral immune response. *FASEB J.* 5:2547–2553, 1992.

128. Nagler, A., L. L. Lanier, and J. H. Phillips. Constitutive expression of high-affinity IL-2 receptors on human CD16-natural killer cells in vivo. *J. Exp. Med.* 171:1527–1533, 1990.

129. Neveu, P. J., and M. LeMoal. Physiological basis for neuroimmunomodulation. *Fundam. Clin. Pharmacol.* 4:281–305, 1990.

130. Newsholme, E. Physical activity and the immune system. C. Bouchard, R. J. Shephard, and T. Stephens (eds). *Physical Activity, Fitness and Health.* Champaign, IL: Human Kinetics Publishers, 1993.

131. Newsholme, E. Glutamine and fat in the overtrained state. *Int. J. Sports Med.*, suppl, in press, 1994.

132. Nieman, D. C. Exercise, infection and immunity. *Int. J. Sports Med.*, suppl., in press, 1994.

133. Nieman, D. C., and S. L. Nehlsen-Cannarella. Effects of endurance exercise on immune response. R. J. Shephard and P. O. Åstrand (eds). *Endurance in Sport.* Oxford: Blackwell Scientific Publications, 1992, pp. 487–504.

134. Nieman, D. C., and S. L. Nehlsen-Cannarella. Exercise and infection. R. R. Watson and M. Eisinger (eds). *Exercise and Disease.* Boca Raton: CRC Press, 1992, pp. 121–148.

135. Nieman, D. C., S. L. Nehlsen-Cannarella, P. A. Markoff, et al. The effects of moderate exercise training on natural killer cells and acute upper respiratory infections. *Int. J. Sports Med.* 11:467–473, 1990.

136. Nieman, D. C., S. L. Nehlsen-Cannarella, K. M. Donohue, et al. The effects of acute moderate exercise on leukocyte and lymphocyte subpopulations. *Med. Sci. Sports Exerc.* 23: 578–585, 1991.

137. Nieman, D. C., D. A. Henson, R. Johnson, et al. Effects of brief heavy exertion on circulating lymphocyte subpopulations and proliferative response. *Med. Sci. Sports Exerc.* 24: 1339–1345, 1992.

138. Nilsson, B. Enzyme-linked immunosorbent assay. *Curr. Opin. Immunol.* 2:898–904, 1990.

139. Nishikawa, K., S. Saito, T. Morii, Y. Kato, and K. Sugamura. Differential expression of the IL-2 receptor beta (p75) chain on human peripheral blood natural killer cells. *Int. Immunol.* 2:481–486, 1990.

140. Noelle, R. J., and C. E. Snow. T-helper cell dependent B cell activation. *FASEB J.* 5:2770–2776, 1991.

141. Noelle, R. J., J. Daum, W. C. Bartlett, J. McMann, and D. M. Shepherd. Cognate interactions between helper T cells and B cells. V. Reconstitution of helper T cells function using purified plasma membranes from activated T_{h1} and T_{h2} helper T cells and lymphokines. *J. Immunol.* 146:1118–1124, 1990.

142. Northoff, H., and A. Berg. Strenuous exercise and cytokine reaction. *Int. J. Sports Med.*, suppl, in press, 1994.

143. Ohashi, Y., T. Takeshita, K. Nagata, S. Mori and K. Sugamura. Differential expression of the IL-2 receptor subunits on various populations of primary peripheral blood mononuclear cells *J. Immunol.* 143:3548–3555, 1989.

144. Oldham, R. K. Natural killer cells: history, relevance and clinical applications. *Nat. Immun. Cell Growth Regul.* 9:297–312, 1990.

145. Ortaldo, J. R. Cytotoxicity by natural killer cells: analysis of large granular lymphocytes. *Methods Enzymol.* 132:445–457, 1986.

146. Ortaldo, J. R., J. Fry, T. Takeshita, and K. Sugamura. Regulation of CD3 lymphocyte function with an antibody against the IL-2R-beta chain receptor: modulation of NK and LAK activity and production of IFN-gamma *Eur. Cytokine Network* 1:27–34, 1990.

147. Oshida, Y., K. Yamanouchi, S. Hayamizu, and Y. Sato. Effect of acute physical exercise on lymphocyte subpopulations in trained and untrained subjects. *Int. J. Sports Med.* 9:137–140, 1988.

148. Pabst, R., and R. M. Binns. Heterogeneity of lymphocyte homing physiology: several mechanisms operate in the control of migration to lymphoid and non-lymphoid organs in vivo. *Immunol. Rev.* 108:83–109, 1989.

149. Pahlavani, M. A., T. H. Cheung, J. A. Chesky, and A. Richardson. Influence of exercise on the immune function of rats of various ages. *J. Appl. Physiol.* 64:1997–2001, 1988.

150. Palacios, R., and G. Moller. T cell growth factor (TCGF) abrogates concanavalin A-induced suppressor cell function. *J. Exp. Med.* 153:360–372, 1981.

151. Papa S., M. Vitale, G. Mozotti, L. M. Neri and F. A. Manzoli. Impaired lymphocyte stimulation induced by long-term training. *Immunol. Lett.* 22:29–33, 1989.

152. Parry-Billings, M., E. Blomstrand, N. McAndrew, and E. Newsholme. A communicational link between skeletal muscle, brain and cells of the immune system. *Int. J. Sports Med.* 11(suppl):S122–S128, 1990.

153. Parry-Billings, M., R. Budgett, Y. J. Koutedakis, et al. Plasma amino acid concentrations in the over-training syndrome: possible effects on the immune system. *Med. Sci. Sports Exerc.* 24:1353–1358, 1992.

154. Payan, D. G., J. P. McGillis, F. K. Renold, M. Mitsuhahi, and E. J. Goetzl. Neuropeptide modulation of leucocyte function. *Ann. N. Y. Acad. Sci.* 496:182–191, 1987.

155. Pedersen, B. K. Influence of physical activity on the cellular immune system: mechanisms of action. *Int. J. Sports Med.* 12:S23—S29, 1991.
156. Pedersen, B. K. The effects of extreme physiological conditions on the immune system. *Int. J. Sports Med.*, suppl, in press, 1994.
157. Pedersen, B. K., and Tvede, N. Immunesystemet og fysisk training. *Ugeskr. Laeger* 155:856–861, 1993.
158. Pedersen, B. K., N. Tvede, L. D. Christensen, K. Klarlund, S. Kragbak, and J. Halkjaer-Kristensen. Natural killer cell activity in peripheral blood of highly trained and untrained persons. *Int. J. Sports Med.* 10:129–131, 1989.
159. Pedersen, B. K., N. Tvede, K. Klarlund, et al. Indomethacin in vitro and in vivo abolishes post-exercise suppression of natural killer cell activity in peripheral blood. *Int. J. Sports Med.* 11:127–131, 1990.
160. Plaut, M. Lymphocyte hormone receptors. *Annu. Rev. Immunol.* 5:621–629, 1987.
161. Raulet, D. H. Effect of IL-2 on thymocytes. *Nature* 314:101–103, 1985.
162. Rey, D. A., H. Besdeovsky, E. Sorkin, and C. A. Dinarello. Interleukin-1 and glucocorticoid hormones integrate an immunoregulatory feedback circuit. B. C. Jankovic, B. M. Markovic, and N. H. Spector (eds). *Ann. N. Y. Acad. Sci.* 496:85–90, 1987.
163. Rhind, S., P. N. Shek, and R. J. Shephard. Relationship between Interleukin receptor alpha and beta chain expression and fitness level. *Int. J. Sports Med.* Paper submitted for publication, 1993.
164. Ricken, K. H., T. Rieder, G. Hauck, and W. Kindermann. Changes in lymphocyte subpopulations after prolonged exercise. *Int. J. Sports Med.* 11:132–135, 1990.
165. Ritz, J., T. J. Campen, R. E. Schmidt, et al. Analysis of T cell receptor gene rearrangement and expression in human natural killer cell clones. *Science* 228:1540–1543, 1985.
166. Robb, R. J. Comparison of low affinity interleukin-2 receptors to a high affinity state following fusion of cell membranes. *Proc. Natl. Acad. Sci. U. S. A.* 83:3992–3996, 1986.
167. Robb, R. J., and W. C. Greene. Internalization of IL-2 is mediated by the beta chain of the high affinity IL-2 receptor. *J. Exp. Med.* 165:1201–1206, 1987.
168. Robertson, A. J., K. C. Ramesar, R. C. Potts, et al. The effect of strenuous physical exercise on circulating blood lymphocytes and circulating serum cortisol levels. *Clin. Lab. Immunol.* 5:53–57, 1981.
169. Robertson, M. J., and J. Ritz. Biology and clinical relevance of human natural killer cells. *J. Am. Soc. Hematol.* 76:2421–2438, 1990.
170. Rocha, B., M. P. Lembezat, A. Freitas, and A. Bandeira. Interleukin 2 receptor expression and interleukin 2 production in exponentially growing T cells: major differences between in vivo and in vitro proliferating T lymphocytes. *Eur. J. Immunol.* 19:1137–1145, 1989.
171. Ross, R. The pathogenesis of atherosclerosis: a perspective for the 1990s. *Nature* 362:801–809, 1993.
172. Sabiston, B. H., W. S. Myles, and M. W. Radomski. Stress-induced changes in the immune system during prolonged physical work. *Aerospace Med.* 51:196–197, 1980.
173. Schedlowski, M., R. Jacobs, G. Stratmann, et al. Changes of natural killer cell activity during acute psychological stress. *J. Clin. Immunol.* 13:119–126, 1993.
174. Schectman, O., R. Elizondo, and M. Taylor. Exercise augments interleukin-2 induction. *Med. Sci. Sports Exerc.* 20:S18, 1988.
175. Schimpff, R.-M., and A.-M. Repellin. Production of interleukin-1-alpha and interleukin-2-alpha by mononuclear cells in healthy adults in relation to different experimental conditions and to the presence of growth hormone. *Hormone Res.* 33:171–176, 1990.
176. Shephard, R. J., and P. N. Shek. Infection and the athlete. *Clin. J. Sports Med.* 3:75–77, 1993.
177. Shimizu, Y., W. Newman, Y. Tanaka, and S. Shaw. Lymphocyte interaction with endothelial cells. *Immunol. Today* 13:106–112, 1992.

178. Shinkai, S., S. Shore, P. N. Shek, and R. J. Shephard. Acute exercise and immune function change. 1. Relationship between lymphocyte activity and subset. *Int. J. Sports Med.* 13:452–461, 1993.

179. Shinkai, S., Y. Kurokawa, S. Hino, et al. Triathlon competition induced a transient immunosuppressive change in the peripheral blood of athletes. *J. Sports Med. Phys. Fitness* 33:70–78, 1993.

180. Siegel, J. P., M. Sharon, P. L. Smith, and W. J. Leonard. The IL-2 receptor beta chain (p70): role in mediating signals for LAK, NK and proliferative activities. *Science* 238:75–78, 1987.

181. Simpson J. A. R., and L. Hoffman-Goetz. Exercise stress and murine natural killer cell function. *Proc. Soc. Exp. Biol. Med.* 195:129–135, 1990.

182. Simpson, J. A. R., and L. Hoffman-Goetz. Exercise, serum zinc, and interleukin-1 concentrations in man: some methodological considerations. *Nutr. Res.* 11:309–323, 1991.

183. Smith, K. A. Interleukin-2. *Sci. Am.* 262:50–75, 1990.

184. Soppi, E., P. Varjo, J. Eskola, and L. A. Likening. Effect of strenuous physical stress on circulating lymphocyte number and function before and after training. *J. Clin. Lab. Immunol.* 8:43–46, 1982.

185. Spinas, G. A., D. Bloesch, M. T. Kaufmann, U. Keller, and J. M. Dayer. Induction of plasma inhibitors of interleukin-1 and TNF-alpha activity by endotoxin administration to normal humans. *Am. J. Physiol.* 259:R993–R997, 1990.

186. Sprenger, H., C. Jacobs, M. Nain, et al. Enhanced release of cytokines, interleukin-2 receptors and neopterin after long distance running. *Clin. Immunol. Immunopathol.* 63:1188–1195, 1992.

187. Steptoe, A., J. Moses, A. Mathews, and S. Edwards. Aerobic fitness, physical activity and psychophysiological reactions to mental tasks. *Psychophysiol.* 27:264–274, 1990.

188. Strober, W., and S. P. James. The interleukins. *Pediatr. Res.* 24:549–557, 1988.

189. Suez, D., and A. R. Hayward. Phenotyping of proliferating cells in cultures of human lymphocytes. *J. Immunol. Methods* 78:49–57, 1985.

190. Surkina, I. D. Stress and immunity among athletes. *Teoriya i Pratika Fizicheskoi Kultury* 3:18. (Translation in *Soviet Sports Rev.* 17:198, 1981.)

191. Suzuki, R., K. Handa, K. Itoh and K. Kumagi. Natural killer (NK) cells as a responder to Interleukin 2 (IL 2). I. Proliferative response and establishment of cloned cells. *J. Immunol.* 130:981–987, 1983.

192. Takeshita, T., Y. Goto, K. Tada, et al. Monoclonal antibody defining a molecule possibly identical to the p75 subunit of interleukin-2 receptor. *J. Exp. Med.* 169:1323–1332, 1989.

193. Talmadge Immunoregulation and immunostimulation of murine lymphocytes by recombinant human interleukin-2. *J. Biol. Response Mod.* 4:18–34, 1985.

194. Taniguchi, T. Interleukin-2 and the IL-2 receptor. *Encyclopedia of Human Biology.* New York: Academic Press, 1991, pp. 527–533.

195. Targan, S., L. Britvan, and F. Dorey. Activation of human NKCC by moderate exercise: increased frequency of NK cells with enhanced capability of effector-target interactions. *Clin. Exp. Immunol.* 45:352–360, 1981.

196. Tavadia, H. B., K. A. Fleming, P. D. Hume, and H. W. Simpson. Circadian rhythmicity of human plasma cortisol and PHA-induced lymphocyte transformation. *Clin. Exp. Immunol.* 22:190–193, 1976.

197. Teodorczyk-Injeyan, J. A., B. G. Sparkes, S. Lalani, W. J. Peters, and G. B. Mills. IL-2 regulation of soluble IL-2 receptor levels following thermal injury. *Clin. Exp. Immunol.* 90:36–42, 1992.

198. Tharp, G. D., and T. L. Preuss. Mitogenic response of T-lymphocytes to exercise training and stress. *J. Appl. Physiol.* 70:2535–2538, 1991.

199. Thiele, D. L., and P. E. Lipsky. The role of cell surface recognition structures in the initiation of MHC-unrestricted "promiscuous" killing by T cells. *Immunol. Today* 10:375–381, 1989.

200. Thorpe, R., M. Wadhwa, C. R. Bird, and A. R. Mire-Sluis. Detection and measurement of cytokines. *Blood Rev.* 6:133–148, 1993.

201. Tigges, M. A., L. S. Casey, and M. E. Koshland. Mechanism of interleukin-2 signalling: mediation of different outcomes by a single receptor and transduction pathway. *Science* 243:781–786, 1989.

202. Tomasi, T. B., F. B. Trudeau, D. Czerwinksi, and S. Erredge. Immune parameters in athletes before and after strenuous exercise. *J. Clin. Immunol.* 2:173–178, 1982.

203. Tonnesen, E., M. J. Christensen, and M. M. Brinkslov. Natural killer cell activity during cortisol and adrenaline infusion in healthy volunteers. *Eur. J. Clin. Invest.* 17:497–503, 1987.

204. Tsudo, M., T. Uchiyama, and H. Uchino. Expression of the Tac antigen on activated normal human B cells. *J. Exp. Med.* 160:612–617, 1984.

205. Tsudo, M., R. W. Kozak, C. K. Goldman, and T. A. Waldmann. Contribution of a p75 interleukin 2 binding peptide to a high affinity interleukin 2 receptor complex. *Proc. Natl. Acad. Sci. U. S. A.* 84:4215–4218, 1987.

206. Tsudo, M., F. Kitamura, and M. Miyaska. Characterization of the interleukin-2 receptor beta chain using three distinct monoclonal antibodies. *Proc. Natl. Acad. Sci. U. S. A.* 86:1982–1986, 1989.

207. Tvede, N., N. K. Pedersen, F. R. Hansen, et al. Effect of physical exercise on blood mononuclear cell subpopulations and in vitro proliferative response. *Scand. J. Immunol.* 29:383–389, 1989.

208. Tvede, N., M. Kappel, J. Halkjaer-Kristensen, H. Galbo, and B. K. Pedersen. The effect of light, moderate and severe bicycle exercise on lymphocyte subsets, natural and lymphokine activated killer cells, lymphocyte proliferative responses and interleukin 2 production. *Int. J. Sports Med.* 14:275–282, 1993.

209. Uhlenbruck, G. Substitution, sport and the immune system. *Int. J. Sports Med.*, suppl, in press, 1994.

210. Uhlenbruck, G., A. Van Mil, K. Dressbach, and O. Koch. Makrophagen und Phagocytose-Funktionteste. *Immunol. Infekt.* 10:122–129, 1982.

211. Uhlenbruck, G., and A. van Mil. *Immunobiologische und andere neue Aspekte der Membranmodulation durch L-carnitine.* Köln: Echoverlags Gmbh, 1993, pp. 1–23.

212. Van Tits, L. J., M. C. Michel, H. Grosse-Wilde, et al. Catecholamines increase lymphocyte beta$_2$-adrenergic receptors via beta$_2$-adrenergic, spleen dependent process. *Am. J. Physiol.* 258:E191–E202, 1990.

213. Verde, T. Short-term exercise and immune function. R. R. Watson and M. Eisinger (eds). *Exercise and Disease.* Boca Raton, FL: CRC Press, 1992, pp. 72–88.

214. Verde, T. J., S. Thomas, P. N. Shek, and R. J. Shephard. Responses of lymphocyte subsets, mitogen-stimulated cell proliferation rates and immunoglobulin synthesis to vigorous exercise in the well-trained athlete. *Clin. J. Sports Med.* 2:87–92, 1992.

215. Verde, T. J., S. Thomas, R. W. Moore, P. N. Shek, and R. J. Shephard. Immune responses and increased training of the elite athlete. *J. Appl. Physiol.* 73:1494–1499, 1992.

216. Verde, T. J., S. Thomas, and R. J. Shephard. Potential markers of heavy training in highly trained distance runners. *Br. J. Sports Med.* 26:167–175, 1992.

217. Verde, T., S. Thomas, P. N. Shek, and R. J. Shephard. The effects of heavy training on two in vitro assessments of cell-mediated immunity in conditioned athletes. *Clin. J. Sports Med.*, 3:211–216, 1993.

218. Verheul, H. A. M., M. Verveld, and E. S. Bos. Immunotherapy through the IL-2 receptor. *Immunol. Res.* 11:42–53, 1992.

219. Völker, K., M. Gracher, T. Wibbels, and W. Hollmann. Uber die Notwendigkeit der Steuerung der Belastungsintensität im Beitensport. J. W. Franz and H. Mellerowicz (eds). *Training und Sport zur Prävention und Rehabilitation in der technisierten Umwelt.* Berlin: Springer Verlag, 1985.

220. Wagner, H., C. Hardt, K. Heeg, et al. NK/T cell interactions during cytotoxic T lymphocyte (CTL) responses. T cell derived helper factor (Interleukin 2) as a probe to analyze CTL responsiveness and thymic maturation of CTL progenitors. *Immunol. Rev.* 51:215–255, 1980.
221. Wallace, C. and D. Keast. Glutamine and macrophage function. *Metabolism* 41: 1016–1020, 1992.
222. Watson, J., and D. Mochizuki. Interleukin-2: A Class of T cells growth factors. *Immunol. Rev.* 51:257–278, 1980.
223. Watson, R. R., S. Moriguchi, J. C. Jackson, L. Werner, J. H. Wilmore, and B. J. Freund. Modification of cellular immune functions in humans by endurance training during beta-adrenergic blockade with atenolol or propranolol. *Med. Sci. Sports Exerc.* 18:95–100, 1986.
224. Weicker, H., and E Werle. Interaction between hormones and the immune system. *Int. J. Sports Med.* 12:30–37, 1991.
225. Weiss, A. Lymphocyte activation. W. E. Paul (ed). *Fundamental Immunology*, 2nd Ed. New York: Raven Press, 1989, pp. 359–384.
226. Weiss, M. J. Fuhrmansky, R. Lulay, and H. Weicker, H. Häufigkeit und Ursache von Immunoglobulinmangel bei Sportlern. *Dtsch. Z. Sportmed.* 35:146–153, 1985.
227. Weksler, M. E., and M. M. Kunts. Use of mitogens in the evaluation of T-lymphocyte function. S. D. Litwin, C. L. Christian and G. W. Siskind (eds). *Clinical Evaluation of Immune Function in Man.* New York: Grune & Stratton, 1976, pp. 151–175.
228. Westerman, J., and R. Pabst. Distribution of lymphocyte subsets and natural killer cells in the human body. *Clin. Invest.* 70:539–544, 1992.
229. Wolpe, S. D., and A. Cerami. Macrophage inflammatory proteins 1 and 2: members of a novel superfamily of cytokines. *FASEB J.* 3:2565–2573, 1989.
230. Yagita, H., M. Nakata, A. Azuma, et al. Activation of peripheral blood T cells via the p75 interleukin-2 receptor. *J. Exp. Med.* 170:1445–1450, 1989.
231. Zänker, K. S. Metabolic interactions—external/internal signals and lymphocyte migration. *Int. J. Sports Med.,* suppl, in press. 1994.
232. Zola, H., R. J. Purling, L. Y. Koh, and M. Tsudo. Expression of p70 chain of the IL-2 receptor on human lymphoid cells: analysis using a monoclonal antibody and high-sensitivity immunofluorescence. *Immunol. Cell Biol.* 68:217–224, 1990.
233. Zola, H., H. Weedon, G. R. Thompson, M. C. Fung, E. Ingley, and A. J. Hapel. Expression of IL-2 receptor p55 and p75 chains by human B lymphocytes: effects of activation and differentiation. *Immunology* 72:167–173, 1991.

8
The Evolution of Research on Motor Development: New Approaches Bringing New Insights

JILL WHITALL, Ph.D.

It is just over 10 years ago that the Exercise and Sport Science Review Series last published a chapter specifically devoted to motor development [11]. Since that time, research in the area has "developed" or "evolved" in a variety of ways, including challenges to existing theoretical frameworks, utilization of alternative methodologies, and expansion of the area's focus. A principal purpose of this chapter is to identify and outline these major changes and new approaches in motor development research. A second purpose is to demonstrate the new insights brought about by these changes by synthesizing selected research on the development of posture and locomotion.

As an introduction to the main purpose of the chapter, it is necessary to define the term motor development and delimit the scope of discussion. Motor development is defined as the changes in motor skill behavior over the life span and the processes that underlie these changes [17]. Adopting this definition immediately illustrates two significant changes in the field of research on motor development that have become instantiated in the last decade. One change is the emphasis on both *product* (i.e., what are the changes in motor behavior) and *process* (i.e., how and why the changes occur). Although it seems obvious that developmental researchers would need and want to understand both product and process of the phenomena under question, this distinction historically has been confusing. (See ref. 17 for a detailed discussion of this point.) The second change illustrated in the definition is the extension of focus from children as exemplified in the chapter by Branta et al [11] to a life span approach in which motor behavior is studied from conception to death. Although some researchers might argue that development is not synonymous with aging, there has been a strong move in developmental psychology to define development as a lifelong process [2, 3]. Researchers interested in motor behavior have followed this lead as reflected in current textbooks [4, 31, 43, 67, 110]. Many researchers study a specific motor skill across the life span rather than studying a variety of motor skills at one age.

Further implications of the above definition of motor development are to recognize that the products of interest are motor *skills* rather than general motor abilities, and that growth, maturation, and learning are all

243

processes or subcategories that contribute to motor development [25]. Thus although there has been much excellent research published on growth and maturation with respect to physical activity [60] and also many experiments concerned with real-time motor learning at different ages [78], this chapter is concerned with motor skill development as an integrated concept that includes (but does not separate) growth, maturation, and learning. Further delimitations (for reasons of space, not conceptualization) are the exclusion of (a) nonhuman research, (b) research published before 1980, and (c) issues dealing with atypical motor skill development, neuropsychological or performance testing, or play. (With regard to nonhuman research, clearly animal research has contributed much to our knowledge about motor development in general and about neurophysiological development in particular. It is not a sound scientific strategy to separate human from animal research, however, it was impossible to include any more material for this chapter. Interested readers are directed, as a starting point, to Bradley and Bekoff [10], who consider relevant animal research with respect to human issues.)

The chapter is organized into four remaining sections. The first outlines the major theoretical and methodological advances that currently characterize the field. Two subsequent sections take up the life span development of posture and locomotion, respectively, and illustrate the advances made by recent research. The attempt here is not to cover every study in the last 15 yr, but to select an illustrative number that give a fairly comprehensive view of current work. Unfortunately, many relevant studies have not been included in this process. Finally, a brief concluding section points out some promising avenues of future research.

THEORETICAL AND METHODOLOGICAL ADVANCES

There is no question that profound theoretical and methodological changes characterize the last decade of research on motor development. These changes have resulted in a "renewed and revitalized" interdisciplinary field of research that some have named "developmental biodynamics" [59], whereas others suggest "developmental kinesiology" [17, 81]. To understand the significance of this revolution it is necessary to review briefly where motor development research was in the early 1980s. (For more detail, see refs. 17, 59, and 89).

As Branta et al. [11] stated in 1984, developmental research over the previous 50 years had primarily led to the agreement that motor skills change in an "orderly manner." In the discipline of kinesiology (physical education), much of the research in the early 1980s revolved around describing the quantitative (product scores) and qualitative (process or movement patterns) changes in fundamental motor skills throughout childhood and adolescence [11]. This work was ethological in nature but, unlike earlier developmental psychologists, who are interested in determining underlying developmental processes, the kinesiologists' work was primarily descriptive and atheoretical. A few researchers, however, did try to base their description on "stage" theory in developmental psychology [73].

Meanwhile, in developmental psychology, the extensive documentation of orderly sequential progressions of posture and movement over the first few years of life had led many to believe that neuromaturation was the primary development process of explanation [33, 62, 79]. Consequently, as psychologists became more interactional in their theoretical orientation, interest in motor development languished behind interest in the psychological changes in perception, cognition, and social and emotional development.

One positive result of the psychologists' interest in perception and cognition actually resulted in an alternative theoretical and methodological approach to studying motor skill development. Following the lead of eminent psychologists such as Piaget and Bruner, many developmentalists began to seek explanations of behavior through hypothetical or abstract processes (perceptual-cognitive processes). Two strands of this approach can be detected. In developmental psychology, a few neo-Piagetians began to study motor skill acquisition as one window to understanding the process of assimilation and accommodation that accompany changes in cognition [63]. Alternatively, in both kinesiology and psychology, many researchers began to model the brain as a computer that receives stimuli, processes the information, and programs a behavioral response. Although much of the motor skill work was directed toward understanding how skills were controlled or learned in adults, some researchers investigated mechanisms in children such as memory [98], response selection and programming [14], and schema formation [78]. A characteristic feature of this approach was the use of experimental paradigms on often very simple (and nonfunctional) skills.

In contrast to either of the two previous psychological paradigms, an alternative route was emerging as a few researchers who came out of a more biological background sought to understand the development of motor skills. These researchers used a neurophysiological (and basically maturational) approach to look at the development of muscle response latencies in a variety of experimental conditions [28].

Thus, at the beginning of the 1980s, motor development research primarily was split between those doing somewhat atheoretical research using descriptive ethological methods, a few doing neurophysiological research (implicitly maturational) using electromyographic (EMG) methodology, and those doing process-oriented research using experimental laboratory-based methods. The watershed for reconceptualizing motor development research came in 1982 with the publication of a paper by Kugler et al. [55]. Although not known as developmental researchers themselves, these three movement scientists extended and elaborated on an earlier paper [54] to include new theoretical ideas about the development of motor control and coordination. In this new conceptualization, three distinct but interrelated themes can be delineated, each of which has contributed to somewhat independent lines of motor development research.

The first theme that emerged from the paper by Kugler et al. [55] was the importance of the work of the Russian physiologist Nicolai Bernstein [6]. As early as the 1930s, Bernstein recognized the enormous task of coordinating multiple degrees of freedom in the body. He suggested that the central nervous system (CNS) input was only part of the whole picture because nonmuscular as well as muscular forces needed to be considered within an interactional process. He argued that coordination arises as an a posteriori or self-organizing synergy of functional specific muscle groups. This line of reasoning stands in sharp contrast to either a traditional maturational or an information-processing viewpoint, where an extensive a priori role is attributed to the CNS.

These ideas had a profound effect on motor development research, as exemplified in the work of Thelen. For example, by using biomechanical measurement techniques, Thelen and her colleagues have challenged the view that neuromaturation of the CNS inhibits reflex action (see ref. 50 for a review of this work). In fact, Thelen has been instrumental in promoting a "systems" approach to motor development that emphasizes the importance and cooperative action of all "maturing" subsystems with no hierarchical priority for the CNS [88, 90, 97]. Out of a Bernsteinian perspective, then, researchers of motor development began to use the measurement techniques of biomechanics and to recognize and consider multiple self-organizing subsystems of the body.

A second and strongly related theme found in Kugler et al. [55] is the argument that principles of continuity and discontinuity in motor development can best be understood by applying generic principles of nonlinear dynamical systems. From a dynamical systems approach, the behavior of a complex system can be characterized by one or more "collective or essential variables" that are representative variables that capture the qualitative change of that system. For example, the relative phasing relationship between the legs has been used as a collective variable to describe the motor skill of walking [93, 106]. By plotting the changes in the collective variable over time, it is possible to determine rules about how the system behaves. These rules form the basis of a theoretical model that may be purely mathematical or, more often, based on a physical model (such as an oscillator) with its known mathematical expression. In the study of rhythmic limb movement, the physical model of coupled nonlinear limit cycle oscillators has been utilized extensively by scientists studying real-time behavior [e.g., 51, 56].

After studying the behavior of the collective variable over time, the next experimental step in a dynamical systems approach is to identify points of transition where the collective variable undergoes a loss of stability and shifts to a new attractive behavioral form (known as an attractor state in dynamical systems language). The region of instability, where a system undergoes a transition, becomes the focus of research as the experimenter tries to find eligible control parameters; that is, parameters of the system whose own incremental change will suddenly cause the system to shift into a new attractive state (showing a change in the collective variable). Thelen [88, 96], for example, has identified the subsystems of postural control and extensor strength as possible rate-limiting developmental control parameters that cause the infant to move from a state of not walking to walking. Ultimately, it is necessary to verify that the identified control parameter(s) do indeed generate a developmental change. One strategy to test this hypothesis is to follow subjects longitudinally and continually measure the control parameter(s) and collective variable to assess the coherence of the changes. A more practical solution is to verify with real-time experiments (sometimes called microgenesis experiments) that supplement the subject with extra or diminished amounts of the control parameter with the idea of causing a positive or negative change in the collective variable, respectively. Again, an example from Thelen's work is her experiment in which babies had ankle weights (equivalent to weight gain) or were placed in water (equivalent to strength gain) with a resulting decrease or increase, respectively, in the stepping actions of the baby [95].

The language and concepts of dynamical systems theory (attractor states, collective variable, transitions, control parameters) have proved quite efficacious to some motor development researchers and have generated fruitful lines of investigation. In addition to Thelen, for example, Clark and her colleagues have used these concepts to demonstrate that young children's gaits exhibit properties similar to those of coupled nonlinear limit cycle oscillators, the model shown to be useful in real-time upper limb movements (see ref. 106 for review of this work). As yet, however, neither Thelen, Clark, nor other developmental researchers have gone to the formal mathematical modeling stage with their work. It is only recently that a few motor development researchers have begun to interact with mathematicians to begin the formal modeling that the dynamical systems theory will allow [e.g., 39].

The two themes from the paper by Kugler et al. [55] discussed so far (Bernstein's ideas and nonlinear dynamical modeling) have become known collectively as the dynamic(al) systems or dynamic pattern approach. (Essentially, the nonlinear dynamic modeling is a formal instantiation of Bernstein's ideas, along with concepts from the German physiologist von Holst [103].) The third theme evident in the paper by Kugler et al. [11] is known under a different name, most commonly that of perception-action or ecological psychology approach and is based on the ecological perception ideas of the American psychologist J. J. Gibson. Gibson [37] argued that the perceptual and motor systems evolved together and need to be studied together. Specifically, he argued that perception is a direct process that occurs as the eyes, head, and body move in space. The incoming information does not require complex calculations, as the information processing theorists presume. People perceive environmental objects directly in relation to their own body, a concept known as affordance. Thus, a set of stairs may afford walking to an adult, but climbing to an infant because of the difference in body scale. As people grow, affordances may change and new movement patterns emerge. This perception-action approach has been developed primarily by developmental psychologists such as Pick [68] and Eleanor Gibson (Gibson's wife). For example, infants have been placed on different surfaces to determine whether the consequent perceptual information will affect the infant's movements (see ref. 35).

Although the perception-action approach has evolved somewhat independently from the Bernsteinian/dynamical systems approach; taken together, they reflect a current approach to motor development research that, although not subsumed under a recognized inclusive name, form a worldview that is very different from previous approaches. No longer is the CNS the fundamental biological (maturation) or psychological (cognitive or information processing) process behind motor development. Rather, the CNS is one of many cooperative subsystems within the organism and its environment that come together to form the emergent behavior. Newell [65] has captured the totality of the new approach in his notion of constraints whereby the organism, task, and environment are a triumvirate influence on developing coordination and control. Organismic constraints (information endogenous to the body) include both structural (e.g., strength) and functional (e.g., prelearned muscle synergy) components, whereas environmental contraints (exogenous to the body) include both physical (e.g., gravity) and social-cultural (e.g., gender bias) components. Completing the triangle and conceptually providing the final organizing information are the parameters of the task itself. Although recognizing the efficacy of this simplistic conceptualization, motor development researchers have not found it easy, of course, to investigate all three corners at once. Nevertheless, there are many efforts to undertake a broader approach by, for example, looking specifically at the mediating effects of various environmental influences such as urban environments [40], psychosocial factors [99], or cultural influences [12].

To summarize, motor development research has evolved considerably over the past 10 years. Concepts and tools provided by the dynamical systems and perception-action schools have taken researchers beyond the descriptive or perceptual-cognitive process-oriented approaches. Ecologically valid studies are now designed to understand the genetic principles of motor development and to unravel the complex interactional process of perceiving information and utilizing the intrinsic properties of the body to accomplish the task at hand. It would be incorrect, however, to imply that all motor development research is now undertaken from these new perspectives. There are many who operate in an atheoretical or maturational perspective and those who are investigating cognitive or information-processing characteristics of subjects over time.

In the subsequent two sections, however, the aim is to provide an overview of how the newer conceptual and methodological approaches have influenced and updated our knowledge of motor development. As exemplars of this work, the sections are devoted to posture and locomotion, respectively. This does not imply that these skills develop separately, but rather that they tend to be studied independently and it is therefore easier to follow the development of each skill (set of skills) over the life span.

POSTURE

For the purpose of this review, posture or postural control will be defined as the ability to gain and maintain bodily orientation to the environment. Although it is impossible to separate this ability from the action of locomotion or, for that matter, from eye-hand coordination tasks, posture has been studied independently and serves as a functional backdrop to other skill development. Three lines of research have provided a window into the development of postural control. First, the use of modern ultrasound technology allowed a glimpse of fetal postural control. Second, from the perception-action perspective, a "moving room or optical flow" experimental paradigm emerged. The moving room produces an optical flow that simulates body sway and, if the visual information is linked to postural muscle synergies, will cause a corresponding directionally specific body sway [58]. Third, from a neurophysiological perspective, a "platform perturbation" experimental paradigm emerged. This paradigm has allowed scientists to study how the postural system regains its orientation to the environment after the center of mass has been destabilized [28]. The section is divided into the three periods of the life span that have been studied in detail: infancy, early childhood, and aging adulthood.

Prenatal to Independently Standing Infants
The postnatal sequential motor milestones of head control, trunk control, rolling, sitting, pull to stand, independent stance, and walking have been documented extensively since the 1930s [62, 79]. This sequence was explained through the role of reflexes and postural reactions as subcomponents that were integrated through the maturation of the CNS. However, no agreement was ever reached as to how or even which neural structures or subcomponents contributed to particular postural milestones [24]. In the last decade, there has been a considerable accumulation of experimental evidence that has both clarified and complicated the overall pic-

ture. An example of this dilemma is illustrated with the new experimental evidence of fetal postural control.

Using ultrasound technology, Prechtl [70] has noted that the fetus shows postural adjustments when it changes its position and orientation in the uterus up to 20 times per hour during the first half of pregnancy. Two movements are employed by the fetus with one initiating a rotation along the longitudinal body axis by a lateral turning of the head or hips and the other, alternating leg movements which produce a somersault if the legs are properly positioned against the uterine wall. Both of these movements reappear in postnatal behavior as the derotative righting reflexes and the stepping reflex, respectively. However, the developmental course is discontinuous because the derotative reflexes reappear several months after birth and the stepping reflex disappears 2–4 mo postnatally. Thus, although we know more about fetal postural adjustment, it is still not clear whether or how these postural adjustments relate to postnatal postural behavior.

According to Prechtl [70], there seems to be a blocking of actual vestibular responses during intrauterine life that prevents the fetus moving every time the mother turns. At birth the vestibular ocular and the Moro reflexes appear quickly but postural control is very weak and, compared with other primates, the human neonate is remarkably poorly adapted to the demands of the extrauterine environment. For example, Prechtl [69] studied the muscle activation of 5-day-old infants and, although neck muscle activity was noticed, there was no evidence of spontaneous activity patterns that would counteract gravity consistently. If spontaneous postural activity patterns are not observed in the neonate, can they be elicited visually by optical flow? Jouen [47] investigated this phenomenon in 3-day-old infants who experienced sequentially activated lights simulating the optical flow created by body movement. He found that 80% of the infants demonstrated a sensitivity to the flow, and 67% of the postural responses were in the same direction as the optical flow. Although this is remarkable evidence of early available postural synergies, the statistics actually mean that expected postural responses were only observed 54% of the time. Thus the capability of the visual system to drive postural reactions in the neonate is not clear-cut. Furthermore, a similarly designed experiment on older infants found that 5-mo-old infants showed no evidence of compensations to optical flow, whereas 7- and 9-mo-olds did [8].

In contrast to an optical display, Sveistrup and colleagues [85] used the moving room stimulus and demonstrated that 5-mo-old independent sitters showed consistent responses to room movement and the sway amplitudes increased in the pull-to-stand infants (8–10 mo) and peaked in the independent walkers (11–14 mo). In this experiment, clear muscle pattern responses were observed that served to pull the infant in the direction of the visual stimulus. However, these responses were more variable than those seen in the platform perturbation experiments by the same authors with children of similar ages and abilities.

Curiously, the more general case has been that platform perturbation experiments have not elicited postural reactions as early as those stimulated in the optical flow experiments. For example, Prechtl [69] used a variation of this paradigm when he placed 5-day-old infants on a board that rotated 15° in the transverse plane. The infants did not respond until 8–10 wk of age, when they showed clear EMG patterns along with head retroflexion and extension of the arms when the head was tilted downward. These responses became consistent by 3 mo of age and coincided with the appearance of voluntary head control. These data indicate that muscle activation of the neck assembles for voluntary action and for response to a physical perturbation at the same time despite evidence that similar synergies may be constrained by visual stimulation alone.

Further evidence of the parallel development of voluntary and response postural control comes from a cross-sectional study of seated infants (4–14 mo) under platform translation conditions [112]. Those children who could not sit independently showed responses only in the neck. Trunk responses became apparent only when the infant gained independent control of the trunk. In fact, responses were not consistently directionally specific until about 8 mo and lack of vision did not seem to affect the responses. Similar results were obtained in longitudinal studies of 2–18-mo-old infants, this time looking at the postural responses of the legs and trunk when standing on the platform [84, 111]. Again, no organized responses occurred at first until the onset of pull-to-stand behavior at around 8 mo. Then directionally specific responses began to emerge, first beginning with lower leg, followed by upper leg, and finally the trunk muscles by late pull-to-stand (10 mo). It should be noted that the trunk muscle activations were not very consistent until about 18 mo. These results are important because they contradict the traditional neuromaturational principles of "proximodistal" development. As noted in the preceding section of this chapter, developmental movement scientists have begun to recognize that the developing nervous system does not act in isolation and that other organismic (environmental, task) constraints may be influential. An example of this thinking is evident in Woollacott's work after conducting the above experiments on newly standing infants.

Woollacott and colleagues observed a large amount of background movement of the joints, which might be explained by a low level of muscle stiffness in the infants. In other words, perhaps muscle strength could be a rate-limiting constraint on the development of postural control. Using biomechanical techniques, they estimated stiffness through the slopes of the torque trace taken at the initiation of the platform perturbation before onset of muscular compensation [111]. They found a drop in muscle stiffness over time that did not support the low stiffness hypothesis. Instead, Woollacott and Sveistrup [111] suggest that the infants' movements are actually a kind of postural "babbling" as they explore postural sensorimotor space.

Concepts such as that of infants exploring postural sensorimotor space are clearly in line with the idea that postural responses are not "hard-wired" neural circuits (reflexive or spontaneous) waiting to be liberated by the growth of the CNS. Rather, postural synergies are carved out of the infant's intrinsic properties but not in a strongly predetermined fashion. This rhetoric contrasts with those who still promote a "predetermined" maturational perspective on postural development. For example, Hirschfeld and Forssberg [46] used the platform perturbation paradigm to look at infants who could sit independently and those who needed support. They found distinct postural synergies for backward sway in all children (but only for 60% of trials) and no distinct responses for forward sway. They suggest that "a basic form of the postural adjustment develops in a predetermined manner before children practice independent sitting" [46, p. 528]. However, this does not explain the 40% of errant backward trials or the forward sway results. Furthermore, Hirschfeld and Forssberg [46] acknowledge that the basic postural synergy pattern is shaped and fine-tuned through practice by multisensory interactions from all activated systems. Two questions arise: (a) how directionally specific should the responses be to claim that they appear to be predetermined and (b) what is the difference between predetermined and "intrinsic" properties, particularly because further fine-tuning is mandated in both cases? It would seem that the same data can be interpreted in different ways according to the theoretical position that one adopts. In a final example, this point is illustrated nicely in a study in which the experimenters designed a functional or ecologically valid perturbation, namely release of support from a sitting position, rather than an artificial perturbation.

Harbourne and colleagues [42] studied infants who could sit with support (at 2–3 mo) and again when they could sit alone momentarily (5 mo). After the infants lost support in the sitting position, the 5-mo-olds showed a decrease in velocity and displacement of the trunk and more directionally appropriate responses compared with the earlier age. Most interestingly, the EMG measures indicated that only 29 of a possible 720 combinations of synergies were identified at the first age, and these were reduced to 13 synergies with 2 predominating by 5 mo. Clearly, an appropriate muscle synergy was "found" over the ensuing months. Both between- and within-subject variability were reduced over time, but the 5-mo olds were still somewhat variable. These data support a dynamical systems interpretation because it seems unlikely that 29 different synergies constitute a "predetermined" synergy; however, one could argue the opposite case, given the 720 possible combinations! Thus, again, the same data can be interpreted in different ways. Although it is not possible to compare across experimental paradigms, there is certainly a suggestion that the more natural perturbation produces more directionally specific muscle responses than the two dominating experimental paradigms in this area of study. Because of the ecological validity of the perturbation, this kind of paradigm appears to have great potential.

In summary, current researchers have demonstrated the development of postural responses to visual and proprioceptive perturbations over the first year of life. One general conclusion is that visual/proprioception directionally specific responses are consistently elicited *in parallel* to functional behaviors of the same muscle groups. This is in contrast to the traditional view of reflexes and postural reactions preceding functional behavior. A second finding is that variability between and within subjects is considerable. Both of these facts argue against an innate, "predetermined" maturational perspective, although there is still debate about interpretation of these data. Finally, there is some confusion between the paradigms regarding when responses are produced and thus how the contributing systems (visual, proprioceptive, vestibular, musculoskeletal) are interacting together. These questions will be difficult to answer without the benefit of an intensive longitudinal study that uses frequent and multiple natural and experimental manipulations. Meanwhile, some attempt at differentiating the contributing systems has taken place in research on older children.

Childhood

For the early developmental researchers, the achievement of independent walking and therefore functional balance resulted in a lack of interest in postural control. The major form of data came from descriptive product-oriented studies of the static or dynamic balance abilities of young children [23]. These studies documented an increasing ability to maintain balance under destabilizing situations, suggesting that maturation and practice were affecting this ability. In the last decade, researchers have begun to investigate this process primarily by utilizing the platform perturbation paradigm.

Experiments with platform perturbations have found that 1.5–3-yr-old children show clearly organized, directionally specific leg muscle responses that are larger in amplitude and longer in duration than those seen in an adult [28, 80]. Also, there often was activation of the antagonist muscles at a slightly longer latency, illustrating a lack of efficiency in muscle response. This age group did not consistently show trunk musculature response, however, illustrating that postural muscle synergies were still being assembled. Interestingly, the 4–6-yr-old children showed leg postural synergies that were consistently slower and more variable in both onset latencies and timing relationships (between distal and proximal muscles) than the younger group. By 7–10 yr of age, however, postural responses were similar to adults. These findings were confirmed in a later study looking at trunk and neck muscles for both age groups [112]. Absence of vision, also, did not affect the 7–10-yr-old children or adults. However, younger children showed a reduction in postural response onset (2–3 yr) and an increase in frequency of the occurrence of monosynaptic responses (2–6 yr). Thus visual cues do not seem necessary to activate postural responses at any age, but there is evidence that vision may be dominant in the younger age groups in that a shift occurs from use of longer latency visual inputs to shorter latency proprioceptive inputs with eyes closed.

The relative influence of the three sensory systems was tested also by asking children 4-yr and older to stand quietly under four sensory conditions that progressively decreased the sensory inputs useful for balance control until only vestibular inputs remained [80]. The 4–6-yr-olds were unable to maintain balance in the latter condition and showed progressively decreasing stability as they lost redundant sensory inputs for postural control. Older age groups were only slightly affected by the vestibular-only condition. Based on their findings, Shumway-Cook and Woollacott suggest that children of 4–6 yr show variability and regression in their postural responses because they are relying less on visual input alone and learning to adapt their responses to changing sensory conditions frequently shifting from one sensory input to another.

Support for these speculations can be found in a behavioral paradigm that investigated the dynamic balance of heel-toe stepping along a balance beam. In a series of experiments, Williams and colleagues [108] tested the balance of 6- and 8-yr-olds while manipulating the visual cues available in terms of body versus environment and peripheral versus central field referents. They found that the 6-yr-olds were not able to use visual information about the body alone but needed to relate this information to the surrounding environment. Six-year-olds also differ from 8-yr-olds by relying more on central visual field referents. In general, there seemed to be a trend away from the need to visually monitor body/environment relationships directly to maintain effective balance at 6 yr toward greater reliance or use of vestibular-proprioceptive information for maintaining dynamic balance control at 8 yr of age.

The parallel findings from neurophysiological and behavioral studies are encouraging, and further support in terms of a postural disorganization in 4–6-yr-olds comes from the work of Riach and Hayes [72], who investigated the anticipation of postural control as children lifted their arms. Unfortunately, very few detailed (and longitudinally valid) studies of functional postural control have been carried out in the behavioral domain across childhood. Thus, it is not possible to map neuromuscular changes with behavioral changes on a developmental continuum.

One of the few functional skills that has been studied across childhood is the skill of rising to stand. Although technically this is really a weight transfer skill between two static postures, the ability to accomplish the skill relies on maintaining control of the body through changing orientation. Furthermore, this research nicely illustrates a very different approach to studying the development of a skill. Van Sant [104] used a prelongitudinal screening paradigm [see 74] to observe and chart the developmental changes in this skill. She found a clear developmental sequence in that young children rotate their trunks and use their arms and legs in an asymmetrical fashion, whereas older children and adults are able to rise symmetrically with no trunk rotation at all. The latter coordination pattern is the most biomechanically efficient pattern and there are interesting questions of how and why children progress (or fail to) through the developmental sequence. Presumably the answer to these questions involves looking at organismic (strength, postural control) as well as task or environmental constraints.

Overall, the research findings on postural control in childhood indicate that young children rely on vision as the primary contributing system, whereas older children have integrated the postural systems and are adultlike in neuromuscular actions. In between these states children show some regression of organization in their neuromuscular actions, although it is not clear from earlier behavioral studies that this proposed reorganization causes a real deterioration in balance performance. More research needs to be undertaken, particularly in relation to this transition age group, around 6 yr. From a dynamical systems perspective, this would now entail a longitudinal study over this age period to determine and measure collective variables and potential control parameters. Unfortunately, few contemporary researchers show much interest in this age in contrast to younger or older age groups.

Aging Adults

The last decade has seen increased attention to the problems of aging and because postural control is obviously a clinically significant problem there has been a consequent increase in research in this area. In general, the results demonstrate a surprisingly small loss of postural ability in otherwise health older adults. Again, Woollacott and colleagues [61, 64, 109, 113] have examined the neuromuscular synergies of older adults using the moving platform paradigm. In cross-sectional research, they noted that the automatic postural responses of 61–78-yr-old adults showed increases in absolute latency of the distal muscles in response to posterior sway only, some inconsistent distal to proximal synergies, an increase in short latency monosynaptic reflexes when subjected to platform rotations and a greater likelihood to activate antagonist muscles. These results are reminiscent of the young children's data and, like the children under 7 years, about half the older adults were less efficient in balancing under conditions of reduced or conflicting sensory information. However, unlike the children, in most instances, the older adults were able to balance in these conditions when given some practice. Falls occurred when the muscle synergies were different from the subject's predominant response or from the strategies of young adults.

On the surface, these results appear to indicate that the "aging" process results in a decline in nervous system function as time progresses. However, when Manchester et al. [61] performed a neurological examination on the older adults in their study, they found that those subjects who lost balance had an indication of borderline peripheral or central nervous system pathology. This supports an alternative hypothesis of aging in that the nervous system can continue to function at a high level until death unless a specific pathological condition causes dysfunction in a specific neural structure.

Finally, Van Sant [104], too, has carried her study of rising-to-stand into the elderly population. Cross-sectional observations of middle-aged and older adults showed that aging did not necessarily produce a regression to the earlier movement patterns shown by children but rather that new and less efficient patterns of the arms and legs appeared (e.g., pushing on the thighs when rising). Thus the elderly appeared to compensate for other factors, perhaps a loss of strength or flexibility, rather than regressing to neurologically and biomechanically easier movement patterns. Correlations with organismic constraints such as strength and fat-free body weight would make these relationships clearer and perhaps further demonstrate that a "healthy" body does not change motor behavior patterns solely as a result of the passing of years.

In general, then, our knowledge so far about "healthy" aging of the postural system is limited because it is difficult to discriminate between compromised and noncompromised organismic constraints. Woollacott's work with intersensory conflict conditions showed that it is possible that sensory integration becomes disorganized for some older adults; however, more controlled experiments would be necessary to investigate whether, for example, vision again becomes the dominant system. Perhaps surprisingly, there seems to have been little work from the perception-action perspective using optical flow perturbations or in designing more ecologically valid perturbation situations.

Summary

Recent studies of the development of postural ability have been undertaken primarily from neurophysiological and perception-action perspectives using two experimental paradigms (but see ref. 71, too). These paradigms, along with ultrasound technology, have significantly added to existing information about the development of postural control and specifically to the role of visual, proprioceptive and vestibular systems in the emergence and aging of postural muscle synergies. All of the research studies cited in this section, however, have been concerned with static rather than dynamic balance situations. In the next section the development of a dynamic balance situation—locomotion—is reviewed. As will be seen, recent research in this area indicates the significance of dynamic balance as a rate-limiting factor in the emergence of certain locomotor patterns of coordination.

LOCOMOTION

The ability to move from one location to another is a fundamental skill for living that can be accomplished by a variety of behavioral motor patterns. Most research, at least by developmental psychologists or neurophysiologists, has focused on walking as the primary motor pattern. More recently there has been a move to study both the antecedent skills to walking and locomotor skills that appear after walking is mastered. Although no single paradigm has dominated this research, the theoretical perspective has been the dynamical systems approach both from a Bernsteinian viewpoint and using nonlinear dynamic modeling principles. In addition, a second line of research has stemmed from the perception-action approach using optical flow as well as affordance paradigms. As with postural ability, the development of locomotion has been studied primarily in infancy, early childhood, and in the aging adult.

Prenatal to Independently Walking Infants
The major postnatal developmental locomotor milestone is the ability to walk independently. This ability is reliably preceded by the appearance and disappearance of simple reflexes such as the step reflex. However, even though most infants will crawl before they walk, the crawl does not seem to be a necessary prerequisite in the same way that sitting precedes standing. Traditional explanations of learning to walk, then, have focused on the sequential appearance of simple reflexes, followed by cortical inhibition of these reflexes, the accomplishment of independent standing, and finally the integration of voluntary or cortical locomotor centers with the subcortical levels to produce a mature walking pattern. Whereas some continue to promote a neuromaturational explanation, others have challenged the predetermined hierarchical CNS control of development beginning with the experimental findings of reflexive or spontaneous movements that appear so similar to subsequent voluntary behavior that they are likely to be a continuous developmental function.

Thus, in prenatal infants, Prechtl [70] has detected alternating flexion and extension movements of the legs during the first half of gestation, whereas Heriza [44] has measured coordinated kicking movements in premature infants as early as 28 wk gestational age, that are identical in shape to newborn movements. In more detailed kinematic [94] and EMG analyses, Thelen and Fisher [92] studied the stepping and kicking actions of 2-wk-old infants. Both actions include the same temporal organization, coactivation of antagonist muscle bursts, and a tight temporal and spatial synchrony among hip, knee, and ankle joints. Thelen and Fisher [92] concluded that these actions were identical, that is, generated by the same neural circuitry, except for the posture in which they are produced. They also noted some similarities to later independent walking. To investigate further the continuity of leg action over the first year, Thelen and Cooke [91] conducted a longitudinal study in which they compared intralimb coordination patterns and EMG in stepping at 1 or 2 mo of age to that of the same infants 1 to 2 mo before independent walking and in the month after the first walking steps. They found that the tight synchrony of intralimb coordination gradually changed into more adultlike patterns in which the knee led the hip in flexion even before the onset of walking, although vestiges of the newborn steps remained. Thus from a dynamical systems perspective it appears as though walking coordination patterns are gradually carved out of the more simple newborn patterns. If this is so, why does the newborn stepping typically disappear whereas the kicking remains?

Thelen et al. [95] proposed that infants discontinue stepping because of the rapid addition of fat in disproportion to muscle strength gain. In a classic experiment, Thelen et al. [95] demonstrated that (a) the infants that gained weight most rapidly between 2 and 6 wk of age also took fewer steps and (b) 4-wk old infants submerged in water (causing an increase in strength-to-weight ratio) dramatically increased their step rate and amplitude, whereas adding weights to their legs had the reverse effect. In dynamical systems terminology the rapid weight gain acts during normal development as a control parameter, shifting the infant from a state of stepping to not stepping. This idea not only challenges the traditional idea of CNS inhibition but also the alternative theory, based on instrumental learning, proposed by Zelazo after he demonstrated that infants who were encouraged to practice stepping did not lose this ability (See refs. 86, 114, and 115 for debate on this issue.) Zelazo's results [116] can be explained easily by the fact that exercising the infants would increase their strength-to-weight ratio. Similarly, the persistence of supine kicking can be explained because the infants can now work partly with gravity instead of needing the strength to work against gravity. Finally, Thelen [87, 93] has demonstrated well-coordinated alternating stepping movements in 7-mo-old infants, who do not normally step, if they are held supported on a small motorized treadmill.

Taken as a whole, the above findings demonstrate the influence of changing non-neural organismic factors such as fat/muscle gain as well as the effect of different contexts (task or environmental constraints) such as postural position or support surface even before the legs are used for voluntary locomotion. In addition, by using kinetic analyses to tease out the use of muscular versus nonmuscular forces, Jensen et al. [49] have demonstrated further that infants change their kicking muscle activation patterns according to their postural position. In other words, the infant's kicks or steps are not predetermined in the nervous system but emerge from the self-assembly of many elements including the neural circuitry, body components, arousal, gravitation, and so on. Thelen [88, 96] contends that any of a number of possible rate-limiting components may actually allow the behavior of independent walking to emerge but in normal development the evidence favors strength and dynamic postural control.

Despite the compelling evidence of Thelen's programmatic research, others still promote a more neuromaturational explanation. Forssberg [27], for example, undertook a longitudinal study of neonates, 1–10 mo-old infants, and independent walkers. In addition to documenting the disappearance of the step reflex, he, too, noted a similarity between 10-mo-old infants during supported stepping and new walking. However, his interpretation (based also on the fact that anencephalic infants can perform similar stepping) is that the neural pattern generator for walking is innate and organized at the brain stem or below. Descending driving systems would then integrate and control the network over the first year of life but adaptive systems for equilibrium control develop over a longer time period and modify the basic pattern generator. It is not clear, however, how this interpretation can account for Zelazo's [116] data or why it is necessary to invoke multiple higher level systems that deterministically control development.

As found in the posture studies, it is very easy to interpret the same data from different theoretical perspectives. For example, in a cross-sectional study, Clark et al. [20] found that new walkers adopted alternating temporal and distance interlimb phasing (i.e., 50% where one foot plants exactly in the middle of the other foot's stride cycle). One could argue that a predetermined neural circuit dictated this alternating pattern or, as Clark et al. [20] prefer, that a bipedal symmetric morphology constrains the system to adopt this as an efficient solution. In any case, the mean interlimb phasing relationships of the new walker were quite variable, indicating a less stable relationship until 3 mo had passed, at which time the variability was adultlike. Similar findings occurred when Clark and Phillips [16] examined infants longitudinally over the first year of walking. These authors analyzed intralimb coordination by using qualitative dynamic techniques (phase plane trajectories) and again the new walkers showed an attraction to the same dynamic solution as the adult, but not until the infants had been walking 3 mo, did the behavior of the system settle into a stable regimen.

Walking stability after 3 mo of experience was also found using the neurophysiological technique of EMG methodology to investigate the underlying muscle activation. Okamoto and Goto [66] found that EMG patterns of the new walker were characterized by co-contraction of antagonist muscles pairs and strong discharge patterns from the rectus abdominis muscle needed to assist in the major postural control problem of the trunk. However, by 3 mo of walking, the infants have achieved a stable pattern of muscle activation that was maintained until about 3 yr before changing again.

Even though these three studies [16, 20, 66] showed that the legs are initially less stable in their coupling, when newly walking infants were supported by hand, they significantly increased their temporal and distance stability [20]. Furthermore, underlying EMG patterns showed more organization and less coactivation with postural stability [66]. This unmasking of underlying coordination by reducing postural demands is evidence to support Thelen's claim that some combination of strength and dynamic balance is the developmental control parameter that allows walking to emerge [88, 96]. It argues, also, against the idea that predetermined higher centers are the sole adaptive mechanisms for equilibrium control [27].

The importance of strength and dynamic balance as rate-limiters has been demonstrated, too, in the emergence of crawling. Longitudinal research by Benson [7] and Freedland and Bertenthal [29] has shown that infants adopt a partial diagonal pattern of interlimb coordination that minimizes the demands of strength and balance and, at the same time, is flexible and dynamically efficient. A different orientation was taken by Goldfield [38], who argued that hand laterality was connected with an infant's first reach and subsequent crawls.

There are many other researchers who have systematically investigated the first year of walking (e.g., [13]), but currently, despite the well-documented knowledge that walking is not fully adultlike until 7 yr of age [83], few have studied walking development after the age of 2. Given all of the changing organismic, task, and environmental constraints that occur over these intervening years it would seem to be a daunting task to detect relationships between changes in the walking pattern and potential rate-limiting or control parameters. At least one group of researchers, however, is clearly trying to map relationships between the environment and the production of walking. These investigators are specifically interested in how perception of the environment interacts with locomotion.

The basic paradigm is to present perceptually different affordances either sequentially or as a choice paradigm and observe how the infants behave. Gibson et al. [36] changed the support surface for infants who were either crawlers or independent walkers. With a rigid (smooth with diagonal lines) versus deformable (water bed) surface, both groups explored the surfaces visually and haptically before traversing, but the walkers explored the water bed for longer and were more wary of traveling on it. To test whether the older walkers were simply wary of any new surface, the same rigid surface was compared with an equally rigid surface, this time covered with black velvet, which presented poor optical information to specify its surface properties. In this set-up, the crawlers were equally wary of the black velvet surface and thus it seemed as though, in the first study, the walkers were seeking information from the deformable surface for an affordance (bipedal balance) that was not yet relevant to the crawlers. A further testing situation indicated that it was haptic rather than visual information that was important to the infant walkers.

These experiments tell us much about how the environment can influence infant movement at different ages (and with different organismic constraints), and other examples such as stair climbability [101] and slope traversability [1] have also shown this interaction. Further revelations concerning vision specifically have come from the use of the moving room paradigm. Stoffregen, et al. [82] studied the effects of global, central, and peripheral optic flow in subjects aged 1 to 5 years, the range that covers the decrease in visual dominance for stance [80]. With global flow, both swaying and falling occurred in stance and locomotion but falling was confined to younger children, as found in the static posture-only studies. Children under 2-yr were susceptible to both frontal and peripheral flow but older children were only affected by peripheral flow. This suggests that children learn to differentiate optic flow so that central flow can be used for steering around obstacles, whereas peripheral flow is left to control postural adjustments.

On the basis of above result, Gibson and Schmuckler [35] argue that the skill of walking will improve as perceptual constraints and action become integrated and refined, with practice, including the ability to differentiate between central and peripheral flow. Thus, if young walkers move through a cluttered environment versus a clear path, they would be expected to have a greater loss of equilibrium from optic flow in the former situation, at least until they had reached an age where differentiated flow was complete. As experiment to test this hypothesis was undertaken using a "moving hallway" with children of 2.7, 8.1, and 17.0 mo of walking experience. Results were as predicted although the older age group (around 2.5 yr) still showed an effect of the cluttered environment. Because few researchers investigate advanced walking it would be interesting to extend this experiment to older children and determine whether changes in perception are correlated with the documented biomechanical changes.

Overall, the research studies in the last decade have demonstrated a developmental continuity of kinematic behavior from prenatal movements to independent walking subserved by functional neuromuscular synergies that are influenced by changing organismic, task, and environmental constraints. No direct test has been made, however, of the assertion that dynamic posture and strength are rate-limiting parameters for the emergence of walking in normally developing infants. Nor has there been much investigation into the acquisition of mature walking in older children.

Childhood
The development of locomotor skills beyond walking has been of little interest to developmental psychologists or neurophysiologists and yet there is much developing during this time period. Primarily from physical education research we know that the locomotor skills appear sequentially in the following order: running (1.5 yr), galloping (2 yr), hopping (3 yr), and skipping (4 yr) [18]. Jumping from 2 ft is also often included as a locomotor skill and this appears at approximately the same time as galloping [75].

What little research occurred before the 1980s was mostly documenting the timetable of appearance. Since then, two major lines of research characterize the period.

One research line documents *qualitative* changes from the inception to a mature state of each skill. These efforts are notable for the use of "component" approach, which describes each body part as having an independent history [74]. This approach stands in contrast to the earlier "whole-body" approach, in which the body components were combined [11]. Many but not all of these more recently documented component sequences have been prelongitudinally screened [77] and some have been longitudinally validated. The following locomotor skills have been partially or fully validated on a relatively large sample of children: hopping [41, 76] and standing long jump [15]. Hypothesized sequences for running and skipping are also available [75].

The very fact that these advanced locomotor skills do not develop in one prescribed "whole-body" pattern is suggestive of a very context-sensitive developmental process. Why do children differ in their developmental profiles? What organismic, task, and environmental constraints aid in this process? To date, no studies have investigated these questions systematically, but several researchers have chosen a method of investigation that ultimately is leading in that direction. For these researchers, the locomotor skills are viewed as attractive but not predetermined muscle synergies (coordinative structures) for which the principles of dynamical systems modeling may apply [18, 106].

The dynamical model that seems to have the most application for studying locomotor limb coordination is that of coupled nonlinear, limit cycle oscillators. For example, Whitall [105] compared the general properties of these oscillators with the temporal and distance phasing relationships of children (ages 2–9 yr) and adults as they ran and galloped. Specifically, the legs were (a) phase-locked (attracted to a specific phase mode of 50% for the run and either 66 or 75% for the gallop); (b) well entrained (showing little variability around the average phasing), and (c) structurally stable (in the sense that adding a 4% weight to one leg had no effect on the phasing of the run and little effect on the gallop). Developmentally, the interesting findings were that these properties appeared even in the youngest children although the 3- and 4-yr-olds were slightly less stable in their phasing patterns. Furthermore, at all ages, the gallop was slightly less stable than the run. Thus the basic organizational properties of the neuromuscular system do not change across age at this behavioral level of analysis even though the actual intralimb kinematics, kinetics, or EMG may.

This organizational principle of a developmentally stable coordination pattern has also been identified in the skill of jumping. Jensen et al. [48] found no differences in coordination patterns of 3- and 4-yr-old standing long jumpers even though differences in actual take-off angles were apparent. In a similar paradigm, Clark et al. [19] filmed 3–9-yr-old children plus three groups of adults—average skill, skilled in volleyball, and skilled in gymnastics—doing the standing long jump and the vertical jump. No differences were found in the leg coordination patterns despite clear differences in the organismic constraints of the groups and the different task demands of the two jumps. Differences were found only in the position and magnitude values, not in the delay to peak extension velocities. Thus, the movements may look qualitatively different but, at a more fundamental level of analysis, show remarkable consistency. Whether this fundamental organization applies to the arm actions as well as the legs is open to question because there are robust developmental changes in the way the arms are coordinated [15]. Of greater interest is the question of how the arms become coordinated with the legs.

Four-limb development was addressed in a 15-yr (from 3–18 yr) longitudinal study on hopping [76]. As with the study on jumping [15], Robertson and Havlerson found relative timing invariances of the hopping leg that was present from the beginning. However, interlimb phasing between the four limbs only gradually became phase-locked. It was suggested that the support leg acts like a forcing oscillator to which the swing leg and the arms eventually become entrained. An interesting feature of this study was the correlation between kinematic data and the developmental component sequences. At least part of the change in developmental level of the separate components is directly analogous to uncoupled and then coupled limit cycle oscillators [73].

A follow-up study by Getchell and Roberton [34] focused on the change between the uncoupled swing leg and the coupled swing leg. In a clever design to eliminate body components as a factor, subjects were found who could hop at one developmental level (Level 2) on one leg and another developmental level (Level 3) on the other. Measures of instantaneous and estimated average whole-body stiffness were far higher for Level 2 than for Level 3. Using a dynamical systems interpretation, Getchell and Roberton [34] hypothesized that regulation of stiffness may be a continuously changing control parameter that, when scaled past some critical value, causes a shift from one hopping organization (uncoupled legs) to another (coupled legs), a reorganization that lowers the stiffness setting.

The above studies focused on intraskill development, which is an interesting developmental phenomenon if one is concerned with how skillfulness is acquired; however, a more fundamental developmental question concerns the interskill developmental milestone. What allows the sequential emergence of these skills? Again, a dynamical systems account of real-time transitions of state has been applied to these developmental transitions [18, 97].

Surprisingly, to date, only the transition of walking to running has been investigated in detail. Two longitudinal studies have compared walking and running in newly running infants and found no differences in interlimb or intralimb coordination based on relative phase except for around the ankle at footstrike [26, 107]. If a shift from walking to running does not occur at the fundamental coordination level, then what prevents a child from running as soon as they can walk? Two possible candidates for rate-limiting constraints are the ability to (a) produce a force of 2 times body weight on one leg and (b) land and balance on single support [18]. Interestingly, Whitall and Getchell [107] found that children who perceptually appeared to be running were still sometimes showing a relative stance time of above 50% (indicating no flight time). Thus strength and dynamic balance requirements are reduced in the initial emergence of running, and these factors are clearly important for acquiring a mature run. Recently Forrester et al. [26] have hypothesized that a related factor in the shift from one gait to another is the ability to manage different energy strategies that characterize specific gait forms. It would seem that kinetic levels of analysis may prove useful for understanding locomotor transitions [34, 49]

In general, information on the development of advanced locomotor skills through childhood is still more descriptive than explanatory. However, the use of dynamical systems concepts, biomechanical methodology, and, in some cases, qualitative dynamics tools has spurred researchers into uncovering developmental principles of organization that appear very similar across different skills. Despite these advances and the rhetoric of the researchers, one avenue of research that has received less attention has been the perception-action approach and, more generally, the role of environmental information. One notable exception to this trend is a recent study by Block [9], who looked at the perceptual affordance characteristics related to a standing long jump. Perhaps other studies of this nature will follow in a similar vein to studies reviewed in the aging adult section below [52, 53].

Aging Adults
Patterns of walking in the elderly showing decreased velocity and concomitant qualitative changes have been well documented (for review, see ref. 22). However, studies that go beyond description to investigating the processes behind these changes are limited. One exception is the work of Gabell and Nayak [32]. These investigators were interested in the stability of gait parameters (notably before the dynamical systems theorists promoted the use of this measure). They hypothesized that increased variability in stride width and double support time would be caused by decreased balance control and that increased variability in step length and stride periods would be attributable to deteriorating gait pattern mechanics. To obtain a pathology-free population, they screened 1187 people over 64 yr of age and selected only 32 older adults. When they compared this healthy population to young adults they found no differences in variability for any

of their measures. The authors concluded that age-related increases in variability of gait parameters must be due to pathology.

These findings support the previously cited theory of aging as a pathological rather than an age-determined process. Further support comes from the perception-action approach of Konczak [52], who used a "moving hallway" to investigate the effect of various patterns of optic flow on old (74 yr) and young (22 yr) adults. Predictable changes in step velocity occurred with conditions of no vision, global, frontal, and peripheral optic flow. However, although it has already been noted that the stationary balance of older adults becomes impaired when exposed to conflicting visual information [61], no age group differences were found in this study. Thus older adults do not seem to rely increasingly on vision for guiding locomotion, as had been predicted. Nor was there a clear-cut dominance of peripheral versus central optic flow as found in older children. Konczak [52] concluded that the perceptual requirements of static and dynamic balance may be different and/or use different modes of control.

A more definitive differences between young and older adults was found in an affordance study on the perception of stair-climbing based on riser height [53]. Konczak et al. [53] found that the young (23 yr) perceived the boundaries of their stair-climbing ability relative to their leg length. However, older subjects (71 yr) perceived their stair-climbing ability relative to leg length *and* to their flexibility and leg strength. Furthermore, the older adults were more accurate in their predictions, presumably because they better perceive their organismic constraints through being motivated by a fear of the consequences of being wrong. This finding very nicely illustrates how perceptions may change over time because of many factors, and how this can influence motor behavior.

These few examples of aging research on locomotion reflect the conclusions from the posture research, namely that "healthy" older adults do not change their motor behavior very much. The interesting study by Konczak et al. [53] suggests that future studies of the elderly should take into account changing perceptions of the subject's organismic constraints as well as perceptions of the motor task itself.

Summary

It is clear that knowledge of locomotor development has increased profoundly in the last 10 yr, and was influenced primarily by concepts and methodologies derived from dynamical systems and perception-action perspectives. Neurophysiological paradigms have been utilized also, and there are still some useful descriptive studies being undertaken in the childhood and aging areas. All of the research studies cited in this section are concerned exclusively with locomotor skills as isolated tasks. However, it should be remembered that locomotion is often combined with other skills such as reaching or carrying in the daily living arena and with throwing, catching, or striking in the sporting arena. Thus an important additional area of research is to determine how the lower limbs can locomote in combination with a multiplicity of upper-limb (often eye-hand coordination) tasks.

Of course, eye-hand coordination itself has been the subject of much research independent of either locomotion or posture. Space does not permit a similar overview of the extensive research on eye-hand coordination. Within this research area, studies range from simple isometric control [100] through visually directed reaching [21, 102] and aiming studies [5] to fundamental motor skills of throwing, catching, and striking [57] with concomitant changes in underlying processes such as knowledge bases [30]. In general, it would be fair to say that cognitive and information-processing approaches continue to contribute to the eye-hand coordination area as well as neurophysiological, dynamical systems, and perception-action approaches. Compared with posture and locomotion studies there seems to be less research on eye-hand coordination in the aging population, too.

CONCLUSION

This review was written to illustrate how motor development research has expanded and changed over the last decade. In doing so, it should be apparent that the research field appears to have grown from a central focus of kinesiologists and physical educators to include an eclectic range of developmental psychologists, neurophysiologists, cognitive and perceptual psychologists, and physical therapists (to name the most prominent orientations in the North American scientific community), all working on similar problems. What are the major conclusions and future directions that can be drawn from this review?

First, it is clear that motor development itself is a very complex process that can no longer be attributed simply to singular concepts like neuromaturation. Multiple cooperating subsystems of the growing organism must be considered along with their interaction with task and environmental constraints. The enormity of this quest is overwhelming, but it speaks to the need for collaboration among researchers who have different areas of expertise, methodologies, and perhaps even conceptual frameworks. For example, those who pursue perception-action integration might collaborate with those who take a dynamical systems and/or biomechanical orientation as well as bringing in neurophysiological techniques or measures of cognition [39]. (There is not room to describe the interesting research on motor development as it relates to cognitive development; for example, the idea that self-produced locomotion promotes changes in perception/cognition of the infant [see, e.g., ref. 7].)

In adopting the new conceptualizations in general and the dynamical systems approach in particular, one distinctly nontrivial matter is that of finding the best measures (collective variables) with which to look at the changing system. Once these are identified, the major task is to look for potential control or rate-limiting parameters and one source for which there is already a considerable amount of information is the growth of various organismic constraints [60]. This information might well be perused more carefully before designing experiments, although it is important to recognize that task and environmental constraints cannot be ignored. Once identified, the potential control parameters require subsequent testing by microgenesis experiments, as discussed earlier. The beauty of these experiments is not only in their potential to inform us of the underlying process of development but also for the applied clinical and educational outcomes that can occur. Essentially, these experiments are actually motor learning studies but with an equal emphasis on the organismic constraints that the person brings with them. That is, there is an emphasis on the developmental history of the organism that will obviously affect future outcomes.

Another consequence of adopting the dynamical systems approach per se is the need to take frequent and multiple measures over a long period of time. This "dense" method of data collection requires a more ideographic data collection procedure than is usually accepted in science. Nevertheless, this is perhaps the only way that we will truly understand the principles of motor development [21].

Based on some of the work presented in this review, one could argue, too, for the approach taken by some investigators of studying one skill only but over a whole life span (e.g., Woollacott's work on postural control). On the other hand, some have clearly chosen to look at a specific period of time, which allows familiarity with the constraints operating during that period while looking at more than one skill (e.g., Thelen's work on infant kicking, stepping, walking, and reaching). There are advantages to both methods, but one suggestion that seems even more important is to combine research on postural control with other skills [45] because posture is so clearly important for all movement and, at least as far as locomotion is concerned, there is much shared use of paradigms and overlapping results.

Finally, it is striking that most of the current published research is on infancy along with some early childhood and aging studies. Although it is true that motor development seems to change more over the first few years than at any other time, this is no excuse for ignoring changes that occur in late childhood, adolescence, or even young adulthood. Perhaps it is time to take a truly life span approach.

In conclusion, this review has described the evolution of research on motor development over the last 15 yr. Clearly there are many researchers in this area, and new insights from the newer approaches abound. Regardless of whether the cross-disciplinary orientations of these researchers ever coalesce under an umbrella term such as developmental kinesiology, it is to be hoped that collaborations will facilitate the acquisition of future knowledge using these new approaches.

REFERENCES

1. Adolph, K. E., M. A. Eppler, and E. J. Gibson. Crawling versus walking infants' perception of affordances for locomotion over sloping surfaces. *Child Dev.* 64:1158–1174, 1993.
2. Baltes, P. B., H. W. Reese, and L. P. Lipsitt. Life-span developmental psychology. *Annu. Rev. Psychol.* 31:65–110, 1980.
3. Baltes, P. B., H. W. Reese, and J. R. Nesselroade. *Life-Span Developmental Psychology: Introduction to Research Methods.* Monterey, CA: Brooks/Cole, 1977.
4. Bard, C., M. Fleury, and L. Hay. *Development of Eye-Hand Coordination across the Life Span.* Columbia, SC: University of South Carolina, 1990.
5. Bard, C., M. Fleury, and L. Hay. Timing and accuracy of visually directed movements in children: control of direction and amplitude components. *J. Exp. Child Psychol.* 50: 102–118, 1993.
6. Bernstein, N. A. *The Co-ordination and Regulation of Movement.* New York: Pergamon Press, 1967.
7. Benson, J. The significance and development of crawling in human infancy. J. E. Clark and J. H. Humphrey (ed). *Advances in Motor Development Research 3.* New York: AMS Press, 1990, pp. 91–142.
8. Bertenthal, B. I., and D. L. Bai. Infants' sensitivity to optical flow for controlling posture. *Dev. Psychol.* 25:936–945, 1989.
9. Block. M. The development of body-scaled information: The case of jumping distances. [Dissertation]. College Park, MD: University of Maryland, 1990.
10. Bradley, N. S., and A. Bekoff. Development of locomotion: animal models. M. H. Woollacott and H. G. Williams (ed). *Development of Posture and Gait across the Lifespan.* Columbia, SC: University of South Carolina Press, 1989, pp. 128–151.
11. Branta, C., J. Haubenstricker, and V. Seefeldt. Age changes in motor skill during childhood and adolescence. *Exerc. Sports Sci. Rev.* 12:467–520, 1984.
12. Bril, B. Motor development and cultural attitudes. H. T. A. Whiting and M. G. Wade (ed). *Themes in Motor Development.* Boston, MA: Martinus Nijhoff, 1986, pp. 297–314.
13. Bril, B., and Y. Breniere. Postural requirements and progression velocity in young walkers. *J. Motor Behav.* 24:105–116, 1992.
14. Clark, J. E. Developmental differences in response processing. *J. Motor Behav.* 14:247–254, 1982.
15. Clark, J. E., and S. J. Phillips. A developmental sequence of the standing long jump. J. E. Clark and J. Humphrey (ed). *Motor Development: Current Selected Research.* Princeton, NJ: Princeton Book, 1985, pp. 73–85.
16. Clark, J. E., and S. J. Phillips. A longitudinal study of intralimb coordination in the first year of independent walking: a dynamical systems analysis. *Child Dev.* 64:1143–1157, 1993.
17. Clark, J. E., and J. Whitall. What is motor development? The lessons of history. *Quest* 41:183–202, 1989.
18. Clark, J. E., and J. Whitall. Changing patterns of locomotion: from walking to skipping. M. H. Woollacott and H. G. Williams (ed). *Development of Posture and Gait across the Lifespan.* Columbia, SC: University of South Carolina Pres, 1989, pp. 128–151.
19. Clark, J. E., S. J. Phillips, and R. Petersen. Developmental stability in jumping. *Dev. Psychol.* 25:929–935.
20. Clark, J. E., J. Whitall, and S. J. Phillips. Human interlimb coordination: the first 6 months of independent walking. *Dev. Psychobiol.* 21:445–456, 1988.
21. Corbetta, D., and E. Thelen. Shifting patterns of interlimb coordination in infant's reaching: a case study. S. P. Swinnen, H. Heuer, J. Massion, and P. Casaer (eds). *Interlimb Coor-*

dination. Neural, Dynamical and Cognitive Constraints. San Diego, CA: Academic Press, 1994, pp. 413–438.

22. Craik, R. Changes in locomotion in the aging adult. M. H. Woollacott and H. G. Williams (eds). *Development of Posture and Gait across the Lifespan.* Columbia, SC: University of South Carolina Press, 1989, pp. 176–210.

23. DeOreo, K. D., and M. G. Wade. Dynamic and static balancing ability of pre-school children. *J. Motor Behav.* 3:326–335, 1971.

24. Fishkind, M., and S. M. Haley. Independent sitting development and the emergence of associated motor components. *Phys. Ther.* 66:1509–1514, 1986.

25. Ford, D. H., and R. M. Lerner. *Developmental Systems Theory, An Integrative Approach.* Newbury Park, CA: Sage, 1992, pp. 52.

26. Forrester, L. W., S. J. Phillips, and J. E. Clark. Locomotor coordination in infancy: the transition from walking to running. G. J. P. Savelsbergh (ed.). *The Development of Coordination in Infancy.* New York: Elsevier, 1993, pp. 359–393.

27. Forssberg. H. Ontogeny of human locomotor control. I. Infant stepping, supported locomotion and transition to independent locomotion. *Exp. Brain Res.* 57:480–493, 1985.

28. Forssberg, H., and L. Nashner. Ontogenetic development of postural control in man: Adaptation to altered support and visual conditions during stance. *J. Neurosci.* 2:545–552, 1982.

29. Freedland, R. L., and B. I. Bertenthal. Developmental changes in interlimb coordination: transition to hands-and-knees crawling. *Psychological Sci.* 5:26–32, 1994.

30. French, K. E., and J. R. Thomas. The relation of knowledge development to children's basketball performance. *J. Sports Psychol.* 9:15–32, 1987.

31. Gabbard, C. *Lifelong Motor Development.* Dubuque, IA: Wm. C. Brown, 1992.

32. Gabell, A., and U. S. L. Nayak. The effect of age on variability of gait. *J. Gerontol.* 39: 662–666, 1984.

33. Gesell, A. *The First Five Years of Life.* New York: Harper and Row, 1940.

34. Getchell, N., and M. A. Roberton. Whole body stiffness as a function of developmental level in children's hopping. *Dev. Psychol.* 25:920–928, 1989.

35. Gibson, E. J., and M. A. Schmuckler. Going somewhere: an ecological and experimental approach to development of mobility. *Ecol. Psychol.* 1:3–25, 1989.

36. Gibson, E. J., G. Riccio, M. A. Schmuckler, T. A. Stoffregen, D. Rosenberg, and J. Taormina. Detection of the traversability of surfaces by crawling and walking infants. *J. Exp. Psychol. Percept. Perform.* 13:533–544, 1987.

37. Gibson, J. J. *An Ecological Approach to Visual Perception.* Boston: Houghton Mifflin, 1979.

38. Goldfield, E. C. Transition from rocking to crawling. *Ecol. Psychol.* 25:913–919, 1989.

39. Goldfield, E. C., B. A. Kay, and W. H. Warren. Infant bouncing: the assembly and tuning of action systems. *Child Dev.* 64:1128–1142, 1993.

40. Goodway, J. The effects of a motor skill intervention on the fundamental motor skills and sustained activity of African American preschoolers who are at-risk. [Dissertation]. Lancing, MI: Michigan State University, 1994.

41. Halverson, L. E., and K. Williams. Developmental sequences for hopping over distance: a prelongitudinal screening. *Res. Q. Exerc. Sport* 56:37–44, 1985.

42. Harbourne, R. T., C. Giuliani, and J. Macneela. A kinematic and electromyographis analysis of the development of sitting posture in infants. *Dev. Psychobiol.* 26:51–64, 1993.

43. Haywood, K. M. *Life Span Motor Development.* Champaign, IL: Human Kinetics, 1993.

44. Heriza, C. B. Comparison of leg movements in preterm infants at term with healthy full-term infants. *Phys. Ther.* 68:1687–1693, 1988.

45. Hirschfeld, H. and H. Forssberg. Development of anticipatory postural adjustments during locomotion in children. *J. Neurophysiol.* 68:542–550, 1992.

46. Hirschfeld, H., and H. Forssberg. Epigenetic development of postural responses for sitting during infancy. *Exp. Brain. Res.* 97:528–540.

47. Jouen, F. Visual-proprioceptive control of posture in newborn infants. B. Amblard, A. Berthoz and F. Clarac (eds). *Posture and Gait: Development, Adaptation and Modulation.* Amsterdam: Elsevier, 1988, pp. 13–22.

48. Jensen, J. L., S. J. Phillips, and J. E. Clark. For young jumpers, differences are in the movement's control not its coordination. *Res. Q. Exerc. Sport,* 65:258–268.

49. Jensen, J. L., B. D. Ulrich, E. Thelen, K. Schneider, R. F. Zernicke. Adaptative dynamics of the leg movement patterns of human infant. I. the effect of posture on spontaneous kicking. *J. Motor Behav.* in press.

50. Kamm, K., E. Thelen, and J. L. Jensen. A dynamical systems approach to motor development. *Phys. Ther.* 70:763–775, 1990.

51. Kelso, J. A. S., and G. S. Schoner. Toward a physical (synergetic) theory of biological coordination. *Springer Proceedings in Physics* 19:224–237, 1987.

52. Konczak, J. Effects of optic flow on the kinematics of human gait: a comparison of young and older adults. *J. Motor Behav.* 23:1992.

53. Koncazk, J., H. J. Meeuwsen, and M. E. Cress. Changing affordances in stair climbing: The perception of maximum climbabilty in young and older adults. *J. Exp. Psychol.* 18:691–697, 1992.

54. Kugler, P. N., J. A. S. Kelso, and M. T. Turvey. On the concept of coordination structures as dissipative structures. I. Theoretical lines of convergence. G. E. Stelmach and J. Requin (eds). *Tutorials in Motor Behavior.* New York: North Holland, 1982, pp. 3–47.

55. Kugler, P. N., J. A. S. Kelso, and M. T. Turvey. On the control and co-ordination of naturally developing systems. J. A. S. Kelso and J. E. Clark (eds). *The Development of Movement Control and Co-ordination.* Chichester, UK: John Wiley & Sons, 1982, pp. 5–78.

56. Kugler, P. N., and M. T. Turvey. *Information, Natural Law and the Self-Assembly of Rhythmic Movement.* Hillsdale, NJ: Erlbaum, 1987.

57. Langendorfer, S. Prelongitudinal screening of overarm striking development performed under two environmental conditions. J. E. Clark and J. H. Humphrey (eds). *Advances in Motor Development Research 1.* New York: AMS Press, 1987, pp. 17–48.

58. Lee, D. N., and E. Aronson. Visual proprioceptive control of standing in human infants. *Percept Psychophys.* 15:529–532, 1974.

59. Lockman, J. J., and E. Thelen. Developmental biodynamics: brain, body, behavior connections. *Child Dev.* 64:953–959, 1993.

60. Malina, R. M., and C. Bouchard. *Growth Maturation and Physical Activity.* Champaign, IL: Human Kinetics, 1991.

61. Manchester, D., M. H. Woollacott, N. Zederbauer-Hylton, and O. Marin. Visual, vestibular and somatosensory contributions to balance control in the older adult. *J. Gerontol.* 44: M118–127, 1989.

62. McGraw, M. B. *The Neuromuscular Maturation of the Human Infant.* New York: Hefner, 1945.

63. Mounoud, P. Action and cognition: cognitive and motor skills in a developmental perspective. M. G. Wade and H. T. A. Whiting (eds). *Motor Development in Children: Aspects of Coordination and Control.* Boston, MA: Martinus Nijhoff, 1986, pp. 373–390.

64. Nashner, L. M., and M. H. Wollacott. The organization of rapid postural adjustments of standing humans: an experimental-conceptual model. R. E. Talbot and D. R. Humphrey (eds). *Posture and Movement.* New York: Raven Press, 1979, pp.

65. Newell, K. M. Constraints on the development of coordination. M. G. Wade and H. T. A. Whiting (eds). *Motor Development in Children: Aspects of Coordination and Control.* Boston, MA: Martinus Nijhoff, 1986, pp. 341–360.

66. Okamoto, T., and Y. Goto. Human infant pre-independent and independent walking. S. Kondo (ed). *Primate Morphophysiology: Locomotor Analyses and Human Bipedalism.* Tokyo: University of Tokyo Press, 1985, pp. 25–45.

67. Payne, V. G., and L. D. Isaacs. *Human Motor Development. A Lifespan Approach.* Mountain View, CA: Mayfield, 1991.

68. Pick, H. L., and C. F. Palmer. Perception and representation in the guidance of spatially coordinated behaviour. M. G. Wade and H. T. A. Whiting (eds). *Motor Development in Children: Aspects of Coordination and Control.* Boston, MA: Martinus Nijhoff, 1986, pp. 135–146.
69. Prechtl, H. F. R. Continuity and changes in early human development. H. F. R. Prechtl (ed). *Continuity of Neural Functions from Prenatal to Postnatal Life.* Oxford: C. D. M. Blackwell, 1984, pp. 1–15.
70. Prechtl, H. F. R. Prenatal motor development. M. G. Wade and H. T. A. Whiting (eds). *Motor Development in Children: Aspects of Coordination and Control.* Boston, MA: Martinus Nijhoff, 1986, pp. 53–64.
71. Reed, E. S. Changing theories of postural development. M. H. Woollacott and H. G. Williams (eds). *Development of Posture and Gait across the Lifespan.* Columbia, SC: University of South Carolina Press, 1989, pp. 3–24.
72. Riach, C. L. and K. C. Hayes. Anticipatory postural control in children. *J. Motor Behav.* 22:250–266, 1990.
73. Roberton, M. A. Describing "stages" in and across motor tasks. J. A. S. Kelso and J. E. Clark (eds). *The Development of Movement Control and Co-ordination.* Chichester, UK: John Wiley & Sons, 1982, pp. 293–308.
74. Roberton, M. A. Changing motor patterns during childhood. J. R. Thomas (ed). *Motor Development during Childhood and Adolescence.* Minneapolis, MN: Burgess, 1984, pp. 48–90.
75. Roberton, M. A. and L. E. Halverson. *Developing Children—Their Changing Movement.* Philadelphia: Lea & Febiger, 1984.
76. Roberton, M. A., and L. E. Halverson. The development of locomotor coordination: Longitudinal change and invariance. *J. Motor Behav.* 20:197–241, 1988.
77. Roberton, M. A., K. Williams, and S. Langendorfer. Prelongitudinal screening of motor development sequences. *Res. Q. Exerc. Sport* 51:724–731, 1980.
78. Shapiro, D. C., and Schmidt, R. A. The schema theory: recent evidence and developmental implications. J. A. S. Kelso and J. E. Clark (eds). *The Development of Movement Control and Co-ordination.* Chichester, UK: John Wiley & Sons, 1982, pp. 113–150.
79. Shirley, M. M. *The First Two Years: Postural and Locomotor Development.* Minneapolis, MN: University of Minnesota Press, 1931.
80. Shumway-Cook, A., and M. H. Woollacott. The growth of stability: postural control from a developmental perspective. *J. Motor. Behav.* 17:131–147, 1985.
81. Smoll, F. L. Developmental kinesiology: toward a subdiscipline focusing on motor development. J. A. S. Kelso and J. E. Clark (eds). *The Development of Movement Control and Co-ordination.* Chichester, UK: John Wiley & Sons, 1982, pp. 319–354.
82. Stoffregen, T. A., M. A. Schmuckler, and E. J. Gibson. Use of central and peripheral optical flow in stance and locomotion in young walkers. *Perception* 16:113–119, 1987.
83. Sutherland, D. H., R. Olshen, L. Cooper, and S. L. Y. Woo. The development of mature gait. *J. Bone Joint Surg.* 62A:336–353, 1980.
84. Sveistrup, H., and M. H. Woollacott. Systems contributing to emergence and maturation of stability in postural development. G. J. P. Savelsbergh (ed). *The Development of Coordination in Infancy.* Amsterdam: Elsevier, 1993, pp. 319–336.
85. Sveistrup, H., E. Foster, and M. H. Woollacott. Changes in the effect of visual flow on postural control across the lifespan. M. H. Woollacott and F. B. Horak (eds). *Posture and Gait: Control Mechanisms.* Eugene, OR: University of Oregon Books, 1992, pp. 224–227.
86. Thelen, E. Walking, thinking and evolving: further comments toward an economical explanation. *J. Motor Behav.* 15:257–260, 1983.
87. Thelen, E. Treadmill-elicited stepping in seven-month-old infants. *Child Dev.* 57:1498–1506, 1986.
88. Thelen, E. Development of coordinated movement: implications for early human movement. M. G. Wade and H. T. A. Whiting (eds). *Motor Development in Children: Aspects of Coordination and Control.* Boston, MA: Martinus Nijhoff, 1986, pp. 107–124.

89. Thelen, E. The role of motor development in developmental psychology: a view of the past and an agenda for the future. N. Eisenberg (ed). *Contemporary Topics in Developmental Psychology.* New York: Wiley, 1987, pp. 3–33.

90. Thelen, E. Self-organizing in developmental processes: can systems approaches work? M. R. Gunnar and E. Thelen (eds). *Systems and Development: The Minnesota Symposia on Child Psychology.* Hillsdale, NJ: Erlbaum, 1988, pp. 77–117.

91. Thelen, E., and D. W. Cooke. Relationship between newborn stepping and later walking: A new interpretation. *Dev. Med. Child Neurol.* 29:380–393.

92. Thelen, E., and D. M. Fisher. Newborn stepping: an explanation for a "disappearing reflex". *Dev. Psychol.* 18:760–775, 1982.

93. Thelen, E., and B. D. Ulrich. Hidden skills: a dynamic systems analysis of treadmill stepping during the first year. *Monogr. Soc. Res. Child Dev.* 56:1991.

94. Thelen, E., G. Bradshaw, and J. A. Ward. Spontaneous kicking in month-old infants: manifestations of a human central locomotor program. *Behav. Neural. Biol.* 32:45–53, 1981.

95. Thelen, E., D. M. Fisher, R. Ridley-Johnson. The relationship between physical growth and a newborn reflex. *Infant Behav. Dev.* 7:39–65, 1984.

96. Thelen, E., B. D. Ulrich, and J. Jensen. The developmental origins of locomotion. M. H. Woollacott and H. G. Williams (eds). *Development of Posture and Gait across the Lifespan.* Columbia, SC: University of South Carolina Press, 1989, pp. 25–47.

97. Thelen, E., J. A. S. Kelso, and A. Fogel. Self-organizing systems and infant motor development. *Dev. Rev.* 7:39–65, 1987.

98. Thomas, J. R. Acquisition of motor skills: Information processing differences between children and adults. *Res. Q. Exerc. Sport* 51:158–173, 1980.

99. Thomas, J. R., and K. E. French. Gender differences across age in motor performance. *Psychol. Bull.* 98:260–282, 1985.

100. Todor, J. I., and J. C. Lazarus. Exertion level and the intensity of associated movements. *Dev. Med. Child Neurol.* 28:205–212.

101. Ulrich, B. D., E. Thelen, and D. Niles. Perceiving affordances: visual guidance of stair climbing. J. E. Clark and J. Humphrey (eds). *Advances in Motor Development Research.* New York: AMS Press, 1991, pp. 1–15.

102. Von Hofsten, C. Structuring of early reaching movements: a longitudinal study. *J. Motor Behav.* 23:280–292, 1991.

103. von Holst, E. *The Behavioral Physiology of Animal and Man.* Coral Gables, FL: University of Miami Press, 1939/1973.

104. Van Sant, A. F. Lifespan development in functional tasks. *Phys. Ther.* 70:788–798, 1990.

105. Whitall, J. A developmental study of the interlimb coordination in running and galloping. *J. Motor Behav.* 21:409–428, 1989.

106. Whitall, J. and J. E. Clark. The development of bipedal interlimb coordination. S. P. Swinnen, H. Heuer, J. Massion, and P. Casaer (eds). *Interlimb Coordination. Neural, Dynamical and Cognitive Constraints.* San Diego, CA: Academic Press, 1994, pp. 391–411.

107. Whitall, J., and N. Getchell. From walking to running: Using a dynamical systems approach to the development of locomotor skills. *Child Dev.* in press.

108. Williams, H., B. McClenaghan, D. Ward, et al. Sensory-motor control and balance: a behavioural perspective. H. T. A. Whiting and M. G. Wade (eds). *Themes in Motor Development.* Boston, MA: Martinus Nijhoff, 1986, pp. 247–264.

109. Woollacott, M. H. Gait and postural control in the aging adult. W. Bles and T. Brandt (eds.). *Disorders of Posture and Gait.* Amsterdam: Elsevier, 1986, pp. 325–326.

110. Woollacott, M. H., and A. Shumway-Cook. *Development of Posture and Gait across the Life Span.* Columbia, SC: University of South Carolina, 1989.

111. Woollacott, M. H., and H. Sveistrup. Changes in the sequencing and timing of muscle response coordination associated with developmental transitions in balance abilities. *Hum. Mov. Sci.* 11:23–36, 1992.

112. Woollacott, M. H., B. Debu, and M. Mowatt. Neuromuscular control of posture in the infant and child: is vision dominant? *J. Motor Behav.* 19:167–186, 1987.

113. Woollacott, M., A. Shumway-Cook, and L. Nashner. Aging and posture control: changes in sensory organization and muscular coordination. *Int. J. Aging Hum. Dev.* 23:97–114, 1986.

114. Zelazo, P. R. The development of walking: new findings and old assumptions. *J. Motor Behav.* 15:99–137, 1983.

115. Zelazo, P. R. "Learning to walk." Recognition of higher order influences? *J. Motor Behav.* 15:251–255, 1983.

116. Zelazo, P. R., N. A. Zelazo, and S. Kolb. Newborn walking. *Science* 177:1058–1059, 1972.

9
Physical Activity, Body Weight, and Adiposity: An Epidemiologic Perspective

LORETTA DiPIETRO, Ph.D., MPH

The influence of regular physical activity on weight regulation is complex. Overweight and obesity are a consequence of a long-term positive energy balance—that is, energy intake exceeds energy expenditure. The relative contributions of overeating, inactivity, or metabolic aberrations on this positive energy balance, however, are not clear [111].

Numerous intervention studies have explored the impact of exercise training of various intensities on the reduction of weight and body fat. Over the past 2 decades, several comprehensive review articles [89, 117, 122, 143] and two meta-analyses [5, 50] have been published on this topic. We can conclude from these reviews that: (a) physical activity affects body composition and weight favorably, by promoting fat loss, while preserving lean mass; (b) the rate of weight loss is positively related to the frequency and duration of the exercise session, as well as the duration of the exercise program, thereby suggesting a dose-response relationship; and (c) whereas the rate of weight loss resulting from increased physical activity is relatively slow, physical activity may nonetheless be a more effective strategy for long-term weight regulation than dieting alone [18, 68].

Less is known, however, about how physical activity patterns affect attained weight and weight gain among the general population; data are especially scarce among younger (<18 yr) and older (>55 yr) age groups, and for minority populations. Indeed, many of the methodological considerations in studying these two variables simultaneously in large-scale observational studies make it difficult to assess the extent of their true association, much less infer a causal relationship.

The purpose of this review is to describe the relation between physical activity, body weight, and adiposity as noted in epidemiologic studies. Accordingly, the discussion is limited to observational studies, among either representative or selected samples of adults, with physical activity as a primary study variable and body weight and/or body fat as outcome variables. Descriptive information on both physical activity and weight patterns among the general population will be presented, and methdological issues pertinent to the interpretation of statistical associations between these two variables will be addressed throughout.

OVERWEIGHT

Prevalence of Overweight

Recent survey data from the third National Health and Nutrition Examination Survey (NHANES III) suggest that overweight (defined as a body mass index [BMI=kg/m^2] ≥ 27.8 for men and ≥27.3 for women) is present in approximately 33% of the adults living in the United States. The overall prevalence of overweight currently is highest in men and women age 50–59 yr (42% and 52%, respectively), and then is progressively lower at older ages [72, 87, 88]. The prevalence of overweight tends to be disproportionally high among minority women and women of lower socioeconomic status and/or lower educational attainment [51, 72, 73, 115]: currently 49% among African-American women and 47% among Mexican-American women.

Trends in Overweight

The prevalence of overweight has increased by approximately 8% among U.S. adults aged 20–74 yr—from 25.4% during the period 1976–1980 to 33.3% during 1988–1991—based on these same NHANES III data. White men and women experienced the greatest increase in prevalence of overweight in these 12 years (8–9%), whereas the increase was slightly less for African-American men (6%) and women (5%) [72].

Between the periods 1976–1980 and 1988–1991, mean BMI increased from 25.3 to 26.3 kg/m^2 among U.S. adults aged 20–74 yr [72]. The greatest increase in BMI during this period was among white women (1.3 kg/m^2) and African-American men (1.1. kg/m^2). Cross-sectional data from the Minnesota Heart Health Program [110] also show a significant age- and education-adjusted increase in mean BMI over 7 years (1980–1987) in their population of adults aged 25–74 yr (0.08 kg/m^2/yr for men, 0.19 kg/m^2/yr for women). The more striking increases in the BMI of the Minnesota population, however, were among people in the upper quartile of the distribution. This was especially true among women, where the increase in BMI was 2–3 times greater than in the lower three quartiles of the distribution. The prevalence of "obesity" (i.e., BMI ≥ 30.2 kg/m^2 for men and ≥29.9 kg/m^2 for women [≥85th percentile]) increased by 0.6% per year among men (P=0.01) and by 1% per year among women (P=0.002). Indeed, 15.1% of the women in this population were considered "obese" in 1981 compared with 21% in 1987.

Risk of Overweight

Among respondents to the NHANES I (1971–1975) Epidemiologic Follow-Up Study (1981–1984) who were not overweight (BMI <27.8 for men and <27.3 for women) at baseline, the risk of becoming overweight during the 10-yr follow-up was similar in men and women and was highest among adults aged 35–44 yr (16.3% among men and 13.5% among women) [142].

The cumulative incidence of major weight gain (≥ 5 kg/m^2), however, was higher in women compared with men and highest among adults aged 25–34 yr (3.9% among men and 8.4% among women). Among those already overweight at baseline, the incidence of a major weight gain was highest among women aged 25–44 yr (14.2%).

Thus, overweight is a common problem among adults in the United States. Trend data further suggest that the population as a group, and particularly women, is becoming heavier with time and that the increase in prevalence of overweight may be most accelerated among those persons who are already overweight or obese. Finally, factors such as socioeconomic status, educational attainment, and marital status may contribute to the excess risk of weight gain among U.S. men and women, especially among African-American women [66, 67, 142].

PHYSICAL ACTIVITY

Definitions

Physical activity is a complex behavior and therefore difficult to define operationally [29]. Problems in the definition and measurement of physical activity limit the knowledge of activity participation levels and, moreover, the knowledge of health consequences associated with an active life-style.

The terms "physical activity," "exercise," and "physical fitness" are often used interchangably in epidemiologic research. Caspersen et al. [25, 29] define physical activity as any bodily movement produced by the skeletal muscles that results in energy expenditure; whereas exercise is described as a subcategory of physical activity behaviors. Accordingly, exercise is defined as "any physical activity which is planned, structured, repetitive, and results in improvements or maintenance of one or more facets of physical fitness." Thus, physical activity and exercise are classified as behaviors, whereas physical fitness is classified as an outcome, related to the ability to achieve certain performance standards or traits [25, 29].

Physical activity can be achieved through occupational activity (e.g., patrolling, lifting or carrying loads), home maintenance activity (e.g. housework, yardwork), or as part of leisure-time pursuits (sports participation, conditioning, walking, golfing, gardening). These behaviors, especially those that are habitual and of lower intensity, are particularly vulnerable to intraindividual variation and inaccurate recall, thereby rendering them difficult to quantify, as well as define. Techniques for assessing physical activity range from very crude current (past week or month) or historical (past year, age cutpoints, or lifetime) self-reported surveys, to very objective, precise, and specific laboratory-based measures, such as calorimetry or doubly labeled water [75]. It follows that the more precise and valid the measurement technique, the less potential there is for misclassification of physical activity level. The more precise measures, however, generally are not feasible in large-scale epidemiologic research; therefore, these studies tend to rely on less costly survey instruments.

Even among survey instruments, physical activity may be measured as the frequency or the volume (frequency × duration) of time spent in various types or various intensities (e.g., light, moderate, vigorous) of activity. Physical activity level then may be expressed as a frequency (%), total time, or kilocalorie expenditure relative to a daily, weekly, or yearly time frame. Although the kilocalorie score for a given time frame may seem the most descriptive of these physical activity indices, it may also be somewhat confusing because 1000 kcal/wk could be achieved in 1 day of intense activity, 4 days of moderate activity, or 7 days of light activity [25]. In addition, information on the important components such as frequency, duration, and intensity may be difficult to gather in large-scale studies and therefore, one or two simple questions about typical physical activity often are used to classify subjects into crude (e.g., low, moderate, or high) levels of participation.

Physical Activity Patterns
In 1991, nearly 60% of the U.S. adult population reported little or no leisure-time physical activity [30]. The prevalence of inactivity (i.e., no reported leisure-time activity [28]) appears to be higher among African-American women [47], older adults [24, 30, 34], and persons of lower educational attainment [30], based on data from several national surveys conducted in the United States. In contrast, the prevalence of regular (i.e., ≥20 min or more per session; ≥3 times a week) and regular and intense (i.e., ≥60% maximal aerobic capacity [$\dot{V}O_2max$]) [28] tends to be higher among whites and increases with level of education [27, 47].

Sociodemographic characteristics such as age, gender, race, and education level are also associated with physical activity choices [24, 46, 47]. Among younger adults (<55 yr), running, team sports, and weight lifting are more common activities among men, whereas participation in aerobics is more prevalent among women [46]. The prevalence of higher-intensity activities declines with age, whereas the popularity of lower-intensity (but sustained) activities such as gardening or golf increases [23, 24, 46]. Walking is the most prevalent activity reported among all sociodemographic strata in the United States [24, 46, 47, 118, 119], Canada [118, 119], and Europe [23]. There are data from the National Health Interview Survey-Health Promotion and Disease Prevention Supplement, however, that suggest that reported regular and intense activity increases with age [24]. This age-related increase may be explained by the fact that, for a given workload, older people work closer to their maximal capacity compared with younger people. Thus, older people are better able to achieve the >60% criterion for intense activity in the National Health Interview Survey.

Trends in Physical Activity Patterns

There are few physical activity surveillance data on large representative samples that use the same tracking methods. Caspersen and Merritt [22, 85] report data from 29 states participating in the Behavioral Risk Factor Surveillance System (BRFSS) that suggest a decline in inactivity (i.e., no reported leisure-time physical activities in the past month) between 1986 and 1990. Unfortunately, when these data were recently stratified by race or level of educational attainment, they show no change in the prevalence of inactivity among nonwhite adults or those with fewer than 12 yr of education [21]. Changes in reported inactivity, however, are apparent in older men (39.5% to 35.6%) and older women (47.3% to 42.9%), as well as younger men (23.4% to 19.3%). These surveillance data also show that reported regular and not intense activity increased between 1986 and 1990 among younger men (38.3% to 42.1%), whereas regular and intense activity increased among older men (11.3% to 16.1%) and older women (7.7% to 11.4%), although this increase may not be apparent among nonwhite adults or people with lower educational attainment.

Data from the University of Minnesota [64], collected between 1957–1960 and 1985–1987 with the Minnesota Leisure-Time Physical Activity survey [122], also suggest that leisure-time physical activity has been increasing for 3 decades among adults living in the upper midwest United States. Among men, the greatest increase occurred before 1975 with modest- and heavy-intensity activity, and was greater for white collar than blue collar workers. Although reported leisure-time activity also increased among women since 1980, the greatest increase was among blue collar women.

In summary, physical activity is a complex behavior and is often difficult to describe. Reported inactivity is highest among the more vulnerable sectors of the population—i.e., those of lower socioeconomic status, lower educational attainment, and, perhaps, older adults. Among those who are physical active, these same sociodemographic factors are important determinants of activity choices and activity patterns. There is encouraging, albeit limited, evidence that the prevalence of reported inactivity is decreasing among some sectors of the general U.S. adult population, with an increasing trend in the prevalence of regular leisure-time activity. There appears to be a widening disparity in activity level by race, however, which may be explained by level of education [21].

It is also important to consider that leisure-time physical activity is only a portion of total activity. The other components of total activity involve occupational activity, household activity, and transportation. Although surveillance data are not available on these other components, one can reasonably assume that energy spent in occupational and housework tasks, as well as in transportation, has progressively declined over time. Therefore, it is possible that overall physical activity has declined despite increases in leisure-time physical activity [96].

OVERWEIGHT, PHYSICAL ACTIVITY, AND CHRONIC DISEASE

The economic cost of obesity in 1986 was estimated at $39.3 billion, or 5.5% of the cost of all illness [32]. Obesity has a major impact on morbidity and mortality in the general population [62, 80, 138] (see 113 for additional references). Moreover, obesity and overweight exacerbate many chronic conditions (hypertension, dyslipidemia, osteoarthritis, and other musculoskeletal problems) [130] and thus may serve as a more basic risk factor in chronic disease etiology. Weight alone may not be as important a factor in chronic disease risk as the distribution of body fat, however. Indeed, the chronic disease risk attributable to obesity may vary by the regional distribution of excess body fat. Recent studies that have focused specifically on fat distribution have demonstrated a greater risk of metabolic complications [19, 37, 39, 44, 109] and coronary heart disease (CHD) [48, 74, 76, 121] with increasing level of abdominal, relative to gluteal or femoral, adiposity.

Physical activity and fitness have been associated with a lower incidence of morbidity and mortality from chronic diseases such as CHD [11, 79, 90] (see 97 for review) cancer [1, 55, 77, 132] (see 10 for additional references), and noninsulin-dependent diabetes mellitus [60, 81, 82], and the evidence suggests that current, rather than past, activity status is the protective factor. Furthermore, there are prospective data suggesting that physical activity is protective even in the presence of established CHD risk factors. Data from the Aerobic Center Longitudinal Study [11] suggest that men with a lower relative level of physical fitness, but with low levels of blood pressure or cholesterol, were still about 2.5 times more likely to die during follow-up than were more fit men with elevated blood pressure or cholesterol. There is also evidence that overweight men and women can benefit from a more active life-style, even in the absence of significant weight loss [11, 60, 82, 86]. This is presumably due to improvements in the metabolic profile (i.e., plasma glucose, insulin, and lipid levels) with physical activity, even in the absence of weight loss [38, 124].

CHD Risk Attributable to Inactivity
The public health impact of a sedentary life-style may be considerable. Based on the pooled results of 43 epidemiologic studies on physical activity and CHD, Powell et al. [97] report a median relative risk for CHD of 1.9 for those persons who were inactive relative to those who reported activity participation of 3 times a week for 20 min/session. This relative risk is similar to those reported in the Coronary Pooling Project [84] for other CHD risk factors; namely, systolic hypertension (RR=2.1), hypercholesterolemia (RR=2.4), and smoking (RR=2.5). Although these four risk factors share a similar relative risk with regard to CHD, there are surveillance data from the Centers for Disease Control to suggest that the prevalence of reported inactivity is much greater in the population than the other three factors [31]. Therefore, because the attributable risk of a given factor is a function

of the risk of disease when the factor is present relative to when it is absent, as well as the prevalence of that factor in the population, the population attributable risk for CHD associated with a sedentary life-style is much greater than the risk attributable to other powerful CHD risk factors such as hypertension, hypercholesterolemia, and smoking [26].

Indeed, the evidence clearly indicates that sedentary behavior is a major risk factor for chronic disease morbidity and mortality. This association is consistently strong, graded, and independent and it is biologically plausible and specific [9], thereby meeting most criteria for inferring a causal relationship. The challenge often encountered in epidemiologic research relying on self-reported measures of physical activity, however, is that of establishing temporal sequencing (i.e., whether sedentary behavior truly precedes the onset of disease). Nonetheless, moderate or high levels of physical activity may provide protection from CHD and this may be evident even among people with already established risk factors.

PHYSICAL ACTIVITY, WEIGHT AND ADIPOSITY

National survey data provide evidence that nearly one-third of adults in the United States are trying to lose weight using a variety of weight loss methods [120]. Although dieting is the most common method of weight loss, the long-term success rate of this strategy seems quite poor [71, 133, 139]. Indeed, only about 10–30% of those who lose weight by dieting maintain their full weight loss over time [106]. Therefore, the physiologic mechanisms linking physical activity or exercise to weight regulation are of considerable interest.

Mechanisms
Adipose tissue is a very abundant and efficient source of fuel, with a high energy reserve per unit of weight. The utilization of fat for fuel is under coordinated metabolic control and can only occur under aerobic conditions [117]. Approximately 30–50% of the fat that is oxidized with exercise comes from the free fatty acids liberated from adipocytes by the hydrolysis of stored triglycerides by hormone-sensitive lipase activity (i.e., lipolysis). With sustained exercise of moderate intensity (<50% $\dot{V}O_2$max), lipids may cover up to 90% of the oxidative metabolism; with of higher intensity (>70% $\dot{V}O_2$max) relies on glycogen as the primary fuel source [117]. This suggests that to maximize relative fatty acid consumption, it is necessary to exercise below the threshold at which glucose begins to replace fatty acids as fuel. With regard to reducing total body fat stores, however, total kilocalorie expenditure during exercise may be more important than the actual fuel source.

Several adaptations leading to improved fat utilization during submaximal exercise occur with exercise training. These adaptations include (a) increased epinephrine-stimulated hydrolysis from subcutaneous adipose tissue [33, 43, 104]; (b) an increase in the capacity of the trained muscle to oxidize lipids [7]; (c) increased hydrolysis of triglycerides within the trained muscle [63]; (d) increased hydrolysis of circulating triglycerides through lipoprotein lipase activity [59]; and (e) decreased insulin concentrations, a primary inhibiting factor to lipid mobilization [7, 8]. There is also evidence that the proportion of energy derived from fatty acids steadily increases with increasing duration of a given exercise bout at a fixed work rate [145]. Thus, a single sustained bout of exercise may be more beneficial with regard to fatty acid consumption than several exercise bouts of shorter duration [3]; however, the effect on energy balance is unclear.

Hypertrophic fat cells may respond more favorably to an exercise intervention than hyperplastic adipose tissue [7]. Indeed, several studies provide evidence that decreases in body fat with exercise training are characterized by a similar decrease in fat cell size, without changes in fat cell number, particularly in men [7, 42, 43]. Moreover, adaptations in energy intake may result in smaller adipose tissue depots, with smaller fat cells [7]. Because abdominal obesity in older men and women is more often composed of hypertrophied fat cells [101, 131], this is encouraging with regard to ameliorating the increased metabolic risk associated with an android pattern of fat distribution with aging.

Additional mechanisms may mediate the pathway between exercise, fat utilization, and weight regulation. These mechanisms include an increase in lean mass [53] and increase in the resting metabolic rate [78, 126] (see 94, 95 for additional references), as well as appetite suppression among those initially overweight and sedentary [93, 146]. Weight loss achieved through increased exercise generally is much lower than expected through the direct expenditure of energy, however, perhaps because of increased caloric intake [124] or decreased physical activity in between exercise bouts [94].

It is also important to consider the contribution of genotype to variations in energy expenditure [13, 14] and body composition [15]. Ravussin et al. [98, 99] found that more than 25% of the variance in 24-hr energy expenditure (adjusted for body composition, age, and gender) was family-dependent (intraclass r=0.26). Heredity may explain as little as 5% of the variance in BMI, but as much as 25% of the variation in percent body fat, and between 25% and 30% of the variation in fat distribution among humans [15]. Furthermore, the role of genotype in the response of a person to exercise training may be considerable. Indeed, as much as 77% of the improvement in aerobic capacity may be a function of genotype [16]. The degree to which heredity influences body composition adaptations to regular exercise, however, is not clear.

Therefore, it seems necessary to determine the optimal exercise prescription that would maximize the oxidation of free fatty acids for such a time that stored body fat is used for fuel in sufficient quantities to alter energy balance. Exercise bouts of moderate intensity, but longer duration seem most efficacious toward this goal, because energy expenditure is maximized. Because many of the aforementioned adaptations to exercise training require time, however, an exercise program may need to be sustained for months and, perhaps years, to result in appreciable weight loss [112]. This may be especially true among the very obese, who initially may not be able to sustain an activity for a sufficient duration. The public health challenge thus lies in promoting an active life-style early in life, which can be maintained throughout adulthood, to prevent substantial weight gain and obesity with age.

Epidemiology
Although the inverse association between physical activity or exercise training and weight has been reported in several cross-sectional epidemiologic studies [27, 35, 46, 52, 54, 56, 114, 135, 137], two meta-analyses [5, 50], and more recent intervention studies [49, 92], there are few longitudinal data on how physical activity affects the risk, or development, of weight gain or overweight in the general population. Comparisons between studies are difficult because of different population characteristics, different criteria for defining overweight or obesity, and varying assessment techniques for physical activity or weight. In addition, the physical activity and weight association often is not the primary study relationship of interest in epidemiologic research. Data on one or the other of these study variables may be collected as part of a constellation of other risk factors for a primary disease outcome, such as CHD, diabetes, or cancer, and thus treated as secondary data. Consequently, information on physical activity or weight is often compromised because of crude indices of physical activity or self-reported, rather than measured, height and weight. Lack of precision in the measurement of physical activity or weight may attenuate the magnitude of their true association, which may explain the relatively low correlations seen between these two variables in large epidemiologic studies.

There is some evidence that the degree of overweight may account for conflicting results among studies. The inverse relationship between physical activity and overweight may be more salient among those highly obese, whereas the activity levels of mildly overweight persons may be indistinguishable from those of persons of normal weight [58, 111, 129].

Cross-sectional Evidence
Several cross-sectional, population-based studies [27, 35, 46, 52, 54, 56, 114, 134, 137] consistently report lower weight or body mass with higher categorical levels of self-reported physical activity. The data suggest that the inverse association may be dependent on the exercise intensity for a given duration, with higher intensity activities maximizing the postexercise negative energy balance (and consequent total energy expenditure) necessary for weight loss [78]. This postexercise increase in energy expenditure may be

negligible among the activity levels of the general population, however, and the stronger associations found between higher-intensity physical activity and weight in these studies may be a consequence of better accuracy in reporting higher-intensity exercise behaviors.

Folsom et al. [52] assessed the association between daily kilocalorie expenditure (using the Leisure-Time Physical Activity survey [122] and several CHD risk factors in a large probability sample of adults aged 25–74 yr from the metropolitan area of Minneapolis-St Paul. Whereas walking, bicycling, light conditioning, and home repair provided the greatest contribution to energy expenditure, in general, leisure-time physical activity level was relatively low in this population: only 34% of the men and 17% of the women expended 2000 kcal or more per week.Total daily kilocalorie expenditure was not significantly associated with the BMI in this population; however, there were small yet significant age-adjusted correlations between daily energy expenditure from heavy activity (≥ 6 kcal/min) and BMI in men ($r = -0.11$; $P < 0.01$) and women ($r = -0.10$; $P < 0.01$).

Data from nearly 19,000 persons (≥ 18 yr) who reported that they were trying to lose weight in the 1989 BRFSS survey, suggest that the prevalence of overweight (BMI ≥ 30 kg/m^2, based on self-reported height and weight) was highest among those reporting no physical activity and lowest among those reporting regular and intense activity ($P < 0.001$) for both men and women [46]. Among persons in all age groups, those who ran or jogged, performed aerobics, or cycled weighed loss ($P < 0.001$) than those who reported no activity, independent of height, race, education, smoking, and caloric restriction. Walking was also associated with lower weight ($P \leq 0.001$) among persons aged 40 yr or older. Moreover, the magnitude of the associations between many of the activities and weight increased with age, up to age 54 yr (Fig. 9.1).

There is potential with the BRFSS data for misclassification of self-reported weight, which may have been differential with regard to physical activity pattern. If sedentary people were more likely to underestimate their weight, however, the results would most likely be biased toward the null. Furthermore, because the questions on physical activity were asked first, well before questions about weight loss in the BRFSS survey, one may assume no bias in the reporting of physical activities by weight status or desire to lose weight.

Physical Activity and Fat Distribution
Physical activity may have a favorable effect on fat distribution as well as on overall adiposity and weight. Indeed, several large cross-sectional studies in Europe [108], Canada [125], and the United States [70, 114, 128, 144] report an inverse association between energy expenditure in physical activity and several somatic indicators of body fat distribution, such as the waist-to-hip ratio (WHR) or waist-to-thigh ratio (WTR).

FIGURE 9.1.

The association between selected activities and mean weight, by age and sex: Behavioral risk factor surveillance system, 1989. Based on multiple linear regression modeling adjusting for age, race, height, education, smoking, and caloric restriction. +Difference in mean weight between those reporting the activity and those reporting no activity. Data are from ref. 46.

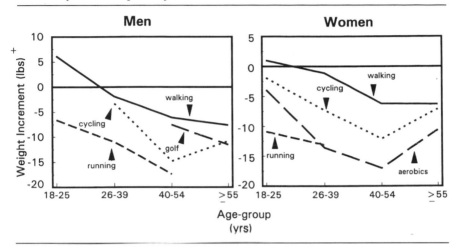

Tremblay et al. [125] analyzed cross-sectional data from 1366 women and 1257 men who participated in the 1981 Canada Fitness Survey [20]. Detailed information was gathered on leisure-time physical activity including type, frequency, duration, and intensity during the previous year [118]. Self-reported activity was then categorized based on intensity level (<5; 5–7; 7–9; and ≥9 metabolic equivalents. Results showed that measured body weights were comparable between activity intensity categories for both men and women. Subjects reporting activity ≥9 metabolic equivalents, however, had a significantly lower WHR (P<0.05) than subjects reporting activities of lower intensity, which was explained primarily by lower waist circumferences. The differences in WHR remained significant after adjustment for total energy expenditure from activities and total skinfold sum. These data suggest that higher-intensity exercise (such as jogging, vs. a lower-intensity activity, such as gardening) is associated with the preferential mobilization of abdominal fat relative to lower body fat.

Seidell and colleagues [108] used the Baecke physical activity survey [4] to calculate index scores for physical activity in sports, work, and leisure time in a cross-sectional population of 538 38-yr-old men from six different European cities. Results from the multiple regression analysis showed a significant inverse association between the sport activity score and the WHR and the WTR. These associations were explained mainly by a lower waist circumference and a greater thigh circumference among those reporting higher levels of sport activity and were independent of body mass index, education, smoking, and mean levels of the dependent variables in the different centers.

Because subcutaneous abdominal fat is much more responsive to epinephrine stimulation with exercise than gluteal fat [140], overweight men may benefit more from regular physical activity or exercise training than women, who tend to deposit excess fat in the more resistant gluteal/femoral region [41, 43, 127]. Therefore, studies of physical activity and fat distribution are particularly interesting in women, especially women with a more android fat pattern (i.e., higher relative abdominal adiposity), which may become more common after a drop in female sex hormone levels with menopause [101].

Cross-sectional data from nearly 41,000 postmenopausal women participating in the Iowa Women's Health Study [70] suggest a simple association between a crude indicator of physical activity and the WHR. This association did not remain significant, however, after adjustment for BMI and several sociodemographic and reproductive factors.

In contrast, among 487 middle-aged women participating in the Healthy Women's Study [144], upper body fat, estimated by the WHR, was inversely associated with weekly kilocalorie score based on the Harvard Alumni Activity Survey [91]. Women in the lowest quartile of energy expenditure (0–500 kcal/wk) had significantly ($P<0.05$) higher mean WHRs (0.78) compared with women in the other three quartiles combined (0.76), after adjustment for BMI. More importantly, however, 3-yr change in physical activity (assessed in a subsample of 108 women) was significantly correlated with change in WHR, after adjustment for change in BMI ($r=0.18$, $P<0.05$). Unfortunately, these analyses were not stratified by menopausal status. A decline in endogenous sex hormone levels will favor abdominal fat accumulation because of increased lipoprotein lipase activity and decreased lipolysis in the abdominal fat depot [100, 102]. Further investigation is needed to establish the association between sex hormone levels, baseline regional fat distribution, and exercise-related weight change in women and men of various ages.

These results suggest a favorable influence of regular, sustained physical activity, particularly activity of moderate to higher intensity, on the chronic disease risk often associated with abdominal, relative to lower body, obesity. However, because large studies on physical activity and fat distribution usually rely on circumference measures or skinfold assessments of subcutaneous fat in the abdomen and lower body, it is not clear whether the intraabdominal (or visceral) fat depot is as easily mobilized with exercise. The use of sophisticated, noninvasive techniques, such as computed tomography or magnetic resonance imaging, which can distinguish intraabdominal from subcutaneous depots generally is not feasible with large study populations.

In summary, the cross-sectional association between higher levels of physical activity and lower body weight or relative abdominal adiposity, although modest, has been demonstrated consistently in a number of different populations. Interpreting cross-sectional data, however, is difficult because the directionality of the association between physical activity and weight or fat distribution cannot be determined. Physical activity patterns and choices may affect weight and fat distribution, just as weight or fat distribution may influence physical activity [18]. Indeed, Seidell et al. [107] propose that among their cohort of European men, the relatively lower levels of sport-related physical activity among those with excess abdominal adiposity may be a consequence of altered muscle morphology because abdominal obesity is associated with increased Type IIb muscle fibers, possibly due to excess levels of glucocorticosteroids. In addition, both adiposity and activity status may be heavily influenced by genetic factors, although Bouchard and colleagues suggest that only about 5% of weight status (i.e, BMI) [15] and approximately 10% of fitness level ($\dot{V}O_2$max, relative to fat-free mass) [17] may be genetically predetermined.

Prevention of Overweight

Longitudinal or cohort studies (i.e., those with forward directionality) may give better information on the etiologic impact of physical activity on the risk of weight or adiposity change over time because, by definition, the exposure (physical activity), measured either prospectively or retrospectively, must precede the outcome. Unfortunately, there is a paucity of longitudinal data that examine the role of physical activity on weight and/or adiposity gain among the general population.

Determinants of significant weight gain ($\geq$ 5 kg/5 yr) were assessed in a large Finnish population, aged 25–64 yr [103]. Subjects were examined at baseline between 1966 and 1972, and then again from 1973 to 1976. The cumulative incidence of significant weight gain over the follow-up was 17.5% among men and 15.1% among women. After adjustment for smoking, caffeine and alcohol intake, health status, and various sociodemographic characteristics, the relative risks (95% confidence intervals) of significant weight gain across baseline categories of self-reported leisure-time physical activity (frequent, occasional, or rare) showed a modest dose-response relationship: 1.0, 1.5 (1.2–2.0), 1.9 (1.5–2.3) in men and 1.0, 1.5 (1.2–2.0), 1.6 (1.2–2.2) in women.

French and colleagues [54] examined several behavioral predictors of body weight in a large cohort of men and women participating in a worksite intervention study. Leisure-time and occupational physical activities were assessed using a 13-item frequency recall [65], with responses for each item ranging from 0 to 5 sessions per week. Walking and high-intensity activities were independently associated with lower weight among both men and women in the cross-sectional analysis. Women who reported high-intensity exercise sessions or walking weighed 5.32 lb and 2.14 lb less, respectively, for each reported session per week than did women who reported no high-intensity or walking activity. Men who reported high-intensity activity weighted 4.25 lb less per session per week than did those who reported no high-intensity activity.

Weight gain over the 2-yr follow-up period averaged 1.37 lb among women and 0.91 lb among men. Reported increases in walking or high-intensity activity between baseline and follow-up were significantly related to attenuated weight gain among both genders, independent of age, education, occupation, smoking, intervention treatment group, and work site. Women who increased their walking or high-intensity activity gained 1.76 lb and 1.39 lb less, respectively, per session increase per week than did women who reported no such activity. Similarly, among men, those who increased their walking gained 0.86 lb less per session increase, whereas men who increased their high-intensity activity gained 3.54 lb less per session increase than did men who reported no walking or high-intensity activity. These results suggest that sustained activity, of moderate to higher intensity, is necessary in attenuating weight gain over time.

Blair et al. (unpublished data) assessed the relationship between changes in physical activity level and fitness level and risk of weight gain in a large cohort of healthy, middle-aged men and women who had at least three preventive medical examinations at the Cooper Clinic. Self-reported physical activity was assessed by a simple survey, which classified respondents into a five-category physical activity index, based on their relative level of walking, running, or jogging during the previous month. Maximal treadmill time (minutes) was the measure of physical fitness level, which was determined by a graded exercise test. Changes in physical activity and fitness level were assessed between the first and second examination (average time interval = 1.8 yr for women and 1.6 yr for men); whereas weight change and change in skinfold sum was determined from the first to the last examination (average time interval = 4.5 yr for women and 4.7 yr for men).

In general, women gained weight over the follow-up period, whereas there was no weight change among the men. Results of the multivariable analyses indicated that improvements in treadmill time from the first to the second examination were independently related to attenuated weight gain, lower odds of a significant weight gain (either >5 kg or >10 kg), and greater reductions in skinfold sums in both men and women; however, reported increases in physical activity level over the follow-up were associated with attenuated weight gain and greater reductions in skinfold sum among men only. A 5-min increase in treadmill time between the first and second examination was associated with a 50% reduction in risk of weight gain of both >5 kg and >10 kg among men; whereas among women, a 5-min increase was associated with a 19% reduction in risk of a >5 kg gain and a 84% reduction in risk of a >10 kg gain.

Data on recreational physical activity (assessed by a single question and classified as low, moderate, or high) and measured body weight were gathered under standardized conditions at baseline and follow-up on a sample more than 9000 male and female repondents to the NHANES I Epidemiologic Follow-up Study (1971–1975 to 1982–1984) [141]. Recreational activity reported at baseline showed little relationship to weight change over the subsequent 10-year follow-up; however, activity reported at the follow-up was strongly related to weight change that had occurred during the study. Men who reported moderate and low levels of activity at the follow-up gained 0.9 and 1.6 kg more, respectively, than did men reporting high levels of activity. Among women, the relationship was slightly stronger: those who reported moderate and low levels of activity gained an average of 1.4 and 1.9 kg more than did women reporting high levels. The level of recreational activity reported at follow-up was also strongly related to severity of weight gain. Indeed, the magnitude of the effect of reported low levels of activity at follow-up increased with increasing severity of weight gain among both genders (Table 9.1). The odds ratios (OR) for gaining >13 kg were 3.1 in men and 3.8 in women.

Williamson et al. [14] also looked at change in activity level and the magnitude of subsequent weight change over the 10 yr of follow-up in this same cohort. Men reporting low activity in both interviews experienced a 4-fold increase in odds of a moderate weight gain (8–13 kg) (OR=3.9, 1.9–7.8) compared with men who reported high levels of activity at both time points, whereas those who reported moderate levels of activity at both interviews doubled their odds of a weight gain of this same magnitude (OR=2.0, 1.0–4.0). Men who decreased their activity between the two interviews increased their odds of an 8–13-kg weight gain more than 3-fold (OR=3.3, 1.7–6.3) relative to those whose activity levels remained unchanged; however, men who reported increased activity also experienced a higher odds of an 8–13-kg weight gain (OR=2.4, 1.2–4.6). Among women, reported recreational activity was strongly related to the odds of a major weight gain (≥13 kg), although the confidence intervals are somewhat wide, presumably because of the small numbers in this weight gain category. Compared with women who consistently reported high levels of activity, those who reported low activity at both interviews had an odds ratio of 7.1 (2.2–23.3) for weight gain ≥13 kg. Those women who decreased their activity level between the two interviews increased their odds of a major weight gain substantially relative to women reporting no change in activity (OR=6.2, 1.9–20.4); but, again, those women whose reported activity level increased also experienced a higher odds of a major weight gain (OR=3.4, 1.0–11.1). These findings were not affected by age or baseline weight status.

TABLE 9.1.
Logistic Regression Estimates of the Relative Odds of Weight Gain Categories by Recreational Physical Activity Levels Measured at Baseline and at Follow-up

Recreational Physical Activity	Men			Women		
	3.1–8.0 kg	8.1–13.0 kg	>13 kg	3.1–8.0 kg	8.1–13.0 kg	>13 kg
			OR (95% CI)[a]			
At baseline						
High	1.0 (–)	1.0 (–)	1.0 (–)	1.0 (–)	1.0 (–)	1.0 (–)
Moderate	0.9 (0.7–1.2)	0.8 (0.5–1.1)	0.9 (0.5–1.4)	0.8 (0.7–1.0)	0.8 (0.6–1.1)	0.7 (0.4–0.9)
Low	1.0 (0.8–1.2)	1.1 (0.8–1.5)	0.8 (0.5–1.2)	0.9 (0.8–1.0)	0.9 (0.7–1.1)	0.9 (0.7–1.2)
At follow-up						
High	1.0 (–)	1.0 (–)	1.0 (–)	1.0 (–)	1.0 (–)	1.0 (–)
Moderate	1.0 (0.8–1.3)	1.4 (0.9–2.1)	1.8 (1.0–3.4)	1.4 (1.1–1.7)	1.2 (0.9–1.7)	2.5 (1.5–4.2)
Low	1.2 (0.9–1.5)	2.3 (1.5–3.5)	3.1 (1.6–6.0)	1.6 (1.3–2.0)	1.8 (1.3–2.5)	3.8 (2.3–6.5)

All estimates are adjusted for nonrecreational physical activity, change in smoking status, and change in drinking status between the baseline and follow-up surveys, morbidity, body mass index and age at baseline, race, education, and duration of follow-up (141).
[a]OR, odds ratio; 95% CI, 95% confidence interval.

In interpreting these seemingly paradoxical findings [141] the authors conclude that a change in physical activity level may be both a cause and consequence of weight gain. Indeed, because changes in self-reported physical activity and weight were assessed concurrently at baseline and follow-up, directionality of the physical activity-weight relationship could not be determined. Longitudinal studies with frequent measurement of physical activity and body weight are necessary to describe adequately the temporal relationship between these two variables among the general population.

Voorips et al. [135] assessed retrospectively the relationship between history of physical activity participation and the development of overweight in a volunteer sample of 45 older (> 70 yr) women. Women were first stratified (lower tertile vs. upper tertile) by self-reported level of current physical activity using one survey (previously validated in this study sample [136], while comprehensive questions about past physical activity in the categories of school, work, home, sports, and during leisure time were asked for several age cutpoints (12, 25, 40, and 55 yr), using a second survey. Responses to questions on past physical activity were rated from 1 to 5, based on the relative contribution of the reported behavior to energy expenditure, and then summed over all categories to derive a total past physical activity score. Information on body weight, body shape, and relative fatness was also collected for these same age cutpoints and combined into a weight index.

There were no statistically significant differences in total past physical activity score between the two groups of women at the different age cutpoints (Fig. 9.2); however, scores for the weight index were significantly higher starting at age 25 among women reporting lower levels of current physical activity compared with their more active counterparts (Fig. 9.3). These data suggest that low levels of current physical activity may be a consequence, rather than a cause, of higher body weight among this group of older women because current differences in body shape or fatness between physically active and relatively inactive older women were already present by age 25 yr and persisted throughout their adult life, even though levels of past physical activity did not differ between the two groups. It is important to remember that two different surveys were used in this study: one to stratify groups by level of current activity, and one to assess past history of physical activity at different ages. Therefore, comparisons between past and current levels of physical activity are difficult to make.

Finally, Klesges and colleagues [69] report data on the relationship between changes in dietary intake, physical activity, and weight change in a small volunteer sample followed for 3 yr. Women (N=152) gained an average of 1.4 kg over the follow-up, whereas men (N=142) gained only about 0.3 kg. Among women, higher work and leisure activity at baseline, as well as increases in work activity, were significantly related to attenuated weight

FIGURE 9.2.

Physical activity score at different ages of 21 currently sedentary and 24 currently physically active elderly women, based on a detailed questionnaire. Values are means ± SD. Data are from ref. 135.

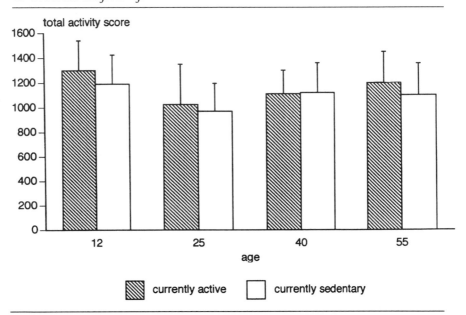

gain over 2 yr, independent of changes in energy intake. However, there were no statistically significant relationships between reported physical activity of any kind and weight change among the men.

Thus, the evidence linking habitual physical activity to the risk of weight gain among the general population or more selected populations is inconclusive. As stated previously, these inconsistent longitudinal relationships may be a consequence of several methodological issues, which make interpreting the data quite difficult.

MEASUREMENT ISSUES

Modest or negligible statistical associations between physical activity and weight may result from a low prevalence of higher-intensity physical activity, or, perhaps, a high prevalence of lower-intensity activities, such as gardening, housework, or leisurely walking, which do not get assessed. Large-scale studies may be limited to one or two questions about specific types of activity (e.g., vigorous or sport-related activity) and many activity surveys may not be sensitive or precise enough to represent accurately the true range for activities engaged in by the general population.

FIGURE 9.3.

Weight index at different ages based on rating of two silhouettes and a comparison of body shape with peers of two groups of elderly women differing in present physical activity. Values are means ± SD. Ratio of sedentary to active women at ages 12, 25, and 55: 19/24, at age 40: 20/23, and at current age: 21/24. *P<.05. Data are from ref. 135.

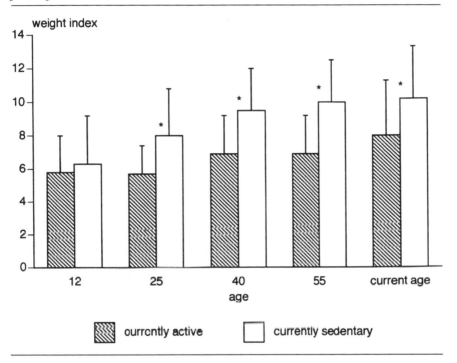

The low correlations often reported between physical activity and weight outcomes may also be a consequence of measurement error due to inaccurate recall. Accuracy in recalling physical activity may vary with gender [105], weight [105], and exercise type and level [6]. Several studies [6, 45, 61, 105] have demonstrated low accuracy in recalling low-intensity behaviors, but higher accuracy with hard or very hard activities. Moreover, structured exercise activities may lend themselves to more accurate and reliable recollection because they are performed within a stable, scheduled time frame that can be referred to readily [25, 29]. Although a fitness indicator such as treadmill time or maximal aerobic capacity ($\dot{V}O_2$max) may provide a more objective and precise marker of habitual physical activity, it is, nonetheless, a performance measure, which may be influenced by genetic predisposition or by weight itself.

In addition, lower-intensity activities may display a great deal of intraindividual variation, and even if a survey queries these types of behaviors, their usual pattern may not be characterized adequately with a one-time assessment. Dannenberg et al. [35] reported substantial seasonal variation in activity patterns in the Framingham Offspring cohort. Furthermore, kilocalorie expenditure was significantly greater in the summer than the winter in both men and women, suggesting seasonal fluctuation in weight as well. Therefore, the time frame of the physical activity assessment becomes extremely important when correlating behavioral patterns to weight outcomes. Activities more easily reported for the past week, or even a typical week in the past month, may not be representative of a year-long or, certainly a life-long, pattern. Thus, multiple assessments are necessary to describe accurately the contribution of physical activity to long-term weight regulation.

Given valid and precise measurement of physical activity patterns, however, the true magnitude of the association between physical activity and weight may vary with regard to gender, especially among younger adult (<45 yr) populations. Blair et al. (unpublished data) report that the impact of increased physical activity on weight gain was stronger among men than women in the Cooper Clinic cohort. Després et al. [36, 43, 127] also provide strong experimental evidence for the resistance to fat loss with exercise training in premenopausal women compared with men, which may relate to a higher proportion of less lipolytically responsive gluteofemoral adipose tissue [40].

In addition, both the direction and the magnitude of the effect of physical activity on weight may vary with regard to age. Few population-based studies have assessed the association between physical activity and weight among older (≥65 yr) men and women. Thus, little is known about the benefits of exercise to weight, adiposity, and subsequent health outcomes among older populations. Data from the 1989 BRFSS survey [46] show that the magnitude of the association between body weight and activities such as walking, running, and aerobics tended to increase with age. Perhaps as the muscle-to-fat ratio declines with age, physical activity will exert a more powerful influence on body composition compared with its influence at younger ages, when the effect of exercise on weight maintenance is often distorted by the influence of increased muscle mass.

On the other hand, selective survival may play a role in attenuating the association between physical activity and weight with age. That is, people most susceptible to putative risk factors may die at earlier ages, diminishing the ability to determine the influence of those factors on surviving populations. Indeed, Marti et al., [81] and Caspersen et al. [23] failed to find statistically significant associations between physical activity and weight among their respective populations of older European men. In addition, there is some evidence that healthy older people may defend their energy balance more robustly than younger people. Goran and Poehlman [57] found that 8 wk of endurance training, although improving cardiorespiratory fitness, did not result in increases in total energy expenditure in their older volunteers because of compensatory decreases in volitional activity between exercise bouts.

Thus, age and gender are important variables in modifying the relationship between physical activity and weight, which may not be apparent when data from different age groups are pooled together. Therefore, large studies comprising younger, middle-aged, and older adults must stratify analyses by age, as well as gender, to obtain a clearer picture of how physical activity and weight may influence each other throughout adulthood.

Finally, a few large studies of physical activity and body weight can control for the confounding influence of caloric intake because diet is as difficult to assess accurately as physical activity. Nonetheless, energy requirements change with increases in activity patterns [2, 12, 146] and statistical analyses must account for changes in food intake and other variables, such as smoking and baseline weight, which may confound the relationship between physical activity and body weight or adiposity.

SUMMARY

Overweight is a common problem in the United States, especially among minority women and persons of lower socioeconomic status and lower educational attainment. Moreover, the prevalence of reported inactivity may be highest in these same population subgroups. Both overweight and sedentary behavior are important risk factors for chronic disease morbidity and mortality; however, there is encouraging evidence that moderate to higher levels of physical activity may provide protection from certain chronic diseases, even among persons with established risk factors.

Several methodological issues preclude the ability to determine accurately the impact of physical activity on body weight and adiposity. These issues include (a) a low prevalence of higher-intensity physical activity in the general population, (b) measurement error with regard to self-reported activity, especially that of lower-intensity, (c) inappropriate time frame of the physical activity assessment, (d) effect modification by age and gender, and (e) failure to adjust for important statistical confounders. Despite these methodological issues, the inverse association between physical activity and weight has been reported in several cross-sectional epidemiologic studies, which consistently report lower body weight, or more favorable distribution of body fat, with higher categorical levels of self-reported physical activity. Directionality of the physical activity and weight relation cannot be determined from these studies, however, and the few longitudinal epidemiologic studies that have assessed the influence of physical activity on the risk of weight gain report inconclusive results. This is possibly because a one-time assessment of physical activity if not adequate in describing the contribution of habitual physical activity on long-term weight maintenance. Therefore, longitudinal population-based studies with multiple assessments of physical activity over long follow-up periods are necessary to determine this relationship.

In any case, the evidence suggests that persons concerned with overweight, or especially the prevention of overweight and obesity, should increase their physical activity. Sociodemographic characteristics such as age, gender, educational level, and weight are associated with physical activity patterns and choices. Therefore, these characteristics should be considered by professionals when implementing physical activity interventions for weight control. Walking is accessible to all segments of the U.S. population. Because walking is convenient, low cost, and safe, and can result in weight loss if done regularly for durations of at least 20–30 min, its relative merits should be stressed in weight reduction and maintenance programs. Furthermore, to reduce the morbidity and mortality associated with overweight, obesity, and sedentary behavior, priority for intervention programs should be directed at persons in the most vulnerable sectors of the population.

ACKNOWLEDGMENTS

I thank Steven N. Blair, Jean-Pierre Després, Ethan R. Nadel, Nina S. Stachenfeld, and John R. Stofan for their comments on the manuscript. This work was supported by National Institutes of Health Grant AG-09872.

REFERENCES

1. Albanes D., A. Blair, and P. R. Taylor. Physical activity and risk of cancer in the NHANES I population. *Am. J. Public Health.* 79:744–750, 1989.
2. Andersson B., X. Xu, M. Rebuffe-Scrive, K. Terning, M. Krotkiewski, and P. Bjorntorp. The effects of exercise training on body composition and metabolism in men and women. *Int. J. Obes.* 15:75–81, 1991.
3. Andrews, J. F. Exercise for slimming. *Proc. Nutr. Soc.* 50:459–471, 1991.
4. Baecke J. A. H., J. Burema, and J. E. R. Frijters. A short questionnaire for the measurement of physical activity in epidemiological studies. *Am. J. Clin. Nutr.* 36:936–942, 1982.
5. Ballor, D. L., and R. E. Keesey. A meta-analysis of the factors affecting exercise-induced changes in body mass, fat mass, and fat-free mass in males and females. *Int. J. Obes.* 5:717–726, 1991.
6. Baranowski T. Validity and reliability of self-report measures of physical activity: an information processing perspective. *Res. Q. Exerc. Sport* 59:314–327, 1987.
7. Bjorntorp P. Adipose tissue adaptation to exercise. C. Bouchard, R. J. Shepard, T. Stephens, J. R. Sutton, and B. D. McPherson (eds). *Exercise, Fitness and Health: A Consensus of Current Knowledge.* Champaign, IL.: Human Kinetics, 1990, pp. 315–323.
8. Bjorntorp, P., M. Fahlen, G. Grimby, et al. Carbohydrate and lipid metabolism in middle-aged, physically well-trained men. *Metabolism* 21:1037–1044, 1972.
9. Blair, S. N., H. W. Kohl III and N. F. Gordon. Physical activity and health: a life-style approach. *Med. Ex. Nutr. Health* 1:54–57, 1992.
10. Blair, S. N., H. W. Kohl, N. F. Gordon, and R. S. Paffenbarger, Jr. How much physical activity is good for health? *Annu. Rev. Public Health* 13:99–126, 1992.

11. Blair, S. N., H. W. Khol III, R. S. Paffenbarger, Jr., et al. Physical fitness and all-cause mortality: a prospective study of healthy men and women. *J. A. M. A.* 262:2392–2401, 1989.
12. Blair, S. N., N. M. Ellsworth, W. L. Haskell, M. P. Stern, J. W. Farquar, and P. D. Wood. Comparison of nutrient intake in middle-aged men and women runners and controls. *Mied. Sci. Sports Exerc.* 13:310–315, 1981.
13. Bogardus, C., S. Lillioja, E. Ravussin, et al. Familial dependence of the resting metabolic rate. *N. Engl. J. Med.* 415:96–100, 1986.
14. Bouchard, C., A. Tremblay, A. Nadeau, et al. Genetic effect in resting and exercise metabolic rates. *Metabolism* 38:364–370, 1989.
15. Bouchard, C., L. Perusse, C. Leblanc, A. Tremblay, and G. Theriault. Heredity, human body fat, and fat distribution. *Int J. Obes.* 12:205–215, 1988.
16. Bouchard, C., M. R. Boulay, J. A. Simoneau, G. Lortie, and L. Perusse. Heredity and trainability of aerobic and anearobic performances: an update. *Sports Med.* 5:69–73, 1988.
17. Bouchard, C., R. Lesage, G. Lortie, et al. Aerobic performance in brothers, dizygotic and monozygotic twins. *Med. Sci. Sports Exerc.* 18:639–646, 1986.
18. Brownell K. D., and A. J. Stunkard. Physical activity in the development and control of obesity. A. J. Stunkard (ed). *Obesity*. Philadelphia: W. B. Saunders, 1980, pp. 300–324.
19. Campbell, A. J., W. J. Busby, C. C. Horwath, and M. C. Robertson. Relation of age, exercise, anthropometric measurements and diet with glucose and insulin levels in a population aged 70 years and over. *Am. J. Epidemiol.* 138:688–696, 1993.
20. Canada Fitness Survey. Fitness and life-style in Canada. Ottawa: Canada Fitness Survey, 1983.
21. Caspersen, C. J., and R. K. Merritt. Leisure-time physical activity trends by race and social status. The Behavior Risk Factor Surveillence System Survey, 1986–1990. *Med. Sci. Sports Exerc.* 26:S80, 1994 (abstract).
22. Caspersen, C. J., and R. K. Merritt. Trends in physical activity patterns among older adults. The Behavior Risk Factor Surveillence System Survey, 1986–1990. *Med. Sci. Sports Exerc.* 24:S26, 1992 (abstract).
23. Caspersen, C. J., B. P. M. Bloemberg, W. H. M. Saris, R. K. Merritt, and D. Kromhout. The prevalence of selected physical activities and their relation with coronary heart disease risk factors in elderly men: the Zutphen Study, 1985. *Am. J. Epidemiol.* 133:1–15, 1991.
24. Caspersen, C. J., and L. DiPietro. National estimates of physical activity among older adults. *Med. Sci. Sports Exerc.* 23:S106, 1991. (abstract).
25. Caspersen, C. J. Physical activity epidemiology: concepts, methods and applications to exercise science. *Exerc. Sports Sci. Rev.* 17:423–473, 1989.
26. Caspersen, C. J. Physical activity and coronary heart disease. *Phys. Sportsmed.* 15:43–44, 1987. (guest editorial).
27. Caspersen, C. J., and R. A. Pollard. Prevalence of physical activity in the United States and its relationship to disease risk factors. *Med. Sci. Sports Exerc.* 19:S6, 1987. (abstract).
28. Caspersen, C. J., R. A. Pollard, and S. O. Pratt. Scoring physical activity data with special consideration for elderly populations. Proceedings of the 21st National Meeting of Public Health Conference on Records and Statistics: Data for an Aging Population, July 13–15, 1987. Hyattsville, MD: U.S. Dept. Health and Human Services, Public Health Service, CDC, NCHS, 1987.
29. Caspersen, C. J., K. E. Powell, and G. M. Christenson. Physical activity, exercise, and physical fitness: definitions and distinctions for health related research. *Public Health Rep.* 100: 126–131, 1985.
30. Centers for Disease Control. Prevalence of sedentary lifestyle–BRFSS, United States, 1991. M. M. W. R. 42:576–579, 1993.
31. Centers for Disease Control. Protective effects of physical activity on coronary heart disease. M. M. W. R. 36:426–430, 1987.
32. Colditz, G. A. Economic cost of obesity. *Am. J. Clin. Nutr.* 55:503s–507s, 1992.

33. Crampes, F., D. Riviere, M. Beauville, M. Marceron, and M. Garrigues. Lipolytic response of adipocytes to epinephrine in sedentary and exercise-trained subjects: sex-related differences. *Eur. J. Appl. Physiol.* 59:249–255, 1989.

34. Crespo, C. J., and J. D. Wright. Prevalence of sedentary lifestyles and frequency of physical activity from the Third National Health and Nutrition Examination Survey. *Med. Sci. Sports Exerc.* 26:S80, 1994. (abstract)

35. Dannenberg, A. L., J. B. Keller, P. W. F. Wilson, and W. P. Castelli. Lesuire time physical activity in the Framingham Offspring Study. Description, seasonal variation, and risk factor correlates. *Am. J. Epidemiol.* 129:76–88, 1989.

36. Després, J.-P., M-C. Pouliot, S. Moorjani, et al. Loss of abdominal fat and metabolic response to exercise training to obese women. *Am. J. Physiol.* 261:E159–E167, 1991.

37. Després, J.-P., S. Moorjani, P. J. Lupien, A. Tremblay, A. Nadeau, and C. Bouchard. Regional distribution of body fat, plasma lipoproteins and cardiovascular disease. *Arteriosclerosis* 10:497–511, 1990.

38. Després, J.-P., A. Tremblay, S. Moorjani, et al. Long-term exercise training with constant energy intake. 3: Effects on plasma lipoprotein level. *Int. J. Obes.* 14:85–94, 1990.

39. Després, J.-P., A. Nadeau. A. Tremblay, et al. Role of deep abdominal fat in the association between regional adipose tissue distribution and glucose tolerance in obese women. *Diabetes.* 38:304–309, 1989.

40. Després, J.-P., A. Tremblay, and C. Bouchard. Sex differences in the regulation of body fat mass with exercise training. P. Bjorntorp and S. Rossner (eds). *Obesity in Europe I.* London: Libbey, 1989, pp. 297–304.

41. Després, J.-P., A. Tremblay, A. Nadeau, and C. Bouchard. Physical training and changes in regional adipose tissue distribution. *Acta Med. Scand. Suppl.* 723:205–212, 1988.

42. Després, J.-P., C. Bouchard, A. Tremblay, R. Savard, and M. Marcotte. Effects of aerobic training on fat distribution in male subjects. *Med. Sci. Sports. Exerc.* 17:113–118, 1985.

43. Després, J.-P., C. Bouchard, R. Savard, A. Tremblay, M. Marcotte, and G. Theriault. The effect of a 20-week endurance program on adipose-tissue morphology and lipolysis in men and women. *Metabolism* 33:235–239, 1984.

44. DiPietro, L., A. M. Ostfeld, and G. L. Rosner. Adiposity and stroke among older adults of low socioeconomic study: the Chicago Stroke Study. *Am. J. Public Health* 84:14–19, 1994.

45. DiPietro, L., C. J. Caspersen, A. M. Ostfeld, and E. R. Nadel. A survey for assessing physical activity among older adults. *Med. Sci. Sports Exerc.* 25:628–642, 1993.

46. DiPietro, L., D. F. Williamson, C. J. Caspersen, and E. Eaker. The descriptive epidemiology of selected physical activities and body weight among adults trying to lose weight: the Behavioral Risk Factor Surveillance System Survey, 1989. *Int. J. Obes.* 17:69–76, 1993.

47. DiPietro, L., and C. J. Caspersen. National estimates of physical activity among white and black americans. *Med. Sci. Sports Exerc.* 23:S105, 1991. (abstract).

48. Donahue R. P., R. D. Abbott, E. Bloom, et al. Central obesity and coronary heart disease in men. *Lancet.* i:821–824, 1987.

49. Duncan, J. J., N. F. Gordon, and C. B. Scott. Women walking for health and fitness. How much is enough? *J. A. M. A.* 266:3295–3299, 1991.

50. Epstein, L. H., and R. R. Wing. Aerobic exercise and weight. *Addict. Behav.* 5:371–388, 1980.

51. Flegal K. M., W. R. Harlan, and J. R. Landis. Secular trends in body mass index and skinfold thickness with socioeconomic factors in young adult women. *Am. J. Clin. Nutr.* 48:535–543, 1988.

52. Folsom, A. R., C. J. Caspersen, H. L. Taylor, et al. Leisure time physical activity and its relationship to coronary risk factors in a population-based sample. The Minnesota Heart Survey. *Am. J. Epidemiol.* 121:570–579, 1985.

53. Forbes, G. B. Exercise and body composition. *J. Appl. Physiol.* 70:994–997, 1990.

54. French, S. A., R. W. Jeffery, J. L. Forster, P. G. McGovern, S. H. Kelder, and J. E. Baxter. Predictors of weight change over two years among a population of working adults: the Healthy Worker Project. *Int. J. Obes.* 18:145–154, 1994.

55. Gerhardsson, M., B. Floderus, and S. E. Norell. Physical activity and colon cancer risk. *Int. J. Epidemiol.* 17:743–746, 1988.

56. Gibbons, L. W., S. N. Blair, K. H. Cooper, and M. Smith. Association between coronary heart disease risk factors and physical fitness in healthy adult women. *Circulation* 67: 977–983, 1983.

57. Goran, M. I. and E. T. Poehlman. Endurance training does not enhance total energy expenditure in healthy older persons. *Am. J. Physiol.* 263:E950–957, 1992.

58. Grilo, C., K. D. Brownell, and A. J. Stunkard. The metabolic and psychological importance of exercise and weight control. A. J. Stunkard and T. A. Wadden (eds). *Obesity: Theory and Therapy, 2nd ed.* New York: Raven Press, Ltd., 1993, pp. 253–272.

59. Haskell, W. L. The influence of exercise on the concentrations of triglycerides and cholesterol in human plasma. *Exerc. Sports Sci. Rev.* 12:205–244, 1984.

60. Helmrich, S. P., D. R. Ragland, R. W. Leung, and R. S. Paffenbarger, Jr. Physical activity and reduced occurrence of non-insulin-dependent diabetes mellitus. *N. Engl. J. Med.* 325: 147–152, 1991.

61. Hopkins, W. G., N. C. Wilson and D. G. Russell. Validation of the physical activity instrument for life in the New Zealand national survey. *Am J. Epidemiol.* 133:73–82, 1991.

62. Hubert, H. B., M. Feinleib, R. M. McNamara, et al. Obesity as an independent risk factor for cardiovascular disease: a 26-year follow-up of participants in the Framingham Study. *Circulation* 67:968–977, 1983.

63. Hurley, B. F., P. M. Nemeth, W. H. Martin, J. M. Hagberg, G. P. Dalsky, and J. O. Holloszy. Muscle triglyceride utilization during exercise: effect of training. *J. Appl. Physiol.* 60: 562–567, 1986.

64. Jacobs, D. R., Jr., L. P. Hahn, A. R. Folsom, P. J. Hannan, J. M. Sprafka, and C. L. Burke. Time trends in leisure-time physical activity in the upper midwest 1957–1987: University of Minnesota Studies. *Epidemiology* 2:8–15, 1991.

65. Jacobs, D. R., Jr, L. P. Hahn, W. L. Haskell, P. P. Price, and S. Sidney. Validity and reliability of a short physical activity history: CARDIA and the Minnesota Heart Health Program. *J. Cardiopulm. Rehab.* 11:448–459, 1989.

66. Kahn, H. S., D. F. Williamson, and J. A. Stevens. Race and weight change in US women: the roles of socioeconomic and marital status. *Am. J. Public Health* 81:319–323, 1991.

67. Kahn, H. S., and D. F. Williamson The contribution of income, education, and change in marital status to weight change among US men. *Int. J. Obes.* 14:1057–1068, 1990.

68. Kayman, S., W. Bruvold, and J. S. Stern. Maintenance and relapse after weight loss in women: behavioral aspects. *Am. J. Clin. Nutr.* 52:800–807, 1990.

69. Klesges, R. C., L. M. Klesges, C. K. Haddock, and L. H. Eck. A longitudinal analysis of the impact of dietary intake and physical activity on weight change in adults. *Am. J. Clin. Nutr.* 55:818–822, 1992.

70. Kaye S. A., A. R. Folsom, R. J. Prineas, J. D. Potter, and S. M. Gapstur. The association of body fat distribution with lifestyle and reproductive factors in a population study of premenopausal women. *Int. J. Obes.* 14:583–591, 1990.

71. Kramer, F. M., R. W. Jeffery, J. L. Forster, and M. Kaye. Long-term follow-up of behavioral treatment for obesity: patterns of weight gain among men and women. *Int. J. Obes.* 13:123–136, 1989.

72. Kuczmarski, R. J., K. M. Flegal, S. M. Campbell, and C. L. Johnson. The increasing prevalence of overweight among US adults. The National Health and Nutrition Examination Surveys, 1960 to 1991. *J. A. M. A.* 272:205–211, 1994.

73. Kumanyika, S. Obesity and black women. *Epidemiol. Rev.* 9:31–50, 1987.

74. Lapidus, L., C. Bengtsson, B. Larsson, et al. Distribution of adipose tissue and risk of cardiovascular disease and death: a 12-year follow-up of participants in the population of women in Gothenburg, Sweden. *Br. Med. J.* 289:1257–1261, 1984.

75. LaPorte, R. E., H. J. Montoye, and C. J. Caspersen. Assessment of physical activity in epidemiologic research: problems and prospects. *Public Health Rep.* 100:131–146, 1985.

300 | *DiPietro*

76. Larsson, B., K. Svardsudd, L. Welin, et al. Abdominal adipose tissue distribution, obesity, and risk of cardiovascular disease and death: a 13-year follow-up of participants in the study of men born in 1913. *Br. Med. J.* 288:1401–1404, 1984.
77. Lee, I-M., R. S. Paffenbarger, Jr., and C. C. Hsieh. Physical activity and risk of developing colorectal cancer among college alumni. *J. N. C. I.* 83:1324–1329, 1991.
78. Lennon, D. F., F. Nagle, F. Stratman, E. Shrago, and S. Dennis. Diet and exercise training effects on resting metabolic rate. *Int. J. Obes.* 9:39–47, 1985.
79. Leon, A. S., J. Connett, D. R. Jacobs, and R. Rauramaa. Leisure time physical activity levels and risk of coronary heart disease and death: the Multiple Risk Factor Intervention Trial. *J. A. M. A.* 258:2388–2395, 1987.
80. Lew E. A., and L. Garfinkel. Variations in mortality by weight among 750,000 men and women. *J. Chronic Dis.* 32:563–576, 1979.
81. Manson, J. E., D. M. Nathan, A. S. Krolewski, M. J. Stampfer, W. C. Willett, and C. H. Hennekens. A prospective study of exercise and incidence of diabetes among US male physicians. *J. A. M. A.* 268:63–67, 1992.
82. Manson, J. E., E. B. Rimm, M. J. Stampfer, G. A. Colditz, W. C. Willett, et al. Physical activity and incidence of non-insulin-dependent diabetes mellitus in women. *Lancet* 338:774–778, 1991.
83. Marti, B., J. Pekkanen, A. Nissinen, A. Ketola, S. Kivela, et al. Association of physical activity with coronary risk factors and physical ability: twenty-year follow-up of a cohort of Finnish men. *Age Ageing.* 18:103–109, 1989.
84. Menotti, A., and F. Seccareccia. Physical activity at work and job responsibility as risk factors for fatal coronary heart disease and other causes of death. *J. Epidemiol. Commun. Health* 39:325–329, 1985.
85. Merritt R. K., and C. J. Caspersen. Trends in physical activity patterns among young adults. The Behavior Risk Factor Surveillence System Survey, 1986–1990. *Med. Sci. Sports Exerc.* 24:S26, 1992. (abstract).
86. Morris, J. N., Clayton, D. G., M. G. Everitt, A. M. Semmence, and E. H. Burgess. Exercise in leisure time: coronary attack and death rates. *Br. Heart J.* 63:325–334, 1990.
87. Najjar M. F., and M. Rowland. Anthropometric reference data and prevalence of overweight, United States, 1976–1980. Vital and Health Statistics (series 11), No. 238. DHHS Publication No. (PHS) 87–1688. Washington, DC: US Government Printing Office, 1987.
88. National Center for Health Statistics. Health, United States, 1989. DHHS Publication No. (PHS) 90–1232. Washington, DC: US Government Printing Office.
89. Oscai, L. B. The role of exercise in weight control. *Exerc. Sports Sci. Rev.* 1:103–123, 1973.
90. Paffenbarger, R. S., Jr., R. T. Hyde, A.. L. Wing. I.-M. Lee, D. L. Jung, and J. B. Kampert. The association of changes in physical activity level and other lifestyle characteristics with mortality among men. *N. Engl. J. Med.* 328:538–545, 1993.
91. Paffenbarger, R. S., Jr., A. L. Wing, and R. T. Hyde. Physical activity as an index of heart attack risk in college alumni. *Am. J. Epidemiol.* 108:161–175, 1978.
92. Pavlou, K. N., S. Krey, and W. P. Steffee. Exercise as an adjunct to weight loss and maintenance in moderately obese subjects. *Am. J. Clin. Nutr.* 49:1115–1123, 1989.
93. Pi-Sunyer, F. X., Effect of exercise on food intake. P. Bjorntorp and B. N. Brodoff (eds). *Obesity.* Philadelphia: J. B. Lippincott, 1992, pp. 454–462.
94. Poehlman, E. T., P. J. Arciero, and M. I. Goran. Endurance exercise in aging humans: effects of energy metabolism. *Exerc. Sports Sci. Rev.* 22:251–284, 1994.
95. Poehlman, E. T. A review: exercise and its influence on resting energy metabolism in man. *Med. Sci. Sports Exerc.* 21:515–525, 1989.
96. Powell, K. E. On basketballs and heartbeats. *Epidemiology.* 2:3–5, 1991. (editorial).
97. Powell, K. E., P. D. Thompson, C. J. Caspersen, and J. S. Hendrick. Physical activity and incidence of coronary heart disease. *Annu. Rev. Public Health* 8:253–287, 1987.
98. Ravussin, E., S. Lillioja, W. C. Knowler, et al. Reduced rate of energy expenditure as a risk factor for body weight gain. *N. Engl. J. Med.* 318:467–472, 1988.

99. Ravussin, E., and B. A. Swinburn. Energy metabolism. A. J. Stunkard and T. A. Wadden (eds). *Obesity: Theory and Therapy, 2nd ed*. New York: Raven Press, 1993, pp. 97–123.

100. Rebuffé-Scrivé, M., P. Mann, and P. Bjorntorp. Effect of testosterone on abdominal adipose tissue in men. *Int. J. Obesity* 15:791–795, 1991.

101. Rebuffé-Scrivé, M. Steroid hormones and distribution of adipose tissue. *Acta Med. Scand. Suppl.* 723:143–146, 1987.

102. Rebuffé-Scrivé, M., J. Eldh, L.-O. Hafstrom, and P. Bjorntorp. Metabolism of mammary, abdominal and femoral adipocytes in women before and after menopause. *Metabolism* 35:792–797, 1986.

103. Rissanen, A., M. Heliovaara, P. Knekt, A. Reunanen, and A. Aromaa. Determinants of weight gain and overweight in adult Finns. *Eur. J. Clin. Nutr.* 45:419–430, 1991.

104. Riviere, D., F. Crampes, M. Beauville, and M. Garrigues. Lipolytic response of fat cells to catecholamines in sedentary and exercise-trained women. *J. Appl. Physiol.* 66:330–335, 1989.

105. Sallis, J. F., W. L. Haskell, P. D. Wood, et al. Physical activity assessment methodology in the Five-City Project. *Am. J. Epidemiol.* 121:91–106.

106. Saris, W. H. M. Long-term results of the treatment of obesity. *J. Drugs Res.* 8:2075–2080, 1983.

107. Seidell J. C. Environmental influences on regional fat distribution. *Int. J. Obes.* 15:31–35, 1991.

108. Seidell, J. C., M. Cigolini, J.-P. Deslypere, J. Charzewska, B.-M. Ellsinger, and A. Cruz. Body fat distribution in relation to physical activity and smoking habits in 38-year-old European men. *Am. J. Epidemiol.* 133:257–265, 1991.

109. Seidell J. C., P. Bjorntorp, L. Sjostrom, H. Kvist, and R. Sannerstedt. Visceral fat accumulation in men is positively associated with insulin, glucose, and C-peptide levels, but negatively associated with testosterone levels. *Metabolism* 39:897–901, 1990.

110. Shah, M., P. J. Hannan, and R. W. Jeffery. Secular trends in body mass index in the adult population communities from the upper mid-western part of the Minnesota Herat Health Program. *Int. J. Obes.* 15:449–453, 1991.

111. Shah, M., and R. W. Jeffery. Is obesity due to overeating and inactivity, or to a defective metabolic rate? A review. *Ann. Behav. Med.* 13:73–81, 1991.

112. Shepard, R. J. Nutritional benefits of exercise. *J. Sports Med.* 29:83–90, 1989.

113. Sjostrom, L. Impacts of body weight, body composition, and adipose tissue distribution on morbidity and mortality. A. J. Stunkard and T. A. Wadden (eds). *Obesity: Theory and Therapy, 2nd ed*. New York: Raven Press, 1993, pp. 13–41.

114. Slattery, M. L., A. Mcdonald, D. E. Bild, et al. Associations of body fat and its distribution with dietary intake, physical activity, alcohol, and smoking in blacks and whites. *Am. J. Clin. Nutr.* 55:943–950, 1992.

115. Sobal, J., and A. J. Stunkard. Socioeconomic status and obesity. A review of the literature. *Psychol. Bull* 105:260–275, 1989.

116. Sparrow, D., G. A. Borkan, S. G. Gerzof, C. Wisniewski, and C. K. Silbert. Relationship of fat distribution in glucose tolerance. Results of computed tomography in male participants of the Normative Aging Study. *Diabetes* 35:411–415, 1986.

117. Stefanick, M. L. Exercise and weight control. *Exerc. Sports Sci. Rev.* 21:363–396, 1993.

118. Stephens, T., and C. L. Craig. Fitness and activity measurement in the 1981 Canada Fitness Survey. T. Stephens and C. L. Craig (eds). *Proceedings of the Workshop on Assessing Physical Fitness and Activity Patterns in General Population Surveys*. Hyattsville, MD: National Center for Health Statistics, 16–20, 1985.

119. Stephens, T., D. R. Jacobs, C. C. White. A descriptive epidemiology of leisure-time physical activity. *Public Health Rep.* 100:147–158, 1985.

120. Stephenson, M. G., A. S. Levy, N. L. Sass, and W. E. McGarvey. 1985 NHIS findings: nutrition knowledge and baseline data for the weight-loss objectives. *Public Health Rep.* 102:61–67, 1987.

121. Stern, M. P., J. K. Patterson, B. D. Mitchell, S. M. Haffner and H. P. Hazuda. Overweight and mortality in Mexican Americans. *Int. J. Obes.* 14:623–629, 1990.
122. Taylor H. L., D. R. Jacobs, B. Schucker, et al. A questionnaire for the assessment of leisure time physical activities. *J. Chronic Dis.* 31:741–755, 1978.
123. Thompson, J. K., G. J. Jarvie, B. B. Lahey, and K. J. Cureton. Exercise and obesity: etiology, physiology, and intervention. *Psychol. Bull.* 91:55–79, 1982.
124. Tremblay, A., J.-P. Després, J. Maheux, et al. Normalization of the metabolic profile in obese women by exercise and low fat diet. *Med. Sci. Sports Exerc.* 23:1326–1331, 1991.
125. Tremblay, A., J.-P. Després, C. Leblanc, et al. Effect of intensity of physical activity on body fatness and fat distribution. *Am. J. Clin. Nutr.* 51:153–157, 1990.
126. Tremblay, A., E. Fontaine, E. T. Poehlman, D. Mitchell, L. Perron, and C. Bouchard. The effect of exercise-training on resting metabolic rate in lean and moderately obese individuals. *Int. J. Obes.* 10:511–517, 1986.
127. Tremblay, A., J.-P. Després, C. Leblanc, and C. Bouchard. Sex dimorphism in fat loss in response to exercise-training. *J. Obes. Weight Regul.* 3:193–203, 1984.
128. Triosi R. J., J. W. Heinold, P. S. Vokonas, and S. T. Weiss. Cigarette smoking, dietary intake, and physical activity: effects on body fat distribution—the Normative Aging Study. *Am. J. Clin. Nutr.* 53:1104–1111, 1953.
129. Tryon, W. W. Activity as a function of body weight. *Am. J. Clin. Nutr.* 36:936–942, 1982.
130. United States Department of Health and Human Services. The Surgeon General's report on nutrition and health. Washington DC: US Government Printing Office. DHHS Publication (PHS) 88–50210, 1988.
131. Vague, J. The degree of masculine differentiation of obesities: a factor determining predisposition to diabetes, atherosclerosis, gout, and uric calculus disease. *Am. J. Clin. Nutr.* 4:20–34, 1956.
132. Vena, J. E., S. Graham, M. Zielezny, M. K. Swanson, R. E. Barnes, and J. Nolan. Life-time occupational exercise and colon cancer. *Am. J. Epidemiol.* 122:357–365, 1985.
133. Volkmar, F. R., A. J. Stunkard, J. Woolston, and R. A. Bailey. High attrition rates in commercial weight reduction programs. *Arch. Intern. Med.* 141:426–428, 1981.
134. Voorrips, L. E., K. A. P. M. Lemmink, M. J. G. van Heuvelen, P. Bult, and W. A. van Staveren. The physical condition of elderly women differing in habitual physical activity. *Med. Sci. Sports Exerc.* 25:1152–1157, 1993.
135. Voorrips, L. E., J. H. H. Meijers, P. Sol, J. C. Seidell, and W. A. van Staveren. History of body weight and physical activity of elderly women differing in current physical activity. *Int. J. Obes.* 16:199–205, 1991.
136. Voorrips, L. E., A. C. J. Ravelli, P. C. A. Dongelmans, P. Deurenberg, and W. A. van Staveren. A physical activity questionnaire for the elderly. *Med. Sci. Sports Exerc.* 23:974–979, 1991.
137. Voorrips, L. E., W. A. van Staveren, J. G. A. J. Hautvast. Are physically active women in a better nutritonal condition than their sedentary peers? *Eur. J. Clin. Nutr.* 45:545–552, 1991.
138. Waaler, H. T. Height, weight and mortality: the Norwegian experience. *Acta Med. Scand. Suppl.* 679:1–56, 1984.
139. Wadden T. A., A. J. Stunkard, and K. D. Brownell. Very low calorie diets: their efficacy, safety, and future. *Ann. Intern. Med.* 99:675–684, 1983.
140. Wahrenberg, H., J. Bolinder, and P. Arner. Andrenergic regulation of lipolysis in human fat cells during exercise. *Eur. J. Clin. Invest.* 21:534–541, 1991.
141. Williamson D. F., J. Madans, R. F. Anda, J. C. Kleinman, H. S. Kahn, and T. Byers. Recreational physical activity and 10-year weight change in a US national cohort. *Int. J. Obes.* 17:279–286, 1993.
142. Williamson, D. F., H. S. Kahn, P. L. Remington, and R. F. Anda. The 10-year incidence of overweight and major weight gain in US adults. *Arch. Intern. Med.* 150:665–672, 1990.

143. Wilmore, J. H. Body composition in sport and exercise: directions for future research. *Med. Sci. Sports Exerc.* 15:21–31, 1983.

144. Wing, R. R., K. A. Matthews, L. H. Kuller, E. N. Meilahn, and P. Plantinga. Waist to hip ratio in middle-aged women. Associations with behavioral and psychosocial factors and with changes in cardiovascular risk factors. *Arteriosclerosis Thrombosis* 11:1250–1257, 1991.

145. Wolfe, R. R., S. Klein, F. Carraro, and J. M. Weber. Role of triglyceride-fatty acid cycle in controlling fat metabolism in humans during and after exercise. *Am. J. Physiol.* 258:E382–E389, 1990.

146. Woo, R., J. S. Garrow, and F. X. Pi-Sunyer. Effect of exercise on sponaneous calorie intake in obesity. *Am. J. Clin. Nutr.* 36:470–477, 1982.

10
Human Skeletal Muscle Metabolism in Health and Disease: Utility of Magnetic Resonance Spectroscopy

JANE A. KENT-BRAUN, Ph.D.
ROBERT G. MILLER, M.D.
MICHAEL W. WEINER, M.D.

The goal of this review is to acquaint the reader with various applications of the magnetic resonance spectroscopy (MRS) technique to the study of human skeletal muscle metabolism. This is intended to be a comprehensive review, beginning with studies of muscle energetics, fatigue, and other "basic" questions, and progressing to studies of the alterations in muscle metabolism produced by disease.

The first in vivo magnetic resonance spectroscopy studies of human skeletal muscle were reported in the early 1980s [37, 47, 51, 135, 139]. Since that time, access to this technique has broadened; its use has now expanded into areas as diverse as those encompassed by the fields of biochemistry, medicine and exercise science. The advantages and limitations of this technique have been delineated. Better methods have been developed. The purpose of this paper is to review, in terms of both breadth and significance of contribution, the body of knowledge that has emerged from the application of MRS to the study of exercising human skeletal muscle. The first part of the review deals with studies of healthy human muscle; the second portion concerns the effects associated with various disease states. The increase in the number of studies of human skeletal muscle that use the MRS technique has been exponential; thus, this review will not be all-inclusive. For an expanded review of clinical MRS studies of skeletal muscle, see ref. 74. To establish a common ground for the discussion of these studies, we will begin with a brief description of the technique of MRS. A full description of the technological development of human MRS is beyond the scope of this review; therefore, papers detailing technique-oriented progress will not be included.

Studies of human skeletal muscle using MRS require a superconducting magnet, a spectrometer, and nonmagnetic exercise equipment (Fig. 10.1). Data are obtained with a nonmagnetic coil, the size and shape of which determine the volume of tissue that will be sampled. MRS uses radiofrequency waves transmitted through the coil in the presence of the static magnetic field to sample the relative concentrations of metabolites containing the nucleus of interest (e.g., phosphorus, carbon, proton). The sensitivity of

FIGURE 10.1.

Typical MRS exercise system. The surface coil is placed on the tibialis anterior mus-
cle in this case. The coil and volume of interest must be located in the isocenter of the
superconducting magnet (dark circle *in center). In addition to the metabolic mea-*
surements obtained with MRS, simultaneous force and electromyographic measure-
ments can also be made during exercise.

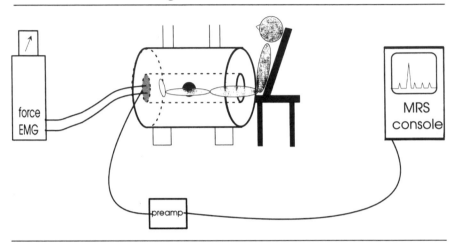

the MRS measurement varies with the nucleus studied. The quality of the
signal depends upon the size of the volume studied, the total data acquisition time, and the adequacy of the radiofrequency shielding in use. Figure
10.2 shows a typical phosphorus (^{31}P) MRS spectrum from resting human
muscle. The frequency (location on the x axis) of each resonance (peak)
relates information regarding the identity of the compound. The area under each peak indicates its relative concentration. In Figure 10.2, the peaks
from inorganic phosphate (P_i), phosphocreatine (PCr), and the three
phosphates of adenosine triphosphate (ATP) are all clearly visible. Peak
areas can be quantitated using curve-fitting programs designed for this
purpose. The data can then be expressed as a simple ratio (e.g., P_i/PCr)
or an estimate of metabolite concentrations can be made. During muscular contractions, PCr decreases and P_i increases; ATP remains unchanged
except during very high-intensity exercise. Adenosine diphosphate (ADP)
is present in the muscle in micromolar concentrations, and is therefore
not visible in the ^{31}P spectrum. Intracellular pH can be determined from
the chemical shift (i.e., the distance) of P_i from PCr. The concentrations
of proton (H^+) and monovalent phosphate ($H_2PO_4^-$) can also be calculated based on P_i and pH. Because MRS is a noninvasive technique, sampling can be continuous. Typical time averaging for a single spectrum is in
the range of 10–60 s.

FIGURE 10.2.

Representative phosphorus spectrum from the resting tibialis anterior muscle of a healthy human. This spectrum was obtained with a 3 cm × 5 cm surface coil taped over the belly of the muscle. Total acquisition time was 5 min. Peaks from inorganic phosphate (P_i), phosphocreatine (PCr) and γ-, α-, and β-adenosine triphosphate (ATP) are clearly resolved. The area under each peak can be estimated using a curve-fitting process, and the relative concentration of each metabolite may then be calculated. Alternatively, the metabolites may more simply be expressed as a ratio (e.g., P_i/PCr). The chemical shift (i.e., distance) between PCr and P_i can be used to calculate intracellular pH.

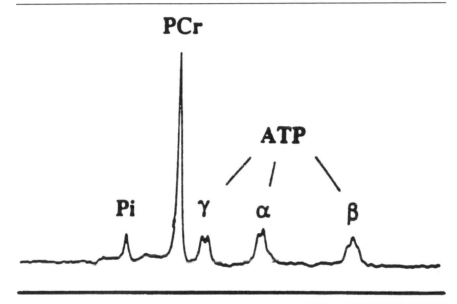

The biggest advantage provided by MRS is the capacity to make repeated, noninvasive measurements of muscle energy metabolism. Data can be collected continuously before, during, and after dynamic or isometric exercise. Under the appropriate conditions, comparisons of metabolic capacity can be made between different populations, and in the same persons before and after an intervention (e.g., exercise training). Of course, there are also disadvantages to this technique, one of which is that the muscle of interest must be located in the isocenter of the magnet. As magnet opening sizes increase, this has become less of a problem. Movement artifact due to muscle contractions can reduce the quality of the MRS signal. Although MRS is useful for measuring relative changes in energy metabolites, absolute quantitation of metabolite concentration is difficult. Likewise, in vivo studies of metabolic regulation in humans are complicated by a lack of information regarding muscle fiber composition, activation, and sample volume. However, studies designed to test theories developed in vitro under more controlled conditions are valuable for determining the consistency with which a theory fits experimental data.

HEALTHY MUSCLE METABOLISM

Muscle Energetics

Most of the early applications of ^{31}P MRS were for the study of intracellular bioenergetics. The metabolites involved in energy production (ADP + PCr + H$^+$ → ATP + creatine) and utilization (ATP → ADP + P$_i$ + energy) are related via the creatine kinase reaction. With certain assumptions, the creatine kinase equilibrium may be used to estimate intracellular [ADP]. In general, the energy state of the muscle is often represented by the ratio PCr/P$_i$ (or, conversely, P$_i$/PCr). Because ^{31}P MRS provides an opportunity to monitor these metabolites continuously and noninvasively, theories previously developed in vitro could be tested with the MRS technique.

Intramuscular oxidative metabolism has been studied using progressive exercise during which a metabolic steady state (i.e., substrate and oxygen are not limiting) is achieved at each work level [37–40]. Chance et al. [38] determined that the relationship between work rate and "energy cost" (expressed as P$_i$/PCr) could be analyzed as a hyperbolic Michaelis-Menten function that represented mitochondrial function. An example of this analysis is presented in Figure 10.3. The creatine kinase equilibrium can be used to estimate cytosolic [ADP] from the changes in P$_i$/PCr. The initial, linear portion of this relationship between work and P$_i$/PCr (or [ADP]) was similar to that observed in isolated mitochondrial preparations, and thus provided in vivo evidence of [ADP] regulation of skeletal muscle oxidative phosphorylation during relatively low work intensities [37]. This relationship is shown in the box in Figure 10.3. In a subsequent study, it was observed that the slope of work versus P$_i$/PCr was increased in trained relative to untrained muscle [40, 75]. In trained muscle, the higher slope of work versus P$_i$/PCr reflected an increased capacity for the mitochondria to keep pace with the progressively increasing demands for ATP. The theoretical relationship between work and P$_i$/PCr was also calculated for conditions where the metabolic controller is not only ADP (e.g., oxygen, P$_i$, NADH).

As a result of the early work of Chance and colleagues, this type of progressive, steady-state exercise protocol has since been used to evaluate muscle performance and oxidative metabolism in healthy subjects and in clinical populations. However, comparisons between different populations, or the same subjects before and after intervention, require adjustments for differences in muscle strength. Thus, comparisons at any given workload require normalization for differences in strength; at the same absolute work-

FIGURE 10.3.

Schematic of the general relationship between power or force and P_i/PCr (or [ADP]) during progressive exercise. As the workload increases, there is a concomitant increase in P_i/PCr as the muscle responds to the increased energy demand. The initial, linear portion of this curve (workload <40% maximum) can be used to estimate the oxidative potential of the muscle (box). In trained compared with untrained subjects, there is less of an increase in P_i/PCr at any given relative workload, thus indicating an improved ability to keep pace with energy needs by means of oxidative phosphorylation. In contrast, in persons with disease that impairs muscle metabolism (either directly or indirectly), the initial slope of work versus P_i/PCr is decreased, indicating a poor capacity for oxidative metabolism.

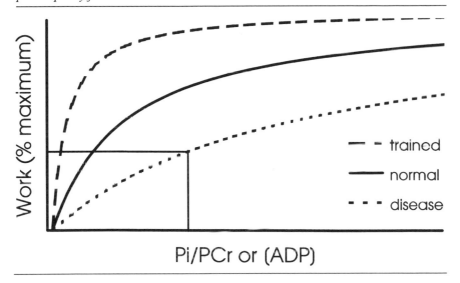

load, a person with a smaller muscle will be working at a much higher relative load. Thus, the metabolic demand will be relatively higher. To adjust for differences in muscle mass, changes in force during exercise can be expressed relative to the preexercise force from a maximum voluntary contraction (MVC). Alternatively, force can be normalized to muscle cross-sectional area (obtained with magnetic resonance imaging [e.g., ref. 123]). Although these adjustments were not always made in the past, future studies should include them to provide for better interpretation of the results.

An important early study undertook the comparison of metabolite concentrations measured with the muscle biopsy technique and with MRS [166]. It was observed that, although total P_i + PCr in the forearm muscle was similar with both techniques, [P_i] was higher and [PCr] was lower in the biopsy relative to MRS measurement. The authors suggested that this difference was due to the hydrolysis of PCr during the time taken to freeze the biopsy sample, and that estimation of metabolite concentrations with MRS may, for this reason, be more accurate in most cases. These investigators also tested the theory of [ADP] control of glycolysis developed from in vitro studies by measuring the independent effects of ischemia (by means of cuff occlusion) and muscle contraction on PCr, P_i, and pH. During exercise, there were significant decreases in PCr (and thus increases in ADP) and pH. However, during ischemia with no exercise, there was a decrease in PCr and a slight increase in pH. The lack of decrease in pH during ischemia indicates that no significant glycolysis occurred. Thus, the onset of glycolysis appeared to be associated closely with the contraction itself; increased [ADP] and [P_i] during ischemia were insufficient to activate it. These results recently have been confirmed in the tibialis muscle [134]. After high-intensity calf exercise (70–90% MVC), the recovery of PCr, P_i, pH, and calculated [ADP] was delayed until the cuff was released. The authors concluded that, despite the presence of strong metabolic stimulators of glycolysis (e.g., P_i, ADP), glycolysis and glycogenolysis did not proceed under ischemic conditions. Thus, these studies suggest that the contractile process itself, rather than the metabolic state of the muscle, is regulating glycolysis under these conditions.

The effects of reduced blood flow on the changes in P_i, PCr, and pH during wrist flexion exercise have been studied in healthy control subjects [165]. A progressive exercise protocol was performed with and without partial cuff occlusion. Flow reduction (40–60%) resulted in higher P_i/PCr and lower pH at each workload in these subjects, consistent with an oxygen limitation under these conditions. These results demonstrated that MRS can detect hypoperfusion during exercise, and therefore is a clinically useful tool for the study of peripheral vascular disease (see below).

Saturation transfer was applied to the study of the kinetics of the creatine kinase reaction during forearm exercise in healthy volunteers [137]. Under steady-state exercise conditions, it was determined that the flux from PCr to ATP was significantly lower than that predicted from in vitro animal experiments. The authors suggested that this discrepancy might have been due to an underestimation of the concentration of ADP. Of further note, the intrinsic spin-lattice relaxation time (T1) for PCr in resting muscle was reported to be 4.76 s, and this value did not change significantly during exercise.

An estimation of the ATP cost of force production was made [32]. High time resolution spectra (1–8 s) were obtained from the gastrocnemius/soleus muscle group during maximal isometric plantarflexion exercise. Muscle cross-sectional area was measured using magnetic resonance imaging (MRI). The rate of ATP production from the creatine kinase reaction was estimated from the rate of PCr decrease at the onset of exercise, the rate of ATP production from oxidative phosphorylation was estimated from the initial rate of recovery of PCr after exercise, and the rate of ATP production from anaerobic glycolysis was estimated based upon the rate of change of pH (with assumptions of buffer capacity and H^+ production per unit ATP turnover). Although a weakness of this study was a lack of information regarding the portion of muscle mass that contributed to force production relative to the muscle volume from which the metabolic data were obtained, this work reflects the potential of MRS for understanding the relative roles for each pathway of ATP production during muscular work.

ATP utilization rates were also estimated during ischemic, electrically stimulated exercise of the wrist flexor muscles during which pH did not fall [30]. Both PCr degradation and resynthesis followed monoexponential time courses. Because PCr resynthesis after exercise is primarily by means of oxidative phosphorylation, maximal ATP synthesis rates from oxidative phosphorylation were then calculated from the rate of PCr recovery after cessation of exercise and release of cuff occlusion. These results demonstrated the feasibility of quantitative noninvasive assessments of muscle oxidative capacity under conditions in which muscle recruitment and nonoxidative sources of ATP production are controlled.

Proton production, efflux, and buffering during exercise and recovery have been studied using ^{31}P MRS. By comparing the recoveries of PCr and pH in healthy subjects, and in [ATP] during ischemic exercise in McArdle's subjects, Kemp et al. were able to estimate an effective intramuscular buffer capacity of 20–30 mmol/liter/pH [69]. The authors then used this estimate to calculate ATP production during exercise and proton efflux during recovery. The results of this analysis suggested that the rate of ATP production is associated with [Pi], and proton efflux from the muscle is pH dependent.

In summary, ^{31}P MRS has proven useful for the noninvasive investigation of the relationship between muscle performance and the supply of energy for this performance. By quantitating the temporal alterations of each metabolic parameter, the nature of the relationship between work and the metabolic pathways may be inferred.

Muscle Fatigue

Muscle fatigue, generally defined as a decline in force-generating capacity, can arise from a variety of causes. The precise mechanisms of muscle fatigue are not known, although it is now clear that the source(s) of fatigue depends in part upon the type of exercise performed. In 1986, Taylor et al. reported one of the early studies of muscle fatigue using ^{31}P MRS [152]. The goal of this study was to determine the effect of ATP depletion during fatigue produced by moderate and high-intensity forearm exercise. High-intensity exercise resulted in a greater change in intramuscular metabolism; PCr depletion exceeded 80% and intracellular pH fell below 6.2. Depletion of ATP was also observed under these extreme conditions. The recovery of PCr, P_i, and pH was slower after high-intensity exercise compared with moderate exercise, and ATP recovery was much slower than that of the other metabolites. These results were interpreted to indicate that intense, fatiguing exercise could lead to severe metabolic depletion associated with slowed recovery.

The relationship between muscle fatigue and metabolism has since been studied during various exercise protocols. Wilson et al. [169] observed a strong linear relationship between fatigue and the increase of monovalent phosphate ($H_2PO_4^-$) during maximum contractions of the wrist flexor muscles in healthy volunteers. Their use of several different exercise protocols provided evidence that the relationship between $H_2PO_4^-$ and fatigue was stronger and more consistent than was the relationship between pH and fatigue. In a different study, intermittent isometric exercise of the adductor pollicis resulted in more gradual changes in metabolites and force compared with sustained exercise [105]. However, during both intermittent and sustained exercise, force was more strongly related to proton [H^+] and [$H_2PO_4^-$] than to either either [PCr] or [P_i]. Therefore, the authors concluded that H^+ and $H_2PO_4^-$ play important roles in the development of muscle fatigue. Similar results were later reported for the less fatigable tibialis anterior muscle [162]. An examination of the recovery of force and metabolites after fatiguing exercise indicated that $H_2PO_4^-$ was most clearly related to maximal force-generating capacity during recovery from fatigue [33]. Cady and coworkers [34] also reported a linear relationship between $H_2PO_4^-$ and fatigue, in this case in the first dorsal interosseous muscle of healthy subjects. No such relationship was observed in a subject with myophosphorylase deficiency who could not utilize muscle glycogen. These researchers noted a dissociation between fatigue and pH, particularly during the recovery period. In a parallel study, they provided evidence that this pH-independent component to fatigue may be related to the slowed rate of force relaxation observed during fatigue, as suggested by a 50% slowing of relaxation in fatigued muscle at a time when pH was unchanged [35]. In summary, these studies suggest that muscle fatigue developed during intense exercise may be due, in part, to an accumulation of metabolic byproducts.

However, in a follow-up study of fatigue exercise at different submaximal force levels, there was no strong relationship between adductor pollicis fatigue and the change in any metabolite [120]. A similar observation was made in the gastrocnemius muscle during progressive exercise to fatigue [170]. By using a rapid MRS scan rate (2 s), another group of investigators was able to detect a nonlinear relationship between plantarflexor fatigue and H^+, P_i, and $H_2PO_4^-$ at the onset of exercise [45]. Thus, these studies suggest that a strong association between fatigue and intramuscular metabolism is not observed under all conditions.

To clarify further the importance of metabolism in fatigue, Baker et al. [13] investigated the roles of metabolic and nonmetabolic factors during fatigue induced with two different types of exercise. MVCs of the ankle dorsiflexors sustained for 2 min and intermittent MVCs performed for 15–20 min resulted in similar levels of fatigue. The sustained MVC was associated with significant increases in P_i, whereas the change in P_i during the intermittent protocol was much less, and force recovery was significantly slower. These results suggested that short-duration fatigue may have been due to metabolic inhibition of the contractile process, whereas long-duration fatigue may be due to nonmetabolic factors such as failure of excitation-contraction coupling. In a subsequent study of the effects of muscle length on energy use during dorsiflexion exercise, the same investigators observed a better relationship between fatigue and both P_i and $H_2PO_4^-$ than between fatigue and H^+ at both optimal and shortened muscle lengths [12]. Finally, the same investigators observed an important metabolic component to fatigue during submaximal, but very rapid, isometric contractions of the dorsiflexors, during which time there was also significant slowing of voluntary force development [109].

In summary, a series of MRS studies of muscle fatigue suggests a role for metabolic inhibition of the contractile process in the development of fatigue during some types of exercise. In general, it appears that fatigue during high-intensity exercise is most likely to be associated with changes in metabolites, whereas fatigue during submaximal exercise also arises from nonmetabolic sources such as impairment of muscular activation (see below).

COMBINING MRS AND ELECTROMYOGRAPHY TO STUDY FATIGUE. It is possible to make simultaneous measurements of metabolism and the electromyographic response to exercise [72, 77, 107, 158]. Combining MRS with surface electromyography (EMG) ultimately will provide a more thorough understanding of the complex events that occur during the development of human muscle fatigue. In 1987, Miller et al. [107] reported the time course of change in force, pH, PCr, the compound muscle action potential (elicited with a twitch stimulus), and the rectified integrated electromyogram (RIEMG) in the adductor pollicis muscle of healthy subjects. During fatigue, force fell by 90%, pH decreased to 6.4, and PCr was nearly depleted. Both neuromuscular efficiency (force/RIEMG) and the compound muscle action potential also decreased during fatigue. There were three phases of recovery after exercise, which suggested three components to fatigue. First, changes in the compound muscle action potential indicated a rapidly recovering alteration of muscle membrane excitation and impulse propagation; second, recovery of PCr and pH suggested a more slowly recovering alteration in the metabolic state of the muscle; and third, the slow recovery of neuromuscular efficiency was consistent with a long-duration impairment of excitation-contraction coupling. The observation of impaired excitation-contraction coupling was further investigated during low-intensity exercise in the adductor pollicis and tibialis anterior muscles [118]. During fatigue, the fall in twitch tension was markedly greater than that of the compound muscle action potential, PCr, or pH, and recovery of twitch tension was quite slow. These results were interpreted to indicate that low-intensity exercise is associated with a nonmetabolic form of fatigue, and that failure of excitation-contraction coupling is possible with this type of exercise.

It has been suggested that changes in the EMG signal during muscle fatigue may be due to feedback from the accumulation of metabolic byproducts within the muscle fatigue. This question has been examined by combining MRS and EMG [21, 158]. During fatiguing exercise of the tibialis anterior muscle, the root-mean-square of the surface EMG signal fell precipitously once PCr decreased below 60–70% of resting level, and pH fell below 6.75 [158]. The median frequency of the EMG signal fell linearly with pH (r=0.82). These results again demonstrated the technical capacity for these measurements, and began an exploration of the relationship between fatigue, metabolism, and the electromyogram. Laurent et al. [79] continued this exploration with a study of the associations between muscle metabolism and the change in mean power frequency of the EMG signal during fatiguing exercise in the calf muscles. They observed significant associations between changes in mean power frequency and both $H_2PO_4^-$ and H^+ during exercise, although the regression coefficients for these associations were not high. The authors concluded that changes in EMG signal during fatigue may be directly or indirectly linked to muscle metabolism. However, the poor (although statistically significant) correlation coefficients suggest that other factors must also play a role in the change in EMG signal during fatigue.

In summary, these studies demonstrate the utility of combining MRS and EMG in studies of muscle performance. Unfortunately, the relative contributions of (a) metabolic inhibition of the contractile process and (b) activation failure to the development of human skeletal muscle fatigue remain unclear. We have recently developed an approach that combines MRS and EMG in an effort to quantitate muscle activation, metabolism, and fatigue during isometric exercise in several clinical populations [72, 77, 108, 140].

Rest-Exercise-Rest Transitions
An early MRS study on the transition from rest to work described the changes in PCr and P_i at the onset of wrist flexion exercise [116]. Four men were studied several times during repetitive bulb-squeezing. While intrasubject variability in the measurement of pH, PCr, and P_i was high (approximately 20–40%), within-subject variability (i.e., repeatability) was quite low (less than 10%) for these measurements. The changes in P_i and PCr during exercise followed an exponential time course, and equilibration occurred after approximately 50 seconds. Proton and ATP were also changed during exercise, but the time course of these changes lagged behind those of P_i and

PCr. The results of this early study demonstrated the utility of monitoring changes in high-energy phosphates at the onset of exercise using ^{31}P MRS. Marsh et al. [91] recently studied the on-off transients from rest to steady-state exercise and back to rest. Under conditions in which ATP and pH did not change, their results indicated that PCr kinetics were best fit by a single, rather than double, exponential. They also observed that the time constant for the decrease in PCr at the onset of exercise was the same as that for the recovery of PCr after exercise (approximately 30 s), and that this time constant was similar to that previously reported for oxygen consumption measured during cycle ergometry. The results of this study suggest that the monoexponential on and off transients for PCr kinetics may be useful for quantitating muscle oxidative capacity. Yoshida and Watari [172] investigated the effect of exercise intensity on PCr and P_i kinetics at the onset of exercise and recovery. They observed that both the PCr and P_i time constants at the onset of exercise were independent of exercise intensity. However, at the end of exercise, the time constant for P_i recovery was slowed by the lower pH generated during higher-intensity exercise.

The effects of a "warm up" on the attainment of steady-state exercise conditions have been investigated [80]. Warming up on a cycle ergometer before performing high-intensity (80% maximum force) plantar flexion exercise resulted in lower steady-state levels of P_i/PCr and higher pH. In separate experiments, a warm-up resulted in less tissue deoxygenation during exercise. Interestingly, submaximal exercise protocol of progressively increasing intensity such as those used by Chance and coworkers [38, 76] resulted in a steady-state P_i/PCr level similar to that obtained in the "warmed-up" condition. Thus, as is the case for whole-body exercise, it appears that the intramuscular metabolic response to the transition from rest to work is dependent upon the initial exercise intensity.

Metabolic Transitions during Exercise
The ability to monitor intramuscular metabolism noninvasively throughout the time course of progressive exercise has led to some interesting observations. The role of peripheral metabolism in the development of ventilatory and lactate thresholds was the focus of a study by Systrom et al. [143]. Fourteen healthy volunteers performed plantar flexion exercise of progressively increasing intensity during which ventilation, venous lactate, and intracellular pH were measured. The results showed the development of an intracellular pH threshold concurrent with the ventilatory and lactate thresholds during this progressive exercise protocol. The authors concluded that the developing acidity in the muscle during exercise may explain the lactate threshold, and could also play an important feedback role for the increase in ventilation at this point. They also suggested that the intracellular pH threshold was consistent with a threshold for glycolytic metabolism.

Marsh et al. expanded upon the topic of intracellular metabolic transition points, or thresholds, in a 1991 study of the wrist flexor muscles of healthy volunteers [92]. Dynamic, progressive exercise was used to elicit gradual changes in work, P_i/PCr, and pH. The results indicated that, at approximately 60% of maximum force, both the log of P_i/PCr and pH demonstrated an abrupt increase in their rates of change. The data were fit to a bilinear model and coincident thresholds were demonstrated. As in the Systrom study [143], these "thresholds" were considered to be consistent with the possibility of a role for intracellular events in causing the ventilatory and lactate thresholds observed during whole-body exercise.

In contrast to the Marsh study, Kent-Braun et al. [76] recently reported the finding of temporally displaced inflection points in P_i/PCr and H^+ during progressive exercise to fatigue. Isometric exercise of the dorsiflexors was used to demonstrate a sequence of three metabolic phases during the transition from rest to fatiguing level of exercise. The length of the first phase, during which energy for contraction was produced primarily by oxidative phosphorylation, was significantly related to the "oxidative potential" of the muscle (i.e., the initial slope of force vs. P_i/PCr). This first phase was followed by a second, intermediate phase during which P_i/PCr was increasing at a more rapid rate, whereas H^+ remained relatively unchanged. The onset of the third phase, during which glycolytic sources of ATP begin to contribute more significantly to energy production, was observed as an inflection in H^+ with continued steady increases in P_i/PCr. It was this third, non–steady-state phase that was associated with muscle fatigue.

In summary, these studies demonstrated the utility of ^{31}P MRS for the study of the relationships between oxidative and glycolytic metabolism during progressive exercise. By comparing the time course of change for metabolites involved primarily in either oxidative or glycolytic metabolism, insight may be gained into the interplay between these pathways. Unfortunately, because of the heterogeneity of fiber types as well as the changes in fiber recruitment during progressive exercise, absolute quantitation of metabolic regulation during this type of exercise is difficult.

Metabolic Recovery from Exercise

Measuring the rate of PCr recovery after exercise provides an index of the oxidative capacity of the muscle that is independent of work level (provided pH does not decrease significantly). Thus, PCr recovery measurements are simpler than comparisons of the metabolic change observed during exercise, where measurements of force and normalization to muscle mass must be performed. The use of PCr recovery rates to indicate the capacity for mitochondrial oxidative phosphorylation was originally based upon biopsy data [58]. A theoretical model for the observed monoexponential recovery of PCr and its relationship to oxidative phosphorylation was developed by Meyer [104], and has subsequently been verified and applied in many MRS studies of human skeletal muscle [e.g., 69, 73, 98]. The effect of mild and intense forearm exercise on the recovery rates of PCr, pH, and ADP indicated that PCr resynthesis rates are markedly influenced by the degree of acidosis that develops during exercise [8]. In fact, in another study of PCr recovery kinetics, it was demonstrated that the relationship between the rate of PCr recovery and the extent of acidosis during exercise is essentially linear [23]. Thus, because of the influence of acidosis on PCr resynthesis, it is important that studies of PCr recovery after exercise be conducted using exercise protocols in which the drop in pH is minimal and similar in all groups being compared. As a result of these early studies, the quantitation of PCr recovery rate has become a valuable tool for the noninvasive assessment of skeletal muscle oxidative capacity in various populations (Fig. 10.4).

Monitoring P_i recovery requires a very rapid sampling rate because the P_i signal is quickly lost in the baseline of the phosphorus spectrum. The recovery of P_i after wrist flexion exercise has been reported to be stoichiometric with that of PCr, except in cases of intense exercise where there may

FIGURE 10.4.

Schematic of PCr recovery after exercise. Phosphocreatine resynthesis after muscular contraction is accomplished primarily by means of oxidative phosphorylation. Individual data are fit to a single exponential and the half-time of recovery is used as an index of oxidative metabolism. This analysis requires exercise conditions in which PCr declines to approximately 50% of initial with no significant decline in intramuscular pH. In trained subjects, PCr recovery is very fast compared with normal subjects. In subjects with disease that affects oxidative capacity, the rate of PCr recovery is slowed.

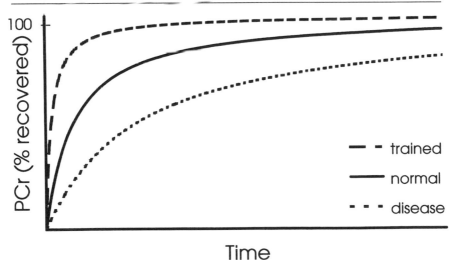

be a loss of adenine nucleotide [23]. The authors suggested that this was evidence for P_i "trapping" in the glycogenolytic pathway. Iotti et al. [59, 60] studied the recovery of P_i after plantar flexion exercise in 10 healthy adults. Similar to Arnold et al. [8], these authors found a dependence of the initial rate of P_i recovery on the extent of acidity developed during exercise. In addition, they reported a bilinear pattern of P_i recovery; the first phase independent of pH and the second, slow phase pH dependent. Unlike reports of PCr recovery, in this study, P_i recovery was not well fit to a monoexponential. Interestingly, the authors interpreted their results to indicate that the recovery of P_i is limited by the rate of P_i transport into the mitochondria, rather than by the rate of mitochondrial oxidative phosphorylation.

Heterogeneity in the MRS Spectrum

Interpretation of muscle performance and metabolic data obtained using MRS has been clouded by the problem of heterogeneity within the MRS sample volume. There are two sources of this heterogeneity: (a) the variable contributions of resting and exercising fibers to the spectrum, and (b) the variable metabolic characteristics of Type I and Type II fibers, both of which contribute to the spectrum. Localization techniques and improved coil design have all but eliminated the first problem. Efforts to reduce the second problem by clarifying the metabolic response of different fiber pools have provided interesting results.

Insight as to the source of heterogeneity in the MRS signal has been obtained by the application of localization techniques that allow nonexercising muscle to be eliminated from the sample. This is accomplished by combining imaging and spectroscopy methods. These techniques can also be used to study the metabolic variability within a single muscle by allowing the investigator to select distinct regions of a single muscle for spectral analysis. For example, the metabolic response of the medial gastrocnemius may thus be compared with that of the lateral gastrocnemius. Superficial and deep portions of the same muscle may also be compared.

Chemical shift imaging in the forearm muscles of healthy volunteers during finger flexion exercise was used to obtain metabolite maps that localized the regions of active muscle during exercise [119]. The magnitude of change in PCr, P_i, and pH was measured in the ^{31}P spectra from each region. By using localization, Jeneson et al. [61] demonstrated heterogeneity within the flexor digitorum profundus muscle during finger flexion with varying numbers of fingers. The use of this technique enabled the investigators to determine the recruitment pattern of this muscle during different exercise protocols. These studies demonstrate the possibility of spatially localizing and then quantitating the heterogeneity of the metabolic response to exercise that is due to variable recruitment patterns.

Resolving the heterogeneity that arises from variable fiber type metabolic characteristics requires a different approach. As mentioned above, the location of the P_i peak relative to PCr can be used to calculate intramuscular pH. During exercise in which there is a decrease in pH, the P_i peak shifts toward PCr. Under conditions where there is a range of pH values in the muscle sample (e.g., because of the different metabolic capacities of Type I and Type II fibers), the P_i peak will broaden. If the decrease in pH in any given pool of fibers is severe enough, the P_i peak can be resolved into two or three peaks (Fig. 10.5). Although fiber typing with this method remains problematic because of the issues of recruitment and sample volume, information can be obtained regarding the relative heterogeneity of a muscle's metabolic response to exercise.

Although the first "splitting" of a P_i peak can be seen in Figure 10.1 of Taylor et al. in 1984 [150], it was not until Park et al. [128] reported the appearance of a "split" P_i peak during exercise at 47% MVC that this phenomenon first received attention. The two P_i peaks were associated with two pools of fibers, one working oxidatively and one working with a greater contribution of energy from glycolytic metabolism. These two pools showed different pH values equivalent to 7.0 and 6.2. The authors concluded that these pools represented the metabolic conditions for Type I (oxidative) fibers in the high-pH pool and Type II (glycolytic) fibers in the low-pH pool. This study was followed by another in 1990 concerning the response of the calf muscles to high-intensity exercise [1]. These investigators used the recovery of P_i as an index of oxidative metabolism and reported that the high-pH pool (Type I fibers) recovered much more rapidly than did the low-pH pool (Type II fibers). This result was consistent with the pH dependence of PCr and P_i recovery described by other investigators (see above). Vandenborne et al. [157] also observed the development of 2–3 P_i peaks in the calf muscles during intense plantar flexion exercise. Each of the P_i peaks was associated with varying degrees of acidosis during exercise. These investigators pursued this result with a study of pH heterogeneity in the soleus, medial gastrocnemius, and lateral gastrocnemius during exercise [156]. Using localization techniques, they documented metabolic heterogeneity, apparently due to fiber type heterogeneity, within a single muscle.

The possibility that the two P_i peaks observed during some exercise studies were due to contribution from active and inactive fibers, rather than from Type I and Type II fibers, was addressed by Mizuno and coworkers [115]. By using tubocurarine to block the recruitment of Type I fibers during intense exercise, these investigators demonstrated that P_i peak splitting could be eliminated. Thus, because exercise under tubocurarine conditions resulted in a pool of active + inactive fibers, and no P_i split was observed, these results were interpreted to indicate that the split P_i peak was a result of a combination of fiber types in the MRS spectrum. Another argument against the split being due to a combination of active + inactive fibers is that P_i would not increase in the inactive fibers during exercise. Therefore, P_i in the inactive fibers would remain undetected, and the ob-

FIGURE 10.5.

Phosphorus MRS spectrum obtained during 60% of maximal exercise intensity and relative occurrence of two major fiber types (ST = slow twitch, FT = fast twitch) determined from biopsies of flexor carpi radialis in healthy volunteers. (Reproduced with permission from the authors and the American Physiological Society.) Note that the subject (top) with a predominance of ST fibers also demonstrated a single P_i peak with a high pH. The intermediate subject (middle) had a mixed fiber composition and showed a splitting of the P_i peak during exercise because of metabolic heterogeneity. The subject with a majority of FT fibers had a single P_i peak with a relatively low pH.

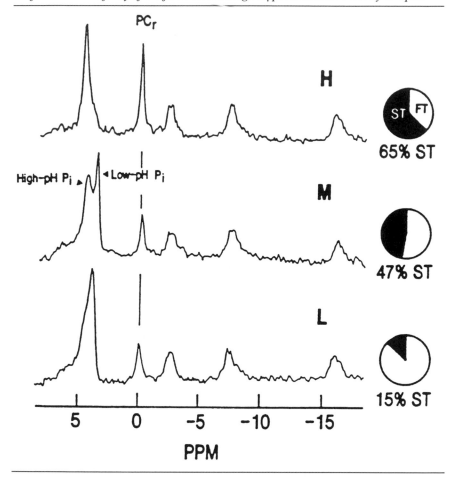

served P_i peak would be single, with the signal coming from the active fibers only. Thus, there is good evidence that P_i peak splitting is due to different fiber types, rather than a combination of active + inactive fibers.

A study of the masseter muscle supported the observation of considerable heterogeneity within a single muscle, even at rest [78]. This is particularly true of the multipennate masseter, which is known to be composed of three histochemically and functionally distinct portions. These investigators reported similar pH and different P_i/PCr at rest in the superficial, intermediate, and deep portions of the masseter muscles of six healthy volunteers. These results reinforce the importance of accurate localization during studies of muscle metabolism using ^{31}P MRS. Bernus et al. [25] observed differences in P_i/PCr at rest in the quadriceps muscles of sprinters, long-distance runners, and sedentary persons. They attributed these differences to varying fiber type composition in these three groups [25].

The influence of fiber type composition on the metabolic response to exercise observed with MRS was the focus of a recent investigation [114]. In this study, the researchers performed both MRS and muscle biopsy analysis of the wrist flexor muscles of a group of untrained volunteers. In addition, rectified surface EMG was monitored during the progressive exercise protocol. Subjects were separated into three groups, depending on their metabolic response to exercise. Those subjects who demonstrated a single P_i peak with high pH during exercise had faster recovery of PCr and P_i after exercise and a predominance of Type I fibers compared with the group with a single P_i peak, low pH during exercise, and a predominance of Type II fibers (Fig. 10.5). Those subjects with a split P_i peak having both a low and a high pH component had intermediate recovery characteristics and a mixed fiber type composition. The results of this study help clarify the variable contribution of different fiber types on the split P_i peak observed during exercise, and indicate that MRS can be sufficiently sensitive to detect different metabolic pools during exercise that are based upon fiber type differences.

Substrate Utilization
The recent application of ^{13}C MRS to studies of muscle glycogen utilization has yielded interesting results, including the first in vivo evidence that there can be significant intramuscular glycogen resynthesis during exercise at low workloads [11, 63, 133]. Glycogen signal intensity was measured in the gastrocnemius muscle of a healthy subject before, immediately after, and after 19 hr of recovery from exercise [11]. This study demonstrated the feasibility of noninvasively measuring glycogen in human skeletal muscle. Carbon MRS was then used to monitor changes in [glycogen] during and after 9 hr of low-intensity exercise [133]. The results showed that, after predepletion of intramuscular glycogen, stores of glycogen may increase during low-intensity exercise.

Using natural abundance ^{13}C MRS, Taylor et al. [146] studied postprandial glycogen synthesis after a fast in eight healthy subjects. In addition to monitoring gastrocnemius muscle glycogen concentration in the 8 hr after the meal, the investigators measured plasma glucose, lactate, triglyceride and insulin concentrations. There was a 17 mmol/liter increase in muscle glycogen during the first 4 hr after the meal. The results suggested an important role for skeletal muscle glycogen synthesis in the maintenance of postprandial glucose homeostasis. In the future, ^{13}C MRS studies of glycogen synthesis and utilization will be beneficial for the study of the role of glycogen depletion in fatigue, as well as the alterations in substrate utilization that occur in diseases involving impaired glycolytic metabolism.

The effect of dietary fasting on muscle metabolism during fatiguing exercise has been examined. Lunt et al. [84] found that, after fasting, changes in both P_i/PCr and pH during maximal wrist flexion exercise were dampened. The authors suggested that the smaller decrease in pH may have resulted from a shift from carbohydrate to fatty acids and ketones. Likewise, a less acid environment may explain the lower P_i/PCr in the fasted state because of the effect of acidosis on the creatine kinase reaction. These results indicate the importance of dietary considerations in studies of muscle metabolism, particularly in studies of disease in which the patients may be malnourished.

The effects on resting phosphorus metabolites of an oral glucose load designed to induce thermogenesis were studied in the calf muscles of five healthy subjects [155]. Glucose ingestion (1 g/kg body weight) resulted in an increase in P_i and a decrease in PCr/P_i in the 68 min following ingestion. There were no changes in ATP or intracellular pH. The investigators concluded that oral glucose intake may result in a reduction of the energy state of the cell. Following this study, Taylor et al. [149] performed a series of experiments to determine the effect of simultaneous glucose and insulin infusion on intracellular pH and phosphates in four healthy subjects. Insulin was infused for 120 min. Constant plasma glucose levels were maintained by simultaneous infusion of glucose. A 10-fold increase in plasma insulin concentration during infusion resulted in a slight decrease in intracellular pH, an increase in intracellular P_i and a decrease in plasma P_i. Phosphocreatine and ATP were unchanged during infusion. These results, similar to those of Thomsen et al. [155], demonstrated that physiologic concentrations of insulin do not lead to increased intracellular pH. The authors concluded that the action of insulin on the cell is not by means of the effects of alkalinization on intracellular enzyme activity [149]. These studies of the effects of glucose ingestion on phosphorus metabolites at rest indicate the need to control for diet immediately before MRS studies of muscle metabolism.

Exercise Training and Athletic Performance

Phosphorus MRS has been used to study the differences in muscle metabolism, particularly oxidative metabolism, between athletes and nonathletes. In an examination of the wrist flexor muscles of elite runners and sedentary persons, incremental exercise to 60% of maximal voluntary force resulted in a smaller decrease in pH and less of an increase in P_i/PCr in the runners compared with the control subjects [127]. This was despite the fact that the muscles studied were not specific to the athletic event. The authors suggested that these results provided evidence of the genetic component to athletic performance. A better capacity for oxidative metabolism in the wrist flexor muscles of rowers relative to sedentary subjects has also been reported [101]. This was observed as a greater slope of power versus P_i/PCr, less of a decrease in pH during exercise, and a more rapid recovery of PCr after exercise. These data were consistent with the capacity for greater oxidative metabolism in the rowers. A similar observation of greater oxidative capacity in the hamstrings muscle of long distance runners compared with control subjects was also reported [171]. Recently, Laurent et al. [81] reported the ability to discriminate between cross-country skiers, downhill skiers, and sedentary persons using a discriminate analysis that combined MRS and whole-body oxygen consumption measures.

The effects of daily activity on the metabolic profile of relatively sedentary people was the subject of a study by Minotti et al. [110]. This was accomplished by comparing the changes in the wrist flexor muscles during exercise in the dominant and nondominant forearms of the same people. There were significantly greater increases in P_i/PCr and decreases in pH in the nondominant relative to dominant arms during exercise in these subjects. There were no differences in blood flow or muscle mass. The authors interpreted these results as evidence for better oxidative capacity in the more active, dominant arms of these healthy subjects in a manner similar to that of a training effect.

It is well known that endurance exercise training will elicit improvements in the capacity of skeletal muscle for oxidative metabolism. Two MRS studies of the effects of wrist flexion training were reported in 1990 [75, 112]. Minotti et al. [112] quantitated the effects of 7 wk of training on the blood flow, muscle mass, endurance, and metabolism of the wrist flexors, as well as whole-body oxygen consumption. After training, there were no differences in muscle cross-sectional area, forearm blood flow, strength, or $\dot{V}O_2$max. There were significant increases in endurance and decreases in P_i/PCr at the same relative exercise intensity after training. The authors concluded that training resulted in improved oxidative capacity in the wrist flexor muscles that was independent of muscle mass, blood flow, or whole-body oxygen consumption. Kent-Braun et al. [75] reported the effects of 8 wk of endurance training on the work performance, resistance to fatigue, and oxidative capacity of the wrist flexor muscles. After training, the subjects demonstrated significantly increased work performance, a slower rate of fatigue, and lower P_i/PCr at the highest workloads. There were no changes in maximum force. The authors concluded that endurance training could lead to increased work capacity, decreased rates of fatigue, and increased oxidative capacity. Before and after training, the relationship between power and P_i/PCr demonstrated the expected hyperbolic transfer function theorized earlier by Chance and coworkers (as illustrated in Fig. 10.3). Thus, these data were consistent with the model of [ADP] control of oxidative metabolism in skeletal muscle during low-intensity, steady-state exercise. In a study of the short-term effects of training, 14 days of intense exercise training of the wrist flexor muscles resulted in improved oxidative metabolism and significant elevations of resting P_i/PCr during the training period [99]. The elevation of P_i/PCr at rest may have been evidence of muscle injury (see below), or the acute adaptation to high-intensity training.

To investigate the mechanisms of peripheral muscle adaptations to chronic hypobaric hypoxia, Matheson et al. [95] studied people who normally reside at high altitudes. They studied both systemic oxygen consumption ($\dot{V}O_2$) in response to cycle ergometry and the metabolic changes in the gastrocnemius muscle during plantar flexion. Their results indicated that the altitude-adapted people, although of only moderately high systemic oxygen capacity, demonstrated a relatively high capacity for oxidative metabolism at the single-muscle level. That is, the decrease in pH and increase in P_i/PCr at fatigue was less in the altitude-adapted subjects compared with both sedentary and power-trained sea level-dwelling subjects. The single muscle metabolic response of the altitude-adjusted people was similar to highly trained aerobic athletes living at sea level. These results indicated that persons living at altitude adapted to the conditions of chronic hypobaric hypoxia with an increased intramuscular potential for oxidative phosphorylation.

Studies of Aging Muscle

Increasing interest has been focused on the intramuscular changes that may occur during the aging process. An early ^{31}P MRS study of skeletal muscle metabolism in aging indicated that there was no difference either at rest or in the metabolic response to exercise in healthy elderly subjects compared with young adults [150]. Since that time, several studies of muscle metabolism and the effects of exercise training in the elderly have been performed. McCully et al. [102] observed that the calf muscles of elderly subjects demonstrated lower PCr/P_i at rest and a slower rate of PCr recovery after exercise compared with young subjects. No difference between young and elderly in the change in metabolites during exercise was observed. A mild exercise training program had no effect on the slowed PCr recovery observed in the elderly. This study was followed by another from the same investigators that compared oxygen consumption, gastrocnemius muscle MRS, and biopsy results in young (mean age=28 yr) and elderly (mean age=66 yr) subjects [98]. Peak oxygen consumption ($\dot{V}O_2$ peak) during cycling, citrate synthase activity, and PCr recovery rates were lower in elderly compared with young subjects. PCr recovery rates were strongly associated with both citrate synthase activity and $\dot{V}O_2$ peak, and citrate synthase activity was well correlated to $\dot{V}O_2$ peak. No correlations were observed between fiber type distribution and any of the other measures. These results indicated that oxidative metabolism was reduced in the elderly, and that MRS and biopsy measurements were well correlated.

The effects of aging and training status have been examined [41]. The ratio of P_i/PCr at rest was not significantly higher in the elderly, but citrate synthase activity was significantly reduced. The slope of P_i/PCr versus power was greater in the older trained and untrained subjects compared with the young, even when corrected for the 10–12% loss of muscle mass observed in the elderly. This slope was inversely related to citrate synthase activity. These results indicated that aging was associated with a loss of muscle mass and metabolic capacity, and that training status only partially offset these losses. In a study of the effects of wrist flexion training in a small number of subjects (n=4, mean age=58 yr), Marsh et al. [90] reported a significant training-induced increase in endurance and delay in the onset of intracellular acidosis during progressive exercise. Blood flow to the muscle (measured using venous occlusion plethysmography) was unaffected by training.

In a different approach to the study of the effects of aging, a comparison of the metabolic response to exercise of children and adults indicated that children have a relatively higher capacity for oxidative metabolism that in part reflects a limited ability to produce ATP anaerobically [174].

In summary, recent studies indicate that reductions in metabolic capacity occur with aging, and that these reductions may be, at least in part, offset with exercise training. The extent to which the aging process itself, rather than deconditioning, leads to these deficits remains to be determined.

Miscellaneous

MYOGLOBIN SATURATION. Deoxymyoglobin can be measured during exercise by using proton MRS [160]. As a result, the adequacy of tissue oxygenation under various conditions can be studied. This relatively new technique will provide an opportunity to study the role of myoglobin saturation and oxygen delivery to the muscle during exercise.

EXERCISE MODE. Transcutaneous nerve stimulation can be used to eliminate the effects of central factors in fatigue on the metabolic measurements made during exercise [77, 96, 108, 141]. Helpern et al. [56] reported progressive decreases in PCr and pH, with similar increases in P_i, during supramaximal stimulation of the tibialis anterior muscle in healthy subjects. The results indicated that the exercise was moderately severe, but well-tolerated in the healthy subjects, demonstrating the feasibility of ^{31}P measurements during stimulated exercise. More recently, Matheson et al. [96] reported the changes in phosphorus metabolites and pH during progressively increasing frequencies and voltages of stimulation. The rectus femoris muscles of 10 healthy subjects were stimulated and the changes in P_i/PCr and pH were measured. The results indicated that optimal stimulation parameters for the study of muscle metabolism during graded, stimulated exercise included maximal intensity (voltage) and progressively increasing frequencies.

The relative efficiency of concentric and eccentric exercise was the focus of a study by Menard et al. [103]. Changes in phosphorus metabolism during low-intensity (15% MVC) concentric, eccentric, and isometric finger flexion exercise were studied in eight healthy individuals. The results indicated that the metabolic cost (expressed as increased P_i/PCr) of concentric exercise was significantly greater than either eccentric or isometric exercise. In fact, the change in P_i/PCr during eccentric and isometric exercise was small over a range of loads. These results were consistent with those reported using whole-body metabolic measurements of oxygen consumption, and likely reflect differences in the activity of the contractile apparatus during each of these types of contraction.

IMAGING STUDIES. Fleckenstein et al. [49] first reported the use of T2-weighted proton images (MRI) to determine the active muscle mass after exercise. This imaging technique exploits the fact that exercise is associated with increased extracellular water. Thus, use of this technique provides localization of active muscle area. The issue of muscle activation and recruitment during exercise can thus be addressed by using a combination of MIR and MRS. For example, DeSuso et al. [44] quantitated the metabolic changes (using MRS) in the active muscle (identified with MRI) during quadriceps exercise. This technique has also been used to monitor the onset and resolution of muscle injury.

FLUID SHIFTS DURING EXERCISE. Recently, proton spectroscopy has been applied to the study of the fluid shifts that accompany exercise [50]. Low-intensity exercise of the gastrocnemius muscle resulted in transient increases in the proton peak representing water, followed by a biexponential decrease after exercise. These changes were consistent with the results of studies using more invasive techniques, as well as MRI observations of increased proton signal intensity after exercise (see above). It was concluded that this increased proton signal intensity reflects changes in water between the vasculature and the muscle during exercise.

MUSCLE INJURY. Elevated P_i/PCr in resting muscle has been reported after exercise thought to induce muscle injury [4, 100]. For example, an increase in the resting level of P_i/PCr in the days after intense eccentric exercise has been reported [100]. Decreased ATP was also observed 24 hr after the exercise protocol. Similar elevations of resting P_i/PCr were observed in a nonexercised group of subjects with neuromuscular disorders that result in muscle tissue necrosis. As a result of these findings, the investigators suggested that resting P_i/PCr may serve as a useful, noninvasive index of muscle injury. However, Kemp et al. [71] recently reported that the resting level of P_i/ATP was not elevated 1–2 days after a 67-mile bicycle ride in the gastrocnemius muscles of 7 healthy volunteers. To determine whether elevated Pi/PCR at rest is indicative of muscle injury, it will be necessary to perform morphological studies in conjunction with MRS studies.

METABOLISM AND SYMPATHETIC ACTIVATION. An investigation of the relationship between intracellular pH and reflex sympathetic nerve activation during exercise was undertaken by Victor et al. [159]. Measurements made during handgrip exercise indicated that the onset of sympathetic outflow coincided with intracellular acidification. Furthermore, the onset of sympathetic outflow was not correlated to changes in [ADP], [PCr], or [P_i]. The authors concluded that accumulation of H^+ resulting from increased glycolysis in the muscle plays an important role in stimulating the reflex sympathetic response during exercise.

SUMMARY. The studies described above indicate the variety of questions that can be addressed using MRS. Increasingly sophisticated methods have been developed that provide excellent sensitivity to changes in the intramuscular environment. As a result, MRS should no longer be considered a "new" technology. In the future, the combination of MRS with other methodologies will provide a more thorough understanding of human skeletal muscle metabolism and performance under various conditions.

MUSCLE METABOLISM IN DISEASE

Metabolic Myopathies

MCARDLE'S SYNDROME. The first MRS study of a metabolic myopathy concerned McArdle's syndrome [139]. Phosphorus MRS indicated no intramuscular acidification in a McArdle's patient during exercise, which was consistent with the absence of glycogen phosphorylase. During ischemic exercise, PCr decreased more in McArdle's than in healthy subjects, which suggested an inability of the muscle to produce sufficient energy from nonoxidative sources. The rate of recovery of PCr after exercise was normal, indicating that oxidative resynthesis of ATP was unimpaired. A subsequent study of three patients with McArdle's disease again showed an abnormally low PCr/P_i after exercise, without acidosis [22]. In these patients, however, there was a slow recovery of PCr in these patients, which suggested impaired oxidative metabolism. Lewis et al. [83] reported that one McArdle's patient developed a muscle contracture during exercise that was accompanied by markedly decreased PCr and increased Pi. Glucose infusion allowed the patient to exercise easily for 7 min with less PCr depletion and P_i accumulation. In control subjects during the same exercise protocol, muscle metabolites changed much more modestly and were not at all affected by the glucose infusion. Jensen et al. investigated a McArdle's patient using cycle ergometry [62]. A high-protein diet and glucose infusion improved muscle energy kinetics in this patient, but intravenous amino acids had no effect. These reports indicate that, in the absence of glycogen phosphorylase, glucose may be used as a source of energy.

PHOSPHOFRUCTOKINASE DEFICIENCY. In one of the first MRS studies of human muscle, Edwards et al. [47] reported that a patient with phosphofructokinase deficiency showed little change during exercise in intracellular pH but a 50-fold increase in the phosphomonoester region (representing phosphorylated intermediates of the glycolytic pathway). Bertocci et al. [27] also investigated the metabolic consequences of exercise in patients with phosphofructokinase deficiency. During maximal effort, ADP in muscle was twice as high and venous ammonia was much greater in patients with phosphofructokinase deficiency compared with control subjects. In contrast, the decrease in PCr and increase in P_i were less in patients compared with control subjects. In a subsequent study, lactate infusion attenuated the fall in PCr and the rise in P_i, ADP, and venous ammonia during exercise [26]. These studies suggest that the diminished oxidizable substrate (i.e., pyruvate) in phosphofructokinase deficiency results in an impaired oxidative capacity because of a decreased rate of oxidative phosphorylation.

MITOCHONDRIAL MYOPATHIES. Phosphorus MRS has also been used to study abnormal mitochondrial function [5, 24, 29, 42, 51, 97, 124, 135]. In an early MRS study, the observation of increased P_i/PCr at rest was consistent with a diagnosis of mitochondrial myopathy in a 16-yr-old boy [51]. In an exercise study of a patient with mitochondrial NADH-coenzyme Q reductase deficiency, an abnormally slow recovery of PCr and pH after exercise was noted [135]. Twelve patients with mitochondrial myopathies demonstrated metabolic abnormalities using ^{31}P MRS [5]. For example, resting PCr/P_i was reduced in most of these patients, and exercise-induced changes of PCr/P_i were abnormal in 5 patients who could perform exercise. The fall in pH during exercise was less severe in the patients than in the control subjects. The rate of PCr/P_i recovery after low-intensity exercise was slow in 11 of the 12 patients. In a case of mitochondrial myopathy due to Complex I deficiency, PCr/P_i and ATP in resting muscle were well within the normal range at rest [29]. However, the decrease of PCr during exercise was greater in this patient than in control subjects. In another report, resting ^{31}P MRS spectra showed elevated P_i in 13 of 17 patients with myopathy compared with controls [97]. A few of these patients also had reduced PCr. These studies demonstrate that ^{31}P MRS of muscle both at rest and during exercise can be of practical value in a clinical setting for the diagnosis of mitochondrial myopathies.

Magnetic resonance spectroscopy was used to demonstrate that coenzyme Q increased exercise tolerance and the rate of postexercise PCr/P_i recovery in a patient with cytochrome oxidase deficiency [124]. In two patients with severe mitochondrial encephalomyopathy due to Complex I and IV deficiency, treatment with coenzyme Q resulted in significant clinical improvement and increased PCr/P_i at rest [24]. In another patient with a defect in Complex III of the electron transport chain, resting PCr/P_i was reduced and the rate of recovery of PCr/P_i after exercise was only 2.5% of normal [48]. After administration of menadione and ascorbic acid, there was a 21-fold increase in PCr/P_i recovery rate relative to pretherapy in this patient. A subsequent MRS study of this patient showed that the patient's condition continued to be stable with this therapy [6]. Elimination of vitamin K3 supplementation followed by vitamin K3 readministration produced deterioration and subsequent improvement in the patient's condition.

Neuromuscular and Neurological Diseases

The use of MRS to study muscle metabolism has provided evidence that, in a number of neuromuscular and neurologic disorders, there are alterations of muscle energy metabolism at rest and during exercise. Some of these changes are nonspecific, and thus are probably not a primary effect of the disease. At rest, patients with denervated muscle had lower PCr/P_i and higher intracellular pH than did control subjects [177]. Phosphorus MRS of patients with Duchenne dystrophy, myotonic dystrophy, postpoliomyelitis, Werdnig-Hoffman disease, and pedal dystonia showed increased ATP/PCr and P_i/PCr in resting muscle [14]. Using ^1H MRS, these investigators also performed quantitative and qualitative fat analysis in human leg muscle and found that the fat/water ratio was greatly increased in primary and secondary muscle disorders. Spectra from diseased muscle showed multiple resonances from polyunsaturated fatty acids, which were not seen in healthy muscle [15].

MUSCULAR DYSTROPHY. Phosphorus MRS studies of boys with Duchenne muscular dystrophy demonstrated higher P_i, intracellular pH, and phosphodiester at rest compared with control subjects [173]. In these patients, PCr was reduced, but ATP was not significantly different from control subjects. As the disease progressed, the patients showed further decreases in PCr and PCr/P_i and increases in P_i and phosphodiester; ATP remained unchanged. These results suggested progressive metabolic deterioration in Duchenne muscular dystrophy [173]. Two other reports documented reduced PCr/ATP and PCr/P_i in resting muscle in patients with Duchenne muscular dystrophy [52, 121]. A signal in the phosphodiester region was consistently recorded in Duchenne muscular dystrophy patients but not in control subjects [121]. A reduction of the total phosphorus signal was the result of muscle fiber loss and it was concluded that muscle fiber ATP concentration was probably normal [52]. Intracellular pH was alkaline was also observed in patients with Duchenne muscular dystrophy compared with control subjects [70].

Studies of female carriers for muscular dystrophy (Becker or Duchenne) showed no significant metabolic differences between carriers and controls in resting muscle [17, 18]. However, during gastrocnemius exercise, carriers had a decreased ability to perform work and a higher P_i/PCr ratio at similar work levels. In addition, the rate of postexercise PCr recovery was lower in carriers. Recently, these investigators reported marked slowing of Pi recovery after lengthening exercise in carriers compared with control subjects. [16] Thus, these studies indicate metabolic abnormalities in the muscles of carriers for muscular dystrophy.

A recent study of myotonic muscular dystrophy found that resting muscle had normal pH, but elevated P_i/ATP, phosphomonoester/ATP, and phosphodiester/ATP [147]. In five siblings with autosomal dominant oculopharyngeal muscular dystrophy, PCr/(PCr+P_i) of the forearm flexor muscles were reduced and pH was elevated compared with control subjects [176]. Exercise caused PCr/(PCr + P_i) and pH to fall rapidly, despite diminished work output. After exercise, PCr/PCr + P_i recovery was normal but pH recovery was slow.

In summary, these reports indicate that there are significant alterations in muscle metabolism at rest and during exercise in various forms of muscular dystrophy.

MULTIPLE SCLEROSIS. Spectroscopy studies conducted during electrically stimulated tetanic contractions provided evidence of excessive muscle fatigue and an exaggerated metabolic response in patients with spastic paraparesis (most of whom had multiple sclerosis [108]). During stimulated contractions of the ankle dorsiflexors, tetanic force fell more in patients than in control subjects, indicating greater fatigability. At the same time, PCr and pH also decreased significantly more in patients compared with control subjects. These observations suggested that alterations in intramuscular metabolism in patients with central nervous system disease may contribute to their excessive fatigability. Consistent with the possibility of diminished muscle function in multiple sclerosis, Kent-Braun et al. [73] observed slowed PCr recovery after dorsiflexion exercise in multiple sclerosis patients compared with control subjects. These results suggested that skeletal muscle oxidative capacity is impaired in some persons with multiple sclerosis. Recently, surface electromyography was combined with ^{31}P MRS to study dorsiflexor muscle activation and metabolism in multiple sclerosis patients during voluntary exercise to fatigue [72]. The results indicated that there was a significant reduction in the activation of the muscle during voluntary exercise in patients with multiple sclerosis. This was detected as significantly smaller changes in P_i/PCr and pH in multiple sclerosis patients compared with control subjects at the same relative force level. This study demonstrated the utility of MRS in detecting incomplete muscular activation during voluntary contractions in patients with a central nervous system deficit.

POSTPOLIO SYNDROME. Intermittent isometric exercise resulted in greater fatigue in postpolio syndrome patients compared with healthy control subjects [140]. Interestingly, the decrease in PCr and pH during exercise at the same relative force level was not different between the groups, despite greater fatigue in the postpolio patients. In conjunction with the delayed force recovery and prolonged tetanic force relaxation also observed in the patients, these data suggested a failure of muscular activation in postpolio syndrome during voluntary exercise. As with the study of multiple sclerosis patients [73], this study demonstrated the utility of MRS measurements for detecting activation failure in neuromuscular and neurological disease during voluntary exercise.

Diseases with Limited Tissue Oxygenation

HEART FAILURE. One of the most prevalent applications of the MRS technique has been for the study of heart disease. Fatigue during activity is a primary limitation for patients with congestive heart failure. Traditionally it has been thought that this limitation was the result of an inadequate increase of cardiac output in response to exercise, which would result in insufficient oxygen delivery to the exercising skeletal muscle. Phosphorus MRS studies of skeletal muscle have demonstrated that skeletal muscle fatigue in heart failure probably caused both by reduced oxygen delivery and intramuscular alterations.

The metabolic response to exercise in control subjects and in patients with congestive heart failure or other types of heart disease has been studied by several groups [2, 3, 66, 85–88, 93, 94, 136, 145, 164, 168]. Although P_i/PCr and pH were similar at rest, heart failure patients had significantly reduced power output at all workloads compared with control subjects [168]. This was associated with a greater increase in P_i/PCr and more acidosis during exercise in the patients compared with control subjects. To determine whether altered energy metabolism was due to reduced blood flow, additional studies using plethysmography were performed [164]. During progressive exercise, patients with heart failure had a greater increase in P_i/PCr at each power level compared with healthy control subjects (similar to the "disease" scenario illustrated in Fig. 10.3). At the same time, forearm blood flow was similar in both groups during exercise. Thus, the greater increase in P_i/PCr during exercise in the patients could not be attributed to a limitation of blood flow. In a similar study, Arnolda et al. [10] studied the blood flow and metabolic response of the gastrocnemius muscles of patients with mild congestive heart failure. The $PCr/(PCr+P_i)$ ratio was lower in patients with heart failure than in control subjects at a similar exercise rate, although pH and blood flow were similar. Cytosolic free ADP concentration was markedly increased in patients with heart failure compared with control subjects at the same workload. Although the maximum workload achieved by heart failure patients was less than half that of control subjects, pH and $PCr/(PCr+P_i)$ were lower in the patients during maximal effort. Therefore, the authors concluded that metabolic abnormalities in skeletal muscle of heart failure patients may contribute to exercise intolerance.

Similarly, other investigators found that PCr utilization and acidosis were significantly greater during forearm flexion exercise in patients with heart failure compared with control subjects, and that these results were not due to impaired blood flow [94]. The rate of PCr recovery after exercise was also reduced in heart failure patients compared with control subjects. In some patients, the P_i peak split during exercise, suggesting a greater heterogeneity in the metabolic response to exercise in heart failure. To further rule out the effects of blood flow, additional studies were performed during tourniquet ischemia [93]. The greater decreases in PCr and pH observed in heart failure patients during nonischemic exercise were also present throughout ischemic exercise. Thus, the excessive metabolic response to exercise observed in heart failure patients was not due to reduced oxygen delivery. The authors concluded that patients with heart failure have a greater reliance on glycolytic metabolism during exercise. In yet another study of patients with congestive heart failure, less work was necessary to produce a similar PCr depletion compared with control subjects [89]. In contrast, PCr recovery rate was similar after both aerobic and ischemic exercise. The authors concluded that the greater PCr depletion produced by ischemic work together with the similar PCr recovery rates indicated metabolic modifications that cannot be explained by reduced blood flow to the muscle. The results of these studies strongly suggest that muscle metabolism is impaired in heart failure and that this impairment is not solely due to reduced perfusion.

To investigate the etiology of the altered skeletal muscle metabolism in heart failure patients, muscle biopsies were compared with those from control subjects. The heart failure biopsy data showed a shift in fiber distribution toward an increased percentage of glycolytic (easily fatigable) Type IIb fibers, atrophy of both Type IIa and Type IIb fibers, and decreased activity of β-hydroxyacyl coenzyme A dehydrogenase when compared with control subjects [85]. However, there were no correlations between the slope of P_i/PCr versus oxygen consumption, fiber type composition, or enzyme activity. These results suggested that heart failure patients develop intrinsic skeletal muscle changes, but that these changes did not contribute significantly to the abnormal skeletal muscle metabolism observed in such patients. Mancini et al. [88] also investigated the prevalence of skeletal muscle atrophy and its relationship to abnormal muscle metabolism and exercise intolerance in patients with heart failure. In association with reduced skeletal muscle mass (noted in 68% of the patients), there was a modest linear correlation between peak oxygen consumption measured during treadmill exercise and muscle volume. Metabolic abnormalities observed using ^{31}P MRS during exercise in the patients with heart failure were consistent with intrinsic reductions in muscle oxidative capacity. Thus, the authors concluded that atrophy contributes modestly to altered muscle metabolism and reduced exercise capacity in heart failure.

The effects of exercise training on skeletal muscle metabolism in heart failure patients has also been studied using ^{31}P MRS. As in healthy subjects [75, 112], wrist flexor training improved the relationship between P_i/PCr and low-intensity workloads in subjects with heart failure [111]. Muscle mass, limb blood flow, and pH were unchanged after training. These results indicated that exercise training can reverse some of the skeletal muscle metabolic abnormalities typically observed in heart failure. Cycle training also attenuated the PCr fall and ADP rise during plantar flexion exercise, improved exercise tolerance, and increased PCr recovery rates in patients with heart failure [2]. Thus, exercise training can substantially correct the defect in oxidative capacity observed in the skeletal muscle of persons with heart failure.

PERIPHERAL VASCULAR DISEASE. During nonischemic foot exercise in severely afflicted patients with peripheral vascular disease, PCr and pH decreased to a greater degree than in control subjects [68]. Intracellular pH and PCr also recovered more slowly in patients with peripheral vascular disease than in control subjects. Phosphocreatine recovery after ischemic exercise correlated significantly with degree of arterial stenosis assessed by Doppler ultrasound and by angiography. This result suggested that the degree of arterial stenosis limits the rate of oxidative phosphorylation in the muscle. In a study of patients with claudication, pain was not related to intracellular pH or concentration of phosphorus metabolites [54]. However, patients with severe claudication had significantly greater decreases in PCr and pH during exercise and slower recovery of PCr and pH after exercise. Surgical correction of the arterial stenosis led to correction of the metabolic abnormalities.

In persons with severe limb ischemia, PCr/P_i was reduced at rest compared with control subjects [175]. Furthermore, in moderately ischemic limbs the rate of metabolite recovery after exercise was slowed. In patients with peripheral arterial occlusive disease, the fall of PCr during exercise was greater than in control subjects [138]. A significant fall of intracellular pH occurred only in the patients with arterial occlusion. The fall of pH correlated closely with a rise in the arteriovenous lactate difference, which suggested that anaerobic production of energy was sufficient to maintain ATP concentration even during claudication pain. In another study of peripheral arterial occlusive disease, pH was not significantly different between patients and control subjects during progressive exercise [167]. However, after exercise, P_i recovery was significantly slower in these patients. There was no significant correlation between recovery rate and ankle-brachial pressure index, but there was a strong negative correlation between recovery rate and angiographic resistance grades. A study of foot muscle metabolism showed that intracellular pH and the ratio of P_i/PCr were significantly higher in the feet of patients with rest pain and were particularly high in those with gangrene or ulceration [55]. In contrast, ankle pressures and transcutaneous O_2 and CO_2 measurements failed to distinguish patients with advanced peripheral ischemia. Together, these studies document the capacity of MRS noninvasively to detect abnormalities in muscle metabolism that result from reduced oxygen delivery due to peripheral vascular disease.

RESPIRATORY FAILURE. Skeletal muscle metabolic abnormalities have also been observed in persons with chronic respiratory failure. During progressive exercise, respiratory failure patients exhibited higher P_i/PCr and lower pH compared with control subjects at the same relative workload [132]. In addition, PCr resynthesis during recovery was slower in the patients than in control subjects. These results suggest an impairment of aerobic capacity in the working skeletal muscle of patients with chronic respiratory failure, probably because of hypoxemia. Thompson et al. [153] found greater and faster PCr depletion and pH decline during exercise in patients with respiratory failure, but normal metabolic recovery. Supplemental oxygen was subsequently shown to produce significant although incomplete improvement in all metabolic parameters, which suggests that oxidative metabolism depends on oxygen delivery in patients with chronic respiratory insufficiency [129].

Other Diseases

AIDS MYOPATHY. Few MRS studies have been performed concerning alterations of muscle metabolism due to HIV disease, AIDS, and AIDS treatments. In one study, no significant differences were observed between AIDS patients (5 of 9 were taking AZT) and control subjects in terms of fatigability, muscle metabolism, or muscle activation [106]. These results provided no support for the hypothesis that fatigue or myalgia in AIDS patients derives from altered muscle metabolism. However, in a study of the calf muscles of HIV patients (all of whom were taking AZT) the recovery of PCr after exercise was significantly delayed in the AZT-treated patients compared with control subjects [163] Thus, these results support the hypothesis that the myopathy associated with chronic AZT administration results from impaired mitochondrial function. Clearly, more work needs to be done in this area to understand the metabolic changes that occur in the muscle of persons with HIV and AIDS.

CHRONIC FATIGUE SYNDROME. A case study of a person who presented with general malaise, fatigue, exertional exhaustion, and muscle pain after severe exercise was reported in 1984 [9]. In this study, exercise of the forearm muscles resulted in severe acidosis, which was proportionally greater than the change in PCr. The authors suggested that the severe acidoisis represented excessive lactic acid formation, resulting from a disorder of metabolic regulation. A muscle biopsy showed scattered necrotic fibers and Type II fiber predominance. More recently, Kent-Braun et al. [77] studied seven patients with "chronic fatigue syndrome" using both submaximal, intermittent exercise and maximal, sustained exercise protocols. In this study, both fatigue and the changes in PCr and pH during ankle dorsiflexion exercise, as well as the recovery of force and metabolites, were similar in patients and control subjects. These results indicated that excessive acidosis was not responsible for the fatigue reported in this condition. Furthermore, both before and at the end of exercise, the patients demonstrated a significantly greater increment in force when a tetanic stimulus was imposed upon a maximal voluntary contraction. This result indicated incomplete voluntary activation of the muscle in chronic fatigue syndrome. The authors concluded that a central failure of muscle activation may play an important role in the fatigue of chronic fatigue syndrome, rather than any defect of muscle endurance or metabolism. Similar to this report was another recent study that found no consistent muscle metabolic defect in chronic fatigue syndrome patients [19].

UREMIA AND DIALYSIS. Uremic muscles have been found to have significantly lower ATP, PCr, and higher P_i concentrations than nonuremic control muscles, but there were no significant differences in pH [122]. Cardoso et al. [36] studied resting gastrocnemius muscle metabolism in three patients with renal insufficiency before and during hemodialysis. During dialysis, intracellular and extracellular P_i fell, ATP did not change, and no significant pyrophosphate accumulation was seen. Several recent studies have documented subnormal oxidative metabolism in uremic patients with increased anaerobic glycolysis as a compensatory mechanism [46, 117, 144, 154]. Most recently, improved oxidative phosphorylation was demonstrated in uremic patients after treatment with recombinant erythropoetin to correct anemia [126, 154]. Higgins et al. [57] reported four patients with asymptomatic chronic hypophosphatemia after renal transplant who demonstrated reduced concentrations of P_i in resting muscle compared with control subjects. Three of these patients had a greater fall of intracellular pH during exercise and delayed recovery of pH following exercise.

THYROID DISEASE. Patients with both hypothyroidism and hyperthyroidism have demonstrated abnormal muscle metabolism [7, 53, 64, 65, 151]. Argov et al. [7] first reported low PCr/P_i at rest, increased PCr depletion during exercise, and delayed postexercise recovery of PCr/P_i in two hypothyroid patients. These results were reproduced in 13 other patients with mild to severe thyroid insufficiency [64]. Other investigators reported reduced ATP, P_i/PCr, and pH in resting muscle of hypothyroid patients compared with control subjects [151]. During exercise, PCr was depleted more rapidly in hypothyroid compared with healthy muscle. Although the recovery of PCr was unimpaired in the hypothyroid subjects, intracellular pH recovered more slowly, which was interpreted to indicate normal oxidative metabolism but abnormal proton handling in the patients. Thus, most patients with hypothyroidism demonstrate altered muscle metabolism at rest and impaired energy metabolism during exercise.

Studies of hyperthyroid subjects showed no abnormality in the ^{31}P MRS spectra at rest [65]. However, after 5 min of exercise there was greater PCr depletion and more acidosis in the nine hyperthyroid subjects compared with control subjects. Phosphocreatine recovery was not significantly different in the patients.

MALIGNANT HYPERTHERMIA. Webster et al. [161] investigated the pathogenesis of malignant hyperthermia in 11 biopsy-positive malignant hyperthermia-sensitive patients compared with 26 control subjects [161]. In the patients, there was a premature drop in intracellular pH during mild aerobic exercise and recovery of pH was slower. The ratio of $PCr/(PCr+P_i)$ also dropped early during exercise, but recovered normally. Olgin et al. [125] also investigated malignant hypothermia-susceptible patients with ^{31}P MRS. At rest, these patients had lower Pr/P_i compared with control subjects. After exercise, the patients showed slower recovery of PCr/P_i. The sensitivity and specificity of MRS for detecting susceptibility for malignant hyperthermia were estimated to be 98%. The MRS studies and halothane/caffeine contracture tests demonstrated an overall agreement for detecting hyperthermia susceptibility of 93%. Recently, Payen et al. [130] advocated using the combination of resting P_i/PCr and phosphodiester/PCr ratios to detect malignant hyperthermia susceptibility, which provided a sensitivity of 93% and specificity of 95%.

DIABETES MELLITUS. Carbon MRS has been used to study noninsulin-dependent diabetes. ^{13}C-glucose infusions were performed to quantitate the rate of incorporation of ^{13}C-glucose into muscle glycogen [142]. The rate of glycogen synthesis was about half in the diabetic subjects compared with healthy subjects. Furthermore, the rate of nonoxidative glucose metabolism was considerably lower in the diabetic subjects compared with control subjects. The synthesis of muscle glycogen appeared to account for most of the total body glucose uptake and all of the nonoxidative glucose metabolism in both patients and control subjects. The authors concluded that muscle glycogen synthesis is the principal pathway of glucose disposal in healthy and diabetic subjects, and that defects in glycogen synthesis may play a role in insulin resistance. Carbon MRS has also been applied to the study of glycogen storage disease [20].

OTHER CLINICAL CONDITIONS. The resting gastrocnemius muscle of a 10-mo-old infant with a rachitic hypotonia was examined during supplementation with vitamin D, calcium, and phosphorus [113]. During early treatment, muscle PCr/ATP ratio increased and muscle strength recovered concomitantly. The response indicated that the synchrony of clinical recovery may relate to the recovery kinetics of energy metabolites.

Studies of the skeletal muscle of low-birth-weight infants at rest and during reflex-induced muscle contractions have been performed [28]. Their relative concentrations of PCr and ATP were reduced at rest compared to larger infants. During reflex-induced isometric contractions, there was a marked decline of $PCr/(PC+P_i)$ and $ATP/(ADP \cdot P_i)$. The authors suggested that in very low-birth-weight infants with hypotonia, there may be a limited reserve for energy production.

The thigh muscles of 21 patients with injury-related chronic anterior cruciate ligament insufficiency were examined using MRS [67]. The quadriceps muscles had reduced cross-sectional area although the knee flexors were not reduced. Phosphocreatine was decreased in the atrophied muscles; this reduction correlated with muscle cross-sectional area. There was no difference in muscular pH.

Eighteen alcoholic patients (10 with and 8 without a recent history of rhabdomyolysis) and 15 healthy, nonalcoholic volunteers were studied using ^{31}P MRS [31]. At rest, phosphorus metabolites were similar in patients and controls subjects. However, during exercise, PCr utilization was greater, pH fell more slowly, and maximal acidosis was less in alcoholic patients with previous rhabdomyolysis than in control subjects. During ischemic exercise, both alcoholic groups exhibited significantly slower and smaller decreases in pH than did control subjects. These findings are consistent with impaired muscle glycolysis or glycogenolysis in both alcoholic groups, which may contribute to the onset of acute rhabdomyolysis.

The long-term effects of heat stroke were investigated in 13 patients 6 mo after their events [131]. There were no differences between patients and control subjects at rest, during exercise, or during recovery. The authors concluded that patients who develop exertional heat stroke do not have a predisposing myopathy.

MRS performed at the site of tender points in the trapezius muscle of patients with a primary fibromyalgia syndrome indicated no metabolic abnormalities [43]. This result was in contrast to a suggestion of changes in high-energy phosphates in biopsies taken from the affected region.

Taylor et al. [148] studied a patient with postexertional muscle pain that was responsive to verapamil. The muscle decreased its high-energy phosphate content and acidified more rapidly than healthy muscle during exercise. Phosphocreatine recovery after exercise was normal. It was suggested that the patient suffers from a defect in calcium handling in the muscle. Direct measurements of Ca^{2+}-ATPase activity in sarcoplasmic reticulum ATPase showed that activity was reduced by 90%.

The muscles of patients with previous histories of exercise hypothermia have been examined using ^{31}P MRS [82]. At rest, there were no differences between hypothermia patients and healthy control subjects. During exercise, [ATP] was not affected except in hypothermia subjects exercising under partial ischemia. During recovery, the return of metabolites to preexercise level was much slower in the hypothermia patients than in control subjects, especially for pH. These results suggested the possibility of a latent myopathy and of a persistent metabolic disorder in these patients.

SUMMARY. These clinical demonstrate the utility of the MRS technique for assisting in the diagnosis and evaluation of treatment effects in a wide variety of diseases that directly or indirectly affect skeletal muscle function. Study of these conditions also provides an opportunity to further our understanding of muscle metabolism and performance in healthy individuals. Many of the metabolic abnormalities observed in these chronic clinical conditions are nonspecific. Exercise training often results in an improvement in muscle performance and metabolic capacity. These results suggest that, in chronic diseases with no primary metabolic abnormality, deconditioning may play an important role in the reduced muscle function that has been observed.

CONCLUSION

The noninvasive study of human skeletal muscle metabolism under various experimental conditions has clarified the relationship between energy supply and demand in exercising muscle. Oxidative and glycolytic metabolism have been the focus of many studies of muscle performance. Investigations of the role of metabolism in the development of muscle fatigue indicated that metabolic inhibition of the contractile process is often, but not always, an important factor in fatigue. The results of these studies have been consistent with theories developed using other techniques, and in many cases new refinements of these theories have been presented. The ability to monitor metabolism continuously has allowed examination of the sequence of metabolic events that occur during various types of exercise.

Perhaps one of the most important clinical uses of MRS in the future will be for the detection of subnormal metabolism in conditions where there is a primary (e.g., myopathy) or secondary (e.g., chronic disease) impairment of muscle function. Likewise, the ability to monitor the efficacy of various therapeutic interventions in a noninvasive manner will be of great value in the treatment of these conditions. Thus, an important future direction of MRS research is akin to a future direction of the field of exercise science in general, wherein a focused effort regarding the evaluation and management of functional capacity is expected.

ACKNOWLEDGMENTS

We thank Daryl Zapata and Suzanne Martin for their assistance in preparing this manuscript. Funding for this work was from National Institutes of Health Grant R01 AG10897, the Muscular Dystrophy Association, and the National Multiple Sclerosis Society.

REFERENCES

1. Achten, E., M. van Cauteren, R. Willem, et al. ^{31}P NMR spectroscopy and the metabolic properties of different muscle fibers. *J. Appl. Physiol.* 68:644–649, 1990.
2. Adamopoulos, A., A. J. S. Coats, F. Brunotte, et al. Physical training improves skeletal muscle metabolism in patients with chronic heart failure. *J. Am. Coll. Cardiol.* 21:1101–1106, 1993.
3. Adamopoulos, S., A. J. S. Coats. Peripheral abnormalities in chronic heart failure. *Postgrad. Med. J.* 67(suppl 1):S74–S80, 1991.
4. Aldridge, R., E. B. Cady, D. A. Jones, G. Obletter. Muscle pain after exercise is linked with an inorganic phosphate increase as shown by ^{31}P NMR. *Biosci. Rep.* 6:663–667, 1986.

5. Argov, Z., W. J. Bank, J. Maris, et al. Bioenergetic heterogeneity of human mitochondrial myopathies: phosphorus magnetic resonance spectroscopy study. *Neurology* 37:257–262, 1987.

6. Argov, Z., W. J. Bank, J. Maris, et al. Treatment of mitochondrial myopathy due to complex III deficiency with vitamins K3 and C: a ^{31}P NMR follow-up study. *Ann. Neurol.* 19: 598–602, 1986.

7. Argov, Z., P. F. Renshaw, B. Boden, et al. Effects of thyroid hormones on skeletal muscle bioenergetics. *J. Clin. Invest.* 81:1695–1701, 1988.

8. Arnold, D. L., P. M. Matthews, G. K. Radda. Metabolic recovery after exercise and the assessment of mitochondrial function in vivo in human skeletal muscle by means of ^{31}P NMR. *Magn. Reson. Med.* 1:307–315, 1984.

9. Arnold, D. L., G. K. Radda, P. J. Bore, P. Styles. Excessive intracellular acidosis of skeletal muscle on exercise in a patient with a post-viral exhaustion/fatigue syndrome. *Lancet* June 23; 1367–1369, 1984.

10. Arnolda, L., M. Conway, M. Dolecki, et al. Skeletal muscle metabolism in heart failure: a ^{31}P nuclear magnetic resonance spectroscopy study of leg muscle. *Clin. Sci.* 79:583–589, 1990.

11. Avison, M. J., D. L. Rothman, E. Nadel, R. G. Shulman. Detection of human muscle glycogen by natural abundance ^{13}C NMR. *Proc. Natl. Acad. Sci. U. S. A.* 85:1634–1636, 1988.

12. Baker, A. J., P. J. Carson, A. T. Green, et al. Influence of human muscle length on energy transduction studied by ^{31}P NMR. *J. Appl. Physiol.* 73:160–165, 1992.

13. Baker, A. J., K. G. Kostov, R. G. Miller, M. W. Weiner. Slow force recovery after long duration exercise: metabolic and activation factors in muscle fatigue. *J. Appl. Physiol.* 74: 2294–2300, 1993.

14. Barany, M., I. M. Siegel, P. N. Venkatasubramanian, et al. Human leg neuromuscular diseases: P-31 MR spectroscopy. *Radiology* 172:503–508, 1989.

15. Barany, M., P. N. Venkatasubramanian, E. Mok, et al. Quantitative and qualitative fat analysis in human leg muscle of neuromuscular diseases by III MR spectroscopy in vivo. *Magn. Reson. Med.* 10:210–226, 1989.

16. Barbiroli, B., K. K. McCully, S. Iotti, R. Lodi, P. Zaniol, B. Chance. Further impairment of muscle phosphate kinetics by lengthening exercise in DMD/BMD carriers. *J. Neurol. Sci.* 119.65–73, 1993.

17. Barbiroli, B., R. Funicello, A. Ferlini, et al. Muscle energy metabolism in female DMD/BMD carriers: a ^{31}P MR spectroscopy study. *Muscle Nerve* 15:344–348, 1992.

18. Barbiroli, B., R. Funicello, S. Iotti, et al. ^{31}P-NMR spectroscopy of skeletal muscle in Becker dystrophy and DMD/BMD carriers. *J. Neurol. Sci.* 188–195, 1992.

19. Barnes, P. R. J., D. J. Taylor, G. J. Kemp, G. K. Radda. Skeletal muscle bioenergetics in the chronic fatigue syndrome. *J. Neurol. Neurosurg. Psychiatry* 56:679–683, 1993.

20. Beckman, N., J. Seelig, H. Wick. Analysis of glycogen storage disease by in vivo 13C NMR: comparison of normal volunteers with a patient. *Magn. Reson. Med.* 16:150–160, 1990.

21. Beliveau, L., J.-N. Helal, E. Gaillard, et al. EMG spectral shift and ^{31}P NMR determined intracellular pH in fatigued human biceps brachii muscle. *Neurology* 41:1998–2001, 1991.

22. Bendahan, D., S. Confort-Gouny, G. Kozak-Ribbens, P. J. Cozzone. ^{31}P NMR characterization of the metabolic anomalies associated with the lack of glycogen phosphorylase activity in human forearm muscle. *Biochem. Biophys. Res. Commun.* 185:16–21, 1992.

23. Bendahan, D., S. Confort-Gouny, G. Kozak-Ribbens, P. J. Cozzone. Pi trapping in glycogenolytic pathway can explain transient Pi disappearance during recovery from muscular exercise. *FEBS Lett.* 269:402–405, 1990.

24. Bendahan, D., C. Desnuelle, D. Vanuxem, et al. ^{31}P NMR spectroscopy and ergometer exercise test as evidence for muscle oxidative performance improvement with coenzyme Q in mitochondrial myopathies. *Neurology* 42:2103–1208, 1992.

25. Bernus, G., J. M. G. DeSuso, J. Alonso, P. A. Martin, J. A. Prat, C. Arus. ^{31}P-MRS of quadriceps reveals quantitative differences between sprinters and long-distance runners. *Med. Sci. Sports Exerc.* 25:479–484, 1993.

26. Bertocci, L. A., R. G. Haller, S. F. Lewis. Muscle metabolism during lactate infusion in human phosphofructokinase deficiency. *J. Appl. Physiol.* 74:1342–1347, 1993.

27. Bertocci, L. A., R. G. Haller, S. F. Lewis, et al. Abnormal high-energy phosphate metabolism in human muscle phosphofructokinase deficiency. *J. Appl. Physiol.* 70:1201–1207, 1991.

28. Bertocci, L. A., C. E. Mize, R. Uauy. Muscle phosphorus energy state in very-low-birthweight infants: effect of exercise. *Am. J. Physiol.* 262:E289–E294. 1992.

29. Bet, L., N. Bresolin, M. Moggio, et al. A case of mitochondrial myopathy, lactic acidosis and complex I deficiency. *J. Neurol.* 237:399–404, 1990.

30. Blei, M. L., K. E. Conley, M. J. Kushmerick. Separate measures of ATP utilization and recovery in human skeletal muscles. *J. Physiol (Lond.)* 465:203–222, 1993.

31. Bollaert, P. E.,B. Robin-Lherbier, J. M. Escanye, et al. Phosphorus nuclear magnetic resonance evidence of abnormal skeltal muscle metabolism in chronic alcholics. *Neurology* 39:821–824, 1989.

32. Boska, M. Estimating the ATP cost of force production in the human gastrocnemius/soleus muscle group using ^{31}P MRS and ^{1}H MRI. *NMR Biomed.* 4:173–181, 1991.

33. Boska, M. D., R. S. Moussavi, P. J. Carson, et al. The metabolic basis of recovery after fatiguing exercise in human muscle. *Neurology* 40:240–244, 1990.

34. Cady, E. B., H. Elshove, D. A. Jones, A Moll. The metabolic causes of slow relaxation in fatigued human skeletal muscle. *J. Physiol. (Lond.)* 418:327–337, 1989.

35. Cady, E. B., D. A. Jones, J. Lynn, D. J. Newham. Changes in force and intracellular metabolites during fatigue of human skeletal muscle. *J. Physiol. (Lond.)* 418:311–325, 1989.

36. Carduso, M., E. Shoubridge, D. Arnold, et al. NMR Monitoring of the energy status of skeletal muscle during hemodialysis using acetate. *Clin. Invest. Med.* 11:292–296, 1988.

37. Chance, B., S. Eleff, D. Sokolow, A. A. Sapega. Mitochondrial regulation of phosphocreatine-phosphate ratios in exercise human muscle: a gated 31P NMR study. *Proc. Natl. Acad. Sci. U. S. A.* 78:6714–6718, 1981.

38. Chance, B., J. S. Leigh, B. J. Clark, et al. Control of oxidative metabolism and oxygen delivery in human skeletal muscle: a steady-state analysis of the work/energy cost transfer function. *Proc. Natl. Acad. Sci. U. S. A.* 82:8384–8388, 1985.

39. Chance, B., J. S. Leigh, J. Kent, et al. Multiple controls of oxidative metabolism in living tissues as studied by phosphorus magnetic resonance. *Proc. Natl. Acad. Sci. U. S. A.* 83: 9458–9462, 1986.

40. Chance, B., J. S. Leigh, J. Kent, K. K. McCully. Metabolic control principles and 31P NMR. *Fed. Proc.* 45:2915–2920, 1986.

41. Coggan, A. R., A. M. Abduljalil, S. C. Swanson, et al. Muscle metabolism during exercise in young and older untrained and endurance-trained men. *J. Appl. Physiol.* 75:2125–2133, 1993.

42. Cortelli, P., P. Montagna, P. Avoni, et al. Leber's hereditary optic neuropathy: genetic, biochemical, and phosphorus magnetic resonance spectroscopy study in an Italian family. *Neurology* 42:1211–1215, 1991.

43. DeBlecourt, A. C., R. F. Wolf, M. H. van Rijswijk, et al. In vivo ^{31}P magnetic resonance spectroscopy (MRS) of tender points in patients with primary fibromyalgia syndrome. *Rheumatol. Int.* 11:51–54, 1991.

44. DeSuso, J. M. G., G. Bernus, et al. Development and characterization of an ergometer to study the bioenergetics of the human quadriceps muscle by ^{31}P NMR spectroscopy inside a standard MR scanner. *Magn. Reson. Med.* 29:575–581, 1993.

45. DeGroot, M., B. M. Massie, M. Boska, J. Gober, R. G. Miller, M. W. Weiner. Dissociation of [H+] from fatigue in human muscle detected by high time resolution ^{31}P-NMR. *Muscle Nerve* 16:91–98, 1993.

46. Durozard, D., P. Pimmel, S. Baretto, et al. ^{31}P NMR spectroscopy investigation of muscle metabolism in hemodialysis patients. *Kidney Int.* 43:885–892, 1993.

47. Edwards, R. H. T., M. J. Dawson, D. R. Wilkie, et al. Clinical use of nuclear magnetic resonance in the investigation of myopathy. *Lancet* i:726–731, 1982.

48. Eleff, S., N. G. Kennaway, N. R. M. Buist, et al. ^{31}P NMR study of improvement in oxidative phosphorylation by vitamins K3 and C in a patient with a defect in electron transport at complex III in skeletal muscle. *Proc. Natl. Acad. Sci. U. S. A.* 81:3529–3533, 1984.

49. Fleckenstein, J. L., L. A. Bertocci, R. L. Nunnally, R. W. Parkey, R. M. Peshock. Exercise-enhanced MR imaging of variations in forearm muscle anatomy and use: importance on MR spectroscopy. *Am. J. Roentgenol* 153:693–698, 1989.

50. Fotedar, L. K., J. M. Slopis, P. A. Narayana, R. M. Peshock. Proton magnetic resonance of exercise-induced water changes in gastrocnemius muscle. *J. Appl. Physiol.* 69(5):1695–1701, 1990.

51. Gadian, D., G. Radda, B. Ross, et al. Examination of a myopathy by phosphorus nuclear magnetic resonance. *Lancet* i:774–775, 1981.

52. Griffiths, R. D., E. B. Cady, R. H. T. Edwards, D. R. Wilkie. Muscle energy metabolism in Duchenne dystrophy studied by ^{31}P NMR: controlled trials show no effect of allopurinol or ribose. *Muscle Nerve* 8:760–767, 1985.

53. Hagspiel, K. D., C. von Weymarn, G. McKinnon, et al. Effect of hypothyroidism on phophorus metabolism in muscle and liver: in vivo P-31 MR spectroscopy study. *J. Magn. Reson. Imag.* 2:527–532, 1992.

54. Hands, L. J., P. J. Bore, G. Galloway, et al. Muscle metabolism in patients with peripheral vascular disease investigated by ^{31}P nuclear resonance spectroscopy. *Clin. Sci.* 71:283–290, 1986.

55. Hands, L. J., M. H. Sharif, G. S. Payne, et al. Muscle ischemia in peripheral vascular disease studied by ^{31}P magnetic resonance spectroscopy. *Eur. J. Vasc. Surg.* 4:637–642, 1990.

56. Helpern, J. A., W. Kao, B. Gross, et al. Interleaved ^{31}P NMR with transcutaneous nerve stimulation (TNS): a method of monitoring compliance-independent skeletal muscle metabolic response to exercise. *Magn. Reson. Med.* 10.50–56, 1989.

57. Higgins, R. M., A. J. Richardson, Z. H. Endre, et al. Hypophosphataemia after renal transplantation: relationship to immunosuppressive drug therapy and effects on muscle detected by ^{31}P nuclear magnetic resonance spectroscopy. *Nephrol. Dial. Transplant.* 5:62–68, 1990.

58. Hultman, E., H. Sjoholm, K. Sahlin, L. Edstrom. Glycolytic and oxidative energy metabolism and contraction characteristics of intact human muscle. In *Human Muscle Fatigue*, Ciba Foundation Symposia No. 82, London: Pitman Medical, 1981, pp 19–40

59. Iotti, S., R. Funicello, P. Zaniol, B. Barbiroli. Kinetics of post-exercise phosphate transport in human skeletal muscle. *Biochem. Biophys. Res. Commun.* 176:1204–1209, 1991.

60. Iotti S., R. Funicello, P. Zaniol, B. Barbiroli. The rate of phosphate transport during recovery from muscular exercise depends on cytosolic [H+]. *Biochem. Biophys. Res. Commun.* 178:871–877, 1991.

61. Jeneson, J. A. L., S. J. Nelson, D. B. Vigneron, et al. Two-dimensional ^{31}P chemical shift imaging of intramuscular heterogeneity in exercising human forearm muscle. *Am. J. Physiol* 263:C357–C364, 1992.

62. Jensen, K.E., J. Jakobsen, C. Thomsen, O. Henrikson. Improved energy kinetics following high protein diet in McArdle's syndrome. A ^{31}P magnetic resonance spectroscopy study. *Acta. Neurol. Scand.* 81:499–503, 1990.

63. Jue, T., D. L. Rothman, B. A. Tavitian, R. G. Shulman. Natural-abundance 13C NMR study of glycogen repletion in human liver and muscle. *Proc. Natl. Acad. Sci. U. S. A.* 86:1439–1442, 1989.

64. Kaminsky, P., B. Robin-Lherbier, F. Brunotte, et al. Energetic metabolism in hypothyroid skeletal muscle, as studied by phosphorus magnetic resonance spectroscopy. *J. Clin. Endocrinol. Metab.* 74:124–129, 1992.

65. Kaminsky, P., B. Robin-Lherbier, P. Walker, et al. Muscle bioenergetic impairment in hyperthyroid man: a study by ^{31}P NMR spectroscopy. *Acta Endocrinol.* 124:271–277, 1991.

66. Kao, W., B. Gross, M. Gheorghiade, et al. Skeletal muscle metabolism at rest and exercise in patients with severe but compensated left ventricular dysfunction—a 31P nuclear magnetic resonance study. *Am. J. Noninvas. Cardiol.* 5:7–11, 1991.

67. Kariya, Y., M. Itoh, T. Nakamura, et al. Magnetic resonance imaging and spectroscopy of thigh muscles in cruciate ligament insufficiency. *Acta. Orthop. Scand.* 60:322–325, 1989.
68. Keller, U., R. Oberhansli, P. Huber, et al. Phosphocreatine content and intracellular pH of calf muscle measured by phosphorus NMR spectroscopy in occulusive arterial disease of the legs. *Eur. J. Clin. Invest.* 15:382–388, 1985.
69. Kemp, G. J., D. J. Taylor, P. Styles, G. K. Radda. The production, buffering and efflux of protons in human skeletal muscle during exercise and recovery. *NMR Biomed.* 6:73–83, 1993.
70. Kemp, G. J., D. J. Taylor, J. F. Dunn, S. P. Frostick, G. K. Radda. Cellular energetics of dystrophic muscle. *J. Neuro. Sci.* 116:201–206, 1993.
71. Kemp, G. J., D. J. Taylor, G. K. Radda, B. Rajogopalan. Bio-energetic changes in human gastrocnemius muscle 1–2 days after strenuous exercise. *Acta. Physiol Scand.* 146:11–14, 1992.
72. Kent-Braun, J. A., K. R. Sharma, M. W. Weiner, R. G. Miller. Effects of exercise on muscle activation and metabolism in multiple sclerosis. *Muscle Nerve,* in press.
73. Kent-Braun, J. A., K. R. Sharma, R. G. Miller, M.W. Winer. Postexercise phosphocreatine resynthesis is slowed in multiple sclerosis. *Muscle Nerve,* 17:835–841, 1994.
74. Kent-Braun, J. A., R. G. Miller, M. W. Weiner. Magnetic resonance spectroscopy studies of human muscle. *Radiol. Clin. North Am.* 32:313–335, 1994.
75. Kent-Braun, J. A., K. K. McCully, B. Chance. Metabolic effects of training in humans: A 31P MRS study. *J. Appl. Physiol.* 69:1165–1170, 1990.
76. Kent-Braun, J. A., R. G. Miller, M.W. Weiner. Phases of metabolism during progressive exercise to fatigue in human skeletal muscle. *J. Appl. Physiol.* 75:573–580, 1993.
77. Kent-Braun, J. A., K. R. Sharma, B. Massie, et al. Central basis of muscle fatigue in chronic fatigue syndrome. *Neurology* 43:125–131, 1993.
78. Lam, E. W. N., A. G. Hannam. Regional ^{31}P magnetic resonance spectroscopy of exercising human masseter muscle. *Arch. Oral. Biol.* 37:49–56, 1992.
79. Laurent, D., P. Portero, F. Goubel, A. Rossi. Electromyogram spectrum changes during sustained contraction related to proton and diprotonated inorganic phosphate accumulation: a ^{31}P nuclear magnetic resonance study on human calf muscles. *Eur. J. Appl. Physiol.* 66:263–268, 1993.
80. Laurent, D., B. Authier, J. F. Lebas, A. Rossi. Effect of prior exercise in Pi/PCr ratio and intracellular pH during a standardized exercise. A study on human muscle using [^{31}P]NMR. *Acta. Physiol. Scand.* 144:31–38, 1992.
81. Laurent, D., H. Reutenauer, J.-F. Payen, et al. Discrimination between cross-country and downhill skiers by pulmonary and local ^{31}PNMR evaluations. *Med. Sci. Sports Exerc.* 25:29–36. 1993.
82. Legros, P., P. Jehenson, J. P. Gascard, G. Kozak-Reiss. Long-term relationship between acute rhabdomyolysis and abnormal high-energy phosphate metabolism potentiated by ischemic exercise. *Med. Sci. Sports Exerc.* 24:298–302, 1992.
83. Lewis, S. F., R. G. Haller, J. D. Cook, R. I. Nunnally. Muscle fatigue in McArdle's disease studied by ^{31}P NMR: effect of glucose infusion. *J. Appl. Physiol* 59:1991–1994, 1985.
84. Lunt, J. A., P. S. Allen, M. Brauer, et al. An evaluation of the effect of fasting on the exercise-induced changes in pH and Pi/PCr from skeletal muscle. *Magn. Reson. Med.* 3:946–952, 1986.
85. Mancini, D. M., E. Coyle. A. Coggan, et al. Contribution of intrinsic skeletal muscle changes to ^{31}P NMR skeletal muscle metabolic abnormalities in patients with chronic heart failurre. *Circulation* 80:1338–1346, 1989.
86. Mancini, D. M., N. Ferraro, M. Tuchler, et al. Detection of abnormal calf muscle metabolism in patients with heart failure using phosphorus-31 nuclear magnetic resonance. *Am. J. Cardiol.* 62:1234–1240, 1988.
87. Mancini, D. M., M. Schwartz, N. Ferraro, et al. Effect of dobutamine on skeletal muscle metabolism in patients with congestive heart failure. *Am. J. Cardiol.* 65:1121–1126, 1990.

88. Mancini, D. M., G. Walter, N. Reichek, et al. Contribution of skeletal muscle atrophy to exercise intolerance and altered muscle metabolism in heart failure. *Circulation* 85:1364–1373, 1992.

89. Marie, P.-Y., J.-M. Escanye, F. Brunotte, et al. Skeletal muscle metabolism in the leg during exercise in patients with congestive heart failure. *Clin. Sci.* 78:515–519, 1990.

90. Marsh, G. D., D. H. Paterson, R. T. Thompson, P. K. Cheung, J. MacDermid, J. M. O. Arnold. Metabolic adaptations to endurance training in older individuals. *Can. J. Appl. Physiol.* 18:366–378, 1993.

91. Marsh, G. D., D. H. Paterson, J. J. Potwarka, R. T. Thompson. Transient changes in muscle high-energy phosphates during moderate exercise. *J. Appl. Physiol.* 75:548–656, 1993.

92. Marsh, G. D., D. H. Paterson, R. T. Thompson, A. A. Driedger. Coincident thresholds in intracellular phosphorylation potential and pH during progressive exercise. *J. Appl. Physiol.* 71:1076–1081, 1991.

93. Massie, B. M., M. Conway, B. Rajagopalan, et al. Skeletal muscle metabolism during exercise under ischemic conditions in congestive heart failure. Evidence for abnormalities unrelated to blood flow. *Circulation* 78:320–326, 1988.

94. Massie, B. M., M. Conway, R. Yonge, et al. Skeletal muscle metabolism in patients with congestive heart failure. Relation to clinical severity and blood flow. *Circulation* 76:1009, 1987.

95. Matheson, G. O., P. S. Allen, D. C. Ellinger, et al. Skeletal muscle metabolism and work capacity: a ^{31}P NMR study of Andean natives and lowlanders. *J. Appl. Physiol.* 70:1963–1976, 1991.

96. Matheson, G. O., D. C. McKenzie, D. Gheorghiu, et al. ^{31}P NMR of electrically stimulated rectus femoris muscle: an in vivo graded exercise model. *Magn. Reson. Med.* 26:60–70, 1992.

97. Matthews, P. M., C. Allaire, E. A. Shoubridge, et al. In vivo muscle magnetic resonance spectroscopy in the clinical investigation of mitochondrial disease. *Neurology* 41:114–120, 1991.

98. McCully, K. K., R. A. Fielding, W. J. Evans, J. S. Leigh, Jr., J. D. Posner. Relationships between in vivo and in vitro measurements of metabolism in young and old human calf muscles. *J. Appl. Physiol.* 75:813–819, 1993.

99. McCully, K. K., J. Kent, B. Chance. Muscle injury and stress measured with 31-P magnetic resonance spectroscopy. Muscle energetics. R. J. Paul, K. Yamada, and G. Elzinge (eds). *Progress in Clinical and Biological Research. Vol. 315.* New York: A. R. Liss, pp. 197–207.

100. McCully, K. K., Z. Argov, B. P. Boden, et al. Detection of muscle injury in humans with ^{31}P magnetic resonance spectroscopy. *Muscle Nerve* 11:212–216, 1988.

101. McCully, K. K., B. P. Boden, M. Tuchler, et al. Wrist flexor muscles of elite rowers measured with magnetic resonance spectroscopy. *J. Appl. Physiol.* 67:926–932, 1989.

102. McCully, K. K., M. A. Forciea, L. M. Hack, et al. Muscle metabolism in older subjects using ^{31}P magnetic resonance spectroscopy. *Can. J. Physiol. Pharmacol.* 69:576–580, 1991.

103. Menard, M. R., A. M. Penn, J. W. K. Lee, et al. Relative metabolic efficiency of concentric and eccentric exercise determined by ^{31}P magnetic resonance spectroscopy. *Arch. Phys. Med. Rehabil.* 72:976–983, 1991.

104. Meyer, R. A. A linear model of muscle respiration explains monoexponential phosphocreatine changes. *Am. J. Physiol.* 254(Cell Physiol 23):C548–553, 1988.

105. Miller, RG, M. D. Boska, R. Moussavi, et al. 31P Nuclear magnetic resonance studies of high energy phophates and pH in human muscle fatigue. *J. Clin. Invest.* 81:1190–1196, 1988.

106. Miller, R. G., P. J. Carson, R. S. Moussavi, et al. Fatigue and myalgia in AIDS patients. *Neurology* 41:1603–1607, 1991.

107. Miller, R. G., D. Giannini, H. S. Milner-Brown, et al. Effects of fatiguing exercise on high-energy phosphates, force and EMG: evidence for three phases of recovery. *Muscle Nerve* 10:810–821, 1987.

108. Miller, R. G., A. T. Green, R. S. Moussavi, et al. Excessive muscular fatigue in patients with spastic paraparesis. *Neurology* 40:1271–1274, 1990.

109. Miller, R. G., R. S. Moussavi, A. T. Green, et al. The fatigue of rapid repetitive movements. *Neurology* 43:755–761, 1993.

110. Minotti, J. R., E. C. Johnson, T. L. Hudson, et al. Forearm metabolic asymmetry detected by ^{31}P NMR during submaximal exercise. *J. Appl. Physiol.* 67:324–329, 1989.

111. Minotti, J. R., E. C. Johnson, T. L. Hudson, et al. Skeletal muscle response to exercise training in congestive heart failure. *J. Clin. Invest.* 86:751–758, 1990.

112. Minotti, J. R., E. C. Johnson, T. L. Hudson, et al. Training-induced skeletal muscle adaptations are independent of systemic adaptations. *J. Appl. Physiol.* 68:289–294, 1990.

113. Mize, C. E., R. J. T. Corbett, R. Uauy, et al. Hypotonia of rickets: a sequential study by P-31 magnetic resonance spectroscopy. *Pediatr. Res.* 24:713–716, 1988.

114. Mizuno, M., N. H. Secher, B. Quistorff. ^{31}P-NMR spectroscopy, rsEMG, and histochemical fiber types of human wrist flexor muscles. *J. Appl. Physiol.* 76:531–538, 1994.

115. Mizuno, M., L. O. Justesen, J. Bedolla, et al. Partial curarization abolishes splitting of the inorganic phosphate peak in ^{31}P NMR spectroscopy during intense forearm exercise in man. *Acta. Physiol. Scand.* 139:611–612, 1990.

116. Mole, P. A., R. L. Coulson, J. R. Caton, et al. In vivo ^{31}P NMR in human muscle: transient patterns with exercise. *J. Appl. Physiol.* 59:101–104, 1985.

117. Moore, G. E., L. A. Bertocci, P. L. Painter. 31P-magnetic resonance spectroscopy assessment of subnormal oxidative metabolism in skeletal muscle of renal failure patients. *J. Clin. Invest.* 91:420–424, 1993.

118. Moussavi, R. S., P. J. Carson, M. D. Boska, et al. Non-metabolic basis of fatigue in exercising human muscle. *Neurology* 39:1222–1226, 1989.

119. Nelson, S. J., J. S. Taylor, D. B. Vigneron, et al. Metabolite images of the human arm: changes in spatial and temporal distribution of high-energy phosphates during exercise. *NMR Biomed.* 4:268–273, 1991.

120. Newham, D. J., E. B. Cady. A [31]P Study of fatigue and metabolism in human skeletal muscle with voluntary, intermittent contractions at different forces. *NMR Biomed.* 3:211–219, 1990.

121. Newman, R. J., P. J. Bore, L. Chan. et al. Nuclear magnetic resonance studies of forearm muscle in Duchenne dystrophy. *Br. Med. J.* 284:1072–1074, 1982.

122. Nishida, A., K. Kubo, M. Uneda, et al. Clinial use of ^{31}P nuclear magnetic resonance spectroscopy for muscle damage in uremia. *Nephron.* 57:489–490, 1991.

123. Nishida, A., H. Nishijima, K. Yonezawa, et al. Phosphorus-31 magnetic resonance spectroscopy of forearm flexor muscles in student rowers using an exercise protocol adjusted for differences in cross-sectional muscle area. *Eur. J. Appl. Physiol.* 64:528–533, 1992.

124. Nishikawa, Y., M. Takahashi, S. Yorifuji, et al. Long-term coenzyme Q10 therapy for a mitochondrial encephalomyopathy with cytochrome c oxidase deficiency: a ^{31}P NMR study. *Neurology* 39:399–403, 1989.

125. Olgin, J., H. Rosenberg, G. Allen, et al. A blinded comparison of noninvasive, in vivo phosphorus nuclear magnetic resonance spectroscopy and the in vitro halothane/caffeine contracture test in the evaluation of malignant hyperthermia susceptibility. *Anesth. Analg.* 72:36–47, 1991.

126. Park, J. S., S. B. Kim, S-K. Park, T. H. Lim. D. K. Lee, C. D. Hong. Effect of recombinant human erythropoietin on muscle energy metabolism in patients with end-stage renal disease: a ^{31}P-nuclear magnetic resonance spectroscopic study. *Am. J. Kidney Dis.* 21:612–618, 1993.

127. Park, J. H., R. L. Brown, C. R. Park, et al. Energy metabolism of the untrained muscle of elite runners as observed by ^{31}P magnetic resonance spectroscopy: evidence suggesting a genetic endowment for endurance exercise. *Proc. Natl. Acad. Sci. U. S. A.* 85:8780–8784, 1988.

128. Park, J. H., R. L. Brown, C. R. Park, et al. Functional pools of oxidative and glycolytic fibers in human muscle observed by ^{31}P magnetic resonance spectroscopy during exercise. *Proc. Natl. Acad. Sci. U. S. A.* 84:8976–8980, 1987.

129. Payen, J-F., B. Wuyam, P. Levy, et al. Muscular metabolism during oxygen supplementation in patients with chronic hypoxemia. *Am. Rev. Respir. Dis.* 147:592–598, 1993.

130. Payen, J.-F., J.-L. Bosson, L. Bourdon, et al. Improved noninvasive diagnostic testing for malignant hyperthermia susceptibility from a combination of metabolites determined in vivo with ^{31}P-magnetic resonance spectroscopy. *Anesthesiology* 78:848–855, 1993.

131. Payen, J.-F., L. Bourdon, H. Reutenauer, et al. Exertional heat-stroke and muscle metabolism: an in vivo ^{31}P MRS study. *Med. Sci. Sports Exerc.* 24:420–425, 1992.

132. Payen, J.-F., B. Wuyam, H. Retenauer, et al. Impairment of muscular metabolism in chronic respiratory failure. A human 31P MRS study. *NMR Biomed.* 4:41–45, 1991.

133. Price, T. B., D. L. Rothman, M. J. Avison, et al. 13C-NMR measurements of muscle glycogen during low-intensity exercise. *J. Appl. Physiol.* 70:1836–1844, 1991.

134. Quistorff, B., L. Johansen, K. Sahlin. Absence of phosphocreatine resynthesis in human calf muscle during ischemic recovery. *Biochem. J.* 291:681–686, 1992.

135. Radda, G. K., P. J. Bore, D. G. Gadian, et al. ^{31}P NMR examination of two patients with NADH-CoQ reductase deficiency. *Nature* 295:608, 1982.

136. Rajagopalan, B., M. A. Conway, B. Massie, G. K. Radda. Alterations of skeletal muscle metabolism in humans studied by phosphorus 31 magnetic resonance spectroscopy in congestive heart failure. *Am. J. Cardiol.* 62:53E–57E, 1988.

137. Rees, D., M. B. Smith, J. Harley, G. K. Radda. In vivo functioning of creatine phosphokinase in human forearm muscle, studied by ^{31}P NMR saturation transfer. *Magn. Reson. Med.* 9:39–52, 1989.

138. Rexroth, W.,W. Semler, F. Guckel, et al. Assessment of muscular metabolism in peripheral aterial occlusive disease using ^{31}P nuclear magnetic resonance spectroscopy. *Klin. Wochenschr.* 67:804–819, 1989.

139. Ross, B. D., G. K. Radda, D. G. Gadian, et al. Examination of a case of suspected McArdle's syndrome by ^{31}P nuclear magnetic resonance. *N. Engl. J. Med.* 304:1338–1342, 1981.

140. Sharma, K. R., J. A. Kent-Braun, M. A., Mynhier, M. W. Weiner, R. G. Miller. Excessive muscular fatigue in the post-polio myelitis syndrome. *Neurology* 44:642–646, 1994.

141. Shenton, D. W., R. B. Heppenstall, B. Chance, et al. Electrical stimulation of human muscle studied using ^{31}P-nuclear magnetic resonance spectroscopy. *J. Orthop. Res.* 4:204–211, 1986.

142. Shulman, G. I., D. L. Rothman, T. Jue, et al. Quantitation of muscle glycogen synthesis in normal subjects and subjects with non-insulin-dependent diabetes by 13C nuclear magnetic resonance spectroscopy. *N. Engl. J. Med.* 322:223–228, 1990.

143. Systrom, D. M., D. J. Kanarek, S. J. Kohler, H. Kazemi. 31P Nuclear magnetic resonance spectroscopy study of the anaerobic threshold in humans. *J. Appl. Physiol.* 68:2060–2066, 1990.

144. Taborsky, P., I. Sotornik, J. Kaslikova, O. Schuck, M. Hajek, A. Horska. ^{31}P magnetic resonance spectroscopy investigation of skeletal muscle metabolism in uraemic patients. *Nephron.* 65:222–226, 1993.

145. Tada, H., H. Kato, T. Misawa, et al. ^{31}P Nuclear magnetic resonance evidence of abnormal skeletal muscle metabolism in patients with chronic lung disease and congestive heart failure. *Eur. Respir. J.* 5:163–169, 1992.

146. Taylor, R., T. B. Price, L. D. Katz, R. G. Shulman, G. I. Shulman. Direct measurement of change in muscle glycogen concentration after a mixed meal in normal subjects. *Am. J. Physiol.* 265(*Endocrinol Metab* 28):E224–E229, 1993.

147. Taylor, D. J., G. J. Kemp, C. G. Woods, J. H. Edwards, G. K. Radda. Skeletal muscle bioenergetics in myotonic dystrophy. *J. Neurol. Sci.* 116:193–200, 1993.

148. Taylor, D. J., M. J. Brosnan, D. L. Arnold, et al. Ca^{2+}-ATPase deficiency in a patient with an exertional muscle pain syndrome. *J. Neurol. Neurosurg. Psychiat.* 51:1425–1433, 1988.

149. Taylor, D. J., S. W. Coppack, T. A. D. Cadoux-Hudson, et al. Effect of insulin on intracellular pH and phosphate metabolism in human skeletal muscle in vivo. *Clin. Sci.* 81:123–128, 1991.

150. Taylor, D. J., M. Crowe, P. J. Bore, P. Styles, D. L. Arnold, G. K. Radda. Examination of the energetics of aging skeletal muscle using nuclear magnetic resonance. *Gerontology* 30:2–7, 1984.

151. Taylor, D. J., B. Rajagopalan, G. K. Radda. Cellular energetics in hypothyroid muscle. *Eur. J. Clin. Invest.* 22:358–365, 1992.

152. Taylor, D. J., P. Styles, P. M. Matthews, et al. Energetics of human muscles: exercise-induced ATP depletion. *Magn. Reson. Med.* 3:44–54, 1986.

153. Thompson, C. H., R. J. O. Davies, G. J. Kemp, D. J. Taylor, G. K. Radda, B. Rajagopalan. Skeletal muscle metabolism during exercise and recovery in patients with respiratory failure. *Thorax* 48:486–490, 1993.

154. Thompson, C. H., G. J. Kemp, D. J. Taylor, J. G. G. Ledingham, G. K. Radda, B. Rajagopalan. Effect of chronic uraemia on skeletal muscle metabolism in man. *Nephrol. Dial. Transplant* 8:218–222, 1993.

155. Thomsen, C., K. E. Jensen, A. Astrup, et al. Changes of high-energy phosphorus compounds in skeletal muscle during glucose-induced thermogenesis in man: a ^{31}P spectroscopy study. *Acta. Physiol. Scand.* 137:335–339, 1989.

156. Vandenborne, K., G. Walter, J. S. Leigh, G. Goelman. pH heterogeneity during exercise in localized spectra from single human muscles. *Am. J. Physiol.* 265(*Cell Physiol* 34): C1332–C1339, 1993.

157. Vandenborne, K., K. McCully, H. Kakihira, et al. Metabolic heterogeneity in human calf muscle during maximal exercise. *Proc. Natl. Acad. Sci. U. S. A.* 88:5714–5718, 1991.

158. Vestergaard-Poulsen, P., C. Thomsen, T. Sinkjaer, M. Stubgaard, A. Rosenfack, O. Henriksen. Simultaneous electromyography and 31P nuclear magnetic resonance spectroscopy—with application to muscle fatigue. *Electroencephalogr. Clin. Neurophysiol.* 85:402–411, 1992.

159. Victor, R. G., L.A. Bertocci, S. L. Pryor, R. L. Nunnally. Sympathetic nerve discharge is coupled to muscle cell pH during exercise in humans. *J. Clin. Invest.* 82:1301–1306, 1988.

160. Wang, Z., E. A. Noyszewski, J. S. Leigh. In vivo MRS measurement of deoxymyoglobin in human forearms. *Magn. Reson. Med.* 14:562–567, 1990.

161. Webster, D. W., R. T. Thompson, D. R. Gravelle, et al. Metabolic response to exercise in malignant hyperthermia-sensitive patients measured by ^{31}P magnetic resonance spectroscopy. *Magn. Reson. Med.* 15:81–89, 1990.

162. Weiner, M.W., R. S. Moussavi, A. J. Baker, et al. Constant relationships between force, phosphate concentration, and pH in muscles with differential fatigability. *Neurology* 40:1888–1893, 1990.

163. Weissman, J. D., I. Constantinitis, P. Hudgins, D. C. Wallace. ^{31}P magnetic resonance spectroscopy suggests impaired mitochondrial function in AZT-treated HIV-infected patients. *Neurology* 42:619–623, 1992.

164. Wiener, D. H., L. I. Fink, J. Maris, et al. Abnormal skeletal muscle bioenergetics during exercise in patients with heart failure: role of reduced muscle blood flow. *Circulation* 73:1127–1136, 1986.

165. Wiener, D. H., J. Maris, B. Chance, J. R. Wilson. Detection of skeletal muscle hypoperfusion during exercise using phosphorus-31 nuclear magnetic resonance spectroscopy. *J. Am. Coll. Cardiol.* 7:793–799, 1986.

166. Wilkie, D. R., M. J. Dawson, R. H. T. Edwards, et al. ^{31}P NMR studies of resting muscle in normal human subjects. *Adv. Exp. Med. Biol.* 170:333–347, 1984.

167. Williams, D. M., L. Fencil, T. L. Chenevert. Peripheral arterial occlusive disease: P-31 MR spectroscopy of calf muscle. *Radiology* 175:381–385, 1990.

168. Wilson, J. R., L. Fink, J. Maris, et al. Evaluation of energy metabolism in skeletal muscle of patients with heart failure with gated phosphorus-31 nuclear magnetic resonance. *Circulation* 71:57–62, 1985.

169. Wilson, J. R., K. K. McCully, D. M. Mancini, et al. Relationship of muscular fatigue to pH and diprotonated Pi in humans: a 31P-NMR study. *J. Appl. Physiol.* 64:2333–2339, 1988.

170. Wong, R., N. Davies, D. Marshall, et al. Metabolism of normal skeletal muscle during dynamic exercise to clinical fatigue: in vivo assessment by nuclear magnetic resonance spectroscopy. *Can. J. Cardiol.* 6:391–395, 1990.

171. Yoshida, T., H. Watari. Metabolic consequences of repeated exercise in long distance runners. *Eur. J. Appl. Physiol.* 67:261–265, 1993.

172. Yoshida, T., H. Watari. ^{31}P-Nuclear magnetic resonance spectroscopy study of the time course of energy metabolism during exercise and recovery. *Eur. J. Appl. Physiol.* 66: 494–499, 1993.

173. Younkin, D. P., P. Berman, J. Sladky, et al. ^{31}P NMR studies in Duchenne muscular dystrophy: age-related metabolic changes. *Neurology* 37:165–169, 1987.

174. Zanconato, S., S. Buchthal, T. J. Barstow, D. M. Cooper. ^{31}P-magnetic resonance spectroscopy of leg muscle metabolism during exercise in children and adults. *J. Appl. Physiol.* 74:2214–2218, 1993.

175. Zatina, M. A., H. D. Berkowitz, G. M. Gross, et al. [31]P Nuclear magnetic resonance spectroscopy: noninvasive biochemical analysis of the ischemic extremity. *J. Vasc. Surg.* 3:411–420, 1986.

176. Zochodne, D. W., W. J. Koopman, N. J. Witt, et al. Forearm P-31 nuclear magnetic resonance spectroscopy studies in oculopharyngeal muscular dystrophy. *Can. J. Neurol. Sci.* 19:174–179, 1992.

177. Zochodne, D. W., R. T. Thompson, A. A. Driedger, et al. Metabolic changes in human muscle denervation: topical ^{31}P NMR spectroscopy studies. *Magn. Reson. Med.* 7:373–383, 1988.

11
Role of Exercise in the Cause and Prevention of Cardiac Dysfunction

JOSEPH W. STARNES, Ph.D
DOUGLAS K. BOWLES, Ph.D.

Exercise-induced ischemia is common in people with coronary artery disease and may lead to myocardial dysfunction lasting for hours or days [39, 82]. Even healthy people engaged in prolonged strenuous exercise may experience impaired performance of the heart that some investigators attribute to cardiac fatigue [26, 91]. On the other hand, chronic exercise training is known to exert a protective effect against the morbidity and mortality associated with ischemic heart disease [75, 80]. Morris et al. [66] have reported that regular physical activity decreases the overall incidence of heart attacks and reduces the risk of dying should a heart attack occur. Furthermore, Douglas et al. [27] have stated that endurance-trained persons have a higher threshold of cardiac fatigue than do their untrained counterparts. Thus, exercise-induced adaptations may do more than improve intrinsic pump performance during exercise [86, 87]; they may also serve to prevent a decline in performance during prolonged or strenuous exercise and to protect the heart against a variety of environmental stresses. A tenable hypothesis for this overlap is that exercise and certain pathological stresses, i.e., ischemia, have some similarities including changes in energy demand–energy supply and perhaps an increased production of oxygen free radicals. To support this hypothesis, this chapter will begin by reviewing several studies reporting that exercise can indeed lead to cardiac dysfunction and will discuss the potential roles of energy supply–energy demand and free radicals as the basis for the dysfunction. Then studies investigating whether exercise training protects the heart against ischemia will be reviewed. Finally, adaptations that likely play key roles in preserving optimum cardica function during severe exercise or pathological stress will be discussed. Exercise-induced adaptations within the coronary vasculature will be emphasized because they are arguably the most important intrinsic myocardial adaptations for protection against the morbidity and mortality associated with ischemic heart disease.

EXERCISE-INDUCED CARDIAC DYSFUNCTION

After a strenuous bout of exercise, some degree of fatigue is often experienced in the involved skeletal muscles and it is common practice to rest these muscles until maximum function is regained. There is now evidence that the heart also can experience a temporary reduction in performance as a result of strenuous exercise, but unlike skeletal muscle, cardiac muscle must continue to perform considerable levels of work during recovery to sustain life. In healthy young adults, the magnitude of the dysfunction is minimal, but could limit performance at the highest intensities of exercise. However, in people with coronary vascular disease, the degree of dysfunction can range greatly, from mild regional dysfunction that does not affect overall global performance to extensive global dysfunction that adversely impacts daily life, depending on the severity of the disease and the intensity or duration of the exercise.

Reports of cardiac fatigue associated with prolonged exercise in healthy persons have been in the literature for at least 30 years. Saltin and Stenberg [85] studied four subjects and found a reduction in submaximum stroke volume after 3 hr of exercise at 75% of maximum oxygen consumption. Potentially this decline could be due to a change in the intrinsic inotropic state or to an indirect factor, such as hypovolumia, which would decrease stroke volume through a decrease in venous return. Saltin and Stenberg found that the decline in stroke volume occurred without any measured change in blood volume and was observed in both erect and supine positions and thus concluded that intrinsic cardiac function was compromised. Although submaximum stroke volume declined, maximum stroke volume was not altered. Assuming that the intrinsic inotropic state was indeed compromised, there are at least two explanations for this apparent discrepancy. Maximum stroke volume was measured 2 hr postexercise; thus, one possibility is that enough rest was allowed for the organ to recover full maximum function. Another possibility is that the hearts were "stunned" as a result of prolonged exercise. The phenomenon of stunning was first recognized several years after Saltin and Stenberg's study and can be defined as contractile dysfunction in the absence of myocardial necrosis [17]. Although stunning has not been linked directly to exercise-induced changes in stroke volume in hearts free of coronary artery disease, stunning is a well-known occurrence after brief periods of ischemia and has recently been implicated in cardiac dysfunction observed after exercise-induced ischemia [37]. An aspect of stunning that is relevant to Saltin and Stenberg's study is that the contractile dysfunction can sometimes be overridden through adequate sympathetic stimulation [7]. Perhaps the effort to attain maximum exercise provided enough of a sympathetic drive to override the contractile dysfunction Saltin and Stenberg observed at submaximum exercise conditions. Although the mechanisms responsible for myocardial stunning have not been unequivocally determined, evidence is accumulating in support of the role of oxygen free radicals [10, 52].

Maher et al. [60] observed diminished contractile characteristics in isolated trabecular muscles of rats after the animals ran for approximately 3.5

hr until exhausted. Specifically, isometric peak tension development was decreased by more than 50% at all muscle lengths tested, the force-velocity relationship was severely depressed, and the inotropic response to exogenous norepinephrine was lower. The large magnitude of the declines implies that the isolated muscle was severely damaged. However, the function of the heart in vivo was not evaluated so the status of the heart before removal from its host is not known. It does not seem plausible for the function in vivo to be declined as much as that reported in vitro, because declines of such magnitude would likely result in death. In fact, based on more recent data (see below) it is likely that in vivo hemodynamics were only modestly affected. The conclusion reached by Maher et al. [60] was that the diminished contractile characteristics were due to alterations within excitation–contraction coupling because tissue levels of norepinephrine and high-energy phosphates were not changed after exercise. Although the general location of the alterations may be correct, the may have been too subtle to seriously affect contractile characteristics in vivo, but they may have rendered the organ more fragile and susceptible to damage as a result of the further stresses of isolating it from the animal and preparing the tissue for in vitro analysis. Subsequent biochemical in vitro studies have also found exhaustion-induced changes within the excitation–contraction system without any depression of mitochondrial energy production capacity [8, 79, 99]. Belcastro and Sopper [8] used an exhaustion protocol similar to that of Maher et al. and reported a depression of myofibrillar ATPase activity at physiological Ca^{2+} concentrations and Pierce et al. [79] found that rats swum to exhaustion had depressed cardiac sarcoplasmic reticulum Ca^{2+} uptake velocities with no change in several sarcolemmal pump activities or sarcolemmal Ca^{2+} binding. Terjung et al. [99] found normal oxidative phosphorylation capacity in cardiac mitochondria isolated from rates after an exhausting exercise bout. It remains uncertain whether the changes observed in vitro are also manifested in vivo. However, the fact that they occurred at all and that other cellular functions were not altered indicates that specific changes did occur.

Additional studies carried out on humans during the 1980s support Saltin and Stenberg's conclusion that strenuous exercise can have a deleterious effect on cardiac function. Using radionuclide angiocardiography, Upton et al. [104] found that 2 hr of submaximal exercise in well-trained men caused a significant decline in cardiac output (13%) and stroke volume (10%) during maximum exercise. They proposed that these declines were due to either fluid loss because end-diastolic volume was decreased, or to actual cardiac fatigue because more than half of the subjects were no longer able to increase ejection fraction (it actually decreased) in response to increased exercise intensity. However, the authors did not measure blood volume and did not discuss the possibility that the decrease in end-diastolic volume could also be due to an intrinsic alteration affecting ventricular relaxation characteristics or diastolic stiffness. Several studies employing echocardiographic assessments have concluded that some degree of cardiac fatigue is associated with prolonged exercise. For example, Niemela et al. [68] studied experienced male ultramarathon runners competing in a 24-hr run, Douglas et al. [27] studied highly trained ultraendurance athletes competing in the Hawaii Ironman Triathlon, and Seals et al. [91] studied healthy untrained men who ran to exhaustion at an intensity equal to about 70% of maximum oxygen consumption. All of these studies found declines in fractional shortening and in the velocity of circumferential fiber shortening immediately after exercise. Although these two commonly used indices of myocardial contractility do not necessarily imply an altered inotropic state because they are influenced by preload and afterload, the above studies also reported indices, such as the ratio of end-systolic pressure/end-systolic left ventricular dimension, which are indicative of intrinsic contractile state because they do consider loading conditions. Importantly, in all three of the echocardiographic studies, indices of intrinsic contractile state were also reported to decline after exercise. Two of the above studies, Niemela et al. [68] and Douglas et al. [27], charted recovery of cardiac function and found that the postexercise abnormalities had returned to normal within 2–3 days.

The study by Seals et al. [91] used untrained subjects and required considerably less exercise duration to cause a greater impairment of cardiac function, suggesting that endurance training protects the heart against fatigue associated with prolonged exercise. Not surprisingly, people with coronary artery disease are even more susceptible to exercise-related impairments in cardiac function. Homans et al. [39] have reported that exercising for only 10 min produces significant postexercise regional dysfunction when coronary blood flow is restricted enough to produce regional ischemia during the exercise bout.

WHAT CAUSES EXERCISE-INDUCED CARDIAC DYSFUNCTION?

The cause of exercise dysfunction associated with prolonged exercise in healthy people is unknown. However, taken as a whole, the papers discussed in the previous section provide considerable circumstantial evidence suggesting that the dysfunction found in a healthy person whose heart has adequate coronary blood flow throughout the exercise is actually a form of myocardial stunning, which is clinically associated with periods of ischemia. Like the in vitro findings of myocardial changes after exhaustion discussed previously [8, 60, 79, 99], stunning has been characterized as affecting myofibrillar calcium responsiveness and sarcoplasmic reticulum calcium uptake, without affecting mitochondrial oxidative phosphorylation [52]. Contractile dysfunction in the stunned myocardium can sometimes be overridden by catecholamines [7], which may have also occurred during maximum exercise in the study by Saltin and Stenberg [85]. Furthermore, stunning does not result in necrosis or permanent cellular damage and resolves itself over the course of several hours to a couple of days in a manner consistent with the postexercise recovery profiles reported by Douglas et al. [27] and Niemela et al. [68]. Finally, exercise is associated with elevated free radical production [1], and there is a strong consensus that a major cause of stunning is free radicals [10, 52]. A recent study by Kumar et al. [51] reported that exhaustive endurance exercise in rats increased the generation of free radicals in the myocardium. Supplementation with the antioxidant vitamin E for 60 days completely abolished the free radical production during exercise and protected the animals from oxidative damage. A considerable length of time may be required for metabolically produced free radicals to have a measurable impact on cardiac function, which may explain why cardiac dysfunction is only noticed after several hours of prolonged exercise in healthy people. However, we stress the point that at this time we can only speculate that these apparent similarities indicate that stunning can occur in the nonischemic heart during prolonged exercise.

A well-known cause of cardiac dysfunction that is common clinically is exercise-induced ischemia. People who are the most susceptible to this problem are, paradoxically, also the ones who will likely receive the most benefit from exercising on a regular basis. These people are those who have developed some degree of coronary artery disease, which is the primary cause of death among middle-aged men. Kannel and Dawber [41] have stated that the pathological changes that lead to atherosclerosis begin in infancy and develop throughout life; thus most people will develop at least a moderate degree of coronary artery disease. Evidence of coronary atherosclerosis was detected in more than 70% of autopsied soldiers killed in action in Korea [29] and in 45% of Vietnam combat casualties [65]. People with coronary artery disease will have less capacity to deliver oxygen to the heart and, thus, may find themselves in a situation where myocardial energy production is insufficient to meet the energy demands. They will benefit from endurance training because key training-induced adaptations include those that improve the energy supply–energy demand balance, thus raising the threshold for the occurrence of ischemia, and serve to protect the heart should an ischemic event occur. The mechanisms for the improved supply-demand relationships will be discussed later in the article.

Adequate oxygen delivery is necessary at all times and at all levels of mechanical work because cardiac muscle relies exclusively on aerobic energy production to maintain an essentially constant concentration of high-energy phosphates ATP and creatine phosphate [5, 94]. This is not the case for skeletal muscle, which incurs a significant decrease in creatine phosphate during high-energy demands [50]. The two muscle types differ in that the heart cannot afford the luxury of an inactive rest period to replete its high-energy phosphate levels; it must beat continuously for the survival of its host. The stored amounts of high-energy compounds in the left ventricle are quite low; approximately 5 μmol/g for ATP and 8 μmol/g for creatine phosphate [94]. This represents only enough energy to support cardiac work for about 15 sec at rest or about 4 sec during maximum work (the actual times will be much shorter, however, because work would cease before total depletion of the high-energy phosphates). Thus, the myocardium relies on a very close temporal matching of oxidative metabolism to changes in metabolic demand. It has very little tolerance for an oxygen debt and even a very brief interruption or lag in oxidative metabolism adversely affects cardiac function.

It has been estimated that there are more than 2,500 capillaries/mm^2 of left ventricle [73]. The amount of oxygen extracted from the blood as it passes through the myocardium is near the physiological maximum even in the resting state; thus increasing the volume of blood flowing through the coronary circulation is absolutely required for myocardial metabolism to produce enough ATP for exercise-induced cardiac work. We [94] and others [70] have reported that over a broad range of cardiac work, oxygen extraction changes very little and coronary flow varies linearly with oxygen consumption. Inadequate blood flow will render the heart ischemic and quickly lead to a decrease in function; thus persons with coronary artery disease are the most susceptible to exercise-induced cardiac dysfunction. The crucial importance of adequate coronary vasodilation during exercise was demonstrated quite clearly in a recent study by Weiss et al. [106] that used isometric exercise in coronary patients. Cardiac energy demand was estimated by the rate-pressure product (heart rate × systolic blood pressure) (HR × SPB) and myocardial energy status was evaluated with phosphorus-31 nuclear magnetic resonance spectroscopy while patients squeezed for 7–8 min with one hand at 30% of maximum grip strength. At rest the energy status (estimated by the creatine phosphate:ATP ratio) in all participants was equal. The exercise resulted in a modest increase in HR × SBP from approximately 10,000 to 13,000 in all groups. In normal subjects this 30% increase did not alter left ventricular energy status, whereas in patients with coronary stenosis the same increase in cardiac work resulted in a significant decline of high-energy phosphates. Proof that these metabolic changes were specifically due to inadequate blood flow was obtained by evaluating the exercise in a group of patients before and after revascularization procedures. These patients displayed the typical exercise-induced decline in energy status before revascularization, but were able to increase cardiac work without compromising energy status after revascularization.

Episodes of exercise-induced ischemia have been reported to result in reversible myocardial dysfunction similar to that which occurs after episodes of coronary artery occlusions causing stunning in resting animals [38, 39, 101]. Postexercise recovery has been described as a triphasic response consisting of an immediate recovery of function associated with reactive hyperemia, subsequent deterioration, and a final slow, gradual improvement over a period of hours or possibly days [37]. Homans et al. [37] recently carried out a study to determine whether the free radical quenchers superoxide dismutase (SOD) and catalase would reduce the extent of myocardial stunning that occurs after 10 min of exercise-induced ischemia in dogs performing treadmill exercise. They found that the infusion of these enzymes had no effect on either the transient rebound function occurring early after exercise or the prolonged period of dysfunction and concluded that postexercise myocardial stunning is unlikely to be mediated by oxygen free radicals. We believe that this is a very important study and it will be used as a "launching pad" for many other studies; however, it suffers from the fact that it is the first and only study in the area. For example, a typical assumption of studies using indirect methods is that if free radicals are involved, adding free radical scavengers will eliminate or attenuate the dysfunction. This is not necessarily the case. SOD plus catalase will indeed quench free radicals and lessen tissue damage if they can get to the free radicals. This may be a problem in the study by Homans et al. because these high-molecular-weight enzymes are too large to penetrate the cell membrane to get to free radicals that may be produced on or inside the cell. Furthermore, the dose of SOD plus catalase used was typical of that used in studies of myocardial ischemia/reperfusion in resting, anesthetized animals. Perhaps a larger dose is required during exercise because of increased clearance or because the quenchers are being overwhelmed by additional free radicals produced at locations other than the heart. The authors made no direct measurements of oxidative stress to determine whether free radical-related changes occurred at the intensity of exercise and degree of coronary constriction employed. Finally, only one intensity of exercise was investigated. Homans et al. point out that there are likely several mechanisms for ischemia-induced cardiac dysfunction and that more severe exercise stress may be required for free radical mechanisms to be involved. Clearly, other studies are needed to eliminate oxygen free radicals unequivocally as a mechanism for cardiac dysfunction after exercise-induced ischemia.

DOES EXERCISE TRAINING INCREASE THE HEART'S TOLERANCE FOR ISCHEMIA?

Whether exercise training produces intrinsic adaptations within the heart that may also contribute to an increased tolerance for severe environmental or pathological stresses has been an actively pursued research question. Many studies have used ischemia as a pathological stressor because it is an all-too-common occurrence. There is evidence that reperfusing the ischemic tissue can induce damage to the tissue that is distinct from the damage due to ischemia per se. However, cell death is inevitable in ischemic tissue without reinstating blood flow; therefore, ischemia/reperfusion damage has significant clinical relevance. Ischemia/reperfusion episodes are clinically common and are increasing in occurrence because of recent advances in medicine such as streptokinase, tissue plasminogen activator, and percutaneous transluminal angioplasty, which are used to reestablish coronary flow in patients with coronary obstruction. In addition, ischemia/reperfusion sequences occur in patients with vasospastic angina [31] and have been reported to occur in people with coronary artery disease during increased physical exertion [46].

Several experimental models have been used to examine the effects of chronic exercise training on myocardial ischemia tolerance, including in vivo coronary occlusion [21, 23, 64], isoproterenol resistance [30, 81], and hypoxia tolerance in vivo [21, 24]. Almost all of the studies in this area have been carried out on the laboratory rat. A particularly useful model to elucidate whether relevant intrinsic adaptations have occurred is the isolated perfused working heart preparation, because it eliminates extrinsic neural and hormonal influences yet allows contractile and hemodynamic function to be measured under controlled loading conditions similar to those in vivo. Because the ultimate goal of any prophylactic measure in myocardial ischemia/reperfusion treatment is the resumption of full contractile function, it seems logical to use contractile pump function as the primary dependent measure in the study of myocardial response to ischemia/reperfusion. In addition, isolated heart preparations allow the use of global ischemia to negate the potential contribution of collateral blood supply, which has been reported to play a major role in reducing infarct size in trained hearts [64]. Thus, this model has several advantages that make it a rigorous measure of intrinsic myocardial tolerance to ischemia. Isolated, perfused heart studies investigating the relationship between state of training and tolerance to ischemia/reperfusion or hypoxia/reoxygenation have used both swim training and treadmill training with differing results. Swim training has been reported to increase functional capacity during ischemia and hypoxia [9, 89], decrease reoxygenation cell lysis [43], and improve functional recovery from cardioplegic ischemia [18]. Earlier treadmill studies have reported no protective effect regarding either hypoxia or low-flow ischemia [32, 77]; however, more recent studies from our laboratory have found that treadmill training does improve recovery after ischemia [12, 14]. In the remainder of this section we will critically review many of the studies mentioned above. Studies from this section are summarized in Table 11.1.

In Situ Studies
Male rats trained on a motor-driven treadmill for 5 days/wk for up to 16 wk at up to 26 m/min for 90 min were reported to have increased tolerance to hypoxia, but not ischemia in situ [21]. Open-chest rats were either venti-

TABLE 11.1.
Summary of Exercise Training Effects on Hypoxic or Ischemic Tolerance

Rat Strain	Training Mode/Protocol	Training Effect Before	Hypoxia or Ischemia	Training Effect After	Heart Size	Reference
Wistar male	Swim/1.33, 3 or 8 hr	NA	Ischemia after 2 min 7 mM Ca²⁺ perfusion	$T_{1/2}$ ↓	↑	Korge and Mannik [47]
Wistar male	Swim/2×2 hr	NA	Hypoxia	↓CK, ↑CF	↑	Kihlstrom [43]
Wistar	Swim/90 min	↑CF NS, ↑Q, SV	Cardioplegic, 20 min	↑CF, ↑Q, ↑SV	↑	Brinkman et al. [18]
SD male	Swim/60 min	NA	Infarct-in situ	↓ infarct	NA	McElroy et al. [64]
Wistar male	Swim/75×2 min	↑SV, PLVSP, dP/dt	12 min, one-way valve	During, ↑SV, PLVSP, La	no Δ	Bersohn and Scheuer [9]
Wistar male	Swim/90 min	Q, no Δ, ↑PLVSP, dP/dt	50% O₂ hypoxia	During, ↑Q PLVSP, dP/dt	no Δ	Scheuer and Stezoski [89]
Wistar male	Run/low, mod and interval	NA	Ischemia after 2 min 7 mM Ca²⁺ perfusion	$T_{1/2}$ ↓ in low and int, ↑ in mod	↑	Korge and Mannik [47]
SD male	Run/21/5% 90 min	No Δ	75-min low-flow ischemia	No Δ, NS ↓ Q in trained	↑	Paulson et al. [77]
SD female	Run/22/5% 60 min +sprint	↑ at inc. afterload	In situ 1-min hypoxia	↑CI	no Δ	Cutilletta et al. [24]
Long Evans male	Run/22/9% 60 min	No Δ	Hypoxia, 5 min	No diff	no Δ	Fuller and Nutter [32]
F344 male	Run/various speeds, 40–60 min	No Δ	Ischemia, 25 min	↑CF ↑Q ↑SV ↑HEP	↑	Bowles et al. [12]

↑, increase; ↓ decrease; NS, not significant; NA, not available; SD, Sprague-Dawley; run, treadmill trained; Q, cardiac output; CI, cardiac index; SV, stroke volume; PLVSP, peak left ventricular systolic pressure; CF, coronary flow; dP/dt, maximal rate of pressure change; Δ, change; CK, creatine kinase release during reoxygenation; La, lactate production; HEP, high-energy phosphates; $T_{1/2}$, half-time to contracture.

lated with 14.72% O_2, 2.75% CO_2, and 82.53% N_2 for hypoxia or total occlusion of the left coronary artery for ischemia. Trained rats were found to have significantly longer times to 50% reduction of maximal rate of pressure change (dP/dt) during hypoxia, but a nonsignificant decrease in time during ischemia. During hypoxia, trained rats maintained higher mechanical work, as indicated by HR × left ventricular systolic pressure (LVSP), at all times and at 50% dP/dt. Myocardial high-energy phosphates (HEP) and lactate were not significantly different between trained and untrained at 50% dP/dt in either hypoxia or ischemia. Lower HEP and higher lactate levels were found in ischemia compared with hypoxia. These results show that when taken to the same functional end point, treadmill-trained rats perform more work during hypoxia, but not ischemia with no subcellular training effects observed. No parameters were measured after reperfusion.

Cutilletta et al. [24] reported that in situ recovery from hypoxia is increased by moderate treadmill training in rats. Training consisted of increased treadmill running for 8 wk until the animals were running 60 min/day at 25 m/min with 1-min sprints at 35 m/min every 10 min. Hemodynamic function was evaluated in situ during and after a 1-min hypoxic bout consisting of ventilation with 95% N_2, 5% CO_2. Recovery of left ventricular systolic pressure was greater in the sedentary group. However, cardiac index tended to be higher in the trained group, with no differences in heart rate; thus stroke volume (SV) appeared to be greater in the trained group. Differences in peripheral vasodilation altering afterload may have allowed greater SV with a lower LVSP in the trained group; therefore inferences about intrinsic myocardial adaptation to training are cautioned.

Swim-trained, male rats (60 min/day, 5 days/wk for 5 wk) show increased capillary:fiber ratios (30%) and reduced infarct size (21.5% vs. 31.3% of left ventricle) in response to left coronary artery occlusion in situ [64]. Increased myocardial vascularity was deemed the major contributor to decreased infarct size due to training. A similar experiment in treadmill-trained dogs found no protective effect of prior training on left coronary artery occlusion-induced infarct size, enzyme release, or collateral development [23], whereas a prior study found increased collateral flow and reduced infarct zone [44]. Thus, conflicting results from in situ coronary occlusion can be obtained because of variances in training-induced vascularity changes.

Isolated, Perfused Heart Studies

Using the isolated working heart, swim-trained rats have shown improved contractile and pump performance *during* hypoxia [89] and ischemia [9]. Improved functional recovery postischemia [18] and protection from hypoxia/reperfusion injury [43] also have been reported.

Scheuer and Stezoski [89] swam male Wistar rats 90 min/day, 5 day/wk until they were well trained and then exposed their isolated hearts to hypoxia in either an isovolumic Langendorff or working heart model. Hypoxia in the isovolumic preparation was obtained by lowering the perfusate pO_2 from >600 torr (gassing with 95% O_2) to ~140 torr (gassing with 20% O_2) for 25 min. To maintain cardiac output in the working heart mode, perfusate pO_2 was lowered only to 350 torr (gassed with 50% O_2) for 10 min. In the isovolumic preparation, coronary flow was higher and left ventricular end-diastolic pressure lower in hearts of trained animals during hypoxia and early recovery. No differences in LVSP or dP/dt were noted. In the working heart mode, trained rats had higher LVSP, dP/dt, cardiac work, and efficiency during aerobic control conditions. *During* hypoxia, all parameters fell in both groups. However, the trained hearts maintained higher levels of LVSP (peak and mean), cardiac output, dP/dt, cardiac work, and efficiency. Cardiac work and efficiency were approximately twice that of sedentary values. Neither model showed differences in $\dot{V}O_2$, lactate production, lactate:pyruvate ratios, residual glycogen, or HEP; thus energy formation was not indicated as the contributing factor to improved function. Full functional recovery was quickly regained upon reoxygenation/reflow in both trained and untrained groups because of the mild nature of the hypoxic insult.

A training-related increase in tolerance to ischemia was demonstrated by Bersohn and Scheuer [9] using the working heart model made ischemic by means of a one-way ball valve inserted into the aortic outflow line. This technique allows myocardial pump function to be evaluated under a high-flow ischemia condition in which coronary flow is reduced about 40%. Hearts from male Wistar swim-trained rats (75 min twice daily, 5 days/wk for 8 wk) exhibited greater stroke volume and left ventricular systolic pressure responses to increased preload during ischemia. In addition, SV, peak LVSP and $-dP/dt_{max}$ were all higher than in the control group, whereas time from onset of systole to $-dP/dt_{max}$ was less. Lactate and lactate:pyruvate ratios were also increased, although total calculated ATP production was not different. Therefore, it was concluded that swim training improves cardiac function *during* an ischemic bout. Again, recovery of contractile function was complete upon restoration of normal coronary perfusion pressure, indicating the mildness of the ischemic bout. Reduced coronary flow (60% control) was maintained for only 12 min.

More recently, Kihlstrom [43] reported that isolated hearts of rats swim-trained for 2 hr twice each day released less creatine phosphokinase and maintained higher coronary flows after a 45-min bout of substrate-free, profound hypoxia (gassed with 95% N_2, 5% CO_2, 0% O_2). Despite a decrease in the antioxidants catalase, glutathione reductase, and subendomyocardial vitamin E, lipid peroxidation was lower both before and after hypoxia/reoxygenation in the trained hearts. Another key antioxidant, reduced glutathione (GSH) was increased by training and fell during hypoxia to levels similar to that of controls, indicating that oxidative stress occurred.

Increasing myocardial GSH content is known to decrease the enzyme release during reperfusion, thus protection of cell lysis with training could be attributed to increased GSH content. No contractile parameters were measured and caution should be exercised when extrapolating enzyme release to functional recovery because the two are not correlated in the isolated heart [76, 92].

Brinkman et al. [18] found that functional recovery after cardioplegic arrest in isolated working rat hearts was significantly improved by swim training. In normoxic conditions, trained hearts had similar cardiac output, stroke volume, and heart rates, whereas coronary flows were increased and aortic flows decreased in trained hearts. After 20 min of normothermic cardioplegia-induced arrest, trained hearts recovered 90% of preischemic cardiac output compared with 71% for sedentary hearts. Cardioplegia-induced arrest in the presence of calcium blockers verapamil and diltiazem increased recovery of cardiac output in the control group from 71% to 87% with no effect on the recovery of trained hearts. This suggests that calcium-handling differences accounted for the improved functional recovery in the trained myocardium.

Hypoxia/reoxygenation tolerance was studied in treadmill-trained rats by Fuller and Nutter [32]. The animals trained for 12 wk at a speed of 22 m/min up a 9% incline for 60 min/day. Treadmill-trained and sedentary controls showed no difference in left ventricular pressure during 5 min of hypoxia (gassed with 10% O_2) in the working heart. Relative to prehypoxic values, cardiac output recovery 10 min after hypoxia was 80% and 82%, in control and trained hearts, respectively. Unfortunately, Fuller and Nutter did not include nonhypoxic time controls to determine whether the 20% drop in posthypoxic function associated with only 5 min of mild hypoxia was due to actual cardiac dysfunction or to an unstable preparation. This is not a trivial matter. If, for instance, the nonhypoxic time controls remained at 100% of function for the 15 min of the hypoxia/reoxygenation period, an 80% recovery by both groups indicates that training had no effect on recovery of function. However, if the nonhypoxic controls dropped to 80% of function over the same 15 min, an 80% recovery by both groups indicates that they recovered fully and the stress was too mild to allow any possible discrimination between the groups.

The effect of training on half-time to contracture ($T_{1/2}$) was measured by Korge and Mannik [47] follow short (2-min) perfusion with 7 mM Ca^{2+} Tyrode solution. Hearts from male Wistar rats either swim trained or treadmill trained at three intensities were compared with hearts from sedentary rats. Only rats from high-intensity swim training (8 hr/day) and moderate-intensity treadmill running (six 4-min bouts at 40 m/min) showed significant changes in relative $T_{1/2}$. Swim-trained hearts decreased, whereas treadmill-trained hearts increased time to contracture. Lactate production was highest in this group; therefore, glycolytic rate during ischemia was deemed beneficial in these hearts, contrary to findings from similar studies of the same group [48].

In a recent study by Bowles et al. [12], male Fischer 344 rats were treadmill trained at one of three intensities: low (20 m/min, 0% grade, 60 min/day), moderate (30 m/min, 5% grade, 60 min/day), or intense (10 bouts of alternating 2-min runs at 16 and 60 m/min, 5% grade). Cardiac function was evaluated both before and after 25 min of global, zero-flow ischemia in the isolated, working heart model. Evaluation of cardiac performance before ischemia revealed that none of these treadmill training protocols affected basic intrinsic cardiac pump performance (normalized per gram of heart). However, after ischemia, cardiac function of the trained rats was significantly better than that of the sedentary rats. Percent recovery of cardiac output (relative to preischemia) was 36.0 ± 7.1 in sedentary and 61.2 ± 6.5, 68.1 ± 9.3, and 73.2 ± 5.0 in low, moderate, and intense training, respectively. A nonischemic control group of sedentary rates maintained 97.3% of cardiac output over this same time period, indicating that the preparation was stable and that almost all of the decreases in function were due to actual ischemia-induced cardiac dysfunction. The lack of an improvement in preschemic cardiac performance is consistent with several other studies using young adult rats [18, 32, 77] and indicates that improved postischemic recovery of cardiac function with training is not dependent on a training-enhanced preischemic pump performance. Coronary flow during initial reperfusion at a constant perfusion pressure was significantly enhanced in the trained groups and correlated with subsequent recovery of cardiac output ($R^2 = 0.613$). Furthermore, the energy status of the trained hearts was considerably better than the control hearts after 45 min of reperfusion. In a subsequent study by the same group [14], these results were confirmed using rats trained according to the moderate exercise intensity. Because these results were obtained using the isolated perfused working heart with equal loading conditions among all hearts, the authors concluded that exercise training results in an intrinsic myocardial adaptation allowing greater recovery of cardiac pump function after global ischemia. However, the exact nature of the intrinsic adaptation has yet to be elucidated clearly.

The only other study to have used the isolated working heart to examine the effect of treadmill training on postischemic functional recovery appears to disagree with the findings of Bowles et al. [12]. Paulson et al. [77] trained rats at 21 m/min, 5% grade for 90 min/day, an intensity similar to that of the low intensity group in the study by Bowles et al. Hearts were evaluated under moderate conditions consisting of 10 cm H_2O preload, 100 cm H_2O afterload and a heart rate of 300 beats per minute, before and after 75 minutes of low-flow (1 ml/min) ischemia. Training was found to have no effect on recovery of cardiac output or work; both groups declined approximately 25% compared with preischemic values. However, during the low-flow ischemic period, the perfusate was supplemented with 22 mM glucose, which amounted to 297 g of glucose being provided during ischemia.High levels of extracellular glucose are known to protect the myocardium from hypoxic damage [6] and extend the time to onset of contracture during ischemia [74]. In addition, their study lacked a nonischemic control group to determine whether a decline in function occurred in the absence of ischemia because of the prolonged perfusion. Thus, a training-induced effect in the study of Paulson et al. [77] may have been masked by the benefit of exogenous glucose to the control hearts or the lack of a time-matched normoxic control group.

As mentioned previously, Bowles et al. [12] observed that trained hearts had improved coronary flow characteristics upon reperfusion after 25 min of ischemia. Because the investigators set perfusion pressure equal in all hearts, this indicates a relative increase in coronary resistance in the sedentary hearts. Recovery of contractile function among all hearts was significantly correlated to total coronary flow during the initial 10 min of reperfusion. The same investigators [14] have also implicated coronary flow limitations as the reason that hearts from sedentary rats were not able to recover intracellular energetic status as well as exercise-trained rats upon reperfusion after 25 min of ischemia. These studies support the earlier finding by Kilhstrom [43] that swim-trained rat hearts had a greater coronary flow response upon reoxygenation, which was associated with lower cellular enzyme release. Also, Homans et al. [39] have observed that a maximum reactive hyperemic response is absolutely required for adequate recovery after exercise-induced ischemia. Thus, it appears that the correlation between initial reperfusion coronary flow and subsequent functional recovery is important and suggests that the integrity of the coronary vasculature is important for maintaining cardiac function. In light of the obvious importance of coronary flow to cardiac dysfunction, coronary vascular adaptations with training will be reviewed briefly later in this chapter.

The potential impact of exercise-induced hypertrophy is relevant because chronic pressure overload studies have reported that cardiac hypertrophy decreases ischemic tolerance [2, 3, 78]. Pressure overload hypertrophy decreased time to onset of contracture and increased the area that could not regain any flow upon reperfusion (no-reflow area) in isolated rat hearts [2, 3]. Phasic overload-induced hypertrophy, as occurs in exercise training, has produced equivocal results. Korge and Mannik [47] report a significant negative correlation between heart size and half-time to contracture during ischemia in both swim-trained and treadmill-trained rat hearts. However, one treadmill-trained group with hypertrophy improved ischemic tolerance. Similarly, swim training is reported to result in both hypertrophy and improved ischemic tolerance [9]. Bowles et al. [12] employed three exercise groups and found that absolute heart weights were similar to nonexercised control groups in one exercise group and increased in the other two exercise groups, yet all training groups showed improved functional recovery. Thus, the mild hypertrophy (~6–10%) noted in two of the exercise groups did not appear to influence myocardial tolerance to ischemia.

In summary, most studies using a variety of training protocols have concluded that exercise training increases the heart's tolerance to ischemia. Furthermore, there is evidence of a positive relationship between intensity of training and ischemic tolerance. In the study by Bowles et al. [12], the most intense training protocol used was associated with the greatest ischemic tolerance. Increased speed and duration of treadmill training have also been reported to provide a greater reduction of the cardiotoxic effects of isoproterenol [30]. Although a direct intensity effect appears to exist, it is important to note that in the study by Bowles et al. even the lowest intensity of training (~75% $\dot{V}O_2$max, 60 min/day) resulted in an approximate twofold improvement in recovery compared with hearts from sedentary rats. Thus, it appears that most of the potential benefit of exercise training is attained at a relatively low threshold of energy expenditure. Although comparisons to human epidemiological studies are tempting, it should be noted that the lowest intensity used by Bowles et al. is more vigorous than many "low-intensity" activities routinely practiced in the human population.

ADAPTATIONS IN ENERGY SUPPLY AND DEMAND WITH TRAINING

Regularly performed aerobic types of exercise produce adaptations that serve to decrease myocardial energy demand and improve its energy supply. The decrease in energy demand is realized by the well-known bradycardia observed at rest and during submaximal exercise intensities [63]. Cardiac output is maintained at the lower heart rate because the longer diastolic period allows greater ventricular filling, which produces a greater stroke volume according to the law of Starling [93]. Because energy demand is primarily determined by the rate-pressure product (HR × SBP), and is only minimally effected by stroke volume, the magnitude of the energy savings approaches the magnitude of the decline in heart rate. Well-conditioned endurance athletes typically have resting and submaximum exercise heart rates at least 30% less than untrained people [63]. From a clinical point of view, this may be the most important adaptation resulting from a program of regular exercise because the associated decrease in energy demand at a given submaximum work intensity puts the person further away from the threshold of myocardial ischemia even in the absence of a change in energy supply. Furthermore, most of the exercise-related bradycardia is realized within the first 4–8 weeks of training [62]. The answer to why the bradycardia occurs so rapidly may at least partially lie in the fact that heart rate is influenced by sympathetic and parasympathetic systems and that outflow from these systems may acclimatize very rapidly to changes in activity patterns and stress.

In addition to the decrease in energy demand, there may be changes in substrate metabolism that provides an improvement in energy supply. There is an increase in stored glycogen content [88], and glucose uptake is significantly enhanced [40] in rat hearts after swim training. The enhanced glucose uptake occurs independently of cardiac workload or the availability of other exogenous substrates, which suggests an adaptation at the level of the glucose transporter [40]. Switching away from fats and lactate and toward glucose as a substrate for energy metabolism improves the energy supply in the following two ways. First, maximum cardiac performance is depressed when hearts are primarily utilizing lactate as an energy source [45, 69] and in vivo situations do indeed occur where lactate is the primary substrate [42, 59]. Second, efficiency of mechanical work becomes progressively less and coronary blood flow needs greater as substrate use shifts toward fat and away from glucose [94]. This is the general trend in substrate utilization during prolonged endurance exercise [42, 59], thus an adaptation that would attenuate the substrate shift would be beneficial to the heart. The explanation for the fat-induced decline in efficiency and increase in coronary flow is that the metabolic routes taken by fats result in more oxygen required for each ATP molecule produced compared with the routes taken by glucose. Potentially the impact could be considerable when one considers that a heart using fatty acid alone would need about 16% more oxygen to produce the same amount of ATP than when using only glucose [94].

A particularly desirable adaptation to exercise training for persons with coronary artery disease (CAD) is an improved capacity of the coronary vascular bed to supply oxygen. A study of Ehsani et al. [28] provided strong, indirect evidence that 1 yr of intense endurance training in patients with CAD will increase coronary blood flow capacity. Evaluation of heart rate, blood pressure, and electrocardiogram responses during a treadmill exercise test indicated that the training program resulted in the achievement of a 22% higher rate-pressure product before ST-segment depression occurred, less ST-segment depression at a given rate-pressure product, and a 20% increase in maximum rate-pressure product. Because the magnitude of ST-segment depression is considered to reflect the severity of myocardial ischemia, this study supports an improvement in myocardial oxygen supply during exercise. In contrast, Detry and Bruce [25] did not find any change in the ST-segment depression and rate-pressure product relationship after 3 mo of exercise training in CAD patients. Perhaps the training intensity and duration employed by Detry and Bruce were insufficient to produce a physiological change within the coronary vaculature. In the next section we will discuss exercise-induced adaptations within the coronary vasculture in more detail.

CORONARY VASCULAR ADAPTATIONS WITH TRAINING

Adaptations within the coronary vasculature may be among the most important to occur as a result of chronic endurance training. With the increased myocardial oxygen demand of exercise comes an obligatory increase in coronary blood flow and, as discussed earlier, an inability to increase flow adequately is a major cause of exercise-induced cardiac dysfunction. Furthermore, several studies [12, 18, 39] have reported that the ability to regain cardiac function after an ischemic insult is dependent on the level of flow that can be achieved. Initial studies focused on the hypothesis that chronic exercise would result in structural adaptations allowing greater coronary flow [36, 97, 98, 100]. In recent years, however, studies have revealed distinct functional adaptations to exercise training at the cellular level [95, 96, 102, 103]. This section provides a brief overview of the training-induced alterations in coronary vascular structure and function. Discussion will be limited to those adaptations intrinsic to the myocardial vasculature, not, for example, adaptations in neural control. Despite this limitation, a thorough overview is beyond the scope of this section. For a more extensive treatment the reader is referred to the recent review by Laughlin and McAllister [55].

Coronary Transport Capacity
Coronary transport capacity is the ability to deliver nutrients to and waste products away from the myocardium. Coronary transport capacity is the product of both total blood flow capacity and capillary exchange capacity [53]. When properly controlled, endurance exercise training consistently produces increases in total coronary blood flow capacity in swim-trained rats [20], treadmill-trained dogs [26, 54, 57, 90], and treadmill-trained pigs [56]. Endurance exercise training increased coronary blood flow during maximal adenosine vasodilation 22% in pigs [56] and 36% in dogs [54]. Capillary exchange capacity is also increased by training in both dogs [54, 57] and pigs [56]. Increases in coronary transport capacity after chronic endurance exercise can occur by an increase in size and/or number of coronary vessels (structural adaptation) or an alteration in vasomotor function of existing vessels (functional adaptation).

Structural Adaptation
Various studies over the past 30 years have shown increased coronary vascularity due to endurance exercise training [4, 58, 98, 100, 106]. Coronary cast weights obtained from swim-trained rats were increased compared with controls and remained significantly elevated after 8 wk of deconditioning [98]. Wyatt and Mitchell [107] used angiography and histology to determine coronary diameter and capillarization in endurance-trained dogs. Endurance training produced a small increase in proximal coronary artery diameter, with no change in capillary density. Coronary diameters normalized

after a 6-wk deconditioning period. Increases in proximal coronary diameter after exercise training have also been noted in rats [35, 36, 54, 97, 98], monkeys [49], and humans [34]. In the latter study, Haskell et al. [34] compared coronary arteriographs of 11 male ultradistance runners with 11 male physically inactive control subjects before and after nitroglycerin administration. Under basal conditions, coronary artery diameters were not different between groups, with the exception of a small, yet significant, increase of right coronary artery diameter in the runners. Following intracoronary nitroglycerin administration, total coronary artery diameter increased significantly more in the runners compared with sedentary control subjects. Because cardiac mass was not different between the groups, this suggests that endurance exercise may result in a greater coronary reserve in the human myocardium. However, because this study was cross-sectional, additional factors, cannot be ruled out. For example, because successful ultradistance runners are quite rare, it is possible that genetic differences may have existed between the two groups. Also, because most of the inactive control subjects had chest pain syndrome, they may have had impaired coronary vasodilatory capacity even when compared with another group of inactive subjects.

Although increases in capillary density have been reported after endurance exercise training [4, 100], it has been found primarily in young rats. In large adult mammals, increased capillarization due to training appears coupled to increased cardiac mass, resulting in a maintained capillary density [55]. Thus, in healthy myocardium, increased capillarization in response to endurance training appears limited to young rodent models [55, 87], whereas increases in large coronary artery and arteriole diameter may be more prevalent in larger mammals. Because 40–50% of total coronary vascular resistance can be accounted for by vessels greater than 100 μm [61], these training-induced increases in large coronary vessel size may contribute, in part, to increased coronary blood flow capacity. However, it also appears that additional factors contribute to increased coronary transport capacity, such as adaptation in functional control of the coronary vasculature.

Functional Adaptation
Endurance exercise training alters the coronary vascular response to various vasoactive agents [11, 26, 54, 72, 83]. Di Carlo et al. [26] found that 4 wk of treadmill training in dogs enhanced in vivo coronary vessel sensitivity to both α-adrenergic constriction and dilation via β_2-agonist and adenosine. However, decreased responsiveness to intracoronary phenylephrine has also been noted in trained, intact dogs [11]. To clarify changes in intrinsic coronary vessel reactivity from neural control influences, studies have been performed in vitro on isolated coronary artery rings from exercise-trained dogs [83] and pigs [13, 72]. Rogers et al. [83] isolated coronary arteries from dogs after 11 wk of treadmill training. Neither α_2-vasoconstriction nor α_2-vasodilation was altered by training. However, concentration-relaxation curves for β-adrenergic agonists were shifted to the right, in-

dicating a decrease in β-adrenergic responsiveness. Vasoconstriction to vasoactive intestinal polypeptide was diminished by training. Oltman et al. [72] examined coronary vasomotor reactivity in vitro using isolated coronary arteries from endurance trained pigs. Isometric contractions to high potassium, platelet growth factor-2α acetylcholine, and endothelin were not affected by training. However, the contractile response to norepinephrine was attenuated and the vasorelaxation to adenosine augmented in proximal coronary arteries from trained animals. These differences were not dependent on the presence of endothelium; thus one can conclude that endurance training altered selective, intrinsic properties of the vascular smooth muscle.

Cellular Adaptation

Endurance training in the pig produces adaptations in coronary vasular cell calcium handling [13, 95, 96, 102]. Calcium influx and/or release from internal stores serves a primary role in both the contraction of smooth muscle to many vasoactive agents and the release of vasoactive substances, such as endothelium-derived relaxing factor, from endothelial cells. Thus, alterations in calcium handling at the cellular level may account, in part, for changes in coronary function due to exercise training. Using the intracellular calcium indicator fura-2, Stehno-Bittel et al. [95, 96] found that coronary vascular smooth muscle cells from trained pigs exhibit a time-dependent decrease in the caffeine-sensitive sarcoplasmic reticulum (SR) calcium store, with no increase in the bulk myoplasmic calcium level. This time-dependent decrease, termed "SR calcium unloading," can be mimicked in cells from sedentary pigs by a low dose of ryanodine, indicating that training alters the function of SR calcium release channels [96]. According to this model, the coronary smooth muscle cells from trained animals slowly unload the SR calcium store, which is then extruded from the cell. Because many vasoconstrictors trigger the release of SR calcium, this SR calcium unloading may attenuated the contractile response to vasoactive agents in the vasculature of trained animals. In addition, when partially depleted, the SR can buffer calcium influx and attenuate the contractile response to vasoconstrictors [15, 22]. Endothelin, a potent vasoconstrictor, produces a transient increase in intracellular calcium, primarily from release of SR calcium stores [105]. Exposure of isolated, coronary smooth muscle cells from trained animals to endothelin results in a diminished intracellular calcium response compared with sedentary controls, supporting the model of "SR calcium unloading" [103]. However, simultaneous measurement of intracellular calcium and contraction in coronary vessels from trained and sedentary pigs shows a training-induced decrease in the calcium response to endothelin with no change in contraction [13]. Thus, the exact role of SR calcium unloading in control of coronary vascular function needs further study.

Since the discovery of a functional role for the endothelium in modulating vascular tone [33], intense study has proven a very vital and complex role of the endothelium in vascular biology. Endothelial cells modulate vascular tone by means of production of both vasoactive constrictors and dilators in response to chemical or mechanical stimuli. Increases in coronary flow produce endothelial-dependent vasodilation in coronary vessels [84]. This flow-induced vasodilation probably occurs as a result of increased intracellular calcium in the endothelium in response to shear stress [19]. Therefore, it would seem plausible that chronic exercise training, with its associated increases in coronary blood flow, could alter endothelial calcium handling and subsequently regulation of coronary tone. Few studies to date have examined the effect of exercise training on coronary endothelial function. In dogs, Rogers et al. [83] found no difference in endothelium-dependent relaxation to intracoronary infusion of α_2-agonist with exercise training. Similarly, proximal coronary arteries from trained pigs show no change in endothelium-dependent relaxation to bradykinin, substance P, or A23187 in vitro [71]. However, isolated endothelial cells from proximal coronary arteries of trained pigs show a diminished intracellular calcium response to bradykinin [16]. Furthermore, endothelium-derived relaxing factor release is increased in distal coronary arteries (70–100 μm diameter) of endurance-trained pigs [67]. Thus, it appears that further investigation in the role of exercise training on endothelial vasoregulation is warranted.

Studies to date provide evidence that chronic endurance exercise training results in adaptation in the coronary vasculature ranging from gross structural remodeling to alterations in cell signaling. Although these changes are complex and sometimes disparate, a model set forth by Laughlin and McAllister [55] provides that a central mechanism of these changes may be an attempt to normalize coronary shear stress associated with increased blood flow during exercise. Finally, because functional response of the coronary vasculature are heterogeneous with regard to vessel size [55], further adaptations to exercise may be revealed as studies on smaller vessels progress.

In summary, there appear to be intrinsic exercise-induced adaptations within the heart that serve the role of preventing cardiac dysfunction during prolonged or strenuous exercise and protecting the heart against a variety of environmental stresses including ischemia and reperfusion. We have discussed the potential roles of intrinsic changes in energy supply–energy demand, antioxidant protection against free radicals, and the coronary vasculature. However, further research is needed to understand better the key intrinsic adaptations that serve to protect the myocardium during stressful conditions.

REFERENCES

1. Alessio, H. M. Exercise-induced oxidative stress. *Med. Sci. Sports Exerc.* 25:218–224, 1993.
2. Anderson, P. G., M. F. Allard, G. D. Thomas, S. P. Bishop, and S. B. Digerness. Increased ishemic injury but decreased hypoxic injury in hypertrophied rat hearts. *Circ. Res.* 67:948–959, 1990.

3. Anderson, P. G., S. P. Bishop, and S. B. Digerness. Transmural progression of morphologic changes during ischemic contracture and reperfusion in the normal and hypertrophied rat heart. *Am. J. Pathol.* 129:152–157, 1987.

4. Anversa, P., R. Ricci, and G. Olivetta. Effects of exercise on the capillary vasculature of the rat heart. *Circulation* 75:I12–I18, 1987.

5. Balaban, R. S. Regulation of oxidative phosphorylation in the mammalian cell. *Am. J. Physiol. Cell Physiol.* 258:C377–C389, 1990.

6. Barry, A. C., G. D. Barry, and J. A. Zimmerman. Protective effect of glucose on the anoxic myocardium of old and young mice. *Mech. Ageing Dev.* 40:41–55, 1987.

7. Becker, L.C., J. H. Levine, A. F. DiPaula, T. Guarnieri, and T. Aversano. Reversal of dysfuction in postischemic stunned myocardium by epinephrine and postextrasystolic potentiation. *J. Am. Coll. Cardiol.* 7:580–589, 1986.

8. Belcastro, A. N., and M. M. Sopper. Calcium requirements of cardiac myofibril ATPase activity following exhaustive exercise. *Int. J. Biochem.* 16:93–98, 1984.

9. Bersohn, M. M., and J. Sheuer. Effect of ischemia on the performance of hearts from physically trained rats. *Am. J. Physiol. Heart Circ. Physiol.* 238:H215–H218, 1978.

10. Bolli, R. Mechanism of myocardial "stunning." *Circulation* 82:723–738, 1990.

11. Bove, A. A., and J. D. Dewey. Proximal coronary vasomotor reactivity after exercise training in dogs. *Circulation* 71:620–625, 1985.

12. Bowles, D. K., R. P. Farrar, and J.W. Starnes. Exercise training improves cardiac function after ischemia in the isolated, working rat heart. *Am. J. Physiol. Heart Circ. Physiol.* 263: H804–H809, 1992.

13. Bowles, D. K., M. H. Laughlin, and M. Sturek. Exercise training alters Ca, not tension, in porcine coronary artery segments. *J. Mol. Cell. Cardiol.* 25 (suppl III):S34, 1993 (abstract).

14. Bowles, D. K., and J. W. Starnes. Exercise training improves metabolic response following ischemia in the isolated, working rat heart. *J. Appl. Physiol.* 76:1608–1614, 1994.

15. Bowles, D. K., and M. Sturek. Effect of SR Ca buffering on intracellular Ca and tension in porcine coronary arteries. *FASEB J.* 7:A757, 1993 (abstract)

16. Bowman, L., M. Sturek, C. L. Oltman, and M. H. Laughlin. Intracellular free calcium in pig coronary artery endothelial and smooth muscle cells. *FASEB J.* 3:A1175, 1989.

17. Braunwald, E., and R. A. Kloner. The stunned myocardium: prolonged, postischemic ventricular dysfunction. *Circulation* 66:1146–1149, 1982.

18. Brinkman, C. J. J., A. van der Laarse, G. J. Los, A. P. Kappetein, J. J. Weening, and H. A. Huysmans. Assessment of hemodynamic function and tolerance to ischemia in the absence or presence of calcium antagonists in hearts if Isoproterenol-treated, exercise-trained, and sedentary rats. *Eur. J. Cardiothorac. Surg.* 2:448–452, 1988.

19. Busse, R., A. Mulsch, I. Fleming, and M. Hecker. Mechanisms of nitric oxide release from the vascular endothelium. *Circulation* 87 (suppl V):V18–V25, 1993.

20. Buttrick, P. M., T. F. Schaible, and J. Scheuer. Combined effects of hypertension and conditioning on coronary vascular reserve in rats. *J. Appl. Physiol.* 60:275–279, 1985.

21. Carey, R. A., C. M. Tipton, and D. R. Lund. Influence of training on myocardial responses of rats subjected to conditions of ischemia and hypoxia. *Cardiovasc. Res.* 10:359–367, 1976.

22. Chen, Q., M. Cannell, and C. Van Breemen. The superficial buffer barrier in vascular smooth muscle. *Can. J. Physiol. Pharmacol.* 70:509–514, 1992.

23. Cohen, M. V. and R. M. Steingart. Lack of effect of prior training on subsequent ischaemic and infarcting myocardium and collateral development in dogs with normal hearts. *Cardiovasc. Res.* 21:269–278, 1987.

24. Cutiletta, A. F., K. Edmiston, and R. T. Dowell. Effect of a mild exercise program on myocardial function and the development of hypertrophy. *J. Appl. Physiol.* 46:354–360, 1979.

25. Detry, J. M. and R. A. Bruce. Effects of physical training on exertional ST-segment depression in coronary heart disease. *Circulation* 44:390–396, 1971.

26. DiCarlo, S. E., R. W. Blair, V. S. Bishop, and H. L. Stone. Daily exercise enhances coronary resistance vessel sensitivity to pharmacological activation. *J. Appl. Physiol.* 66:421–428, 1989.

27. Douglas, P. S., M. L. O'Toole, W. D. B. Hiller, K. Hackney, and N. Reichek. Cardiac fatigue after prolonged exercise. *Circulation* 76:1206–1213, 1987.

28. Ehsani, A. A., G. W. Heath, J. M. Hagberg, B. E. Sobel, and J. O. Holloszy. Effects of 12 months of intense exercise training on ischemic ST-segment depression in patients with coronary artery disease. *Circulation* 64:1116–1124, 1981.

29. Enos, W. F., R. H. Holmes, and J. Beyer. Coronary artery disease among United States soldiers killed in action in Korea. *J. A. M. A.* 152:1090–1093, 1953.

30. Faltova, E., M. Mraz, J. Parizkova, and J. Sediv. Physical activity of different intensities and the development of myocardial resistance to injury. *Phys. Bohemoslov.* 34:289–296, 1985.

31. Ferrari, R., C. Ceconi, S. Curello, et al. Oxygen free radicals and myocardial damage: protective role of thiol-containing agents. *Am. J. Med.* 91:95S–105S, 1991.

32. Fuller, E. O., and D. O. Nutter. Endurance training in the rat. II. Performance of isolated and intact heart. *J. Appl. Physiol.* 51:941–947, 1981.

33. Furchgott, R. F. and J. V. Zawadzki. The obligatory role of endothelial cells in the relaxation of arterial smooth muscle by acetylcholine. *Nature* 288:373–376, 1980.

34. Haskell, W. L., C. Sims, J. Myll, W. M. Bortz, F. G. St. Goar, and E. L. Alderman. Coronary artery size and dilating capacity in ultradistance runners. *Circulation* 87:1076–1082, 1993.

35. Haslam, R. W. and R. B. Cobb. Frequency of intensive, prolonged exercise a determinant of relative coronary circumference index. *Int. J. Sports. Med* 3:118–121, 1982.

36. Haslam, R. W. and G. A. Stull. Duration and frequency of training as determinants of coronary tree capacity in rats. *Res. Q. Exerc. Sports* 45:178–184, 1974.

37. Homans, D. C., R. Asinger, T. Pavek, et al. Effect of superoxide dismutase and catalase on regional dysfunction after exercise-induced ischemia. *Am. J. Physiol Heart Circ. Physiol.* 263: H392–H398, 1992.

38. Homans, D. C., D. D. Laxson, E. Sublett, P. Lindstrom, and R. J. Bache. Cumulative deterioration of myocardial function after repeated episodes of exercise-induced ischemia. *Am. J. Physiol. Heart Circ. Physiol.* 256:H1462–H1471, 1989.

39. Homans, D. C., E. Sublett, X. Dai, and R. J. Bache. Persistence of regional left ventricular dysfunction after exercise-induced myocardial ischemia. *J. Clin. Invest.* 77:66–73, 1986.

40. Kainulainen, H., P. Virtanen, H. Ruskoaho, and T. E. S. Takala. Training increases cardiac glucose uptake during rest and exercise in rats. *Am. J. Physiol. Heart Circ. Physiol.* 257: H839–H845, 1989.

41. Kannel, W. B., and T. R. Dawber. Atherosclerosis as a pediatric problem. *J. Pediatr.* 80: 544–554, 1972.

42. Keul, J. Myocardial metabolism in athletes. B. Pernow, B. Saltin (eds). *Muscle Metabolism during Exercise.* New York: Plenum, 1971, pp. 447–455.

43. Kihlstrom, M. Protection effect of endurance training against reoxygenation-induced injuries in rat heart. *J. Appl. Physiol.* 68:1672–1678, 1990.

44. Knight, D. R., and H. L. Stone. Alteration of ischemic cardiac function in normal hearts by exercise. *J. Appl. Physiol.* 55:52–60, 1983.

45. Kabayashi, K., and J. R. Neely. Control of maximum rates of glycolysis in rat cardiac muscle. *Circ. Res.* 44:166–175, 1979.

46. Kolibash, A. J., C. A. Bush, R. A. Wepsic, D. P. Schroeder, M. R. Tetalman, and R. P. Lewis. Coronary vessels: spectrum of physiological capabilities with respect to providing rest and stress myocardial perfusion, maintenance of left ventricular function, and protection against infarction. *Am. J. Cardiol.* 50:230–238, 1982.

47. Korge, P., and G. Mannik. The effect of regular physical exercise on sensitivity to ischemia in the rat's heart. *Eur. J. Appl. Physiol.* 61:42–47, 1990.

48. Korge, P., and G. Mannik. The effect of physical exertions on heart sensitivity to ischemia and metabolic conditioning of these changes. *Int. J. Sports Med.* 11:387–392, 1990.

49. Kramsch, D. M., A. J. Aspen, B. M. Abramowitz, T. Kreimendahl, and W. B. Wood. Reduction of coronary athereosclerosis by moderate conditioning exercise in monkeys on an atherogenic diet. *N. Engl. J. Med.* 305:1483–1489, 1981.

50. Krisanda, J. M., T. S. Moreland, and M. J. Kushmerick. ATP supply and demand during exercise. E. S. Horton, and R. L. Terjung (eds). *Exercise, Nutrition, and Energy Metabolism.* New York: Macmillan, 1988, pp. 27–44.

51. Kumar, C. T., V. K. Reddy, M. Prasad, K. Thyagaraju, and P. Reddanna. Dietary supplementation of vitamin E protects heart tissue from exercise-induced oxidant stress. *Mol. Cell. Biochem.* 111:109–115, 1992.

52. Kusuoka, H., and E. Marban. Cellular mechanisms of myocardial stunning. *Annu. Rev. Physiol.* 54:243–256, 1992.

53. Laughlin, M. H. Coronary transport reserve on normal dogs. *J. Appl. Physiol.* 57:551–561, 1984.

54. Laughlin, M. H. Effects of exercise training on coronary transport capacity. *J. Appl. Physiol.* 58:468–476, 1985.

55. Laughlin, M. H. and R. M. Mcallister. Exercise training-induced coronary vascular adaptation. *J. Appl. Physiol.* 73:2209–2225, 1992.

56. Laughlin, M. H., K. A. Overholser, and M. J. Bhatte. Exercise training increases coronary transport reserve in miniature swine. *J. Appl. Physiol.* 67:1140–1149, 1989.

57. Laughlin, M. H., and R. J. Tomanek. Myocardial capillarity and maximal capillary diffusion capacity in ET dogs. *J. Appl. Physiol.* 63:1481–1486, 1987.

58. Leon, A. S., and C. M. Bloor. Effects of exercise and its cessation on the heart and its blood supply. *J. Appl. Physiol.* 24:485–490, 1968.

59. Lassers, B. W., L. Kaijser, M. L. Wahlqvist, and L.A. Carlson. Myocardial metabolism in man at rest and during prolonged exercise. B. Pernow and B. Saltin (eds). *Muscle Metabolism during Exercise.* New York: Plenum, 1971, pp. 457–467.

60. Maher, J. T., A. L. Goodman, R. Francesconi, W. D. Bowers, L. H. Hartley, and E. T. Angelakos. Responses of rat myocardium to exhaustive exercise. *Am. J. Physiol.* 222:207–212, 1972.

61. Marcus, M. L., W. M. Chilian, H. Kanatsuka, K. C. Dellsperger, C. L. Eastham, and K.G. Lamping. Understanding the coronary circulation through studies at the microvascular level. *Circulation* 82:1–7, 1990.

62. Mary, D. A. S. G. Exercise training and its effect on the heart. *Rev. Physiol. Biochem. Pharmacol.* 109:61–144, 1987.

63. McArdle, W. D., F. I. Katch, and V. L. Katch. *Exercise Physiology.* Philadelphia: Lea & Febiger, 1991, pp. 292–325.

64. McElroy, C. L., S. A. Gissen, and M. C. Fishbein. Exercise-induced reduction in myocardial infarct size after coronary artery occlusion in the rat. *Circulation* 57:958–962, 1978.

65. McNamara, J. J., M. A. Molot, J. F. Stremple, and R. T. Cutting. Coronary artery disease in combat casualties in Vietnam. *J. A. M. A.* 216:1185–1187, 1987.

66. Morris, J. N., R. Pollard, M. G. Everitt, and S. P. W. Chave. Vigorous exercise in leisure-time: protection against coronary heart disease. *Lancet* Dec. 6:1207–1210, 1980.

67. Muller, J. M., P. R. Myers, M. A. Tanner, and M. H. Laughlin. The effect of exercise training on sensitivity of porcine coronary artery resistance arterioles to bradykinin. *FASEB J.* 5:A658, 1991 (abstract).

68. Niemela, K. O., I. J. Palatsi, M. J. Ikaheimo, J.T. Takkunen, and J. I. Vuori. Evidence of impaired left ventricular performance after an uninterrupted competitive 24 hour run. *Circulation* 70:350–356, 1984.

69. Noakes, T. D., L. H. Opie. Substrates for maximum mechanical function in isolated perfused working rat heart. *J. Appl. Cardiol.* 4:391–405, 1989.

70. Nuutinen, E. M., K. Nishiki, M. Erecinska, and D. F. Wilson. Role of mitochondrial oxidative phosphorylation in regulation of coronary blood flow. *Am. J. Physiol. Heart Circ. Physiol.* 243:H159–H169, 1982.

71. Oltman, C. L., and M. H. Laughlin. Endothelial dependent responses of proximal coronary arteries isolated from exercise training pigs. *J. Mol. Cell. Cardiol.* 25 (suppl III):S36, 1993 (abstract).

72. Oltman, C. L., J. L. Parker, H. R. Adams, and M. H. Laughlin. Effects of exercise training on vasomotor reactivity of porcine coronary arteries. *Am. J. Physiol. Heart Circ. Physiol.* 263:H372–H382, 1992.

73. Opie, L. H. *The Heart.* New York: Grune & Stratton, 1984, p 154–165.

74. Owen, P., S. Dennis, and L. H. Opie. Glucose flux regulates onset of ischemic contracture in globally underperfused rat hearts. *Circ. Res.* 66:344–354, 1990.

75. Paffenbarger, R. S. Physical activity as an index of heart attack risk in college alumni. *Am. J. Epidemiol.* 108:163–175, 1978.

76. Park, Y., D. K. Bowles, and J. Kehrer. Protection against hypoxic injury in isolated-perfused rat heart by ruthenium red. *J. Pharmacol. Exp. Ther.* 253:628–635, 1990.

77. Paulson, D. J., S. J. Kopp, D. G. Peace, and J. P. Tow. Improved postischemic recovery of cardiac pump function in exercised trained diabetic rats. *J. Appl. Physiol.* 65:187–193, 1988.

78. Peyton, R. B., P. V. Trigt, G. L. Pellom, R. N. Jones, J. D. Sink, and A. S. Wechsler. Improved tolerance to ischemia in hypertrophied myocardium by preischemic enhancement of adenosine triphosphate. *J. Thorac. Cardiovasc. Surg.* 84:11–15, 1982.

79. Pierce, G. N., M. J. B. Kutryk, K. S. Dhalla, R. E. Beamish, and N. S. Dhalla. Biochemical alterations in heart after exhaustive swimming in rats. *J. Appl. Physiol.* 57:326–331, 1984.

80. Rechnitzer, P. A., H. A. Pickard, A. V. Paivio, M. S. Yuhasz, and D. Cunningham. Long-term follow-up study of survival and recurrence rates following myocardial infarction in exercising and control subjects. *Circulation* 45:853–857, 1972.

81. Riggs, C. E., C. W. Landis. G. T. Jessup, and H. W. Bonner. Effects of exercise on the severity of isoproterenol-induced myocardial infarction. *Med. Sci. Sports* 9:83–87, 1977.

82. Robertson, W. S., H. Feigenbaum, W. F. Armstrong, J. C. Dillon, J. O'Donnell, and P. W. McHenry. Exercise echocardiography: a clinically practical addition in the evaluation of coronary artery disease. *J. Am. Coll. Cardiol.* 2:1085–1091, 1983.

83. Rogers, P. J., T. D. Miller, B. A. Bauer, J. M. Brum, A. A. Bove, and P. M. Vanhoutte. Exercise training and responsiveness of isolated coronary arteries. *J. Appl. Physiol.* 71:2346–2351, 1991.

84. Rubanyl, G. M., J. C. Romero, and P. M. Vanhoutte. Flow-induced release of endothelium-derived relaxing factor. *Am. J. Physiol. Heart Circ. Physiol.* 250:H1145–H1149, 1986.

85. Saltin, B., and J. Stenberg. Circulatory response to prolonged severe exercise. *J. Appl. Physiol.* 19:833–838, 1964.

86. Schaible, T., A. Malhotra, G. Ciambrone, P. Buttrick, and J. Scheuer. Combined effects of hypertension and chronic running program on rat heart. *J. Appl. Physiol.* 63:322–327, 1987.

87. Schaible, T. F. and J. Scheuer. Effects of physical training by running or swimming on ventricular performance of rat hearts. *J. Appl. Physiol.* 46:854–860, 1979.

88. Scheuer, J., S. Penpargkul, and A. K. Bhan. Experimental observations on the effects of physical training upon intrinsic cardiac physiology and biochemistry. *Am. J. Cardiol.* 33:744–751, 1974.

89. Scheuer J. A. and S. Stezoski. Effect of physical training on the mechanical and metabolic response of the rat heart to hypoxia. *Circ. Res.* 30:418–429, 1972.

90. Scheel, K. W., L. A. Ingram, and J. L. Wilson. Effects of exercise on the coronary collateral vasculature of beagles with and without coronary occlusion. *Circ. Res.* 48:523–530, 1981.

91. Seals, D. R., M. A. Rogers, J. M. Hagberg, C. Yamomoto, P. E. Cryer, and A. A. Ehsani. Left ventricular dysfunction after prolonged strenuous exercise in healthy subjects. *Am. J. Cardiol.* 61:875–889, 1988.

92. Seiler, K. S., J. P. Kehrer, and J. W. Starnes. Effect of perfusion pressure at reoxygenation on reflow and function in isloated hearts. *Am. J. Physiol. Heart Circ. Physiol.* 262:H1029–H1035, 1992.

93. Starling, E. H. *The Linacre Lecture on the Law of the Heart.* London: Longmans, Green and Co., 1918.

94. Starnes, J. W., D. F. Wilson, and M. Erecinska. Substrate dependence of metabolic state and coronary flow in perfused rat heart. *Am. J. Physiol. Heart Circ. Physiol.* 246:H799–H806, 1985.

95. Stehno-Bittel, L., M. H. Laughlin, and M. Sturek. Exercise training alters Ca release from coronary smooth muscle sarcoplasmic reticulum. *Am. J. Physiol. Heart Circ. Physiol.* 259:H643–H647, 1990.

96. Stehno-Bittel, L., M. H. Laughlin, and M. Sturek. Exercise training depletes sarcoplasmic reticulum calcium in coronary smooth muscle. *J. Appl. Physiol* 71:1764–1773, 1991.

97. Stevenson, J.A., V. Feleki, and P. Rechnitzer. Effect of exercise on coronary tree size in the rat. *Circ. Res.* 15:265–269, 1964.

98. Tepperman, J., and D. Pearlman. Effects of exercise and anemia on coronary arteries in small animals as revealed by the corrosion-cast technique. *Circ. Res.* 9:576–584, 1961.

99. Terjung, R. L., G. H. Klinkerfuss, K. M. Baldwin, W. M. Winder, and J. O. Holloszy. Effects of exhaustive exercise on rat heart mitochondria. *Am. J. Physiol.* 225:300–305, 1973.

100. Tomanek, R. J. Effects of age and exercise on the extent of the myocardial capillary bed. *Anat. Rec.* 167:55–62, 1970.

101. Tomoike, H., D. Franklin, D. McKown, W. S. Kemper, M. Goberek, and J. Ross, Jr. Regional myocardial dysfunction and hemodynamic abnormalities during strenuous exercise in dogs with limited coronary flow. *Circ. Res.* 42:487–496, 1978.

102. Underwood, F. B., M. H. Laughlin, and M. S. Sturek. Altered control of calcium in coronary smooth muscle cells by exercise training. *Med. Sci. Sports Exerc.* 26: 1994, in press.

103. Underwood, F. B., M. B. Laughlin, and M. S. Sturek. Exercise training decreases coronary smooth muscle free calcium responses to endothelin. *Physiologist* 35:214, 1992 (abstract).

104. Upton, M. T., S. K. Rerych, J.R. Roeback, G. E. Newman, J. M. Douglas, A. G. Wallace, and R. H. Jones. Effect of brief and prolonged exercise on left ventricular function. *Am. J. Cardiol.* 45:1154–1160, 1980.

105. Wagner-Mann, C., and M. S. Sturek. Endothelin mediates Ca influx and release in porcine coronary smooth muscle cells. *Am. J. Physiol. Cell Physiol.* 260:C771–C777, 1991.

106. Weiss, R. G., P. A. Bottomly, C. J. Hardy, and G. Gerstenblith. Regional myocardial metabolism of high-energy phosphates during isometric exercise in patients with coronary artery disease. *N. Engl J. Med.* 323:1593–1600, 1990.

107. Wyatt, H. L., and J. Mitchell. Influences of physical conditioning and deconditioning on coronary vasculature of dogs. *J. Appl. Physiol.* 45:619–625, 1978.

12
Free Radicals and Exercise: Effects of Nutritional Antioxidant Supplementation

MITCHELL KANTER, Ph.D.

The human body possesses a remarkable ability to adapt to the various external and internal stresses that are constantly placed on it. If a particular stress is habitually introduced to the body, adaptations tend to occur to help the body deal with the stress. Chronic physical exercise constitutes such a stress, and the adaptations that occur in response to habitual exercise, including enhanced cardiovascular function [113], changes in body composition [82] and blood pressure [129], improved glucose tolerance [48], and numerous biochemical changes at the cellular level [52, 53] serve to make an organism stronger and, presumably, more resistant to the stresses of daily living.

Despite the number of positive adaptations that occur as a result of habitual activity, however, there are few well-controlled studies demonstrating that exercise, in and of itself, promotes longevity or resistance to various disease conditions. In light of this phenomenon, some researchers have postulated that physical exercise may evoke an event or series of events that may "damage" an organism, and effectively offset the positive adaptations to exercise. Free radical generation, by means of an increased electron flux through the cytochrome chain or transient muscle hypoxia [24, 58], and subsequent lipid peroxidation, may represent these damaging events.

It is now well understood that there are hazards of life in an oxygen-rich environment, including toxicity of molecular oxygen and its derivatives, superoxide anion (O_2^-), singlet oxygen, hydrogen peroxide (H_2O_2), and the hydroxyl radical ($OH^\bullet$) [78]. The potency of this oxygen toxicity is vividly demonstrated when animals are placed in an atmosphere of 100% oxygen and succumb within 60 hr because of progressive dyspnea and hypoxemia resulting from pulmonary edema [83].

To protect against the damage associated with oxidant stress, aerobic organisms possess a free radical defense mechanism consisting of the metalloenzymes superoxide dismutase (which removes O_2^-), catalase, and various peroxidases (which remove H_2O_2), and a variety of nutritional antioxidant compounds. Although these defense systems appear to detoxify free radicals effectively under basal conditions, there is a large body of literature suggesting that the elevated metabolism concomitant with physical exercise may outstrip the body's natural defense mechanisms [47, 51, 79, 98, 99], and that active people might benefit from exogenous antioxidant supplementation [27, 28].

375

The enzymatic defense systems are discussed in detail in another section of this text. This review will focus on a number of potential nutritional antioxidant defenses, including vitamins E and C, beta carotene, coenzyme Q_{10}, and various minerals and herbs. Before discussing antioxidant supplementation, the chemistry of free radical production and lipid peroxidation and their relationship to physical exercise will be reviewed.

THE CHEMISTRY OF FREE RADICAL PRODUCTION AND LIPID PEROXIDATION

Atomic and molecular orbitals can maximally hold two electrons, and atoms and molecules tend to be most stable when they contain a pair of electrons in their outer orbital. A free radical is defined as a species capable of independent existence that contains one or more unpaired electrons in an orbital [46]. The presence of unpaired electrons tends to produce highly reactive species that can interact with numerous biological molecules, and set in motion a series of damaging free radical reactions.

Free radical chain reactions occur in three distinct steps [15]. The first stage is an initiation process, when free radicals are generated. The second, or propagation, stage involves the conservation of free radicals when a radical gives one electron to, takes one electron from, or simply adds on to a nonradical, thus producing a new radical [46]. The third and final stage, termination, results in the destruction of free radicals when two radicals bond to produce a stable nonradical.

As stated previously, free radical proliferation can promote damage to numerous biological systems. Proteins and DNA are often more prevalent targets of damage than are lipids, and lipid peroxidation often occurs later in the injury process. Nevertheless, lipid peroxidation is the most studied of the biologically relevant free radical chain reactions [46].

Lipid peroxidation is a continuous physiological process occurring in cell membranes. The process acts as a membrane renewal factor, as well as in the synthesis of prostaglandins and leukotrienes [86]. Excessive activation of the process, however, has been implicated as a mechanism in the development of various disease conditions. Lipid peroxidation is defined as the oxidative deterioration of polyunsaturated fats [126]. It involves the reaction of oxygen and polyunsaturated lipids to form lipid free radicals and semistable hydroperoxides, which in turn promote free radical chain reactions [15] (see Fig. 12.1).

The presence of double bonds in polyunsaturated fatty acids makes them particularly susceptible to peroxidation. A double bond weakens the carbon–hydrogen bond, making allylic hydrogens susceptible to abstraction by small amounts of initiators [24]. Once formed, these lipid free radicals enter the propagation phase of perioxidation, and undergo approximately

FIGURE 12.1.
Schematic representation of lipid peroxidation.

Initiation:	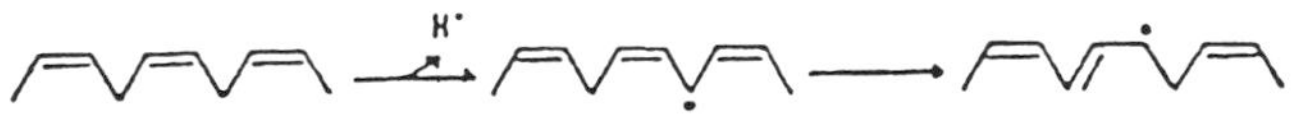

Propagation: $R^{\bullet} + O_2 \longrightarrow RO_2^{\bullet}$

$RO_2^{\bullet} + RH \longrightarrow ROOH + R^{\bullet}$

Termination: $2 R^{\bullet} \longrightarrow R\text{-}R$
$2 ROO^{\bullet} \longrightarrow O_2 + ROOR$
$ROO^{\bullet} + R \longrightarrow ROOR$

8–14 propagation cycles [139]. It is during this propagation cycling period that the bulk of the tissue damage occurs.

Aside from the deterioration of membrane lipids, free radicals can cause changes in membrane protein structure, which can lead to alterations in enzyme activity [24]. Mitochondrial and sarcoplasmic reticulum membranes contain a high proportion of unsaturated fats, and a preponderance of iron associated with their cell membranes. Consequently, both organelles appear to be highly susceptible to perioxidative damage [126]. Swelling and lysis of mitochondrial membranes, as well as alterations in the activities of NADH-cytochrome c reductase and the succinoxidase system of heart and liver mitochondria have been associated with lipid perioxidation damage [15]. In addition, breakdown of lysosomal membranes, which leads to the release of proteolytic enzymes [36], erythrocyte hemolysis in vitamin E deficiency, and edema seen with anthracycline toxicity [35] have all been attributed to peroxidative destruction.

Role of Oxygen in Free Radical Production
There are various pathways for the production of free radicals in living systems; one principal pathway involves the enzymatically controlled reduction of molecular oxygen via the cytochrome chain. Molecular oxygen is paramagnetic because it contains two unpaired electrons with parallel spin states. These unpaired electrons may not reside in the same orbital because two electrons must have antiparallel spins to do so. To reduce oxygen fully it is necessary for election spin inversion to occur. Because this is a slow process, the problem can be obviated by the successive addition of single electrons. This univalent pathway of oxygen reduction is favored by living systems; however, the products of this pathway are an oxidized organic compound and two superoxide radicals [83].

The oxygen molecule can accept four electrons at most, and thus form water. However, the addition of one, two, or three electrons to oxygen transiently leads to the production of superoxide (O_2^-), hydrogen peroxide (H_2O_2), and hydroxyl-radical OH•, respectively (see Table 12.1).

Although enzymes have evolved that accomplish the divalent and tetravalent reduction of molecular oxygen without generally releasing free radical intermediates [38], it has been demonstrated that reactive intermediates are formed as a result of normal cellular respiration. For example, Britton et al. [12] estimated that in organisms in which superoxide dismutase (an antioxidant enzyme) activity was inhibited, 17% of the oxygen consumed by these organisms resulted in O_2^- production. Boveris and Chance [13] have estimated that in intact organisms between 2 and 5% of the total electron flux through the cytochrome chain results in superoxide production. Furthermore, the rate of mitochondrial H_2O_2 production is apparently dependent on the metabolic state of the organelle [76].

Importance of Iron in Free Radical Generation

The role of the superoxide anion in the initiation of peroxidation reactions has been a subject of extensive investigation because the radical by itself does not appear to be directly involved in the initiation of lipid peroxidation [15]. In 1934, Haber and Weiss [44] proposed the generation of the highly reactive hydroxyl radical (OH•) by the following reaction:

$$O_2^- + H_2O_2 \rightarrow OH^\bullet + OH^- + O_2$$

Although this reaction is thermodynamically feasible, kinetically it is so slow that it is practically nonexistent in living systems [83]. More recent studies have indicated that the basic assumption of the Haber-Weiss reaction is correct; however, the presence of a catalyzing agent (most likely iron) is necessary to drive the reaction. Numerous investigators have proposed the generation of hydroxyl radical via an "iron-catalyzed Haber-Weiss reaction" as follows [84]:

$$O_2^- + Fe^{3+} \rightarrow O_2 + Fe^{2+}$$

$$Fe^{2+} + H_2O_2 \rightarrow Fe^{3+} + OH^- + OH^\bullet$$

$$\text{Net: } O_2^- + H_2O_2 \rightarrow O_2 + OH^- + OH^\bullet$$

TABLE 12.1.
Univalent Reduction of Molecular Oxygen

O_2 + 1 electron → superoxide anion (O_2^-)
O_2 + 2 electrons → hydrogen peroxide (H_2O_2)
O_2 + 3 electrons → hydroxyl radical (OH•)
O_2 + 4 electrons → water (H_2O)

Another highly reactive and potentially significant species that has been postulated to be formed as a product of the Haber-Weiss reactions is singlet oxygen [83].

The generation of highly reactive free radicals from moderately reactive free radicals and the apparent necessity of metals in catalyzing many of these reactions have implications in living systems, particularly during exercise. For example, the body tends to handle metals carefully by keeping them bound within proteins [123]. During exercise that promotes protein degradation, metals may be bound to protein carriers more loosely, if at all [59]. When coupled with the increased oxygen consumption associated with physical activity, the organism may be more susceptible to free radical-mediated damage during or after physical exercise.

Finally, it should be pointed out that non–oxygen-dependent reactions can produce free radicals in living systems as well. For example, mechanical processes such as the forces involved in joint compression have been shown to produce free radicals [124]. In fact, Jenkins [59] has suggested that activity-related joint trauma may result from free radicals induced by a combination of joint compression, inflammation, and reperfusion injury.

EXERCISE AND FREE RADICAL GENERATION

Numerous studies conducted during the past 20 years have strongly suggested that free radical production is increased as oxygen consumption increases [1, 2, 23, 58, 67, 68, 107, 108, 118]. McCord [83] has estimated that for every 25 oxygen molecules reduced by cytochrome oxidase, one oxygen molecule is reduced by ubisemiquinone to produce a free radical; Loschen et al. [76] have demonstrated that the rate of hydrogen peroxide formation in mitochondria is linked directly to the energy coupling mechanism.

Exercise may promote free radical production in a number of ways. The 10–20-fold rise in oxygen consumption that can occur during exercise can certainly promote free radical generation. In addition, increases in catecholamine levels [18] and lactic acid production [25], and an elevated rate of hemoglobin autooxidation [92] during and after exercise may increase free radical production. Recent research by Salo et al. [110] suggests that exercise-induced hyperthermia may be a trigger for oxidative stress by promoting mitochondrial uncoupling, loss of respiratory control, and, ultimately, free radical proliferation. Furthermore, the transient hypoxia and reoxygenation that may occur in muscles and joints during exercise [89] can enhance oxidative stress. In this ischemia–reperfusion model, lipid peroxidation is enhanced when an event that promotes an excess of electron donors (i.e., reduced NAD) is followed by an event that leads to an excess in electron acceptors (i.e., molecular oxygen). Strenuous exercise promotes an analogous scenario.

Nevertheless, not all studies have demonstrated evidence of free radical production during physical exercise, or support the role of oxidant stress in the development of exercise-induced tissue damage. Saxton et al. [112] monitored plasma and skeletal muscle markers of free radical-mediated damage in men subjected to alternate bouts of concentric and eccentric muscle actions. Plasma markers (thiobarbituric acid-reactive substances and diene-conjugated compounds) and skeletal muscle markers (malondialdehyde [MDA] and protein carbonyl derivatives) did not, for the most part, change immediately after exercise, prompting the authors to conclude that oxygen free radicals apparently are not involved in exercise-induced muscle damage. Similar conclusions have been reached by Dernbach et al. [26] in rowers after 4 wk of intensive training, and Sahlin et al. [107] after either repetitive static exercise (two-legged intermittent knee extensions) or dynamic exercise (cycling at 60% $\dot{V}O_2$max) bouts in men. Viguie et al. [133] reported increases in blood markers indicative of oxidant stress in young healthy subjects after prolonged submaximal exercise; however, there was no evidence that the exercise altered blood antioxidant status or promoted damage to cells.

Finally, recent studies have reported that the increased leukocyte invasion into damaged skeletal muscle that occurs in the 4–6 hr after strenuous exercise may promote oxidative stress as well [119]. A study by Duarte et al. [31] suggested that inhibition of leukocyte invasion by administration of colchicine after exercise can transiently diminish oxidant stress. These data do not imply that leukocyte inhibition after exercise is a desired condition; in fact, the investigators suggest that some species of leukocytes actually play an important role in the recovery of damaged skeletal muscle after strenuous exercise. However, these findings do raise a number of questions regarding exercise-induced free radical production. Do free radicals actually promote exercise-induced tissue injury, or are they merely the products of such injury? Additional studies are needed to answer these and several other questions about the significance of free radical production during and after physical activity.

POSSIBLE JUSTIFICATION FOR THE USE OF NUTRITIONAL ANTIOXIDANTS

The possible role of nutritional antioxidants in minimizing the risk of developing diverse disease conditions such as cardiovascular disease [104, 121], certain forms of cancer [8], diabetes [19], and cataracts [127] has received increased attention in recent years. Furthermore, numerous researchers have suggested that people involved in acute or chronic physical exercise programs may benefit from antioxidant supplementation as well. Although habitual physical training has been shown to enhance various antioxidant enzymes [41, 60, 65, 87, 98, 105] and presumably make a person less susceptible to free radical damage, it is postulated that nutritional antioxidant supplements can augment endogenous defenses [25, 99]. It has also been suggested that the "nonhabituated" exerciser, whose physical activity is sporadic in nature, might derive a greater benefit from nutritional supplements than the trained exerciser, in part because of their less well developed antioxidant enzyme system.

Acute physical activity has been shown to tax endogenuous antioxidant systems. Ohno et al. [98] have demonstrated increased erythrocyte glutathione reductase activity in previously sedentary men following submaximal cycling activity. Glutathione reductase is involved in the reduction of oxidized glutathione, and elevated activity is thought to be indicative of increased free radical generation. Similarly, Pincemail et al. [102] reported elevated plasma tocopherol levels in subjects after strenuous activity and suggested that enhanced antioxidant mobilization occurs in response to a free radical challenge. Reports such as these strengthen the assertion that physical exercise may increase exogenous antioxidant requirements.

MECHANISM OF ACTION OF NUTRITIONAL ANTIOXIDANTS

Although numerous compounds with known antioxidant properties exist in many of the food products that we eat, such as rice, oats, and various spices, the most well-researched nutritional antioxidants have been the fat-soluble vitamin E and beta carotene, and the water-soluble vitamin C. Of these nutrients, vitamin E is generally considered to be the most important antioxidant in biological systems because of its association with cell membranes [7]. Vitamin E is actually a generic term for tocopherols and tocotricnols [130]. Of the eight naturally occurring vitamin E derivatives, α-tocopherol has the highest biological activity [136], and the greatest free radical scavenging ability [96]. Vitamin E acts as an antioxidant in a number of different ways. It can act directly on various oxygen-derived free radicals, and it scavenges the potentially damaging singlet oxygen [34]. Vitamin E also serves as an antioxidant indirectly by protecting beta carotene and by sparing selenium usage. Regarding the relationship between vitamin E and selenium (a mineral important to the structure of glutathione peroxidase, an antioxidant enzyme), it has been demonstrated that increased availability of dietary selenium can partially allay the symptomatic responses to certain vitamin E deficiencies [141] and that there is complimentary overlap in the protective effects of the two nutrients. Nevertheless, it is clear that selenium cannot substitute for tocopherol activity, and tocopherols cannot substitute for dietary selenium requirements.

For the most part, vitamin E deficiency is extremely rare in human beings, unless a preexisting medical condition (such as intestinal malabsorption syndrome) is present [77]. Most information regarding vitamin E deficiency symptoms have been gleaned from animal studies and human infant data after dietary intakes high in polyunsaturated fat and iron [141]. Rats fed a vitamin E-deficient diet exhibit a decrease in mitochondrial respiratory control, a 40% decline in endurance capacity, and increased lipid peroxide formation after exhaustive physical exercise [23].

On the other hand, vitamin E toxicity is not widely reported, and intakes as high as 200 times the recommended daily allowance have been ingested without apparent complications [4]. This knowledge has prompted some investigators to suggest higher vitamin E intakes by persons consuming a high polyunsaturated fat diet [14], and intakes in excess of 10 times the current recommended daily allowance of 15 IU have been recommended for persons engaged in habitual physical exercise [55].

Vitamin C (ascorbic acid) is an essential nutrient in humans and it plays a role in the synthesis of collagen, hormones, and neurotransmitters [80]. It also serves as an important antioxidant and free radical scavenger [5, 37], and because individual physiological demand for vitamin C can be influenced by a number of environmental factors (temperature, smog, cigarette smoke, exposure to heavy metals, etc.) [141], many researchers believe that physically active people require greater than recommended daily allowance intakes of ascorbate. However, there are data indicating that chronic, multigram intakes of vitamin C can produce a number of physiologic disturbances. Reports of increased renal stone formation [11], increased thrombocytosis and decreased coagulation time [114], gastrointestinal disturbances [20], and erythrocyte hemolysis [88] suggest that megadose supplements of vitamin C are not warranted. It has also been demonstrated that in the presence of iron, vitamin C can act as a potent prooxidant [50]. A recent report by Herbert [50] suggests that the iron-overload–induced cardiac death of three athletes may have been precipitated by megadose intakes of vitamin C, and that a genetic predisposition among some people to the development of iron overload should limit daily vitamin C intake to no more than 500 mg for the general population.

Beta carotene is one of more than 400 carotenoid compounds that exist in nature [73]. It is the most widely distributed of the carotenoids, and its antioxidant characteristics are well documented [3, 56]. However, it is far from the only carotenoid with purported antioxidant capabilities. Recent work suggests that other carotenoid compounds such as lycopene, which is primarily found in tomatoes, and lutein, a principal carotenoid in green leafy vegetables, may possess potent antioxidant function as well [39]. The primary antioxidant role of beta carotene is to quench the highly reactive singlet oxygen species.

Coenzyme Q_{10} (CoQ_{10}) or ubiquinone, is a "vitamin-like substance" whose role in electron transport chain function is well established. CoQ_{10} also has purported antioxidant properties [69]. Numerous studies conducted in Japan suggest that CoQ_{10} can be beneficial in alleviating symptoms associated with heart disease [140], and Katagiri et al. [70] reported that CoQ_{10} could diminish the extent of ischemia-induced cellular damage. Beyer et al. [6] reported that CoQ_{10} levels were elevated in the hearts of chronically exercise-trained rats. However, the effects of CoQ_{10} supplementation on exercise-induced lipid peroxidation and skeletal muscle damage have been mixed. Rats supplemented with CoQ_{10} displayed diminished serum creatine kinase and lactate dehydrogenase activities after downhill running [116], but similar effects were not demonstrated in human subjects after an exhaustive bout of cycling [142]. It is presently unknown what the optimal dosage of CoQ_{10} is that will merely raise blood levels of the compound. Based on current research, the potential of CoQ_{10} as a protective nutrient for physically active people is speculative at best.

Numerous other micronutrients have antioxidant properties, or serve as structural components of compounds with known antioxidant functions. Copper and zinc are part of the structure of cytosolic superoxide dismutase, and manganese is part of the mitochondrial superoxide dismutase enzyme. Iron is a necessary component of the enzyme catalase, and selenium is an important component of glutathione peroxidase (see Table 12.2). Various of these nutrients may be diminished with physical training [30, 45]; however, large doses of certain minerals may promote toxocity symptoms. High zinc intakes may diminish high-density lipoprotein levels, and can inhibit copper absorption [85]. Similarly, physiological levels of ascorbate may interfere with the binding of copper to the superoxide dismutase enzyme [59]. Although it has been demonstrated that deficiencies of individual nutrients (selenium, for example [61]) can increase an animal's susceptibility to exercise-induced lipid peroxidation, more research regarding the interactions of nutrients is warranted before indiscriminate mineral supplementation is undertaken by anyone, regardless of their physical activity habits.

Finally, a number of natural antioxidants in foods are currently being tested in biological systems for potential protective effects against oxidant stress. Numerous plant oils, grains, beans, and spices contain compounds that prolong the shelf life of foods [94]. Whether or not these compounds

TABLE 12.2.
Micronutrients Necessary for Antioxidant Enzyme Production

Cytosolic superoxide dismutase
  Copper
  Zinc
Mitochondrial superoxide dismutase
  Manganese
Glutathione peroxidase
  Selenium
Catalase
  Iron

TABLE 12.3.
*Purported Natural Antioxidants**

Plant
  Oil seeds (e.g., sesame)
  Grains (e.g., rice)
  Beans (e.g., soybeans)
  Vegetables
  Fruits
  Bark and nuts (e.g., tannins)
Spices (e.g., sage, black pepper, rosemary, thyme)
Seaweeds
Protein hydrolysates

*Adapted from Namiki [94].

are absorbed in the body and provide protective effects at the cellular level remains to be seen. To date, there are no compelling data indicating that physically active people would benefit by supplementing with any of these compounds (see Table 12.3).

POTENTIAL ERGOGENIC EFFECTS OF ANTIOXIDANT SUPPLEMENTS

Researchers and athletes have been interested in the possible ergogenic effects of individual nutrients for many years. During the past three decades or so, two nutrients with antioxidant properties that have been studied extensively for their potential to enhance physical performance are vitamins E and C. Although most studies conducted to date suggest that vitamin supplementation in the absence of a preexisting deficiency will not likely improve one's ability to perform physical work, it should be remembered that the effects of any given micronutrient may be overshadowed by the physiological effects of a bout of exercise. According to Gerster [39], it would take an estimated sample size in excess of 5000 subjects to detect the effects on performance of a single micronutrient supplement.

Early studies suggested that vitamin C supplements might be beneficial for active individuals because of the large sweat loss of the vitamin that was purported to occur [103]. However, studies by Robinson and Robinson [106] and others failed to substantiate significant sweat vitamin C losses. Later studies using regimens of acute [10, 71] or chronic [40, 72] vitamin C supplementation failed to demonstrate improvements in either strength or endurance performance measurements.

A recent study demonstrated that vitamin C infusion at relatively high rates (0.9 mmol/min) improves basal whole body glucose disposal in healthy aged and diabetic subjects [100]. Furthermore, a significant relationship was shown to exist between plasma vitamin C levels and whole-body glucose uptake. It remains to be seen whether similar changes (that are apparently indicative of improved insulin action) can be duplicated in healthy exercising subjects after vitamin C infusion, and the implications that this may have on the diminution of oxidant stress and on whole-body carbohydrate storage, usage, and resynthesis.

Although it is known that vitamin E supplementation can raise serum and muscle levels of the vitamin in both rats and humans, the possible ergogenic effects associated with supplementation are equivocal. Studies using daily intakes of vitamin E ranging from 300 IU/day [75] to 1600 IU/day [125] have failed to show alterations in aerobic performance of swimmers. However, a recent study of Simon-Schnass and Pabst [117] suggested that physical performance in high-altitude mountain climbers (as measured by alterations in the anaerobic threshold and in expired pentane production during cycle ergometry) could be improved with the inclusion of vitamin E supplements (400 mg/day for 10 wk) in the diet. Therefore, the potential ergogenicity of vitamin E supplements in atmospheric conditions imposed by altitude cannot be ruled out.

A study using a supplement consisting of 200 IU of vitamin E and 100 mg of CoQ_{10}, as well as inosine and cytochrome c, failed to show a performance benefit in trained triathletes who performed a combined running and cycling exercise bout to exhaustion. It should be pointed out, however, that a relatively small (n=11) sample size coupled with very large intersubject variation may have affected the results of this study [120].

Finally, a recent study conducted by Novelli et al. [97] suggested that glutathione ingestion could improve the swimming endurance time of mice. However, no follow-up studies have been conducted, and this effect has not been replicated in human subjects.

ANTIOXIDANT SUPPLEMENTATION AND EXERCISE-INDUCED LIPID PEROXIDATION

As stated previously, a key issue regarding the antioxidant needs of the active person is whether or not a well-nourished person, with no known nutrient deficiencies, would benefit by supplementing above and beyond recommended dietary intakes. Numerous animal studies, including those by Gohil et al. [43] and Davies et al. [23], have demonstrated that vitamin E deficiencies can impair physical performance, and Salminen et al. [109] have shown increased susceptibility to lipid peroxidation in rats fed a vitamin E-deficient diet. However, it should be pointed out that most studies assessing the nutritional status of active human subjects have found little or no evidence of antioxidant vitamin deficiencies, as measured by blood analysis.

In studies conducted with apparently well-nourished subjects, data regarding the effects of antioxidant supplementation on exercise-induced lipid peroxidation and muscle tissue damage have been equivocal. Numerous studies have demonstrated that antioxidant vitamin supplements can be beneficial for lowering markers indicative of oxidant stress and lipid peroxidation [28, 68, 74, 99, 122, 126]. However, a near-equal number of studies have failed to show protective effects of antioxidants in preventing tissue damage and lipid peroxidation [49, 64, 135, 137].

Studies Involving Vitamin E Supplementation
Early research conducted by Dillard et al. [28] in the 1970s reported that breath pentane concentration (a marker of whole-body lipid peroxidation) could be attenuated by daily ingestion of 1200 IU of vitamin E for 2 wk before submaximal exercise bout. More recent work by Simon-Schnass and Pabst [117] with mountain climbers performing work at altitude demonstrated a similar effect on breath pentane production in climbers consuming vitamin E, and Sumida et al. [122] reported that ingestion of 300 mg of vitamin E for 4 wk could attenuate the rise in serum MDA levels after an exhaustive exercise bout. Recent work by Canon et al. [16] and Meydani et al. [90, 91] in active older subjects substantiates the benefits of vitamin E supplementation (800 IU/day for 48 days [91]) for diminishing exercise-induced lipid peroxidation.

The aforementioned study by Sumida et al. [122] also demonstrated that vitamin E supplementation could diminish serum levels of mitochondrial glutamic oxaloacetic transaminase isoenzyme and β-glucuronidase (thought to be indicative of tissue damage) after exercise. However, studies by Warren et al. [135] in rats, and Kanter and Eddy [64] and Helgheim et al. [49] in human subjects failed to corroborate the findings of diminished serum enzyme appearance after physical exercise in vitamin-supplemented subjects. These contradictory findings may have been due in part to the different modes of exercise employed in the various studies (i.e., high-intensity vs. moderate-intensity exercise; concentric vs. eccentric muscle actions), or to the possibility that exercise-induced injury may be a multifactorial process in which free radicals are involved only in a particular phase of damage [59]. Regardless, contradictory findings such as these lend credence to the statement by Tiidus et al. [128] that "the proposed link between exercise, free radicals . . . and an increased dietary need for vitamin E may be premature."

Studies Involving Vitamin C Supplementation
There are few studies in which vitamin C has been used as the sole antioxidant nutrient before a bout of exercise. In most cases in which vitamin C has been administered, it was given as part of a mixture including other nutrients as well. Further complicating the issue is the fact that most species of animals are capable of synthesizing vitamin C [137]. Therefore, most vitamin C deficiency studies involving animals have been confined to the guinea pig, which does not synthesize the vitamin, although numerous sup-

plementation studies involving other species have been carried out. A recent study by Gohil et al. [43] demonstrated that vitamin C supplementation did not improve the reduction in aerobic capacity induced in rats by placing them on a low vitamin E diet.

In humans, plasma vitamin C levels have been reported to be depressed in runners after a 21-km race [42]. In addition, a recent study by Peters et al. [101] suggested that runners who consumed a 600 mg vitamin C supplement daily for 3 wk before a 42-km race incurred fewer upper respiratory tract infections than did runners who were not supplemented. However, Peters et al. did not measure any markers indicative of free radical-mediated lipid peroxidation, so the antioxidant potential of vitamin C for marathon runners cannot be assessed based on the results of this study. Similarly, a study by Kaminski et al. [63] reported less muscle soreness in subjects who consumed 3 g of vitamin C for 3 days before and 4 days after strenuous calf muscle exercises. However, it is impossible to ascribe a particular mechanism or rationale for these results in the absence of measurements indicative of lipid peroxidation or free radical generation

A recent study by Jakeman and Maxwell [57] demonstrated that 3 wk of pretreatment with 400 mg/day vitamin C, followed by 7 days of continued vitamin use after 60 min of eccentric box-stepping exercise promoted faster recovery of the subjects' maximal voluntary contraction measurements, and less muscle damage. Although the authors proposed that the supplement protected against free radical injury (without having measured any free radical markers), these data nonetheless support the role of vitamin C as a protective nutrient against exercise-induced tissue damage.

Studies Involving Antioxidant Vitamin Mixtures and Other Antioxidant Compounds

Several studies have assessed the effects of antioxidant nutrient mixtures on exercise-induced lipid peroxidation and skeletal muscle damage. Although these studies make it impossible to ascertain the potential benefits of individual antioxidant nutrients, and rarely address the issue of nutrient–nutrient interactions that may affect the observed results, they can help to shed light on the general effects of antioxidant supplementation in exercising subjects.

Kanter et al. [68] studied the effects of ingesting vitamin C (1000 mg/day), vitamin E (800 IU/day), and beta carotene (30 mg/day) for 6 wk before bouts of submaximal (60% $\dot{V}O_2$max) and near-maximal (90% $\dot{V}O_2$max) running exercise. Although the supplement did not prevent an exercise-induced increase in lipid peroxidation, subjects who consumed the vitamins demonstrated significantly lower levels of breath pentane and serum MDA at rest and after both exercise bouts after the supplementation period. These data suggest a protective effect of the antioxidant vitamin mixture.

However, a follow-up study by Kanter and Eddy [64] using the same vitamin mixture failed to demonstrate a protective role of the supplement in lowering markers of lipid peroxidation, skeletal muscle soreness, and muscle damage. The mode of exercise employed in the latter study was downhill running. This prompted the researchers to suggest that the type of exercise performed may impact on the potential protective benefits of antioxidant supplements. Submaximal and near-maximal running on a level treadmill requires a greater cumulative oxygen consumption than does a bout of downhill treadmill running. Based on these data, one could speculate that antioxidant vitamin use may be appropriate for activities in which metabolic activity is high, and less beneficial when activities involving greatly elevated mechanical stress (weight lifting, etc.) are performed.

Numerous other studies that have used antioxidant mixtures or other antioxidant compounds before physical exercise have been conducted. Viguie et al. [132] used a vitamin mixture similar to that used by Kanter et al. in the aforementioned studies, and reported an enhancement of the blood glutathione redox system in human subjects who ingested the supplement before downhill treadmill running. Glutathione redox cycling is a major intracellular antioxidant system that prevents the accumulation of hydroperoxides. Similar results have been reported by Sastre et al. [111] after exhaustive exercise in human subjects given a single dose of 1 g of glutathione plus 2 of vitamin C, or in rats administered doses of either glutathione, vitamin C, or N-acetyl-L-cysteine for 1 wk before exercise. N-Acetyl-L-cysteine previously has been shown to diminish the cardiotoxic effects associated with antracycline drug administration, purportedly as a result of its antioxidant properties [131].

Dragan et al. [29] found a decrease in serum MDA levels in cyclists training for 2 hr/day while consuming supplements containing selenium, vitamin E, glutathione, and cysteine. However, the results of this study are in question because the subjects did not ingest the various supplements in a randomized fashion, creating the possibility of bias error. No follow-up studies using similar supplements have been performed to date.

The potential of dietary carbohydrate supplementation during physical activity as a means of suppressing exercise-induced oxidant stress has been studied as well. Although previous studies have suggested that various energy nutrients, such as dextrose, may be potent stimulators of lipid peroxidation in rats [93], Ji et al. [62] demonstrated that carbohydrate ingestion during prolonged submaximal (70% $\dot{V}O_2$max) exercise diminished the rise in blood GSH concentration, presumably indicating a decrease in exercise-induced lipid peroxidation. Further research is necessary to corroborate these findings and to elucidate a possible mechanism for this effect.

METHODOLOGICAL CONCERNS

Interpretation of the results of studies regarding the effects of antioxidant supplementation on exercise-induced lipid peroxidation and skeletal muscle damage is clouded somewhat by the fact that all of the available methods for measuring free radical generation and lipid peroxidation in living systems have been questioned for their lack of specificity, sensitivity, and reproducibility [138]. Presently, the only method that can directly detect the presence of free radicals is electron paramagnetic resonance (EPR). However, the use of EPR in in vivo studies is in its relative infancy, and few studies have measured EPR signals in exercising human tissue.

Most of the studies that have attempted to measure oxidant stress after exercise in animals and humans generally have measured blood and tissue markers purportedly indicative of lipid peroxidation. One of the most prevalently studied markers of lipid peroxidation has been MDA production by means of the thiobarbituric acid assay. However, Halliwell and Chirico [46] and others have questioned the use of the thiobarbituric acid assay in tissue extracts and body fluids, citing its lack of sensitivity and specificity. Wong et al. [138] have suggested the use of liquid chromatography as a means of alleviating some of the methodological error inherent in the spectrophotometric procedure.

Similarly, Halliwell and Gutteridge [47] have stated that, although the ultraviolet absorption of conjugated dienes can be a useful method for measuring unsaturated fatty acid oxidation in in vitro studies, it is difficult to measure in biological studies because of the presence of other substances, such as heme proteins, purines, and pyrimidines that absorb strongly at the same wavelength. Furthermore, the presence of conjugated diene products in animal diets has been suggested [46], further calling into question its use in biological studies.

Another technique that has been used to measure lipid peroxidation in animals is the measurement of expired hydrocarbon gases such as pentane and ethane. Pentane is formed by the oxidation of linoleic acid; ethane is an oxidation product of linolenic acid [27]. Although the production of hydrocarbon gases constitutes a noninvasive means of measuring whole-body lipid peroxidation in in vivo studies, the gases are considered to be minor end-products of lipid peroxidation, and their production may reflect an increased availability of metal ions, rather than increased initiation of peroxidation [47].

New, promising methods include the production of urinary markers of DNA oxidation such as thymine glycol and thymidine glycol [17, 115], single photon counting of chemiluminescence [59], and the use of monoclonal antibody techniques [32]. However, few exercise studies performed to date have utilized these methods, and more research is required before any particular marker can be considered the method of choice in studies measuring lipid peroxidation in biological samples. Until more reliable markers are identified, Halliwell and Gutteridge [47] suggest the use of two or more different assays to increase one's ability to interpret the results of studies attempting to assess the extent of oxidant stress in human and animal studies.

Finally, the measurement of serum enzymes such as CK and LDH are often used as indicators of skeletal muscle damage in studies designed to measure the relationship between oxidant stress and tissue damage in human subjects [66, 67, 81]. However, large intersubject variability in serum CK and LDH changes have been reported by many investigators [21, 22, 95]. Factors that promote this variability include the age, gender, body composition, and race of the subjects [54]. The mode, intensity, and duration of exercise can also affect the alterations in serum enzyme levels. It has been suggested that serum enzyme changes may not be an accurate predictor of skeletal muscle damage [22, 33], and Evans and Cannon [33] have intimated that the postexercise rise in serum enzymes may represent a manifestation of skeletal muscle damage, but may not be a quantitatively accurate indicator of it.

CONCLUSIONS

A large body of literature strongly suggests that free radical-mediated reactions are increased as a result of physical exercise. Potential mechanisms responsible for the purported rise in radical activity include an elevation in oxygen consumption, increased neutrophil activation, or a rise in ischemia–reperfusion reactions. Free radical reactions can cause damage to lipid membranes, proteins, DNA, and other cellular constituents.

The potential of nutritional antioxidants for reducing the damaging effects of free radicals has been studied primarily as a means of preventing chronic, age-related diseases. Although a preponderance of recent data indicates that persons who consume supplemental doses of antioxidant nutrients (particularly vitamins E and C) tend to display a lower risk of developing various disease conditions, it should be remembered that these data were gleaned from epidemiological studies, and not under controlled experimental conditions. This does not imply that the current data are flawed, just incomplete [134]. Further experimental studies are necessary to establish a true cause-and-effect relationship between increased antioxidant intake and reduced disease risk.

With respect to physical activity, a number of questions regarding the possible benefits of antioxidants for active people remain to be elucidated. Although it is well established in animal studies that antioxidant deficiencies can exacerbate tissue damage, the effects of supplementation in healthy, well-fed people are not as clear-cut. Numerous studies suggest that increased antioxidant intake is beneficial for the active person; however, a near equal number of studies indicate no positive effects. Future studies should assess the long-term effects of antioxidant supplementation by physically active people. In most studies, supplements are provided for periods ranging from a few days to 8 wk. Such relatively short time courses may not be sufficient to ascertain the effects of a supplement. Conversely, it would be of interest to know the effects of long-term, chronic supplementation versus an acute, bolus dose of an antioxidant. It is necessary for an athlete to take large doses of a supplement for long periods, or can or she "load up" in the days or hours before or after a competition? These questions have not been addressed in a systematic fashion.

Other issues that need to be addressed include the possible synergies that exist between antioxidant nutrients, and the effects that these synergies may have on optimal dosage recommendations. If a person ingests multiple nutrients, does he or she need to ingest as much of each nutrient as they would if they ingested individual antioxidant nutrients? Furthermore, the effects of environmental stressors on the antioxidant requirements of active people should be assessed. Does a person who exercises habitually in an urban environment with poor air quality require a greater daily intake of antioxidant nutrients than does a person who exercises in a rural environment?

Finally, one should bear in mind the limitations of current methods used to assess exercise-induced lipid peroxidation and skeletal muscle damage when analyzing the results of antioxidant supplementation experiments. The development of more sensitive blood and tissue markers should help to clarify many of the contradictions in the current literature, and make it easier to provide recommendations to active people regarding their nutritional antioxidant requirements.

REFERENCES

1. Alessio, H. M. and A. H. Goldfarb. Lipid peroxidation and scavenger enzymes during exercise: adaptive response to training. *J. Appl. Physiol.* 64:1333–1336, 1988.
2. Alessio, H. M., A. H. Goldfarb, and R. G. Cutler. MDA content increases in fast and slow-twitch skeletal muscle with intensity of exercise in a rat. *Am. J. Physiol.* 255:C874–C877, 1988.
3. Bendich, A. Carotenoids and the immune response. *J. Nutr.* 119:112–115, 1989.
4. Bendich, A. and L. J. Machlin. Safety of oral intake of vitamin E. *Am. J. Clin. Nutr.* 48:1088–1089, 1988.
5. Bendich, A., L. J. Machlin, O. Scandurra, G. W. Burton and D. D. M. Wayner. The antioxidant role of vitamin C. *Adv. Free Radical Biol. Med.* 2:419–444, 1986.
6. Beyer, R. E., K. Nordenbrand, and L. Ernster. The function of coenzyme Q in free radical production and as an antioxidant: a review. *Chem. Scripta* 27:145–153, 1987.
7. Bjorneboe, A., G. A. Bjorneboe and C. A. Drevon. Absorption, transport and distribution of vitamin E. *J. Nutr.* 120:233–242, 1990.
8. Block, G., B. Patterson, and A. Subar. Fruit, vegetables, and cancer prevention: a review of the epidemiological evidence. *Nutr. Cancer* 18:1–29, 1992.
9. Brady, P. S., L. J. Brady, and D. E. Ullrey. Selenium, vitamin E and the response to swimming stress in the rat. *J. Nutr.* 109:1103–1109, 1979.
10. Bramich, K., and L. McNaughton. The effects of two levels of ascorbic acid on muscular endurance, muscular strength and on VO$_2$max. *Int. Clin. Nutr. Rev.* 7:5–9, 1987.
11. Briggs, M. H., P. Garcia-Webb, and P. Davies. Urinary oxalate and vitamin C supplements. *Lancet* 2:201, 1973.
12. Britton, L., D. P. Malinowski, and I. Fridovich. Superoxide dismutase and oxygen metab-

olism in streptococcus faecalis and comparisons with other organisms. *J. Bacteriol.* 134:229–235, 1978.

13. Boveris, A., and B. Chance. The mitochondrial generation of hydrogen peroxide. *Biochem. J.* 134:707–718, 1973.
14. Buckingham, K. W. Effect of dietary polyunsaturated/saturated fatty acid ratio and dietary vitamin E on lipid peroxidation in the rat. *J. Nutr.* 115:1425–1435, 1985.
15. Bus, J. S. and J. E. Gibson. Lipid peroxidation and its role in toxicology. J. R. Bend, E. Hodgson, and R. M. Philpot (eds). *Reviews in Biochemical Toxicology, Vol. 1.* New York: Elsevier-North Holland, 1979, p. 125.
16. Cannon, J. G., S. F. Orencole, R. A. Fielding, et al. Acute phase response to exercise: interaction of age and vitamin E on neutrophils and muscle enzyme release. *Am. J. Physiol.* 259:R1214–R1219, 1990.
17. Cathcart, R., E. Schwiers, R. L. Saul, and B. N. Ames. Thymine glycol and thymidine glycol in human and rat urine: a possible assay for oxidative DNA damage. *Proc. Natl. Acad. Sci. U. S. A.* 81:5633–5637, 1984.
18. Cohen, G. and R. Heikkila. The generation of hydrogen peroxide, superoxide and hydroxyl radical by 6-hydroxydopamine dialuric acid and related cytotoxic agents. *J. Biol. Chem.* 249:2447–2450, 1974.
19. Collier, A, R. W. Wilson, H. Brodley, J. A. Thomson, and M. Small. Free radicals type II diabetes. *Diabetic Med.* 7:27–30, 1990.
20. Coulehan, J. L., L. Kapner, S. Eberhard, F. J. Taylor, and K. D. Rogers. Vitamin C and upper respiratory illness in Navajo children: preliminary observations. *Ann. N. Y. Acad. Sci.* 258:513–519, 1974.
21. Clarkson, P. M., W. C. Byrnes, K. M. McCormick, and P. Triffletti. Muscle soreness and serum creatine kinase activity following isometric, eccentric and concentric exercise. *Int. J. Sports. Med.* 7:51–56, 1986.
22. Clarkson, P. M., and C. Ebberling. Investigation of serum creatine kinase variability after muscle damaging exercise. *Clin. Sci.* 75:257–261, 1988.
23. Davies, K. J. A., A. T. Qaintanilha, G. A. Brooks, and L. Packer. Free radicals and tissue damage produced by exercise. *Biochem. Biophys. Res. Commun.* 107:1198–1205, 1982.
24. Demopulos, H. B. The basis of free radical pathology. *Fed. Proc.* 32:1859–1865, 1973.
25. Demopoulos, H. B., J. P. Santomier, M. L. Seligman, and D. D. Pietronigro. Free radical pathology: rationale and toxicology of antioxidants and other supplements in sports medicine and exercise science. Katch, F. I., (ed). *Sport, Health and Nutrition.* Champaign, IL: Human Kinetics Publishers, 1986, pp. 139–189.
26. Dernbach, A. R., W. M. Sherman, J. C. Simonsen, K. M. Flowers and D. R. Lamb. No evidence of oxidant stress during high-intensity rowing training. *J. Appl. Physiol.* 74:2140–2145, 1993.
27. Dillard, C. J., E. E. Dumelin and A. L. Tappel. Effect of dietary vitamin E on expiration of pentane and ethane by the rat. *Lipids* 12:109–114, 1976.
28. Dillard, C. J., R. E. Litov, R. E. Savin, E. E. Dumelin and A. L. Tappel. Effects of exercise, vitamin E, and ozone on pulmonary function and lipid peroxidation. *J. Appl. Physiol. Respirat. Environ. Exercise Physiol.* 45:927–932, 1978.
29. Dragan, I., V. Dinu, E. Cristea, M. Mohora, E. Ploesteanu, and V. Stroescu. Studies regarding the effects of an antioxidant compound in top atheletes. *Rev. Roum. Physiol.* 28:105–108, 1991.
30. Dressendorfer, R. H., C. E. Wade, C. L. Keen, and J. H. Scatf. Plasma mineral levels in marathon runners during a 20-day road race. *Phys. Sportsmed.* 8:97–100, 1982.
31. Duarte, J. A. R., H. J. Appell, F. Carvalho, M. L. Bastos, and J. M. C. Soares. Endothelium-derived oxidative stress may contribute to exercise-induced muscle damage. *Int. J. Sports Med.* 14:440–443, 1993.
32. Esterbauer, H., R. G. Shaver, H. Zollner. Chemistry and biochemistry of 4-hydroxynonenal MDA and related aldehydes. *Free Radic Biol. Med.* 11:81–128, 1991.

33. Evans, W. J., and J. C. Cannon. The metabolic effects of exercise-induced muscle damage. J. O. Holloszy (ed). *Exercise and Sports Sciences Reviews,* Vol. 19. Baltimore: Williams & Wilkins, 1991, pp. 99–125.

34. Fahrenholtz, S. R., F. H. Doleiden, A. M. Trozzolo, and A. A. Lamola. On the quenching of singlet oxygen by alpha-tocopherol. *Photochem. Photobiol.* 20:505–509, 1974.

35. Ferrans, V. J. Overview of cardiac pathology in relation to anthracycline cardiotoxicity. *Cancer Treat. Rep.* 62:955–961, 1978.

36. Fong, K., P. B. McCay, J. L. Poyer, B. B. Kelle, and H. Misra. Evidence that peroxidation of lysosomal membranes is initiated by hydroxyl free radicals produced during flavin enzyme activity. *J. Biol. Chem.* 248:7792–7798, 1973.

37. Frei, B., L. England and B. N. Ames. Ascorbate is an outstanding antioxidant in human blood plasma. *Proc. Natl. Acad. Sci. U. S. A.* 86:6377–6381, 1989.

38. Fridovich, I. Superoxide dismutase in biology and medicine. A. Autor (ed). *Pathology of Oxygen.* New York: Academic Press, 1982, p. 1.

39. Gerster, H. Function of vitamin E in physical exercise: a review. *Z. Ernahrungswiss* 30:89–97, 1991.

40. Gey, G. O., K. H. Cooper, and R. A. Bottenberg. Effect of ascorbic acid on endurance performance and athletic injury. *J. A. M. A.* 211:105–111, 1970.

41. Girten, B., C. Oloff, P. Plato, E. Eveland, A. J. Merola and L. Kazarian. Skeletal muscle antioxidant enzyme levels in rats after simulated weightlessness, exercise and dobutamine. *Physiologist* 32:S59–S60, 1989.

42. Gleeson, M., J. D. Robertson and R. J. Maughan. Influence of exercise on ascorbic acid status in man. *Clin. Sci.* 73:501–505, 1987.

43. Gohil, K., L. Packer, B. De Lumen, G. A. Brooks, and S. F. Terblanche. Vitamin E deficiency and vitamin C supplements: exercise and mitochondrial oxidation. *J. Appl. Physiol.* 60: 1986–1991, 1986.

44. Haber, F., and J. Weiss. The catalytic decomposition of hydrogen peroxide by iron salts. *Proc. R. Soc. Lond.* A147:332–337, 1934.

45. Hackman, R. M., and C. L. Keen. Changes in serum zinc and copper levels after zinc supplementation in running and nonrunning men. F. I. Katch (ed). *Sport, Health, and Nutrition.* Champaign, IL: Human Kinetics, 1986, pp. 89–99.

46. Halliwell, B. and S. Chirico. Lipid peroxidation: its mechanism, measurement and significance. *Am. J. Clin. Nutr.* 57 (suppl):715S–725S, 1993.

47. Halliwell, B. and J. M. C. Gutteridge. *Free Radicals in Biology and Medicine.* Oxford: Clarendon Press, 1985, pp. 162–164.

48. Heath, G. W., J. R. Gavin, J. M. Hinderliter, J. M. Hagberg, S. A. Bloomfield and J. O. Holloszy. Effects of exercise and lack of exercise on glucose tolerance and insulin sensitivity. *J. Appl. Physiol.* 55:512–517, 1983.

49. Helgheim, I., O. Hetland, S. Nilsson, F. Ingjer and S. B. Stromme. The effects of vitamin E on serum enzyme levels following heavy exercise. *Eur. J. Appl. Physiol.* 40:283–289, 1979.

50. Herbert, V. Does Mega-C do more good than harm, or more harm than good? *Nutr. Today* Jan/Feb: 28–32, 1993.

51. Higuchi, M., L. J. Cartier, M. Chen and J. O. Holloszy. Superoxide dismutase and catalase in skeletal muscle: adaptative response to exercise. *J. Gerontol* 40:281–286, 1985.

52. Holloszy, J. O. Biochemical adaptations in muscle. *J. Biol. Chem.* 212:2278–2284, 1967.

53. Holloszy, J. O., and E. F. Coyle. Adaptations of skeletal muscle to endurance exercise and their metabolic consequences. *J. Appl. Physiol.* 56:831–837, 1984.

54. Hortobágyi T., and T. Denahan. Variability in creatine kinase: methodological, exercise, and clinically related factors. *Int. J. Sports Med.* 10:69–80, 1989.

55. Horwitt, M. K., C. C. Harvey, D. J. Dahm, and M. T. Searcy. Relationship between tocopherol and serum lipid levels for determination of nutritional adequacy. *Ann. N. Y. Acad. Sci.* 203:233–236, 1972.

56. Isler, O. (ed). *Carotenoids.* Basel: Berkhauser Verlag, 1971.

57. Jakeman, P. and S. Maxwell. Effect of antioxidant vitamin supplementation on muscle function after eccentric exercise. *Eur. J. Appl. Physiol.* 67:426–430, 1993.
58. Jenkins, R. R. Free radical chemistry: relationship to exercise. *Sports Med.* 5:156–170, 1988.
59. Jenkins, R. R. Exercise, oxidative stress, and antioxidants: a review. *Int. J. Sports Nutr.* 3:356–375, 1993.
60. Jenkins, R. R., R. Friedland and H. Howald. The adaptation of the hydroperoxide enzyme system to increased oxygen use. *Med. Sci. Sport Exer.* 14:148, 1982 (abstract).
61. Ji, L. L., F. W. Stratman, and H. A. Lardy. Antioxidant enzyme response to selenium deficiency in rat myocardium. *J. Am. Col. Nutr.* 11:79–86, 1992.
62. Ji, L. L., A. Katz, R. Fu, M. Griffiths, and M. Spencer. Blood glutathione status during exercise: effect of carbohydrate supplementation. *J. Appl. Physiol.* 74:788–792, 1993.
63. Kaminski, M., and R. Boal. An effect of ascorbic acid on delayed-onset muscle soreness. *Pain* 50:317–321, 1992.
64. Kanter, M. M. and D. E. Eddy. Effect of antioxidant supplementation on serum markers of lipid peroxidation and skeletal muscle damage following eccentric exercise. *Med. Sci. Sports Exerc.* 24:S17, 1992 (abstract).
65. Kanter, M. M., R. L. Hamlin, D. V. Unverferth, H. W. Davis and A. J. Merola. Effect of exercise training on antioxidant enzymes and cardiotoxicity of doxorubicin. *J. Appl. Physiol.* 59:1298–1303, 1985.
66. Kanter, M. M., L.A. Kaminsky, J. L. Laham-Saeger, G. R. Lesmes and N. D. Nequin. Serum enzyme levels and lipid peroxidation in ultramarathon runners. *Ann. Sports Med.* 3:39–41, 1986.
67. Kanter, M. M., G. R. Lesmes, L. A. Kaminsky, J. La Ham-Saeger, and N. D. Nequin. Serum creatine kinase and lactate dehydrogenase changes following an eighty kilometer race: relationship to lipid peroxidation. *Eur. J. Appl. Physiol.* 57:60–63, 1988.
68. Kanter, M. M., L.A. Nolte, J. O. Holloszy. Effects of an antioxidant vitamin mixture on lipid peroxidation at rest and postexercise. *J. Appl. Physiol.* 74:965–969, 1993.
69. Karlsson, J. Heart and skeletal muscle ubiquinone or CoQ_{10} as a protective agent against radical formation in man. *Adv. Myochem.* 1:305–318, 1987.
70. Katagiri, T., N. Konno, T. Yanagishita, et al. Protection of ischemic myocardial injury by coenzyme-Q10—mechanism of action. K. Folkers, Y. Yamamura (eds). *Biomedical and Clinical Aspects of Coenzyme Q, Vol. 5.* Amsterdam: Elsevier Science, 1986, pp. 167–177.
71. Keith, R. E. Vitamins in sport and exercise. J. E. Hickson and I. Wolinsky (eds). *Nutrition in Exercise and Sport,* Boca Raton, FL: CRC Press, 1989, pp. 233–253.
72. Keren, G., and Y. Epstein. The effect of high dosage vitamin C intake on aerobic and anaerobic capacity. *J. Sports. Med.* 20:145–148, 1980.
73. Krinsky, N. Antioxidant functions of beta carotene. *Vit. Nutr. Information Service Backgrounder.* 1:1–4, 1989.
74. Kumar, C. T., V. K. Reddy, M. Prasad, K. Thyagaraju and P. Reddanna. Dietary supplementation of vitamin E protects heart tissue from exercise-induced oxidant stress. *Mol. Cell. Biochem.* 111:109–115, 1992.
75. Lawrence, J. D., R. C. Bower, W. P. Riehl and J. L. Smith. Effects of alpha tocopherol acetate on the swimming endurance of trained swimmers. *Am. J. Clin. Nutr.* 28:205–208, 1975.
76. Loschen, S., A. Azzi, and L. Flohe. Mitochondrial H_2O_2 formation: relationship with energy conservations. *FEBS Lett.* 33:84–87, 1973.
77. Losowsky, M. S., and P. J. Leonard. Evidence of vitamin E deficiency in patients with malabsorption or alcoholism and the effects of therapy. *Gut* 8:539–543, 1967.
78. Lown, J. W., A. V. Joshua, and H. H. Chen. Reactive oxugen species leading to lipid peroxidation and DNA lesions implicated in the cytotoxic action of certain antitumor antibiotics. D. C. H. McBrien and T. F. Slater (eds). *Free Radicals Lipid Peroxidation and Cancer.* London: Academic Press, 1982, p. 305.
79. Machlin, L. J. and A. Bendich. Free radical tissue damage: protective role of antioxidant nutrients. *FASEB J.* 1:441–445, 1987.

80. Mangels, A. R., G. Block, C. M. Frey, et al. The bioavailability to humans of ascorbic acid from oranges, orange juice and cooked broccoli is similar to that of synthetic ascorbic acid. *J. Nutr.* 123:1054–1061, 1993.

81. Maughan, R. J., A. E. Donnelly, M. Gleeson, P. H. Whiting, K. A. Walker and P. J. Clough. Delayed-onset muscle damage and lipid peroxidation in man after a downhill run. *Musc. Nerve* 12:332–336, 1989.

82. McArdle W. D. and J. R. Magel. Weight management: diet and exercise. J. Bland and N. Shealy (eds). *The Medical Aspects of Clinical Nutrition.* New Canaan, CT: Keats, 1983.

83. McCord, J. M. Superoxide, superoxide dismutase and oxygen toxicity. *Rev. Biochem. Toxicol.* 1:109–124, 1979.

84. McCord, J. M. and E. D. Day, Jr. Superoxide dependent production of hydroxyl radical catalyzed by iron-EDTA complex. *FEBS Lett.* 86:139–142, 1978.

85. McDonald R., and C. L. Keen. Iron, zinc, and magnesium nutrition and athletic performance. *Sports Med.* 5:171–184, 1988.

86. Meerson, F. Z., V. E. Kagan, Y. P. Kozlov, L. M. Belkins, and Y. V. Arkhipenko. The role of lipid peroxidation in pathogenesis of ischemic damage and the antioxidant protection of the heart. *Basic Res. Caridol.* 77:465–476, 1982.

87. Mena, P., M. Maynar, J. M. Gutierrez, J. Maynar, J. Timon, J. E. Campillo. Erythrocyte free radical scavenger enzymes in professional bicycle racers: adaptation to training. *Int. J. Sports Med.* 12:563–566, 1991.

88. Mengel, C. E., and H. L. Greene. Ascorbic acid effects on erythrocyte. *Ann. Intern. Med.* 84:490–494, 1976.

89. Merry, P., B. L. Kidd, A. Claxson, and D. R. Blake. Synovitis of the joint is an example of reperfusion injury. P. C. Beaumont, B. L. Kidd, A. Claxson, and D. R. Blake (eds). *Free Radicals, Metal Ions and Biopolymers.* London: Richelieu Press, 1989, pp. 199–215.

90. Meydani, M. Protective role of dietary vitamin E on oxidative stress in aging. *Age* 15:89–93, 1992.

91. Meydani, M. W. J. Evans, G. Handelman, et al. Protective effect of vitamin E on exercise-induced oxidative damage in young and older adults. *Am. J. Physiol.* 264:R992–R998, 1993.

92. Misra, H. L., and I. Fridovich. The generation of superoxide radical during the autoxidation of hemoglobin. *J. Biol. Chem.* 247:6960–6964, 1972.

93. Mooradian, A. D., M. P. Habib, F. Dickerson. Effect of simple carbohydrates, casein hydrolysate, and a lipid test meal on ethane exhalation rate. *J. Appl. Physiol.* 76:1119–1122, 1994.

94. Namiki, M. Antioxidants/antimutagens in food. *Food Sci. Nutr.* 29:273–300, 1990.

95. Newham, D. J., D. A. Jones, S. E. J. Tolfree, and R. H. T. Edwards. Skeletal muscle damage: a study of isotope uptake, enzyme efflux and pain after stepping. *Eur. J. Appl. Physiol.* 55:106–112, 1986.

96. Niki, E., A. Kawakami, M. Saito, Y. Yamamoto, J. Tsuchiya and Y. Kamiya. Effect of phytyl side chain of vitamin E on its antioxidant activity. *J. Biol. Chem.* 260:2191–2196, 1985.

97. Novelli, G. P., G. Bracciotti, and S. Falsini. Spin-trappers and vitamin E prolong endurance to muscle fatigue in mice. *Free Radic. Biol. Med.* 8:9–13, 1990.

98. Ohno, H., Y. Sato, K. Yamashita, R. Doi, K. Arai, T. Kondo, and N. Taniguchi. The effect of brief physical exercise on free radical scavenging enzyme systems in human red blood cells. *Can. J. Physiol. Pharmacol.* 64:1263–1265, 1986.

99. Packer, L. Vitamin E, physical exercise, and tissue damage in animals. *Med. Biol. Helsinki* 62:105–109, 1984.

100. Paolisso, G., A. D'Amore, V. Balbi, et al. Plasma vitamin C affects glucose homeostasis in healthy subjects and in non-insulin-dependent diabetics. *Am. J. Physiol.* 266 (Endocrinol. Metab. 29):E261–E268, 1994.

101. Peters, E. M., J. M. Goetzsche, B. Grobbelaar and T. D. Noakes. Vitamin C supplementa-

tion reduces the incidence of postrace symptoms of upper-respiratory-tract infection in ultramaration runners. *Am. J. Clin. Nutr.* 57:170–174, 1993.

102. Pincemail, J., C. Derby, G. Camus, F. Pirnay, R. Bouchez, and L. Massaux. Tocopherol mobilization during intensive exercise. *Arch. Int. Physiol. Biochem.* 94:S43–S44, 1986.

103. Poda, G. A. Vitamin C for heat symptoms? *Ann. Intern. Med.* 91:657, 1979.

104. Rimm, E. B., M. J. Stampfer, A. Ascherio, E. G. Giovannucci, G. A. Colditz, W. C. Willett. Vitamin E consumption and the risk of coronary heart disease in men. *N. Engl. J. Med.* 328:1450–1456, 1993.

105. Robertson, J. D., R. J. Maughan, G. G. Duthie, and P. C. Morrice. Increased blood antioxidant systems of runners in response to training load. *Clin. Sci.* 80:611–618, 1991.

106. Robinson, S., and A. H. Robinson. Chemical composition of sweat. *Physiol. Rev.* 34:202–220, 1954.

107. Sahlin, K., S. Cizinsky, M. Warholm, and J. Hoberg. Repetitive static muscle contractions in humans—a trigger of metabolic and oxidative stress? *Eur. J. Appl. Physiol* 64:228–236, 1992.

108. Salminen, A., and V. Vihko. Lipid peroxidation in exercise myopathy. *Exp. Mol. Pathol.* 38:380–388, 1983.

109. Salminen, A., H. Kainulainen, A. U. Arstila, and V. Vihko. Vitamin E deficiency and the susceptibility to lipid peroxidation of mouse cardiac and skeletal muscles. *Acta Physiol. Scand.* 122:565–570, 1984.

110. Salo, D. C. C. M. Donovan and K. J. A. Davies. HSP70 and other possible heat shock or oxidative stress proteins are induced in skeletal muscle, heart and liver during exercise. *Free Radic. Biol. Med.* 11:239–246, 1991.

111. Sastre J., M. Asensi, E. Gasco, et al. Exhaustive physical exercise causes oxidation of glutathione status in blood: prevention by antioxidant administration. *Am. J. Physiol.* 263(Regulatory Integrative Comp. Physiol. 32):R992–R995, 1992.

112. Saxton, J. M., A. E. Donnelly, H. P. Roper. Indices of free-radical-mediated damage following maximum voluntary eccentric and concentric muscular work. *Eur. J. Appl. Physiol.* 68:189–193, 1994.

113. Scheuer, J., and C. M. Tipton. Cardiovascular adaptations to training. *Annu. Rev. Physiol.* 39:221–239, 1977.

114. Schrauzer, G. N., and W. H. Rhead. Ascorbic acid abuse: effects on long term ingestion of excessive amounts on blood levels and urinary excretion. *Int. J. Vitamin Nutr. Res.* 43: 201, 1973.

115. Shigenaga, M. K., C. J. Gimeno, and B. N. Ames. Urinary 8-hydroxy-2'-deoxyguanosine as a biological marker of *in vivo* oxidative DNA damage. *Proc. Natl. Acad. Sci. U. S. A.* 86:1440–1445, 1989.

116. Shimomura, Y., M. Suzuki, S. Sugiyama, Y. Hanaki and T. Ozawa. Protective effect of coenzyme Q10 on exercise-induced muscular injury. *Biochem. Biophys. Res. Commun.* 176: 349–355, 1991.

117. Simon-Schnass, I. and H. Pabst. Influence of vitamin E on physical performance. *Int. J. Vit. Nutr. Res.* 58:49–54, 1988.

118. Sjodin, B., Y. Hellsten Westing and F. S. Apple. Biochemical mechanisms for oxygen free radical formation during exercise. *Sports Med.* 10:236–254, 1990.

119. Smith, J. K., M. B. Grisham, D. N. Granger, and R. J. Korthus. Free radical defense mechanisms and neutrophil infiltration in postischemic skeletal muscle. *Am. J. Physiol.* 256:H789–H793, 1989.

120. Snider, I. P., T. L. Bazzarre, S. D. Murdoch and A. Goldfarb. Effects of Coenzyme Athletic Performance System as an ergogenic aid on endurance performance to exhaustion. *Int. J. Sports Med.* 2:272–286, 1992.

121. Stampfer, M. J., C. H. Hennekens, J. E. Manson, G. A. Colditz, B. Rosner and W. C. Willett. Vitamin E consumption and the risk of coronary disease in women. *N. Engl. J. Med.* 328:1444–1449, 1993.

122. Sumida, S., K. Tanaka, H. Kitao, and F. Nakadomo. Exercise-induced lipid peroxidation and leakage of enzymes before and after vitamin E supplementation. *Int. J. Biochem.* 21:835–838, 1989.

123. Sutton, H. C. and C. Winterbourn. On the participation of high oxidation states of iron and copper in Fenton reactions. *Free Radic. Biol. Med.* 6:53–60, 1989.

124. Symons, M. C. R. Formation of radicals by mechanical processes. *Free Radic. Res. Commun.* 5:131–139, 1988.

125. Talbot, D., and J. Jamieson. An examination of the effect of vitamin E on the performance of highly trained swimmers. *Can. J. Appl. Sport Sci.* 2:67–69, 1977.

126. Tappel., A. Lipid peroxidation damage to cell components. *Fed. Proc.* 32:1870–1875, 1973.

127. Taylor, A. Cataract: relationships between nutrition and oxidation. *J. Am. Coll. Nutr.* 12:138–146, 1993.

128. Tiidus, P. M., W. A. Behrens, R. Madere and M. E. Houston. Muscle vitamin E levels following acute submaximal exercise in female rats. *Acta Physiol. Scand.* 147:249–250, 1993.

129. Tipton, C. M., Exercise training and hypertention. R. Terjung (ed). *Exercise and Sport Sciences Reviews.* Lexington, MA: Collamore Press, 1984, pp. 245–306.

130. Traber, M. G., W. Cohn, D. P. R. Muller. Absorption, transport and delivery to tissues. L. Packer and J. Fuchs (eds). *Vitamin E in Health and Disease.* New York: Marcel Dekker, Inc. 1993, pp. 35–51.

131. Unverferth, D., R. Magorien, C. Leier, and S. Balcerzak. Doxorubicin cardioxotocity. *Cancer Treat Rev.* 9:149–159, 1982.

132. Viguie, C. A., L. Packer and G. A. Brooks. Antioxidant supplementation affects indices of muscle trauma and oxidant stress in human blood during exercise. *Med. Sci. Sports Exerc.* 21:S16, 1989 (abstract).

133. Viguie, C. A., B. Frei, M. K. Shigenaga, B. N. Ames, L. Packer, G. A. Brooks. Antioxidant status and indexes of oxidative stress during consecutive days of exercise. *J. Appl. Physiol.* 75:566–572, 1993.

134. Voelker, R. Recommendations for antioxidants: how much evidence is enough? *J. A. M. A.* 271:1148–1149, 1994.

135. Warren, J. A., R. R. Jenkins, L. Packer, E. H. Witt, and R. B. Armstrong. Elevated muscle vitamin E does not attenuate eccentric exercise-induced muscle injury. *J. Appl. Physiol.* 72:2168–2175, 1992.

136. Willson, R. L. Free radical protection: why vitamin E, not vitamin C, beta-carotene or glutathione. R. Porter and J. Whelan (eds). *Biology of Vitamin E.* Ciba Foundation Symposium 101. London: Pitman Books Ltd., 1983, pp. 19–44.

137. Witt, E. H., A. Z. Reznick, C. A. Viguie, P. Starke-Reed, and L. Packer. Exercise, oxidative damage and effects of antioxidant manipulation. *J. Nutr.* 122:766–773, 1992.

138. Wong, S. H. Y., J. A. Knight, S. M. Hopfer, O. Zaharia, C. N. Leach, F. W. Sunderman. Lipoperoxides in plasma as measured by liquid-chromatographic separation of malondialdehyde-thiobarbituric acid adduct. *Clin. Chem.* 33:214–220, 1987.

139. Wu, G., R. Stein, and J. Mead. Autooxidation of fatty acid monolayers absorbed on silica gel: II rates and products. *Lipids* 12:971–984, 1978.

140. Yamamura, Y. A study of the therapeutic uses of coenzyme Q. G. Lenaz (ed). *Coenzyme Q.* Chichester: Wiley, 479–505, 1985.

141. Zapsilas, C. and R. Anderle Beck. *Food Chemistry and Nutritional Biochemistry.* New York: John Wiley & Sons, 1985, pp. 273–286.

142. Zuliani, U., A. Bonetti, M. Campana, G. Cerioli, F. Solito, and A. Novarini. The influence of ubiquinone (CoQ_{10}) on the metabolic response to work. *J. Sports Med. Phys. Fit.* 29: 57–62, 1989.

13
Sports Medicine Aspects of Cervical Spinal Stenosis

ROBERT C. CANTU, M.D., F.A.C.S., F A C S M

Before the advent of computed tomography (CT) and, more recently, magnetic resonance imaging (MRI) scanning, the presence of cervical spinal stenosis was defined by bony measurements. In 1956, Wolf et al. [23], using randomly selected asymptomatic subjects who underwent lateral cervical spine radiographs at a fixed target distance of 72 inches to eliminate magnification error, established normal values of the sagittal diameters of the cervical spine. Sagittal diameter canal height was defined as the anteroposterior diameter measured from the posterior aspect of the vertebral body to the most anterior point on the spinolaminar line (see N in Fig. 13.1). Wolfe and colleagues found the average anteroposterior diameter was 22 mm at C-1, 20 mm at C-2, and 17 mm from C-3 to C-7. General consensus evolved in the radiologic literature that between C-3 and C-7 when magnification is corrected for that canal heights are normal above 15 mm [1, 2] and spinal stenosis is present below 13 mm [8, 11].

In 1986, Torg et al. [22] and, in 1987, Pavlov et al. [17], described a new method to assess cervical spinal stenosis radiographically using a ratio method to eliminate the need to correct for radiographic magnification error. The height of the spinal canal, as measured from the midpoint of the posterior surface of the vertebral body up to the spinolaminar line, is the numerator and the denominator is the height of the corresponding midvertebral body (see Fig. 13.1). A vertebral canal/vertebral body ratio of less than 0.80 was defined as "significant spinal stenosis."

Recently the Torg ratio as a means to define spinal stenosis has been cast in doubt. First the Kerlan Jobe Orthopedic Clinic found the incidence of spinal stenosis using the Torg "ratio" to be 33% in 124 professional and 100 rookie football players [16].

More recently, Herzog et al. [10] found in 80 asymptomatic professional football players that 49% had abnormal ratios below 0.80 at one or more cervical levels. They also found the ratio to be highly unreliable in determining spinal stenosis with a positive predictive value of only 12%. They found that their athletes had normal canal heights (numerator) but often massive vertebral bodies (denominator), which brought the ratio to less than 0.80. They concluded "if an abnormal Torg ratio is detected, further evaluation is necessary before an athlete can be diagnosed as significantly spinal stenotic" [10].

FIGURE 13.1

N = numerator height of spinal canal; D = denominator height of vertebral body.

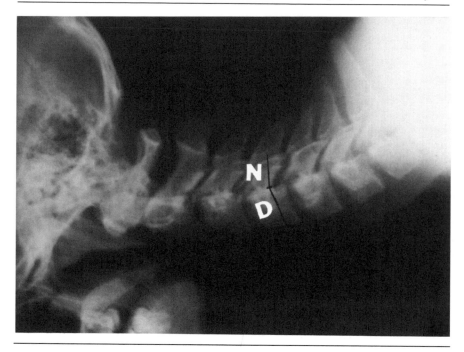

More recently, I have proposed [3, 6] that currently only diagnostic technologies that view the spinal cord itself, such as MRI, contrast-positive CT (CT+), or myelography, should be used to establish the diagnosis of cervical spinal stenosis. Only these technologies and not an x-ray or x-ray ratio assess the size of the neural tissue in relation to the size of the spinal canal. The size of the cervical spinal cord, although usually 9–10 mm in diameter, has been reported to vary between 5 and 11.5 mm [12, 21]. Thus, true stenosis may be present with low to normal canal measurements and a large spinal cord.

I have also advanced the concept of "functional spinal stenosis" [3, 6] as defined by the loss of the "functional reserve" of cerebrospinal fluid (CSF) around the cord or actual deformation of the spinal cord (see Figs. 13.2 and 13.3). Only the MRI, CT+ or myelogram clearly shows whether the spinal cord has a normal functional reserve: the space around the cord largely filled with a protective cushion of cerebrospinal fluid between the cord and the spinal canal's interior walls lined by bone, disc, and ligament. In addition, these technologies can also determine whether the spinal cord is deformed by an abnormality such as disc protrusion or rupture, bony osteophyte, or posterior buckling of the ligamentus flavum.

FIGURE 13.2.

MRI provides an anatomically exact method for assessing cervical spinal stenosis. The cervical spine MRI shown suggests a wide cushion of CSF in a patient with normal functional reserve. The dark area above the arrow represents the CSF.

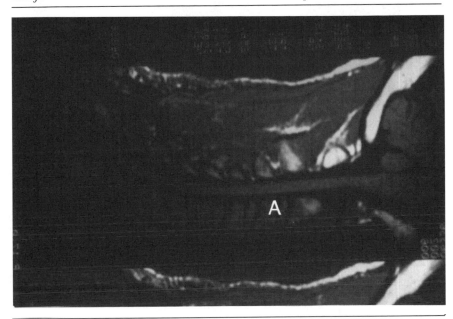

RETURN-TO-PLAY CRITERIA FOR CONTACT OR COLLISION SPORTS AFTER CERVICAL SPINE OR CORD INJURY

Sprain or Strain

Most cervical injuries will involve a ligament sprain, muscle strain, or contusion. With such injuries, there is no neurological or osseous injury and return to competition can occur when the athlete is free of neck pain with and without axial compression, range of motion is full, and the strength of the neck is normal. Cervical x-rays should show no subluxation or abnormal curvatures. If the athlete has a neck profile of maximal weight that he or she can pull with the neck in flexion, extension, and to each side, it is preferable the athlete not return to competition until he or she is asymptomatic and can perform to the level of his or her pre-injury profile.

Cervical Spine Fracture

Stable fractures that have healed completely will allow the player to return by the next season. If there is a one-level anterior or posterior fusion for a fracture, athletes are usually allowed to go back when the neck pain is gone, the range of motion is complete, muscle strength of the neck is normal, and

FIGURE 13.3.

Cervical spine MRI showing functional spinal stenosis with loss of CSF around and even indentation and deformity of the spinal cord [1].

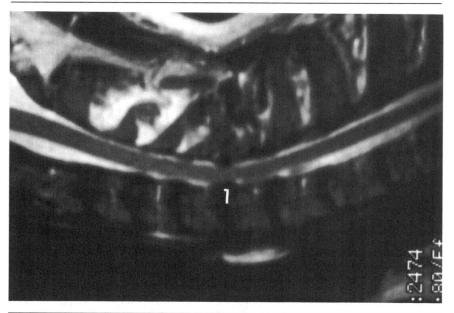

the fusion is solid. In any athlete with a fractured neck, proper warnings against contact or collision sports is advisable until it is certain that the patient is completely healed.

Where there are multilevel fusions or a fusion involves C1-2 or C2-3, return to contact collision sports is contraindicated, but the athlete could participate in a noncontact sport at low risk of neck injury such as tennis.

RETURN-TO-PLAY CRITERIA AFTER A BURNER

Roughly half of so-called "burners" or "stingers" in football at the high school level involve a brachial plexus stretch injury. The majority at the college and professional level involve a cervical nerve root "pinch" phenomenon within the neural foramen. Because the dorsal root ganglion occupies most of the space with the foramen and lies underneath the subluxing facet, it often takes the brunt of the injury and symptoms may be purely sensory in a dermatomal distribution (see Fig. 13.4).

These injuries are unilateral and when not associated with any cervical pain or limitation of cervical movement, if all motor, if present, and sensory symptoms clear within seconds to minutes, the athlete may safely return to

FIGURE 13.4.
Cross-section of spinal canal and its contents. C4-5, disc; VR, ventral ramus; DR, dorsal ramus; NF, nerve foramen; VR, ventral root; RG, dorsal root ganglion; SF, superior facet.

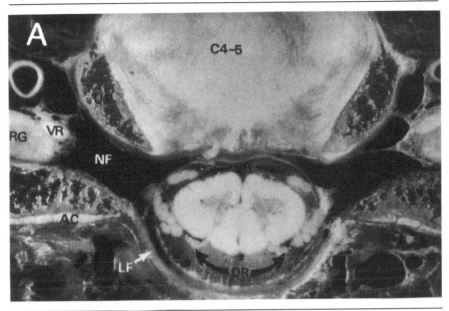

competition. This is especially true if the athlete has had similar symptoms before. If there are any residual symptoms, or neck pain, or incomplete range of motion, or suspicion of a neck injury, return should be deferred.

RETURN-TO-PLAY CRITERIA AFTER TRANSIENT QUADRIPLEGIA

What factors predispose athletes to quadriplegia and when should athletes be withheld from future participation in contact or collision sports after an episode of transient quadriplegia? What are the appropriate circumstances to allow return after transient quadriplegia and what are *relative* and *absolute* contraindications for return? In presenting and discussing three case histories seen in my practice, these questions will be answered.

Case Histories
Case 1 involved a 27-year-old National Football League linebacker who experienced transient upper and lower extremity paralysis and numbness after tackling a 225-lb opponent. The patient made contact sufficient to dent the forehead portion of his helmet and appeared to sustain an axial load injury with some hyperextension. Paralysis lasted 4 min, then, over the next

10–20 min, motor and sensory function returned beginning in the lower extremities. On arrival at the hospital, the patient was complaining of a burning sensation across his neck and shoulders. He denied any loss of consciousness and there was no loss of bowel or bladder function.

On physical examination, higher cortical functions were intact. Motor examination results were 5/5 throughout and reflexes were 2+ and symmetric except the ankles, which were 1+ and symmetric. Plantar response was downgoing bilaterally. Sensory examination results were positive to light touch and pinprick. The cerebellum was intact on examination.

Plain films of the cervical spine showed no evidence of fracture, dislocation or subluxation, or degenerative disc disease. The canal height measured within normal limits: 15 mm at C-3 and C-4 and 20 mm at C-6. Torg ratios were C-3=15/24=0.63, C-4=15/22=0.68, C-5=17/20=0.85, C-6=20/22=0.91. MRI showed no evidence of fracture, canal compromise, or contusion. Flexion and extension views of the spine showed no instability. Cervical CT and MRI showed a functional reserve of CSF around the cord.

Case 2 involved a 23-year-old hockey player, drafted into the National Hockey League, who was injured while filming a team advertisement. Bending at the waist with his neck flexed, he unexpectedly collided with another player. The top of the patient's helmet struck the other player's abdomen. The patient's neck was relaxed because he was not expecting impact. Each player had taken one stride before the impact. The patient had immediate neck pain and felt something was wrong with his arms and legs. He fell to his side and rolled over on the ice onto his back. After 1 min, he was aware that he could move his fingers in his gloves and his toes in his skates. A pins-and-needles sensation extended into both hands and, to a lesser extent, his torso and legs. He was aware of a rigid painful neck within minutes. When he moved his head, a shocklike sensation travelled down his spine to his buttocks. It was about 4 or 5 min before he could rise from the ice. Neurological symptoms persisted at highest intensity for approximately 5 min, then gradually subsided, first in his legs and then his arms. It was 2 wk before all paresthesias had disappeared. Other than a brief concussion in 1984, when his helmeted head struck the boards, he denies any significant prior injury.

Two weeks after injury, the patient had normal range of neck motion. No radiating symptoms could be elicited by compression of his spinous processes or by mild axial loading (negative Spurling's maneuver). No neurologic deficit was detected. Strength and tone were normal throughout. Plantar responses were downgoing. No clonus or abnormal reflexes were present. Upper extremity reflexes were 1+ and lower extremity reflexes were 2+. Gait proved normal and no sensory loss for pinprick, vibration, or position sense was found.

Plain films showed no evidence of degenerative disc disease, subluxation, or fracture. The height of the canal at all levels exceeded 15 mm. Torg ratios measured C-3=17/24=0.71; C-4=15/23=0.65; C-5=15/26=0.68; C-

6=16/23=0.70. MRI revealed mild disc bulging at C3–4 but did not show spinal cord encroachment and did show a functional reserve of CSF around the cord at all levels. Myelogram and CT+ showed slight disc bulging at C3–4 but also CSF around the spinal cord at all levels, including C3–4.

The athlete in Case 3 first injured his neck as a high school football player in 1987. Upon making what he remembers to be a head-up tackle, he fell to his side and was unable to get up or roll onto his back. Sensation and motor movement were absent from the neck down. Gradually, motor function and sensation returned, first in his feet and then his hands. He could not move his head because of cervical spasm, and any attempts do so produced jabs of pain running from his neck to his head. After several minutes, he was able to stand and walk off the field unassisted, although his legs felt very weak. His neck was rigid on the sidelines and he did not return to play. No x-rays were taken at that time and no medical attention was sought. The patient played the following week with a neck collar. He reported that his neck was rigid and thus he performed poorly. He did not play for the next 2 wk because of continued rigidity and severe neck pain. Three weeks after the injury, because of persistent neck pain and stiffness, he sought medical attention at a sports medicine facility. There, cervical spine x-rays were taken. Although canal heights and Torg ratios were not measured, subsequent review of these films revealed canal heights of 12 mm, consistent with spinal stenosis and abnormal Torg ratios at C-4=12/25=0.48 and C-5=12/24=0.50. Two weeks thereafter, the patient returned to competition, his neck pain and stiffness relieved. He played his senior season without further cervical symptoms.

The following fall, as a college freshman on full athletic scholarship, the patient squatted to make a tackle, hitting face to face and chest to chest. With head tilted up, his facemask made first contact. He fell backward on the ground, unable to move and without sensation from the neck down. Over the next few minutes, movement began to return to his right side and patchy sensation to his left side. He was transported to the hospital, where physical examination showed cranial nerves to be intact. There was a Brown-Sequard syndrome with right-sided hemisensory loss and a nearly flaccid left side. Muscle strength was 4/5 on the right except the intrinsic muscles of the hand, which were 3/5. Biceps reflex was 1+ and symmetric, triceps reflex was 2+ on the right and absent on the left, knee jerk reflex was 2+ on the right and absent on the left, ankle jerk reflex was 2+ on the right and 1+ on the left. There were 3 beats of clonus in both ankles.

X-rays, CTs, and MRIs were taken. The films revealed cervical stenosis and posterior disc herniation at C-3 to C-4 with displacement of cord and thecal sac to the right. Torg ratios measured C-2=20/23=0.87; C-3=13/23=0.52; C-5=12/24=0.50; C-6 and C-7 could not be read. Edema was found within the spinal cord from C-2 to C-5. Surgery was performed without complications, but the patient remained paralyzed immediately afterward. A second exploration did not find bleeding. The patient went to rehabilitation and remained in a wheelchair for 8 mo before walking. Presently, he has recovered to a spastic quadriparetic state.

DISCUSSION

All three athletes in these cases suffered a bout of transient quadriplegia. Although such an event may occur after hyperextension or hyperflexion, it most frequently occurs with axial load injury to the cervical spine, as described by Torg [22]. In all cases, the symptoms were consistent with variations of the central spinal cord syndrome as described by Schneider et al. [20].

Cervical spinal stenosis is known to increase the risk of permanent neurological injury [13–15]. Firooznia et al. [9] presented three case reports of patients who became quadriplegic after only "minor trauma." In all three patients, radiological studies revealed "marked stenosis of the spinal canal." Some debate exists, however, over the definition of spinal stenosis. In the past, the anteroposterior (AP) diameter of the spinal canal, measured from the posterior aspect of the vertebral body to the most anterior point on the spinolaminar line, determined the presence of stenosis. General consensus has been that between C-3 and C-7 canal heights are normal above 15 mm and spinal stenosis is present below 13 mm [1]. Resnick says CT and myelography are "the most sensitive diagnostic modalities" in determining spinal stenosis [19]. He points out that roentgenography fails to appraise the width of the cord and is not useful when stenosis results from ligamentous hypertrophy or discal protrusion. Ladd and Scranton [11] state that the AP diameter of the spinal canal is "unimportant" if there is total impedance of the contrast medium. They argue that metrizamide-enhanced myelogram is needed for the injured athlete because CT alone fails to reveal neural compression adequately. Thus, spinal stenosis cannot be defined by bony measurements alone. "Functional" spinal stenosis, defined as loss of the CSF around the cord or, in more extreme cases (i.e., Case 3), deformation of the spinal cord, whether documented by CT+, MRI, or myelography, is a more accurate measure of stenosis [3]. The term "functional" is taken from the radiological term "functional reserve" as applied to the protective cushion of CSF around the spinal cord in a nonstenotic canal [10]. In a recent study in which MRI was used to document the presence or absence of spinal stenosis in 11 athletes rendered quadriplegic, 6 had functional stenosis [3]. Furthermore, in the data from the National Center for Catastrophic Sports Injury Research, cases of quadriplegia without spine fracture have been seen only when functional spinal stenosis is present. Also, complete recovery of neurological function after initial neurological deficit after spine fracture or dislocation has been seen only in the absence of functional spinal stenosis.

Of the three athletes presented, only Case 3 was documented as having cervical spinal stenosis as determined by AP diameter alone (12 mm at C-4 and C-5). In both Cases 1 and 2, the narrowest AP diameter measured 15 mm. In Case 1, CT and MRI showed no abnormalities and did show a functional reserve of CSF around all levels of the cord. In Case 2, CT, MRI, and myelogram all showed slight disc bulging at C3–4 but again showed a reserve of CSF around the cord at all levels. After the second injury, in case 3, the patient was shown to suffer functional cervical spinal stenosis. CT and MRI also showed spinal cord edema and displacement of the cord secondary to disc herniation.

Torg ratios were abnormal for all three athletes, with minimum ratios of 0.63 for Case 1, 0.65 for Case 2, and 0.40 for Case 3. This ratio (canal height/vertebral body AP diameter) of less than 0.80 has been defined as spinal stenosis [3]. For Cases 1 and 2, this ratio is misleading because the large vertebral bodies, not a narrow canal, produced ratios less than 0.80. This is consistent with other reports that an abnormal Torg ratio is a poor predictor of true functional stenosis [10]. Although the ratio leads to many false-positive results (positive predictive value at 12%) [10], it rarely is normal when true stenosis documented by MRI is present (sensitivity = 92%) [10]. Thus, an abnormal ratio in an athlete with spinal cord symptoms means that evaluation with MRI, myelogram, or CT+ should be done.

Given an athlete who has suffered transient quadriplegia, what criteria should be followed for his or her return to contact sports? Case 1 is an example of an athlete who has no contraindications for returning, except for the fact that one episode of transient quadriplegia may make him more likely to have a second than an athlete who has never had these symptoms. This athlete had complete neurological recovery and full range of cervical spine movement. AP diameter was normal at all levels; CT and MRI showed no evidence of functional stenosis. Thus, there were no neurological, mechanical, symptomatic, or structural (functional spinal stenosis) contraindications for return to competition. Understanding that he may be at slightly greater risk for a second event, the athlete returned to competition and has had no further symptoms.

Case 2 involved an athlete who has two relative contraindications for returning to play, namely, mild disc bulging at C3-4 and the fact that the impact that produced the transient quadriplegia seemed relatively minor (head-to-abdomen contact from one step apart). Because myelogram and CT did not show functional stenosis and his cervical films were normal, once his neurological symptoms cleared and his cervical strength and range of motion returned to normal, there was not an absolute contraindication to return to play. After consideration of the relative contraindications, this athlete chose not to return to professional hockey.

Case 3 is an example of an athlete with an absolute contraindication for return. In addition to a stenotic canal according to AP diameter (12 mm), he had functional stenosis on CT and MRI with cord displacement and edema and lack of reserve CSF around the cord at all levels secondary to disc herniation. Because studies were not performed after his initial injury, it is not known whether he had a cord displacement at that time, but the stenosis was present. This should have been evaluated by MRI, myelogram, or CT+, and the presence of functional stenosis should have terminated his football career after the initial episode of transient quadriplegia. If he had not had severe spinal stenosis, it is probable his subsequent disc herniation would have produced radicular symptoms alone instead of severe spinal cord injury.

Given an athlete with cervical spinal stenosis, what is the mechanism of injury causing transient or permanent neurologic deficit? Eismont et al. [7] state that such athletes are "remarkably susceptible to hyperextension injuries known to produce maximal narrowing (up to 2 mm) of the ventrodorsal diameter of the spinal canal." Torg and others [22] note that hyperextension causes "an inward indentation of the ligamentum flavum," which can compress the cord. Penning [18] described a "bony pincers" mechanism in hypoextension in which the cord is compressed between the vertebral body and the closest portion of the spinolaminar line of the inferior vertebra. The athlete in Case 3 appeared to suffer a hyperextension injury, making contact with the facemask, and it was spinal stenosis that predisposed him to neurological injury. The athletes in Cases 1 and 2 suffered axial load injuries. The blow in Case 1 was severe enough to dent the helmet. In Case 2, although the force of the blow was not great, the contact was not expected and therefore the athlete's neck muscles were relaxed, causing greater transmission of forces directly on the spine instead of being dissipated in the muscles.

CONCLUSION

These three athletes present a spectrum of when to allow return to competition in contact or collision sports after an episode of transient quadriplegia. It is important to realize that normal canal size on lateral x-ray does not preclude the possibility of functional spinal stenosis—an absolute contraindication for return. For this diagnosis, myelogram, CT+, or MRI is needed.

REFERENCES

1. Alexander, M. M., C. H. Davis, and C. H. Field Hyperextension injuries of the cervical spine. *Arch. Neurol. Psychiatr.* 79:146–150, 1958.
2. Boijsen, E. The cervical spinal canal in intraspinal expansive processes. *Acta Radiol.* 42:101–115, 1954.
3. Cantu, R. C. Functional cervical spinal stenosis: a contraindication to participation in contact sports. *Med. Sci. Sports Exerc.* 25:316–317, 1993.

4. Cantu, R. C. Letter to the editor. *Med. Sci. Sports Exerc.* 25:1082–1084, 1993.

5. Cantu, R. C. Cervical spinal stenosis: challenging an established detection method. *Phys. Sports Med.* 21:57–63, 1993.

6. Cantu, R. V., and R. C. Cantu. Guidelines for return to contact sports after transient quadriplegia. *J. Neurosurg.* 80:592–594, 1994.

7. Eismont, F. J., S. Clifford, M. Goldberg, et al. Cervical sagittal spinal canal size in spinal injury. *Spine* 9:663–666, 1984.

8. Epstein, J. A., R. Carras, R. A. Hyman, et al. Cervical myelopathy causd by developmental stenosis of the spinal canal. *J. Neurosurg.* 51:362–367, 1979.

9. Firooznia, H., J. Ahn, M. Rafii, et al. Sudden quadriplegia after a minor trauma. The role of pre-existing spinal stenosis. *Surg. Neurol.* 23:165–168, 1985.

10. Herzog, R. J., J. J. Weins, M. F. Dillingham, and M. J. Sontag. Normal cervical spine morphometry and cervical spinal stenosis in asymptomatic professional football players. *Spine* 16:178–186, 1991.

11. Ladd, A. L., and P. E. Scranton. Congenital cervical stenosis presenting as transient quadriplegia in athletes. *J. Bone Joint Surg.* 68:1371–1374, 1986.

12. Lamont, A. C., J. Zachary, and P. W. Sheldon. Cervical cord size in metrizamide myelography. *Clin. Radiol.* 32:409–412, 1981.

13. Matsuura, P., R. L. Waters, R. H. Adkins, S. Rothman, W. Gurbani, and I. Sie. Comparison of computerized tomography parameters of the cervical spine in normal control subjects and spinal cord-injured patients. *J. Bone Joint Surg.* 71:183–188, 1989.

14. Mayfield, F. H. Neurosurgical aspects of cervical trauma. *Clinical Neurosurgery, vol II*. Baltimore: Williams & Wilkins, 1955.

15. Nugent, G. R. Clinicopathologic correlations in cervical spondylosis. *Neurology* 9:273–281, 1959.

16. Odor, J. M., R. G. Watkins, W. H. Dillin, S. Dennis, and M. Saberi. Incidence of cervical spinal stenosis in professional and rookie football players. *Am. J. Sports Med.* 18:507–509, 1990.

17. Pavlov, H., J. S. Torg, B. Robie, et al. Cervical spinal stenosis: determination with vertebral body ratio method. *Radiology* 164:771–775, 1987.

18. Penning, L. Some aspects of plain radiography of the cervical spine in chronic myelopathy. *Neurology* 12:513–519, 1962.

19. Resnick, D. Degenerative disease of the spine. *Diagnosis of Bone and Joint Disorders*. New York: W. B. Saunders Co., 1981, pp. 1408–1415.

20. Schneider, R. S., E. Reifel, H. Crisler, et al. Serious and fatal football injuries involving the head and spinal cord. *J. A. M. A.* 177:362–367, 1961.

21. Thijssen, H. O., A. Keyser, M. W. Horstink, et al. Morphology of the cervical spinal cord on computed myelography. *Neuroradiology* 18:57–62, 1979.

22. Torg, J. S., H. Pavlov, S. E. Genuano, et al. Neuropraxia of the cervical spinal cord with transient quadriplegia. *J. Bone Joint Surg.* 68A:1354–1370, 1986.

23. Wolfe, B. S., M. Khilnani, and L. Malis. The sagittal diameter of the bony cervical spinal canal and its significance in cervical spondylosis. *J. Mt. Sinai Hosp.* 23:283–292, 1956.

14
Aging and Body Composition: Biological Changes and Methodological Issues

SCOTT GOING, Ph.D.
DANIEL WILLIAMS, Ph.D.
TIMOTHY LOHMAN, Ph.D.

There is little doubt that significant changes in body size and composition that have important effects on health and functional capacity occur with aging. A substantial body of literaure is available that describes a number of trends, among them an increase in body weight and body fat in middle and early old age, and a loss of stature [1, 24, 101, 164] and a decrease in body weight [1, 24, 109], the weight of vital organs [20], muscle mass [44], and skeletal tissues [94] in old age. Although qualitatively these changes in size and composition are well known, the rate and ultimately the magnitude to which they are expressed at different ages are not well described [23, 44, 80].

Our aim in this paper is to review aging-related changes in body composition with an emphasis on biological changes and methodological concerns related to the accurate assessment of body composition in the elderly. As will be apparent, there are few body composition reference data available on the elderly. Consequently, much of the available information is based on studies of hexa- and heptagenarians. Moreover, most of the data come from cross-sectional studies of relatively inactive persons, and thus are likely to provide biased estimates of "aging." We know of no longitudinal studies in which changes in activity levels with aging have been related to changes in body composition. For this reason, we also review the results of recent exercise studies that provide strong, albeit indirect evidence of the contribution of inactivity versus aging to the loss of body tissues at older ages.

An important limitation in studies of body composition in older men and women is the need to rely on indirect assessment methods. As is discussed, the assessment of body composition in the elderly presents an interesting dilemma since changes in the aging body potentially affect the techniques that are used to detect them. This methodological dilemma, combined with the lack of longitudinal data, has resulted in uncertainty regarding quantitative estimates of body composition in older men and women. The potential assessment errors have been demonstrated using both anatomical [27, 92, 93] and chemical models [6, 68] of body composition. In this review we focus primarily on chemical models because methods based on chemical models continue to be the most practical methods for most situations.

MODELS AND METHODS

Body composition analysis can be conducted on the elemental, molecular, cellular, tissue system, and whole-body levels [160]. Each level is distinct and the components within each level are distinct, although there are associations within and between the various levels [69]. Significant work is now underway to better describe the relations between levels and how they may change with aging and disease [69].

Historically, chemical models, based on a limited number of cadaver studies [18, 46, 48, 77, 103, 165], have been the foundation of body composition research. In what has proven to be a major advance, the relatively recent development of total body neutron activation analysis (TBNAA) has made it possible to assess human body elemental composition in vivo [66, 67, 69, 135]. With the appropriate instrumentation, 11 elements, accounting for >99% of body weight, can be measured, and when combined with an estimate of body water, a variety of models can be derived [146, 160]. Thus, this nuclear analytical technique has enabled, as far as is possible in living humans, a direct quantitative assessment of chemical composition. The preliminary results suggest that there are no age dependencies in the quantitative associations between the elemental and molecular (chemical) levels of composition [69]. However, additional research in larger groups of carefully defined subjects is needed to verify these findings and to refine equations to calculate higher levels of body composition in elderly men and women.

The complexity, radiation exposure, and expense of TBNAA have limited its use to studies of relatively small numbers of subjects at a few specialized facilities in the United States and abroad. Consequently, most investigators will continue to employ more accessible laboratory and field methods and simpler models of body composition. Thus, there is a need to continue to develop and refine methods for use in a variety of research and clinical settings. It is in this capacity and others that TBNAA will play an important and unique role.

A variety of simpler indirect approaches for estimating body composition have been employed [44]. Undoubtedly the most common approach has been to consider the body as having two compartments, namely, the fat and fat-free body masses, which are derived from the chemical analysis of human cadavers by dissolving away the lipid in organic solvent [46, 48, 103]. In this approach, the fat-free body mass (FFM) includes all mineral, protein, and water plus all other body constituents other than lipids. The lean body mass (LBM) and body cell mass are two related compartments that have also been measured. Although the terms FFM and LBM have been used synonymously, LBM as originally proposed [9] is equal to FFM plus some lipids such as phospholipids in cell membranes defined as essential fat. Hence, LBM is larger than FFM by an equivocal amount estimated to be about 2–3% of body weight [10]. The body cell mass, which excludes lipids and the extracellular water and minerals, is smaller than FFM and LBM, and is wholly contained within them [105]. The choice of which compartment to measure depends largely on the investigators' purpose and the available methods. Because body cell mass is potentially a better index of the metabolically active tissue, it may be more useful than FFM and LBM for defining nutrient and energy requirements. However, it is more difficult to estimate, and as a result it is not often used.

Simple, direct methods for measuring body fat remain elusive. Consequently, body fat is usually calculated from body weight and FFM once FFM is known. Because the FFM is a heterogeneous compartment, it cannot be measured directly, so its estimation must rely upon a model.

The three most widely applied methods for dividing the body into fat and fat-free masses are densitometry, hydrometry, and potassium (^{40}K) spectroscopy. These methods and others based on the two-component model are similar in the sense that they rely upon a known and stable relationship between the compartment of interest (FFM) and the measured constituent. For example, FFM can be estimated by hydrometry by first estimating total-body water (TBW) using isotopically labeled water dilution. FFM is then calculated from TBW on the basis of the average hydration of FFM, which is typically considered to be about 73% [44, 111]. Similarly, FFM can be calculated from total-body potassium (TBK), which can be estimated by ^{40}K counting (TBK = ^{40}K/0.00012 g of ^{40}K per g of TBK) [42, 47, 112] or measurements of total exchangeable potassium [44]. Once TBK is known, FFM is calculated from the average concentration of potassium in FFM; in men, FFM = TBK, g/2.66 g, K per kg FFM and in women, FFM= TBK, g/2.55 g, K per kg FFM. The validity and accuracy of both hydrometry and potassium spectroscopy depend largely on the appropriateness of the conversion constants for the subjects for whom they are applied. As will be evident, the K/FFM ratio varies with age and the usual constants are not appropriate for use in elderly men and women. Similarly, the water fraction of FFM may change with aging, although the magnitude of this change is less certain. The derivation of more valid constants has proved difficult.

The densitometric approach depends on the relationship between whole-body density and the respective densities of the body compartments, regardless of how they are defined. The general principle is that density varies inversely with body fat, or

$$F = f(1/D) \qquad (1)$$

where *F* is the ether-extractable lipid fraction of weight and f is the function describing the relationship between fat and density. For simple, useful solutions of Equation 1 to be derived, an additional assumption is required, i.e., that the densities of other compartments (e.g., FFM) are constant. The well-known Siri equation [139], based on the two-component model, represents the simplest solution of Equation 1, wherein body fat is calculated from body density (D_b) and assumed densities of 0.9 and 1.1 kg/L for the fat [40], and fat-free fractions [9] according to the equation

$$1/D_b = F/D_F + FFM/D_{FFM} \qquad (2)$$

where $1/D_b$ is body mass, set equal to unity, divided by body density(D_b), and F/D_F and FFM/D_{FFM} are the fractions of body mass that are fat and fat-free divided by their respective densities. In the simplest chemical model, FFM is composed primarily of water (W), protein (P), and mineral (M) compartments, and D_{FFM} (1.1 kg/L) is derived from the proportions of W, P, and M divided by their respective densities

$$D_{FFM} = W/D_W + P/D_P + M/D_M \qquad (3)$$

Thus, for D_{FFM} to be constant, the proportions of W, P, and M must be constant or they must vary in such a way that D_{FFM} does not change. In the densitometric approach, any deviation of D_b from D_{FFM}(1.1 kg/L) is assumed to be due to the addition of body fat.

The two-component approach has at least two important limitations that sometimes confound the interpretation of estimates of body composition in elderly men and women. As mentioned, the FFM is a heterogeneous compartment and by combining all nonfat tissues into one compartment, the distinct physiologic functions of the various tissues are obscured. As a result of the differential loss of its constituents, the relationships among the FFM and related compartments, e.g., body cell mass, may change with aging, and the FFM may no longer provide a sufficiently precise representation of these other compartments. Also, age-related loss of FFM constituents invalidates the assumption that the chemical composition of the FFM is the same in older persons as it is in younger persons [6, 68, 92]. Several authors [34, 110] have suggested that age-related changes in the proportions of W, P, and M result in a lower D_{FFM}, which results in overestimation of body fat and underestimation of FFM by hydrodensitometry. These errors in densitometrically estimated fat and FFM represent a potentially important limitation of past studies designed to assess age-related changes in the amount and composition of FFM. Although methods are available for reliable and accurate estimation of the absolute amounts of body water and mineral, it has proved difficult to estimate changes in the proportions of the constituents of the FFM because of the difficulty in obtaining an accurate and independent estimate of FFM.

Alternative Approaches
An alternative to the use of the two component model in the elderly is to use a measurement technique that does not require the assumption of an

invariant fat-free composition. The relatively recent development of dual-energy absorptiometry makes available a technique that may satisfy this requirement. Techniques such as the [153]Gd-based dual-photon absorptiometry and dual-energy x-ray absorptiometry (DXA) are based on the fact that the attenuation of low- and high-energy radiation in bone and soft tissue is very different. For this reason, and because the ratio of the attenuation of low and high energy in soft tissue is linearly related to percent fat, these techniques can be used to simultaneously estimate bone and soft tissue composition in wide range of people with different proportions of mineral in the FFM. Preliminary studies in predominately young adults have been promising [62, 95, 99]. However, despite initial enthusiasm, some questions have been raised concerning the accuracy of regional estimates of composition by DXA [128, 144], and validation is needed in the elderly.

A second alternative to the two-component model approach is to derive estimates of FFM from measurements of several constituents of the FFM. By using TBNAA, which is based on the detection of γ radiation given off by unstable isotopes created by delivering a moderated beam of fast neutrons to the subject, it is possible to measure several elements of the FFM simultaneously and derive what is probably the most accurate estimate of FFM with current technology [28, 67, 135]. As mentioned previously, few such facilities exist and the application of TBNAA is limited by expense and radiation exposure to the subjects. Fortunately, simpler multiple component methods have been developed that utilize measurements of body density by underwater weighing, body water by isotope dilution, and bone mineral by DXA to derive FFM [6, 50, 68, 166, 168]. Recent work has shown that this approach yields estimates of FFM that are not different from FFM estimated by a more complex model based on TBNAA [66]. Also, Friedl et al. [50] have shown that it is possible to derive more accurate estimates of body composition using multiple component models despite the potential problem of "propagation of errors" from multiple measurements. It is likely that these simple multiple component models will prove quite useful in the study of age-related changes in body composition in healthy "young" elderly but they have yet to be used to any significant degree in older populations. Their application is limited in very old men and women by the problems of underwater weighing in this age group. With further development, DXA may prove to be the most useful technique in this population because it can be used to estimate multiple body compartments (lean soft tissue mass, fat mass, and bone mass) without the use of hydrodensitometry [68, 95].

AGE-RELATED CHANGES IN FFM

Estimates of the rate of decline in FFM with age are largely based on data from cross-sectional studies. These estimates are limited by secular changes and sampling variation across age groups and thus are probably biased. Longitudinal data can be used to assess changes more accurately and establish whether there are sex differences and whether the decline deviates from linearity. Estimates of the rate of loss of FFM also are affected by the assessment method as will be evident below.

Cross-sectional Studies

A loss in body potassium with age has been well documented in several large databases [2, 49, 112]. Forbes [44], using cross-sectional data from several studies, estimated that men lose 45 g of potassium (155 g to 110 g) from young adulthood to 80 yr of age, and women lose 20 g of potassium over the same period (100 g to 80 g). If one assumes that potassium is constant in the FFM throughout life then the loss of potassium suggests a 30% loss in FFM in men and a 20% loss in women. Furthermore, if one assumes a linear decrease over six decades, then the average rate of loss is 5% per decade for men and 3.5% for women [44].

Estimates of FFM loss per decade based on cross-sectional measurements of body density, body water, and nitrogen are generally less than estimates based on body potassium. Forbes [44] has compiled data from several studies and calculated a 3% decline per decade in FFM for men and a 2% decline for women. The results from the recent cross-sectional studies of Frontera et al. [51] and Snead et al. [144] using body density from underwater weighing to estimate changes in FFM show a decline from 2.0 to 4.1 kg per decade, with men losing more than women. On a relative basis these losses vary from a 6% to a 4% loss of FFM per decade between ages 45 and 78 yr.

Longitudinal Studies

Forbes and Reina [49], using body potassium, estimated that by age 65–70 yr the average man has lost 12 kg of FFM in comparison to the average FFM at age 25; for women the loss is 5 kg. These observations were based on data from a few subjects measured numerous times over many yr and two measurements made on many subjects over a 5–10-yr span. Forbes [43] presented additional body potassium data from longitudinal analyses and concluded that the average rate of loss in men is 3 kg of FFM per decade. Forbes [44] also observed two subjects for 27 yr and found that one person lost FFM at a rate of 3% per decade and the other at a rate of 0.4% per decade. Part of the difference between the two subjects may be explained by an exercise program in which the latter subject engaged.

The most extensive longitudinal data on men were collected by Flynn et al. [41, 42] in two studies in which body potassium was measured by whole-body counting. In Table 14.1 we have recalculated the rate of decline in body potassium per decade based on her data for each 7-yr period for each of four cohorts at different initial ages. In general, Flynn's data confirm the results of Forbes [43], demonstrating a 3.0-kg loss in FFM per decade from 30 to 70 yr of age. There is considerable variation in estimates both within

TABLE 14.1.
Reanalysis of Longitudinal Changes in Body Potassium (g/yr) in Men[a]

	Age Group, yr				
	Changes in body potassium over a 7-yr interval				
	32–39	*40–47*	*48–55*	*56–63*	*64–71*
Cohort I (n=31)	.76	.32			
Cohort II (n=42)		1.31	0.48		
Cohort III (n=37)			1.32	0.86	
Cohort IV (n=28)				1.23	1.33
Mean K/decade, kg	9.6	8.2	9.0	10.4	13.3
Mean FFM/decade, kg	2.9	3.1	3.4	3.9	5.0

[a]FFM = K,g/2.66 g, K/kg,FFM. Data are from ref. 41.

cohorts and between cohorts and thus, no significant differences among age groups (Table 14.1). For women, Flynn et al. [42] found significant losses in body potassium after the age of 50 but no loss at younger ages. The limited number of women studied, however, prevents generalizations from a comparison between men and women.

CHANGES IN SUBCOMPONENTS OF FFM

An important focus for future research is the identification of the decline in the subcomponents of FFM including the water, protein, and mineral components of a chemical model and the muscle-free lean compartment of an anatomical model. The potential differential change in FFM subcomponents has important implications for both functional capacity and errors related to the assessment of composition based on traditional chemical models. Steen [148] estimated that by age 70 yr, 40% of muscle mass is lost in comparison with early adulthood. This large loss of muscle mass is much greater than the loss of components of the nonmuscle mass such as the liver, kidneys, and lungs. Unfortunately, methodological, theoretical, and statistical limitations of past research prevent definitive conclusions regarding the magnitude, rate, and variation in the loss of protein, water, muscle, and muscle-free lean tissue mass with age. Thus, in the following sections, we present our best estimates derived from selected studies in the literature. The refinement of these estimates is an important focus for future research in body composition assessment.

Protein and Muscle Loss
Cohn et al. [29] have provided evidence of protein loss in 135 men and women, 20–80 yr of age, using neutron-activation analysis for the measure-

ment of total-body nitrogen and whole-body counting for the measurement of total-body potassium (Table 14.2). In this cross-sectional study, the total-body protein (N $\times$ 3 6.25) was estimated along with the muscle and non-muscle protein masses. Based on this study, the total-body protein of men and women aged 30–39 and 40–49 yr appears less than the 20–24-yr-old group, and a further decline is suggested in the 60–64 and 70–79-yr-old groups; however, small subject numbers per group limit the degree of confidence in the mean estimates. A slower loss of nitrogen than potassium is evident in the greater differences with age in potassium (from 155 to 119 g, or -23%) than nitrogen (from 2.06 kg to 1.78 kg or -14%) in men. In women the difference in potassium (decline from 95 g to 71 g, -25%) for young versus older groups is similar to the difference in nitrogen (1.45 kg to 1.15 kg, -21%).

Ellis [37] reported that protein mass declined with age, based on cross-sectional data, from 13.1 kg in 20–29-yr-old men to 11.4 kg in 70–79-yr-old men (13% loss). Protein was estimated from total-body nitrogen using TB-NAA (Table 14.2). In 20–29-yr-old women, protein mass was 9.3 kg and in 70–79-yr-olds, protein mass was 20% lower (7.4 kg). Deurenberg et al. [34] estimated the protein loss in men to be 4% per decade (after 40 yr of age). In women they suggest the rate of loss is a little less (3% per decade). The cross-sectional data of Ellis [37] and Cohn et al. [29] support Deurenberg's estimate for women; however, their work suggests a nonlinear loss with age in men. Unfortunately, there are no longitudinal data using TBNAA; hence, the estimates given in Table 14.3 are largely based on data from Cohn et al. [29] and Ellis [37]. Additional work is needed to address the ap-

TABLE 14.2.
Comparison of Estimates of Total-Body Protein at Different Ages from Three Investigators

| Age group, yr | Protein Mass, kg | | | | | |
| | Cohen et al. [29] | | Deurenberg et al. [34] | | Ellis [37] | |
	Male	Female	Male[a]	Female[b]	Male	Female
20–29	12.9	9.1	–	–	13.1	9.3
30–39	11.8	8.9	–	–	11.8	9.2
40–49	12.0	8.5	11.9	8.4	11.8	8.8
50–59	11.9	7.8	11.4	8.1	11.8	8.3
60–69	11.3	7.5	11.0	7.9	11.6	7.9
70–79	11.1	7.3	10.5	7.6	11.4	7.4
80–89	–	–	10.0	7.4	9.4	–

[a]Assumed 40-yr-old man with body weight = 78.8 kg and FFM = 60.8 kg [37], and estimated protein loss of 4%, 8%, 12%, 16% at 50, 60, 70, and 80 yr of age [34].
[b]Assumed 40-yr-old woman with body weight = 64.4 kg and FFM = 42.8 kg [37], and estimated protein loss of 3%, 6%, 9% and 12% at 50, 60, 70, and 80 yr of age [34].

TABLE 14.3.
Estimated Total-Body Protein at Different Ages

	Protein, kg	
Age group, yr	Men	Women
20–29	13.0	9.2
30–39	11.9	9.0
40–49	11.9	8.6
50–59	11.8	8.2
60–69	11.5	7.8
70–79	11.2	7.4
80–89	9.6	7.0

[a]Based on data from Cohn et al. [29] and Ellis [37].

parent loss in nitrogen in men from 20–29 to 30–39 yr of age (possible sampling difference) and the large loss in men from 70–79 to 80–89 yr of age, which is based on data from fewer than 8 subjects [37]. The estimates of Deurenberg et al. [34] are not included in Table 14.3 because of their indirect derivation.

A change in K/FFM and K/N with age has been well documented by several investigators. The results of these studies suggest that the decline in body potassium with age is greater than the decline in nitrogen. Cohn et al. [29], for example, report the K/N ratio decreases by 6% in women and 11% in men. In the same subjects the K/FFB decreased by 9.3% in women and 10.8% in men. Ellis [37] found a 15.0% decrease in K/FFM from 2.47 to 2.10 g/kg in men and only a 3.3% decrease in women (2.06 to 1.99 g/kg). Womersley et al [170] estimated the K/FFM in older men at 2.42 g/kg as compared to 2.66 g/kg for younger men. For older women they found a K/FFM of 2.67 g/kg versus 2.40 g/kg for younger women. Pierson et al. [114] found a significant effect of body fatness on estimates of potassium using whole-body ^{40}K counting and revised their initial estimates of change in K/FFM based on a large cross-sectional sample [112]. In men, K/FFM decreased from 2.80 g/kg for a 20-yr-old man to 2.42 g/kg for a 70-yr-old man. In women, the regression of K/FFM on age was not significant; however, the decline they found from 2.50 to 2.35 g/kg in young versus older women is in agreement with other studies. Thus, the available cross-sectional data suggest a substantial decrease in K/FFM for men and a somewhat smaller decrease for women (Table 14.4). This differential loss of potassium versus FFM has been attributed to a greater loss of muscle than nonmuscle lean mass [29, 112].

Because a greater percent of body potassium is in muscle than in nonmuscle tissue, it is believed that the greater loss of potassium with age indicates that muscle loss, especially for men, is characteristic of the aging

TABLE 14.4.
Percent Decrease in K/FFM from Young Adulthood to Old Age

	Percent decrease in K/FFM	
Investigator	Male	Female
Cohn et al. [29]	10.8%	9.3%
Pierson et al. [114]	13.6%	6.0%
Ellis [37]	15.0%	3.3%

process. Women, in contrast, appear to lose less muscle mass. This notion is supported by data from Steen [148], who found that men lost 7% of their body potassium over the ages of 76–81 yr, whereas women showed no change. Better estimates of the rate of loss in muscle and nonmuscle lean tissue in men and women from 40 to 80 yr of age is an important goal for future investigation. A mixed longitudinal design such as that of Flynn et al. [41] would be an excellent way to investigate this question.

EFFECTS OF EXERCISE ON MUSCLE MASS. Much of the work documenting changes in muscle mass with age has been done with largely sedentary populations. Whether the rate of decline in muscle and protein is similar in active people is uncertain. The question of how exercise training may influence the rate of loss of muscle mass from 40 to 80 yr of age in both men and women has not been addressed in carefully controlled mixed longitudinal studies. However, one can speculate based on short-term training studies that the rate of loss may be decreased and that some or much of the loss in muscle mass may be prevented with exercise training. Significant increases (5–11% increase) in muscle cross-sectional area (using computed tomography [CT] scans) as a result of weight training have been reported in young men [90], older men aged 60–72 yr [51], and in a frail, institutionalized population of 6 men and 4 women between 86 and 96 yr of age [39]. These studies have stimulated greater interest in the long-term effects of exercise on maintenance of muscle mass at all ages. Forbes [45] recently reviewed the results of a number of studies of the effect of exercise on FFM and found only small changes attributable to exercise (about 2 kg). Methodological limitations have been a major aspect of past research for estimation of muscle mass. With the recent development of DXA, CT and nuclear magnetic resonance techniques to measure regional body composition, it is now possible to obtain better quantitative estimates of muscle and lean tissue mass in adult populations. In our laboratory, using DXA methodology to estimate regional and total mass lean tissue mass, increases in arm lean (4%), leg lean (4%), and trunk lean (1%) were found after an 18-mo program of weight training three times a week in premenopausal women [88]. Although the DXA methodology may yield reliable estimates of change in lean tissue mass in young adults, its validation in older adults has been questioned [144]. Snead et al. [144] found that whole-body fat content was underestimated by DXA as compared with densitometry in older but not in younger subjects. They attributed this underestimation to errors in estimating abdominal fatness, which increases with age, because fat packets placed over the thigh were accurately detected as fat but only partially detected as fat when added to the trunk. It is possible that recent changes in software will correct for these effects [85].

A final consideration in estimating changes in body composition with exercise in the elderly is the individual variation in response to exercise. Bouchard [16, 17] has shown a large variability in aerobic capacity with training attributable to a genetic × environmental interaction. Similar variation in weight loss and fat loss among subjects undergoing reduced caloric intake has been reported [16, 17], and in regard to the training response to exercise, Fiatarone et al. [39] found thigh muscle areas changed from +30% to −8% in the 10 elderly subjects after 8 wk of exercise. Thus, individual variation in the effects of exercise on the loss of muscle mass is an area that needs to be investigated.

Body Water
Water accounts for approximately 50–60% of body weight and ~73% of FFM, making it the most abundant chemical in the body. On that basis alone, knowledge of the total amount of water in the body is basic to a full description of human body composition. It has added significance because water plays a crucial role in the regulation of cell volume, nutrient transport, waste removal and disposal, and temperature regulation. As will be evident, additional information on the changes in body water with aging is needed, particularly in old age, to improve equations for estimating body composition in the elderly [6]. Also, clinicians have a need for better information because elderly persons placed on diuretics are at increased risk for dehydration and its attendant fluid and electrolyte problems. When administered concomitantly, water-soluble drugs may have undesired therapeutic or even toxic effects if the dosages are not adjusted properly [148].

Casual observation of older people has led to the belief that there is a general loss of water from the tissues of the body with advancing age. Numerous cross-sectional studies of men and women using a variety of diluents to estimate TBW seem to support this observation [129, 134, 161]. In perhaps the most comprehensive review of human studies, Watson et al. [161] analyzed TBW volumes for 458 men and 265 women obtained from 30 dilution studies in the literature. Based on these data, Schoeller [129] has estimated that TBW declines by about 0.3 kg/yr in men beginning sometime after age 30 until reaching a nadir after age 70. In contrast, in women, TBW is relatively constant until age 70, after which there is a decline of 0.7 kg/yr [129, 161]. The apparently different trend in women may be due to the effect of cyclical hormonal changes on water balance in pre-menopausal women, especially because in most studies, estimations of TBW were not limited to the follicular phase of the menstrual cycle when water balance is least affected, although other investigators have noted this minimal change in TBW in women [12, 61, 105].

Although the results of Watson et al. [161] and others [52, 110, 173] suggest an age-related decline in TBW, cross-sectional data, by their nature, are susceptible to sampling artifact and their generalizability is uncertain. Schoeller's [129] estimate of the loss of body water in men, for example, suggests that approximately 13 liters of water are lost by age 80 yr. However, a loss of this magnitude is unlikely, given the magnitude of the reported decline in muscle and body cell mass. Given the variation in body weight across samples, it is difficult to derive an estimate of the rate of water loss with aging. Indeed, some investigators have shown no significant aging trend when differences in body weight are statistically controlled. However, considered together, the results of several studies suggest that a loss of 4–6 liters is probable.

In an attempt to control the influence of size differences among age groups, TBW as a fraction of body weight is often compared (Table 14.5). In young adults water accounts for about 60% of total mass in men and about 50% in women. The aqueous fraction of body weight (TBW/WT) declines in both men and women throughout early adulthood and middle age to about 55% or less in men and 45% or less in women, a trend that probably reflects increasing body fat more than a change in TBW [129, 161]. Unlike TBW, the rate of decline in TBW/WT is greater in women than men [113]. After age 70–75, TBW/WT may increase as body weight and body fat declines. As noted earlier, most study designs have been cross-sectional and it is difficult to judge whether this trend is truly due to aging, although there is at least one published study with repeat measurements of men and women between ages 70 and 81 yr that supports the pattern of decreased TBW in kilograms and an increase in water as a percent of body weight [151].

Because the intracellular water (ICW) is closely related to the body cell mass, it is of great interest to determine the degree to which the loss of water with aging is due to changes in the intracellular and extracellular compartments. On this point there is some conflicting evidence. Pierson et al. [113], for example, have reported a relatively stable extracellular water (ECW), a decline in ICW, and an increase in the ECW/ICW ratio with age in both men and women. The loss of skeletal muscle with aging, with its high ICW content, and its replacement by adipose tissue (~3% ICW), presumably explains the decline in ICW in both sexes.

In contrast to the findings from this cross-sectional study [113] and others [52, 82, 137], Steen et al. [151], in a longitudinal study, found the decrease in TBW from age 70 to 81 yr was mostly due to a decrease in ECW in

TABLE 14.5.
Total-Body Water as a Percent of Body Weight and Fat-Free Body Weight

Reference	Age, yr	Sex	N	Diluent	TBW/WT	TBW/FFW
110	20–29	M	4	A	.555	.842 (.776)
	30–39	M	23	A	.539	.743 (.752)
	40–49	M	35	A	.527	.698 (.756)
	50–59	M	30	A	.516	.692 (.756)
	60–69	M	26	A	.527	.696 (.771)
	70–79	M	21	A	.540	.700 (.768)
	80–89	M	4	A	.558	.712 (.792)
173	16–30	F	94	A	.517	.721
	30–40	F	26	A	.493	.680
	40–50	F	27	A	.486	.760
	50–60	F	21	A	.441	.801
137	20–29	M	5	A	.409	–
	30–39	M	14	A	.538	–
	40–49	M	23	A	.544	–
	50–59	M	31	A	.545	–
	60–69	M	43	A	.506	–
	70–79	M	45	A	.518	–
	80–89	M	27	A	.484	–
	90–99	M	5	A	.532	–
161	20–29	M	171	*	.605	–
	30–39	M	93	*	.578	–
	40–49	M	59	*	.570	–
	50–59	M	68	*	.564	–
	60–69	M	33	*	.565	–
	70–79	M	23	*	.540	–
	80–90	M	3	*	.563	
	20–29	F	100	*	.496	–
	30–39	F	48	*	.488	–
	40–49	F	37	*	.475	–
	50–59	F	43	*	.471	–
	60–69	F	19	*	.455	–
	70–79	F	5	*	.470	–
	80–89	F	5	*	.520	–
29	20–29	M	24	^3H_2O	.590	.762 (.699)
	30–39	M	10	^3H_2O	.563	.759 (.671)
	40–49	M	10	^3H_2O	.555	.804 (.711)
	50–59	M	10	^3H_2O	.548	.807 (.733)
	60–69	M	10	^3H_2O	.521	.788 (.694)
	70–79	M	9	^3H_2O	.505	.853 (.707)
	20–29	F	10	^3H_2O	.536	.767 (.693)
	30–39	F	10	^3H_2O	.498	.756 (.717)
	40–49	F	10	^3H_2O	.490	.783 (.723)
	50–59	F	10	^3H_2O	.437	.813 (.779)
	60–69	F	14	^3H_2O	.452	.846 (.750)
	70–79	F	8	^3H_2O	.445	.848 (.731)
68	19–34	F	55	^3H_2O	–	.721
	≥65	F	61	^3H_2O	–	.712

TABLE 14.5—*continued*
Total-Body Water as a Percent of Body Weight and Fat-Free Body Weight

Reference	Age, yr	Sex	N	Diluent	TBW/WT	TBW/FFW
6	65–94	M	35	^3H_2O	.570	.743
	65–94	F	63	^3H_2O	.510	.744
65	22–39	M	12	^2H_2O	–	.710
	65–84	M	30	^2H_2O	–	.726
	22–39	F	19	^2H_2O	–	.707
	65–84	F	32	^2H_2O	–	.723

A = antipyrine
* Data from several sources combined, using A, ^3H_2O, and ^2H_2O.

both men and women. The explanation for this discrepancy is not immediately clear but may be due to differences in survival characteristics, differences in nutrition or lifestyles, or difficulties measuring ECW. Thus, although most evidence from cross-sectional studies suggests a decrease in ICW with aging, it cannot be concluded with certainty that this is an obligatory change in elderly persons.

At this time it is unclear whether the apparent decline in absolute TBW results in a lower water concentration of the FFM in older adults (Fig. 14.1). The results from the direct chemical analysis of six nonedematous adults aged 25–63 yr at the time of death suggest that the hydration of the FFM is constant at about $73 \pm 3\%$ [75, 77]. However, the number of analyses is small and there are no data from subjects more than 63 yr old at the time of death. Although the results from several cross-sectional studies with healthy elderly men and women also indicate no consistent change with age (Table 14.5), indirect in vivo methods show considerable interindividual variation and the sensitivity of the analyses is probably no better than 1–2%.

A major limitation in assessing age-related changes in the water fraction of the FFM (TBW/FFM) has been the difficulty in obtaining an accurate, independent estimate of FFM. This fact is illustrated in the data from Cohn et al. [29], who measured fat-free solids using TBNAA and TBW by isotope dilution in subjects aged 20–80 yr. The average water fraction of the FFM with subjects grouped by decade ranged from about 69 to about 73% in men and about 69 to about 78% in women when FFM is estimated as the sum of the muscle, nonmuscle, and bone mineral masses, and there was no significant trend with age. However, the TBW/FFM ratio is considerably higher (ranging from about 76 to 85% in men and women) when FFM is estimated from total body potassium, especially in the older subjects. Consequently, the comparison between young and old groups of men and women falsely suggests that TBW/FFM is about 5–10% higher in elderly men and women, presumably because the K/FFM ratio is lower in older subjects and FFM is underestimated when the young adult constant is applied.

FIGURE 14.1.

Hydration of the fat-free mass (TBW/FFM) in men and women at different ages. The dashed line is equal to the assumed FFM water concentration of 73.4%. Data are from Refs. 6(♦), 29(◇), 37(■), 65(□), and 82(●).

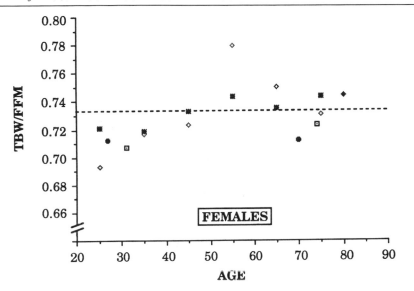

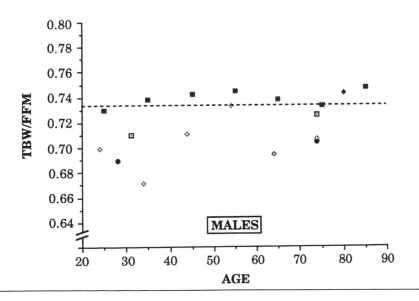

In another study in which independent estimates of TBW (isotope dilution) and FFM were obtained (fat-soluble gas), Lesser and Markofsky [82] reported an increase in the FFM hydration from 69 to 70% in 59–89-yr-old men compared with 17–39-yr-old men. The hydration of the FFM was about 70% in both young (16–38 yr) and old (59–89 yr) women. The results of this study using a more direct method to estimate body fat and then FFM support the findings of Cohn et al. [29] of only small changes in TBW/FFM when FFM is estimated from several FFM solids estimated simultaneously.

Taking a different approach to estimate TBW/FFM, some investigators have used multiple component models that include TBW to calculate FFM [60, 65, 68]. Although the estimates of TBW and FFM are not entirely independent, by estimating FFM from multiple constituents including water, the errors inherent in assuming an invariant FFM are overcome, resulting in more accurate estimates of FFM to evaluate its hydration. Using measures of body density, bone mineral, and TBW to estimate FFM, Baumgartner et al. [60] and Hewitt et al. [65] reported an increase in the hydration of the FFM in older women compared with younger control subjects, although the water concentrations in the two studies were somewhat different, equaling $72.3 \pm 1.7\%$ in the study by Hewitt et al. [65] and $74.4 \pm 3.9\%$ in the study by Baumgartner et al. [6]. A similar increase was also observed in old versus young men with older men having TBW/FFM ratios of $72.6 \pm 1.1\%$ [65] and $74.3 \pm 4.5\%$ [60]. Despite the apparent agreement in the direction of change in TBW/FFM in these two studies it should be noted that Baumgartner et al. [6] compared their results to the assumed concentration in young men and women and did not measure directly the TBW in young adults. Also, the variability in FFM water content was considerably greater in the study by Baumgartner et al. [6] compared with Hewitt et al. [65]. Nevertheless, these results are in agreement with direct chemical analysis of animal tissues, which demonstrates a significant 1% increase in hydration of fat-free tissues [172] and it is possible that the hydration of FFM does increase by a small amount with normal aging.

Bone Mineral
Bone loss is a universal consequence of aging. This fact has been demonstrated in numerous studies using both direct assessment methods such as postmortem analysis of sawed long bones [102], weighing and ashing of dry, defatted skeletons [155, 156], measurements of the density on cubes cut from vertebral bodies [5], in vivo biopsy studies [11, 91], and a variety of indirect methods, including radiography [53], single (SPA) and dual (DPA) photon absorptiometry, [96–98], DXA [95], TBNAA [29, 34], and CT [21]. Destructive techniques obviously are not appropriate for longitudinal and large-scale studies. Hence, as is true of other components of body composition, most estimates of bone loss are based on indirect techniques and cross-sectional rather than longitudinal data.

Considered in toto, the available data support several generalizations (Tables 14.6 and 14.7). Men, for example, generally have higher greater bone mineral mass and density than women and lose less bone with aging. The onset of bone loss varies with site and with the complex interaction of calciotropic hormones, nutrition, and physical activity. Sites with proportionately high amounts of trabecular bone may lose mineral earlier than sites higher in cortical bone. At all sites there is little change until age 40. Thereafter, a consistent decrease in bone mineral density (BMD) occurs. In women, there is an accelerated loss at about the time of menopause, but the effect is modified by the estrogen status of the woman and body weight. In men, the loss is fairly linear.

By virtue of its availability, and its requirement of soft tissue homogeniety, most studies have used single-photon absortiometry to assess forearm bone loss at sites relatively high in compact (cortical) bone. The results of cross-sectional studies suggest that appendicular bone loss in men begins at about 50–60 yr and proceeds at a rate of about 0.3%/yr [98]. Women may begin their decline slightly earlier, and lose about 1% per yr between ages 45 and 75 yr, after which the rate is similar to that in men [98]. The more recent development of DPA and DXA has made possible estimates of bone loss from irregularly shaped bones high in trabecular bone mass such as the vertebrae and femoral neck as well as whole-body analysis. The results of studies with this technology have demonstrated considerable variability in the rates of bone loss at various sites in the axial skeleton [145]. Although not supported by all studies, there is evidence that the loss of trabecular bone begins earlier than compact bone, and most studies suggest that trabecular bone loss in the spine in women accelerates for about 5 yr at menopause followed by a slower decline [3, 4, 79, 125, 126]. Data from Mazess et al. [97] suggest that apparently healthy women by age 70 yr experience about a 20% decrease in vertebral BMD and a 25–40% decrease at the femoral neck and trochanteric regions. In healthy men [96], the decrease in spine (~3%) and femur (~20–30%) BMD by age 70 is less than in women, a fact that helps to explain the lower prevalence of osteoporosis in men.

Few longitudinal data are available to verify estimates of bone loss from cross-sectional studies. In a recent longitudinal study by Aloia et al. [4], the rates of decline in forearm and spine BMD were reasonably similar to the estimates given by Mazess et al. noted above [96–98]. Nevertheless, additional longitudinal studies are needed, especially studies with repeat measurements at several sites in the same subjects so that the differential loss of bone in different regions of the skeleton can be determined. Moreover, the addition of measurements by total-body mineral by TBNAA and DXA would help establish the relationship between regional and total-body bone loss.

The skeleton contains the vast majority of the minerals in the body. For this reason and because of the relative difficulty in estimating nonosseous

TABLE 14.6.
Bone Mineral Density (BMD) (g/cm²) at Different Ages in Men[a]

Age, yr	Radius (Shaft)	Distal Radius	Humerus	Spine (L2–L4)	Femur (Neck)	Whole Body
20–29	.885	.600	1.200	1.26	1.09	1.23
30–39	.895	.588	1.188	1.26	0.98	1.22
40–49	.880	.608	1.181	1.31	0.97	1.21
50–59	.880	.614	1.189	1.21	0.92	1.23
60–69	.790	.516	1.122	1.25	0.89	1.20
70–79	.811	.536	1.114	1.21	0.85	1.16
80–89	.751	.578	0.980	1.24	0.76	1.16
Δ (%)	0.144 (16%)	.036 (6%)	0.22 (18%)	0.070 (5%)	0.33 (30%)	0.070 (6%)

[a]Data are from refs. 89, 96, and 98. Radius and humerus BMD estimated using SPA, spine and femur BMD estimated using DPA, and whole-body BMD estimated using DXA. Δ = Peak BMD – oldest age group BMD.

TABLE 14.7.
Bone Mineral Density (BMD) (g/cm²) at Different Ages in Women[a]

Age, yr	Radius (Shaft)	Distal Radius	Humerus	Spine (L2–L4)	Femur (Neck)	Whole Body
20–29	.774	.539	1.056	1.24	1.00	1.20
30–39	.769	.564	1.074	1.27	0.99	1.14
40–49	.763	.494	1.033	1.21	0.86	1.12
50–59	.706	.482	.943	1.09	0.81	1.08
60–69	.610	.402	.748	0.99	0.75	1.04
70–79	.575	.402	.707	0.97	0.72	1.00
80–89	.538	.388	.644	—	—	—
90–99	.521	.392	.639	—	—	—
Δ (%)	0.253 (33%)	0.172 (30%)	0.435 (40%)	0.300 (24%)	0.280 (28%)	0.200 (17%)

[a]Data are from refs. 89, 97, and 98. Radius and humerus BMD estimated using SPA, spine and femur BMD estimated using DPA, and whole-body BMD estimated using DXA. Δ = Peak BMD − oldest age group BMD.

minerals, studies of changes in the mineral content of FFM with aging typically measure only osseous minerals. From the studies of bone mineral noted above it is clear that the assumption of a constant mineral concentration in the FFM across different ages is unlikely to be true (Tables 14.6 and 14.7). Although the relative contribution of minerals to the total FFM is small, variability in FFM mineral content with aging potentially has a substantial impact on D_{FFM} by virtue of the density of mineral, which is very high relative to the other constituents of the FFM. The magnitude of the effect remains controversial and it depends on the rate of whole-body mineral loss with aging. Norris et al. [110] and Weredin and Kyle [163], for example, estimated D_{FFM} may decline to ~1.06 kg/L from the assumed 1.1 kg/L in an older person with osteoporosis. In contrast, Deurenberg et al. [34], using the estimate of bone loss from Mazess [94], estimate the D_{FFM} at age 70–79 yr to be 1.092 kg/L in women and 1.102 kg/L in men. The estimates from Norris et al. [110] and Weredin and Kyle [163] are unlikely, given more recent data [37], and may be explained by the investigators' assumption that the mineral fraction of FFM changes proportionately with the decline in absolute mineral mass, which may not be true. Ultimately, estimates of D_{FFM} depend on the assumed magnitude of bone loss, the relative decline in other FFM constituents, and the degree to which bone loss at a given site reflects the decline in total-body minerals. It is apparent from Tables 14.6 and 14.7 that there is considerable variability in estimates of the changes in regional and whole-body BMD. Indeed, regional and whole-body estimates of BMD are moderately intercorrelated at best [4], and it is unclear how well changes in BMD reflect changes in whole-body mineral mass.

EFFECTS OF ACTIVITY ON BONE MASS. Concern for the problem of osteoporosis has led to a variety of investigations of the effects of physical activity on bone mass. Although it is clear from "disuse studies" that physical inactivity can result in significant mineral loss, whether or not an increase in activity above habitual levels leads to an increase in bone mineral remains to be proved. The results of numerous cross-sectional studies have demonstrated that the bone mass of active men and women is higher than that of their more inactive peers [145]. Although the results of these studies have been put forth as indirect evidence of an effect of activity on bone, cross-sectional studies are subject to selection bias and cannot substitute for longitudinal study designs. Studies of athletes engaged in chronic repetitive activity such as tennis and baseball pitching [71, 104] support the notion that regular exercise promotes bone growth as evidenced by greater bone width and mineral density in the dominant versus nondominant arms of these athletes. In the absence of well-designed longitudinal studies, these studies provide some of the best evidence that exercise may increase BMD.

Intervention studies aimed at increasing BMD are few and have given conflicting results. There has been no systematic attempt to define the type, frequency, intensity, and duration of exercise most effective for improving bone mass. Moreover, many of the available studies have been confounded by poor study designs including nonrandomization, inadequate control of confounding variables, and poor subject compliance. Longitudinal measurements of radial BMD have been made in several training studies resulting in reports of significant increases, decreases, and no change in radial BMD [141–143, 164]. One problem has been that often exercise programs have been employed that were not designed specifically to stress the bone site being measured, which may help explain the conflicting results. White et al. [164], for example, found no change in forearm BMD in postmenopausal women after 6 mo of dancing, whereas in another study 9 mo of running resulted in a significant increase in the BMD of the calcaneous [169]. Accordingly, the site selected for measurement may be critical to the results.

Dalsky et al. [31], in a relatively recent study, have reported what may be the most impressive results. In their study of exercise in postmenopausal women, these authors observed a 5.2% increase in lumbar vertebrae BMD after 9 mo of weight-bearing and resistance exercise. No change in BMD was observed in a nonrandomized control group. These results have led some authors to speculate that resistance exercise may be more potent than weight-bearing exercise for promoting bone accretion. Pruitt et al. [121] have recently presented data to support this hypothesis, demonstrating an increase in lumbar BMD of 1.6% in early postmenopausal women after 9 mo of weight-training exercise. In contrast, Rockwell et al. [127] reported a 4% decline in lumbar BMD after 9 mo of weight training in a group of premenopausal women. The different results may be age-related, although sample sizes in both studies were small and both studies were potentially confounded by selection bias due to nonrandomization. In our own work we have studied the effects of weight training on BMD in 105 premenopausal women randomly assigned to exercise and control groups [88]. Lumbar vertebrae BMD was increased approximately 2% after 4.5 mo of weight training in the exercise group and unchanged in control subjects. Repeat measurements after 12 and 18 mo of weight training showed that lumbar vertebrae remained significantly higher than pretraining values, although some regression toward baseline BMD had occurred. Thus it appears that weight-training exercise lasting 5–9 mo may promote increases in BMD on the order of ~2% in premenopausal women and that with continued training the gain in BMD is maintained. Whether similar increases are possible in other age, race, and gender groups remains controversial and the specific exercise prescription (type, frequency, intensity, and duration of exercise) that is most beneficial for bone accretion remains unresolved.

ASSESSMENT ERRORS AND VARIATION IN FFM COMPOSITION

The relative importance of changes in the various constituents of the FFM with aging to errors in estimating body composition in older men and women remains unclear. Several investigators have addressed this issue by assessing the contribution of variation in the water and mineral fractions of the FFM to percent fat errors calculated as the difference between two-component and multicomponent model estimates of percent fat. Since the more complex models presumably give a more accurate estimate of percent fat any difference between estimates from the two-component and multi-component models is attributed to the inadequacy of the simpler model.

Both Mazess et al. [99] and Wang et al. [159] have compared percent fat from whole-body DPA and a three-component model (fat, fat-free lean, and bone) with estimates from the Siri two-component model [139]. In both studies there was excellent average agreement (within ~1–2%) between the two techniques. However, large individual errors of up to about 13% occurred that were significantly correlated with whole-body bone mineral expressed as a percent of FFM (r=0.90)[100] and body weight (r=0.65, men; r=0.68, women [159]. Wang et al. [159] estimated that variation in the density of the FFM explained 90% of the variation between the two methods; however, their estimate of this association was inflated by the use of an incorrect formula to calculate D_{FFM} [86, 87]. Based on their empirical results (percent fat error = 27.3 − 4.5 × bone mineral/FFM), Mazess et al. [99] estimated a 30% loss of bone mineral such as occurs with aging would result in 9.5% increase (overestimate) of apparent percent fat. However, their assumption that a 30% decrease in bone mineral leads to an equivalent change in D_{FFM} is not necessarily correct. Based on their theoretical analysis, Lohman and Going [87] estimate that a 30% change in M/FFM leads to a somewhat smaller error, on the order of about 4%.

Total body water was not measured in the studies by Mazess et al. [99] and Wang et al. [159] and so the contributions of variation in both TBW and mineral could not be evaluated. Baumgartner et al. [6] and Williams et al. [168] measured TBW, bone mineral, and body density and compared estimates of percent fat from densitometry and the Siri equation [139] and two four-component models based on body density, TBW, and bone mineral (BM). In their sample of men and women aged 49–82 yr, Williams et al. [168] found that both the aqueous and bone mineral fractions of FFM were independently related to the differences in the two estimates of percent fat (Δ%fat). In men, TBW/FFM (~53%) accounted for more of the variance in Δ%fat than BM/FFM (~25%), whereas in women, BM/FFM (~66%) explained more of the variance than TBW/FFM (~6%). In contrast, Baumgartner et al. [6] found that TBW/FFM (r^2=0.68) but not BM/FFM (r^2=0.03–0.10) was significantly related to Δ%fat in both men and women aged 65–94 yr. The reason for the discrepancy is not clear but may be related to the somewhat different four-component models used to calculate percent fat or the greater variability observed in TBW estimates in the Baumgartner study [6]. A reanalysis of the data from Williams et al. using the Baumgartner et al. four-component model also resulted in significant and independent relationships between both TBW/FFM and BM/FFM Δ%fat [168]. Thus, it would appear that variation in both the aqueous and mineral fractions of FFM contribute to percent fat estimation errors in older persons, although their relative importance may be different in men and women.

DENSITY OF FFM

The effect of age-related variation in body water (W), mineral (M) and protein (P) on the density of the fat-free mass (D_{FFM}) and ultimately on estimation of body fat can be assessed from Equation 3 if the proportions of the FFM constituents and their respective densities are known. Unfortunately, data from longitudinal studies with measurements of W, M, and P in the same subjects at different ages are unavailable. Hence, we estimated average FFM composition and density for men (Table 14.8) and women (Table 14.9) at different ages using cross-sectional data from Cohn et al. [29] and Ellis [37]. In this analysis we used the reported body water values based on tritium dilution and calculated protein from total-body nitrogen (TBN) (protein = TBN × 6.25) [67] and bone ash (BA) from total-body calcium (BA = TBCa/0.34) [67], which were measured using TBNAA. Total-body mineral was derived from bone ash (mineral = BA × 1.279) assuming that osseous mineral was 4.36% greater than bone ash due to the loss of labile components during heating [6] and that the ratio of cell mineral (M_c) to bone ash is 0.235 (g M_c/ g BA) [19]. Fat-free mass was calculated as the sum of masses of W, M, and P.

The estimates of FFM composition and density are given in Table 14.8 for men and in Table 14.9 for women. Based on these data, in men, the overall loss of water, protein, and mineral from 20–29 to 70–79 yr of age is estimated to be 5.6 kg (-12%), 1.7 kg (-13%), and 0.95 kg (-10%), respectively. The largest decreases occur from ages 70–79 to 80–89 yr resulting in approximately 20%, 28%, and 17% declines in W, P, and M by age 80–89 yr, although it must be noted that the sample size for 80–89-yr-old men is very small and the generalizability of the data is uncertain. Relatively small changes are estimated in the respective fractional contributions of W, P, and M to total FFM and as a result D_{FFM} remains stable with aging. In women, W, P, and M decrease from ages 20–29 to 70–79 yr by 4.4 kg (-14%), 1.8 kg (-20%) and 0.80 g (-23%). Although there is a trend for D_{FFM} to decrease with increasing age, D_{FFM} estimated from these data is higher than the typically assumed 1.1 kg/L in the younger women and declines to about 1.1 kg/L by age 50–59 yr, thereafter remaining stable.

Deurenberg et al. [34] have reported a similar analysis using data from a number of sources to estimate the loss of W, M, and P with aging and then derive the theoretical change in D_{FFM}. Their estimates of D_{FFM} are given in Tables 14.8 and 14.9 for comparison with our results. They estimated mineral loss from the change in BMD with aging and assumed that water loss was proportional to muscle loss and that protein was lost at the same rate as muscle. The validity of these assumptions is questionable because total body mineral may change at a slower rate than regional BMD. Moreover, the total body K/W ratio decreases with aging by about 10% in men and women and the total body N/K ratio increases by 6% (women) to 13% (men), suggesting that body cell mass (muscle) is lost at a faster rate than total-body water and protein [29, 37]. In support of this notion, Cohn et al. [29] have suggested that a selective loss of muscle protein occurs with aging, estimated at about 40–45% in men and women, whereas by comparison nonmuscle protein changes very little (3–15%), especially in men (−3%). Consequently, the decline in muscle mass and protein overestimates the loss of total protein.

Despite the different assumptions, our estimates of D_{FFM} based on elemental composition at different ages and those from the theoretical analysis of Deurenberg et al. [34] are essentially equal for men (Table 14.8). The results of both analyses suggest little change in FFM hydration with aging and a decline in protein concentration, which is offset by an increase in the proportional contribution of mineral to total FFM. Thus, D_{FFM} is maintained close to the assumed 1.1 kg/L and the potential percent fat estimation errors associated with densitometry and the two component model (e.g., the Siri equation) are of minor consequence. The results in women are substantially different. Although the results of both analyses suggest an absolute decline in D_{FFM} of about 0.01 kg/L, Deurenberg et al. [34] found

TABLE 14.8.
Composition and Density of Fat-Free Mass (FFM) in Men

Age, yr	Mass[a]				D_{FFM}	
	FFM, kg	Water, kg (%)	Minerals, kg (%)	Protein, kg (%)	kg/L	kg/L [34]
20–29	63.52	45.95 (72.3)	4.59 (7.2)	12.98 (20.4)	1.107	–
30–39	58.10	41.95 (72.2)	4.37 (7.5)	11.78 (20.3)	1.108	–
40–49	60.61	44.25 (73.0)	4.35 (7.5)	12.01 (19.8)	1.104	1.100
50–59	60.78	44.65 (73.5)	4.31 (7.1)	11.82 (19.4)	1.102	1.101
60–69	57.50	41.50 (72.2)	4.22 (7.3)	11.78 (20.5)	1.107	1.101
70–79	55.72	40.30 (72.3)	4.14 (7.4)	11.28 (20.2)	1.108	1.102
80–89	49.80	36.60 (73.5)	3.80 (7.6)	9.40 (18.9)	1.104	1.102

[a]Values in parentheses are percentages of total FFM. Estimates of FFM composition and density are based on average data from Cohn et al. [29] and Ellis [37]. Estimates of D_{FFM} are from Deurenberg et al. [34] for comparison.

TABLE 14.9.
Composition and Density of Fat-Free Mass (FFM) in Women

Age, yr	Mass[a]				D_{FFM}	
	FFM, kg	Water, kg (%)	Minerals, kg (%)	Protein, kg (%)	kg/L	kg/L [34]
20–29	44.20	31.55 (71.5)	3.44 (7.8)	9.16 (20.7)	1.112	–
30–39	44.46	32.05 (72.0)	3.40 (7.6)	9.06 (20.4)	1.109	–
40–49	43.37	31.35 (72.4)	3.32 (7.6)	8.65 (19.9)	1.108	1.100
50–59	42.84	31.60 (73.8)	3.10 (7.2)	8.14 (19.0)	1.101	1.099
60–69	39.08	28.50 (72.9)	2.86 (7.3)	7.72 (19.8)	1.104	1.095
70–79	37.16	27.15 (73.2)	2.64 (7.1)	7.32 (19.7)	1.102	1.092

[a]Values in parentheses are percentages of total FFM. Estimates of FFM composition and density are based on average data from Cohn et al. [29] and Ellis [37]. Estimates of D_{FFM} are from Deurenberg et al. [34] for comparison.

that D_{FFM} declined to 1.09 kg/L at age 80, resulting in up to a 3% overestimation of body fat depending on whole-body density, whereas our results suggest that D_{FFM} is about 1.1 kg/L at older ages and, if anything, minor underestimates of body fat may occur.

Prior theoretical analyses suggest a much larger decline in D_{FFM} (kg/L) than reported herein but those estimates are generally not supported by more recent data. Estimates of D_{FFM} derived from estimates of elemental composition (potassium, nitrogen, and calcium) reported in a more recent paper by Cohn et al. [30] are essentially identical to the estimates of D_{FFM} reported herein. Also, empirical results from recent studies [68, 168] in middle-aged and elderly men and women showing estimates of percent fat based on densitometry (Siri or Brozek equations) differed, on average, by only 1–2% compared with more complex models that adjust for variation in bone mineral and body water support the notion of only small changes in D_{FFM} with aging. Additional research is needed to resolve the question of whether the D_{FFM} changes substantially with aging.

AGE-RELATED CHANGES IN FAT AND FAT DISTRIBUTION

Definitive descriptions of how total fat and fat distribution change in aging humans are limited by a paucity of body composition data in the oldest elderly, a dearth of longitudinal data, and wide differences in total and regional body fat assessment techniques. Because of the methodological discrepancies across studies, the varying estimates of the direction and magnitude of age-related changes in body fat are presented below in detail. Despite a preponderance of mostly unstandardized and somewhat nonspecific anthropometric assessment techniques, age-related changes in body fat distribution have been more consistently described than changes in total body fat. Studies of age-related alterations in energy balance, which underscore the importance of increased physical activity and exercise for mitigating changes in body fat and fat distribution, are also reviewed because changes in energy balance tend to obscure the effects of aging per se. As discussed, more comprehensive and better controlled studies using reliable and more accurate body fat assessment methodologies are needed to determine the efficacy of exercise training for altering body fat, fat distribution, and ultimately metabolic risk factors for coronary heart disease and noninsulin-dependent diabetes mellitus in older populations.

TOTAL-BODY FAT

The results of studies examining aging-related changes in body fat suggest two somewhat contrasting patterns of change. There is either an increase in body fat in early old age followed by a reduction in body fat in later old age, or there is a gradual and continuous increase in body fat with advancing age. Possible explanations for the existence of these different patterns include inconsistencies in study design (e.g., cross-sectional vs. longitudinal), body fat assessment techniques, and subject sampling methods.

The possibility of an increase in body fat followed by a decrease is suggested by anthropometric data. The data from the second National Health and Nutrition Examination Survey (NHANES II) show that the triceps and subscapular skinfolds within a given percentile generally increase in thickness from 18 to 54 yr of age, and that from age 55 to age 74, there is either a leveling off or a decline in the skinfold thickness (Figs. 14.2 and 14.3) [108]. Unfortunately, skinfold data for elderly adults above 74 yr of age were not collected in NHANES II. Such data would be clinically relevant because the most dramatic declines in functional capacity occur at these ages [149].

Normative skinfold data are available for elderly Welsh [19] and French [32] populations. Collectively, the European data show a continued decline in skinfold thicknesses from 75 to ≥85 yr of age. However, the age- and sex-specific values corresponding to a given percentile are systematically lower in the European compared with the American populations, and therefore, the European data cannot be used as reference norms for elderly Americans. At least part of the difference may be due to the use of different skinfold calipers because the Harpenden skinfold calipers used in the European studies give systematically lower values than the Lange calipers used in the U.S. population survey [86]. The development of national skinfold norms for U.S. subjects aged 75 yr and older would be useful for determining nutritional adequacy and risk for chronic disease morbidity and mortality in elderly Americans.

Population-based measurements of height and weight are also available, and the body mass index (BMI, kg/m^2), derived from height and weight, is

FIGURE 14.2.

Values corresponding to the 25th, 50th, and 75th percentiles for triceps and sub-scapular skinfold thicknesses by age and race in U.S. men [108].

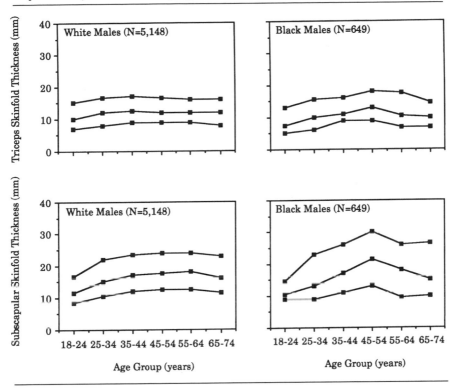

routinely used as an anthropometric approximation of total-body fat. Interestingly, the NHANES II data for BMI do not correspond well with the skinfold data and, in general, show less consistent trends across age groups [108]. However, the usefulness of BMI as a simple index of body fat is limited in studies of human aging. Age-related reductions in vertebral bone mineral [95, 97], coupled with increases in the prevalence of kyphosis [149], contribute to a loss of height with advancing age, which may be interpreted as body fat gains in the context of BMI. In contrast, reductions in bone mineral [95, 97] and skeletal muscle masses [42] with advancing age would reduce BMI independent of actual changes in body fat. Thus, changes in BMI may be a particularly misleading index of changes in body fat in older subjects.

Skinfold thicknesses, although useful and perhaps more specific than BMI, also have important limitations for assessing age-related changes in body fat. For instance, it remains possible that the trend for less skinfold

FIGURE 14.3.

Values corresponding to the 25th, 50th, and 75th percentiles for triceps and sub-scapular skinfold thicknesses by age and race in U.S. women [108].

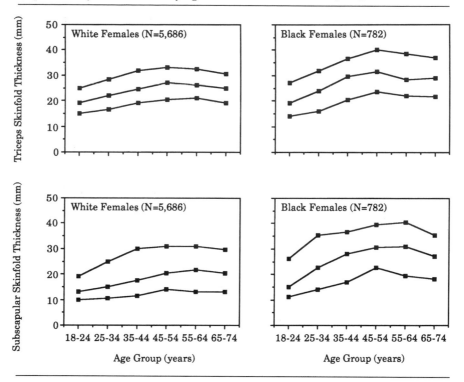

thickness after age 54 may be more indicative of a shift in body fat from sub-cutaneous to visceral depots [7, 38] rather than a reduction in total-body fat. Given the scarcity of data in the oldest elderly, and the limitations of an-thropometric indexes of body fat, it is difficult to define age-related trends with a convincing degree of certainty.

A recent cross-sectional study reporting estimates of body fat percentage derived from bioelectric impedance analysis (BIA) in 514 subjects ranging in age from 29 to 96 yr also supports the notion that body fat may decline in old age [138]. Higher body fat percentages were observed in both men and women age 40–64 yr as compared with their older (≥85 yr) counterparts. However, as with other studies, the generalizability of the estimates of body fat are limited by the small number of subjects aged ≥85 yr and the poten-tial for subject selection bias across the age groups. Also, the validity of the BIA-derived estimates of body fat is unclear because the authors do not re-port whether subject hydration status or the use of diuretics was controlled.

The authors presumably used the BIA instrument manufacturer's (RJL Systems, Inc., Detroit, MI) equations, which may not be age-specific. The lower percent fats of the oldest subjects may not be representative of healthy older subjects because the subjects were nursing home residents.

In addition to the skinfold and BIA data, there is some additional evidence supporting an increase in body fat in early old age followed by a reduction in later old age from cross-sectional studies using multiple component models to estimate body fat. Ellis [37] has reported mean body fats of 27.1% in 20–29-yr-old women, 42.1% in 50–59-yr-old women, and 36.7% in 70–79-yr-old women. Although sample size was small (N=64) and many of the older women were recruited for an osteoporosis study, the estimates of body fat were derived from a multiple-component model incorporating ^3H_2O dilution to estimate total-body water and TBNAA to estimate total-body mineral and total-body protein. As a result, the estimates of body fat from that study are not confounded by possible age-related differences in bone mineral, body water, or protein. Rico et al. [124] have also recently shown that DXA-derived estimates of body fat were significantly (P<0.005) lower in a group of 61 women aged 81 ± 4 yr as compared with a group of 63 women aged 65 ± 4 yr.

Although skinfold norms, BIA-derived estimates of body fat, and some multiple-component model-derived estimates of body fat percentage suggest that body fat increases in early old age followed by a reduction in body fat in later old age, the evidence is limited by its cross-sectional nature. In the absence of longitudinal data, an alternative explanation for the secondary reduction in body fat in later old age is that the sampling of older subjects may be biased by a longer survival of leaner as opposed to fatter subjects.

An important limitation in determining how fatness changes with age is the necessary reliance on indirect techniques to estimate body fat in vivo. In contrast to the results discussed above, data from direct cadaver analysis suggest a different trend for body fatness with aging. Based on data from Clarys et al. [27] from the analysis of 25 Belgian cadavers (aged 55–94 yr at the time of death), we have previously reported a significant positive correlation ($r = 0.41$, P = 0.04) between age and anatomically dissected body fat percentage [54]. Body fat was about 4.4% higher for every decade increase in age. However, these data are not without limitations because stratification for possible gender differences was not reported and because 12 of the subjects had died of coronary heart disease. Thus, it is unclear whether the trend for increased body fat is the result of aging or chronic disease. Studies with large samples of healthy, free living adults are potentially more generalizable than cadaver studies, particularly when multiple component models of body composition are employed.

Cross-sectional body density (R. A. Boileau, personal communication, 1994) [36] and ^{40}K γ spectroscopy [42, 49] data as well as longitudinal ^{40}K γ spectroscopy data [42, 49] suggest that body fat increases continuously with advancing age. Durnin and Womersley [36] estimated body fat percentage from body density and the Siri two-component equation [139] in 209 men and 272 women aged 16–72 yr. These data support the qualitative trend of gradually higher body fat percentages at older ages. In men and women, the average body fat percentage was higher in each successive age group from age 16 through age 72. However, because the data were stratified by age groups with discrepant interval widths, it is difficult to quantify the difference in body fat with increasing age.

In an effort to replicate the qualitative trends identified by Durnin and Womersley [36] and to better quantify the relationship between age and body fat percentage, we analyzed data from R. A. Boileau et al. at the University of Illinois who have measured body density in 458 white men (N=229) and women (N=229) aged 40–81 yr (R. A. Boileau, personal communication, 1994). The mean ± SD values for density-derived (two-component model) estimates of body fat percentage (percent fat) were 26.4 ± 6.5 in men and 35.8 ± 7.3 in women. The relationship between body fat percentage and age is shown in Figure 14.4 for men and in Figure 14.5 for women. Body fat percentage was significantly (P<0.0001) correlated with age in both men and women. Based on the regression slopes, the age-related differences in percent fat were roughly +2.2 ± 0.4% fat per decade in men (Fig. 14.4) and +3.6 ± 0.4% fat per decade in women (Fig. 14.5).

Although the data are cross-sectional, the age-related differences in the Illinois data compare favorably with longitudinal estimates of changes in body fat percentage in 564 men and 61 women with initial ages ranging

FIGURE 14.4.

Relationship between densitometrically determined estimates of body fat percentage (% Fat) and age in 229 white men (R. A. Boileau, personal communication, 1994).

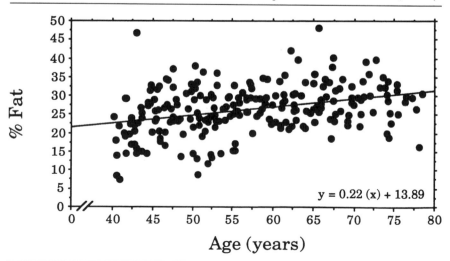

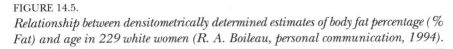

FIGURE 14.5.

Relationship between densitometrically determined estimates of body fat percentage (% Fat) and age in 229 white women (R. A. Boileau, personal communication, 1994).

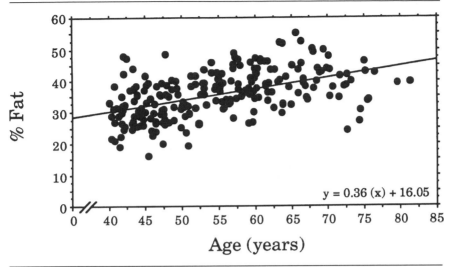

from 28 to 60 yr [42]. Rates of change in body fat percentage over 18 yr were determined from repeated estimates of total-body potassium from ^{40}K γ spectroscopy. The average rate of increase in body fat over the 18 yr of follow-up was 3.0% fat per decade in men and 5.2% fat per decade in women. Taken together, the qualitative and quantitative agreement between the cross-sectional densitometric (R. A. Boileau, personal communication, 1994), and longitudinal ^{40}K γ spectroscopic [42] data suggest that there may be a continuous and relatively linear increase in body fat percentage with advancing age.

As noted earlier, estimation of body fat from densitometry requires an assumption of a constant density of the fat-free tissues [139]. Likewise, body fat estimates from ^{40}K γ spectroscopy alone assume a constant potassium concentration of the fat-free tissues [47]. Given the uncertainty of these assumptions, it remains possible that the trend for a continuous rise in body fat with advancing age suggested by these methods is an artifact of a systematic overestimation of body fat in older subjects [34]. Alternatively, it has been suggested that the interindividual variability in the composition of the fat-free mass increases with age [6]. Thus, if the individual under- and overestimates of body fat from densitometry and ^{40}K γ spectroscopy were to increase nonsystematically with advancing age, then the true magnitude of the relationship between body fat and aging may be underestimated when based on a two-component model of body composition.

Additional studies, with estimates of body fat based on a multiple component model, are required to corroborate the findings of the two-component model-based techniques [36, 42, 49] (R. A. Boileau, personal communication, 1994). In this regard, the recent DXA-derived estimates of body fat in 815 men and women aged 15–83 yr [123] and the estimates of body fat from ^3H_2O dilution and TBNAA in 87 men aged 20–89 yr [37] are significant, with both studies demonstrating progressively higher body fat with increasing age, which confirms the results of the two-component models [36, 42, 49] (R. A. Boileau, personal communication, 1994). In addition, the average age-related difference in body fat of +2.2% per decade in men based on the work of Ellis [37] with a multiple-component model was identical to that estimated herein (Fig. 14.4) with the Illinois densitometric data based on the two-component model (R. A. Boileau, personal communication, 1994).

Clearly, a definitive quantitative description of how body fat changes with advancing age has yet to be done. It will require a large, prospective cohort of adults with repeated body fat estimates, based probably on a multiple-component model of body composition. Although it is plausible that body fat increases in early old age and subsequently declines, longitudinal data are need to confirm the existence of such a trend. In contrast, more of the presently available evidence suggests that body fat increases in a relatively continuous fashion with advancing age.

BODY FAT DISTRIBUTION

Body fat distribution is a generalized term that has been used to refer to the anatomical localization of body fat in central or peripheral, upper or lower body and subcutaneous or visceral sites. Skinfold thicknesses and DXA have been used most commonly to describe age-related changes in central fat distribution, whereas body circumferences have been extensively used to characterize upper-body fat distribution. Skinfold thicknesses, DXA, and body circumferences do not differentiate between subcutaneous and visceral fat. Thus, more complex methodologies, such as magnetic resonance imaging and CT, are required to determine internal or visceral fat distribution.

Central Fat Distribution
In older men and women, skinfold measurements on the trunk are more highly correlated with estimates of total-body fat than are limb skinfolds [25, 26]. These data have been interpreted as indirect evidence that there may be a redistribution of subcutaneous fat from the limbs to the trunk with increasing age [80]. Cross-sectional and longitudinal skinfold data further support the possibility that body fat becomes more centralized with advancing age. We found truncal skinfold thicknesses to be more highly correlated with age than were limb skinfolds in 207 men and women aged 34–84 yr [166]. Our cross-sectional relationships between age and skinfold thicknesses in middle-aged and older adults [166] agree with the longitu-

dinal data of Chien et al. [22] demonstrating significantly greater 12-yr increases in truncal as compared with limb skinfold thicknesses in middle-aged men and women.

DXA has also been used to describe differences in the centralization of body fat between premenopausal and postmenopausal women. Ley et al. [83] reported a significantly greater proportion of total fat on the trunk in postmenopausal as compared with premenopausal women (42.1 ± 4.5% vs. 38.3 ± 5.3%, P < 0.001). These authors [83] also defined upper and lower regions of interest within the trunk and presented evidence that the greater proportion of total fat located on the trunk in the older post-menopausal women is confined to the abdominal region, although this finding must be interpreted cautiously because DXA may have a limited ability to determine truncal fat accurately in the thoracic region [128, 144]. Despite this technical limitation, the relatively high reliability of DXA [128] suggests that DXA may be useful for determining intervention-related changes in fat distribution. Indeed, Haarbo et al. [57] were able to detect a significant protective effect of estrogen replacement therapy for preventing the increasing centralization of body fat, as determined by DXA, in post-menopausal women.

Upper-Body Fat Distribution
In addition to the apparently greater age-related increase in central versus peripheral stores of body fat, many studies using body circumferences suggest that there is an increase in upper-body fatness with advancing age [63, 107, 136, 147, 152]. In contrast to the studies of central or visceral fat distribution, upper-body fat distribution has been described in large and potentially more representative samples of older and aging adults. However, the use of circumferences to determine fat distribution is limited by the lack of standardization of measurement sites [73], the inability of circumferences to differentiate between fat and fat-free tissues [13], and the confounding influence of the increased sagging of the abdominal viscerae with advancing age [15].

The results of cross-sectional studies examining the relationship between age and body circumference ratios suggest that upper- to lower-body fat distribution increases with age in men and women, although possible gender differences may be obscured by the use of different measurement sites and populations. For instance, Muller et al. [107] found age to be more highly correlated with the waist-to-hip ratio (WHR) in 228 women as compared with 421 men aged 17–95 yr (*r*=0.55 vs. *r*=0.36), whereas Sönnichsen et al. [147] found age to be more highly correlated with the WHR in 158 men as compared with 147 women aged 17–78 yr (*r*=0.44 vs. *r*=0.33). Muller et al. [107] sampled white, middle-class Americans and measured the "waist" circumference at the minimal girth between the ribs and the iliac crest and the "hip" circumference at the maximal gluteal protusion. In contrast, Sönnichsen et al. [147] sampled a German population and measured the "waist" circumference at the level of the umbilicus and the "hip" circumference at the level of the greater trochanter. These studies [107, 147] illustrate the difficulties associated with interpreting results across studies due to the lack of a standardized definition of the WHR.

There are other, more general problems associated with the use of the WHR as an index of upper-body fat distribution that limit its value. For instance, age-related differences in the WHR could result from greater waist girths, lower hip girths, or a combination of both. Therefore, Heitmann's [63] cross-sectional description of differences in waist circumference by decade in 35–65-yr-old Danish men (N=1524) and women (N=1463) is perhaps more representative of age-related differences in upper-body fat distribution. The average decade-to-decade difference in waist circumference was +1.9 cm in men and +2.0 cm in women, with waist circumference measured midway between the ribs and the iliac crest [63]. Although these data suggest an increase in upper-body fat distribution with advancing age, they are limited by their cross-sectional nature.

More compelling evidence that upper-body fat distribution increases with advancing age is provided by two notable longitudinal studies in which changes in the waist circumference were reported [136, 152]. Shimokata et al. [136] have reported 5-yr changes in waist circumference in 263 male and 123 female participants of the Baltimore Longitudinal Study of Aging with ages ranging from 45 to 86 yr of baseline. Waist circumference was measured at the minimal girth between the ribs and the iliac crest. The mean increase in waist circumference over 5 yr was 2.0 cm in men and 0.6 cm in women. Changes in waist circumference but not the hip circumference accounted almost entirely for the 5-yr changes in the WHR. In a cohort study of much longer duration, Stevens et al. [152] reported 25-yr changes in abdominal circumference measured at the level of the umbilicus in a biracial cohort of 197 Charleston Heart Study participants with ages ranging from 47 to 74 yr at baseline. Similar to the 5-yr changes in waist circumference [136], the average 25-yr increases in abdominal circumference were greater in men than in women (5.4 vs. 4.6 cm in whites and 8.1 vs. 2.3 cm in blacks). Thus, body circumference data suggest that the distribution of body fat in the upper body, or more specifically the lower trunk or abdominal region, increases with advancing age. Although circumferences have been shown to be predictive of abdominal and intraabdominal fat [133, 162], circumferences are not highly accurate predictors of visceral fat [33]. Therefore, more complex methods are needed to determine age-related changes in internal fat distribution.

Internal (or Visceral) Fat Distribution
A number of cross-sectional studies using CT to differentiate subcutaneous from visceral fat are suggestive of an age-related internalization of body fat [7, 13, 15, 38, 131]. The results from CT studies also highlight the potential problems of a simple interpretation of age-related changes in lower

truncal circumferences as changes in abdominal fat because, in addition to increased visceral fat, they demonstrate lower amounts of intraabdominal lean tissue [13] and a greater sagging or protrusion of abdominal viscerae [15] in older as compared with younger subjects. Currently, the CT data are limited to cross-sectional studies of mostly male subjects.

Although longitudinal changes in waist [136] and abdominal [152] circumferences suggest that the accumulation of total (subcutaneous + visceral) abdominal fat with advancing age may be greater in men than in women, the limited cross-sectional CT data for women [7, 38] suggest that men and women may have similar age-related differences in visceral fat. For example, Enzi and coworkers [38] found similar, inverse correlations between age and the ratio of CT-derived estimates of subcutaneous to visceral adipose tissue volumes in men and women aged 20 to >60 yr ($r=-0.65$ in men and $r=-0.61$ in women, P <0.001 for both). Moreover, in a reanalysis of data from their earlier study [7], Baumgartner et al. [8] report slightly higher mean differences in the CT-derived estimates of the visceral proportion of total abdominal fat in women as compared with men (+2.7% per decade vs. +2.2% per decade). Although longitudinal studies are needed to better describe and quantify the accumulation of intraabdominal fat associated with aging in men and women, the substantial cost and radiation dose associated with CT limits its widespread application.

Age-related changes in body fat distribution, including a redistribution from the limbs to the trunk and from subcutaneous to visceral depots, have been more consistently demonstrated than have age-related increases in total-body fat. However, the conclusion that visceral adiposity increases with advancing age is limited by a lack of longitudinal data using accurate and specific methods for assessing intraabdominal fat. Because of the strong relationship between total and truncal adiposity [14], and given the current limitations of accurately assessing total-body fat in older subjects, it is not possible to say with certainty whether the age-related increases in truncal fat distribution are independent of increases in total-body fat.

Body Fat, Physical Activity, and Exercise
An increase in total-body fat and truncal fat may not be an inevitable result of the aging process. An imbalance between energy intake and energy expenditure is the major determinant of body fat storage, and there are data to suggest that differential changes in energy intake and expenditure resulting in an energy surfeit could account for the increasing amounts of body fat with advancing age.

Hoffman [70] has suggested that the increased accumulation of body fat with advancing age may result primarily from an age-related decline in energy expenditure [70], which is supported by Goran and Poehlman's [55] finding of an inverse correlation ($r=-0.64$, P = 0.018) between total daily energy expenditure assessed by doubly labeled water ($^2H_2{}^{18}O$) and densitometrically determined estimates of fat mass in elderly subjects. In contrast, there have been reports from cross-sectional [171] and longitudinal [41] studies of nonsignificant correlations between age-related changes in energy intake and body fat. It must be noted that the relationship between energy intake and body fat in older adults may be obscured by dietary intake reporting bias. Recent data suggest that older adults may underreport energy intake [74]. A similar conclusion was reached by Lichtman et al. [84] in their study of persistent obesity in "diet-resistant" middle-aged subjects [84].

In the absence of comprehensive longitudinal studies with measurements of body fat and energy intake and expenditure, it is difficult to determine the relationship between changes in energy balance and changes in body fat with advancing age. However, in both cross-sectional and longitudinal studies, energy intake has consistently been shown to decline with advancing age [70], and in one longitudinal study, energy intake was shown to decline while body weight increased in older adults [59]. If this does indeed occur, then it is conceivable that energy expenditure declines to a greater extent than energy intake.

Poehlman and Horton [117] have extensively reviewed the age-related changes in the contribution of resting metabolic rate, physical activity, and the thermic effect of feeding to total energy expenditure. In general, resting metabolic rates [76, 157] and physical activity levels [100, 122, 130] have been reported to decline with increasing age. In contrast, clear age-related differences in the thermic effect of feeding have not been demonstrated [117]. Although it is difficult to quantify definitively age-related changes in energy balance, it appears that the accumulation of body fat with advancing age may, in part, result from a reduction in energy intake that is insufficient to balance an even greater reduction in energy expenditure.

BODY FAT IN ACTIVE AND INACTIVE OLDER ADULTS. Physical activity is a modifiable, behavioral component of the total daily energy expenditure that can be studied as a whole or as a combination of exercise training and nontraining-related activity. Some studies have attempted to determine the effect of physical activity on the body composition of elderly subjects by comparing the total fat and fat distribution of physically active or exercise-trained older subjects to that of their sedentary or untrained peers. Such comparisons have demonstrated that physically active or exercise-trained older subjects have lower body fat percentages [58, 118, 158], lower truncal skinfold thicknesses [78, 81], and smaller waist circumferences [81] than their age- and sex-matched sedentary or untrained peers. Although these studies suggest that exercise and physical activity may reduce the age-related increases in total and truncal adiposity, they may be limited by subject selection bias because healthier subjects with lower amounts of total and truncal fat may simply be more likely to exercise regularly.

EXERCISE TRAINING. Conflicting results have been observed regarding the effect of exercise training on body fat percentage in older adults. For instance, reductions [106, 120, 132], no change [116], and an age-related increase in body fat percentage over 10 yr despite continued endurance training [119] have been reported in older adults. Conclusions regarding the effects of exercise on total-body fat in older adults may be limited by the use of densitometry-derived estimates of body fat percentage in these studies. Exercise and aging may independently affect the components of the fat-free mass (e.g., bone mineral), thereby changing the assumptions underlying the conversion of body density to percent fat with advancing age or increased exercise. In a similar regard, because training may affect fat-free tissues within specific regions (e.g., bone mineral and skeletal muscle), accurate methods of assessing regional composition are needed to quantify training-related changes in fat distribution. CT has been used in only one training study in older adults in which a 25% reduction in CT-derived estimates of intraabdominal fat following 6 months of endurance training in older white men was reported [132]. A somewhat smaller reduction in subcutaneous abdominal fat and much smaller reductions in chest, buttocks, and thigh fat were also observed, which suggests that endurance exercise may result in a preferential loss of body fat from visceral depots in older men.

Recent endurance [115, 116] and resistance [120] exercise training studies in older adults suggest that exercise may ameliorate the age-related decline in resting metabolic rate. In addition, endurance training has been shown to result in a higher level of habitual physical activity in older adults [60]. Furthermore, it has recently been demonstrated that endurance training increases fat oxidation rates in older adults [116]. Taken together, these studies suggest that exercise may reduce body fat in older subjects by increasing energy expenditure and by increasing the use of fat as a metabolic substrate.

At present, the exercise training literature in older adults is limited by a relative lack of data on female subjects and methodological concerns, including the use of nonrandomized, poorly controlled study designs and the limitations of available technology for assessing body fat and fat distribution. Future studies using more reliable and accurate techniques for assessing body fat and fat distribution are required. The extent to which increased physical activity may be used to reduce total body fat or truncal fat has yet to be firmly established. Furthermore, it is not yet known whether favorable changes in coronary heart disease and noninsulin-dependent diabetes mellitus risk factors result from reductions in total-body fat or truncal fat in elderly adults, nor is it clear what threshold of training is needed to produce health benefits for this population.

ASSESSMENT STRATEGIES AND CHALLENGES

From the foregoing discussion it is evident that body fat increases with aging, although the magnitude and variability of the increase, and to some degree, the direction of change in old age is unclear. This situation has arisen because of a lack of longitudinal data in older men and women, and the difficulty in separating changes due to aging per se from environmental factors such as a decline in physical activity. The limitations of indirect assessment techniques and the potential errors associated with the two-component model have also contributed to difficulty interpreting much of the available data. As noted, loss of mineral and protein and the associated decline in D_{FFM} may lead to an overestimation of body fat by traditional techniques, especially in women, although there is conflicting evidence on this point. The successful resolution of questions regarding age-related changes in FFM, total fat, and fat distribution will require extensive validation efforts to improve both the models and the accuracy of accessible methods for obtaining accurate estimates of body composition in older men and women.

Two strategies are possible to minimize the potential errors in estimates of percent fat associated with variability in FFM composition. The ideal procedure is to combine measures of body density with measures of body water and bone mineral and estimate body composition using an equation based on a four-component model of body composition. This approach eliminates the need for assumptions regarding the proportionalities among the constituents of the FFM. Alternatively, body density can be combined with measures of body water [140] or bone mineral [86] and estimates of body fat based on three-component models can be derived. Although presumably more accurate than the two-component equations, these equations do assume a constant protein-to-mineral or protein-to-water ratio and individual deviations from the assumed ratios introduces error, albeit less than the two-component model. Whether body water or bone mineral is measured depends on which constituent is likely to vary most within the population being studied.

Although the multicomponent (three- or four-component model) approach is preferred, it is often not possible to measure water and mineral because of lack of equipment, time constraints, or expense. In this situation, percent fat can be estimated from density alone using modifications of the Siri equation [139] derived from estimates of FFM composition in the population of interest. Estimates of FFM fractional composition and D_{FFM} have been published for older white men and women by Deurenberg et al. [34], and based on those data they have also derived adjusted equations for estimating body fat from body density. Our estimates of D_{FFM} given in Tables 14.8 and 14.9 could be used with Equation 2 to derive similar equations. Although, on average, these adjusted equations are expected to give more accurate estimates of body fat in older persons, this approach assumes that the Siri equation systematically overestimates body fat as a function of increasing age and, as we have shown, this point remains to be clearly established. Moreover, the substantial range in differences between the two-component and multiple-component model-derived estimates of body fat suggests systematic age- and sex-specific adjustments to the Siri equation may be of limited value for improving estimates of body fat in individual subjects. Indeed, we have recently shown [167] that age and sex together explain only 17% of the variation in the difference between estimates of percent fat from two- and four-component models.

Presently, it is unclear whether a three-component (fat, mineral, and soft tissue lean) model, such as can be derived with DXA, can be used as a surrogate for a four-component model (fat, mineral, water, and protein) in older adults. Recent work with DXA has emphasized two potential problems. As explained by Roubenoff et al. [128], potential hydration-related errors in the estimated soft tissue lean mass are propagated to the estimated fat component of body mass. Also, DXA may underestimate body fat in older subjects with greater proportions of total fat located on the trunk due to the inability of DXA to estimate soft tissue composition in regions under- and overlying bone. In this regard, the truncal thoracic region may be particularly problematic because the limited number of bone-free soft tissue pixels increases the number of extrapolations from adjacent soft tissue regions to those regions under- and overlying bone [128, 144]. Further studies are needed to quantify the extent to which hydration status and interindividual variation in fat distribution, as assessed by independent techniques, are related to body fat estimation errors from DXA in older subjects. Despite these possible limitations, DXA remains promising for monitoring changes in body fat associated with aging and intervention because of its high reliability [128]. Furthermore, the recent findings of Svendsen et al. [154] suggest that DXA coupled with anthropometry may eventually be used to predict visceral adiposity in older adults without the substantial cost and radiation exposure associated with CT.

Practical, Field-Based Methods

Because of the potential errors associated with densitometry and the two-component model, and the present uncertainties surrounding DXA as a criterion estimate of body composition [128], there is a need for valid and generalizable equations for predicting four-component (fat, water, mineral, and protein) model-derived estimates of body composition from simple, practical techniques that can be applied on a population level in older subjects. At present, it is difficult to recommend the use of common skinfold equations such as the Jackson and Pollock [72] and Durnin and Womersley [36] equations because of the inaccuracies associated with the conversion of body density to body fat percentage in older adults [6, 65, 166, 167, 168]. Although the Williams et al. [166] skinfold equations, based on a four-component model, may provide more valid estimates of percent fat, the generalizability of the selected sites remains undetermined.

Skinfold thickness measurements to estimate body fat in older men and women have also been criticized because measurement error has been shown to be higher in older subjects [25], skinfold compressibility may vary by site [93] and age [56], and changes in body fat distribution have been associated with aging [13, 15, 22, 38, 131]. Because of these limitations and the lack of skinfold equations developed with a multiple-component criterion, there are no exact descriptions of age-related changes in total body fat in U.S. and other populations.

BIA may be a useful, alternative practical technique for body composition estimation in older populations because of the ease of administration and the relatively low measurement error [23]. We have recently found that BIA measurements predicted a multiple-component criterion estimate of body composition with lower prediction errors than either skinfold thickness or near infrared interactance measures in a sample of middle-aged and older adults [167]. Our findings highlight the potential usefulness of BIA in older populations. If these new BIA equations [167] can also be cross-validated in other samples of older adults, then they would represent an important extension to previously published BIA equations for older adults based on the two-component model [35]. In addition, Svendsen et al. [153] found that BIA significantly improved the anthropometric prediction of estimates of body fat percentage derived from DXA in 75-yr-old men and women. Thus, BIA may prove to be a useful addition to skinfold thicknesses in future population-based studies of older adults.

SUMMARY

There is no doubt that body composition changes with aging. Some general trends have been described, including an increase in body weight and fat mass in middle age followed by a decrease in stature, weight, FFM, and body cell mass at older ages. Losses in muscle, protein, and bone mineral contribute to the decline in FFM; however, the onset and rates of decline remain controversial. Most data are available for men and women <80 yr and we know relatively little about the normal status and the changes that occur in body composition in elderly men and women. This situation has developed in part because the changes that occur in various body constituents with aging confound the estimation of body composition by traditional techniques. Hence, there is a need for longitudinal reference data in persons 80 yr of age, both to describe the normal status and to develop valid prediction equations for estimating body composition in older men and women in settings outside the laboratory. This should be possible using new technologies and approaches based on multiple component models of body composition. An understanding of the normal changes in body composition with increasing age, the normal variation in these changes, and their health implications is important for the health, nutritional support, and pharmacologic treatment of elderly men and women in the United States. The information is especially important because elderly men and women, in terms of both numbers and health care dollars, represent the most rapidly expanding segment of the U.S. population.

ACKNOWLEDGMENTS

We thank Dr. Richard Boileau, Dr. Mary Slaughter, Mr. Ralph Geeseman and colleagues in the Physical Fitness Research Laboratory, Department of Kinesiology, at the University of Illinois, Urbana-Champaign for generously sharing body density data collected on 458 men and women; and Laurie Milliken for help with the figures. Support for some of the authors' work reported herein was received from the National Institute on Aging (Grant AG06180), the National Institute for Arthritis and Musculoskeletal Diseases (Grant AR39559), and the National Heart, Lung, and Blood Institute (Grant HL07034).

REFERENCES

1. Abraham, S., C. L. Johnson, M. F. Najjar. Weight and height of adults 18–74 yr of age. Rockville, MD: National Center for Health Statistics, 1979. Vital and health statistics series 11 (DHEW publication [PHS] 79-1659).
2. Allen, T. H., E. C. Anderson, and W. H. Langham. Total body potassium and gross body composition in relation to age. *J. Gerontol.* 15:348–357, 1960.
3. Aloia, J. F., A. Vaswani, K. Ellis, K. Yuen, and S. H. Cohn. A model for involutional bone loss. *J. Lab. Clin. Med.* 106:630–637, 1985.
4. Aloia, J. F., A. Vaswani, P. Ross, and S. H. Cohn. Aging bone loss from the femur, spine, radius, and total skeleton. *Metabolism* 39:1144–1150, 1990.
5. Arnold, J. S. Quantification of mineralization of bone as an organ and tissue in osteoporosis. *Clin. Orthopaedics* 17:167–175, 1960.
6. Baumgartner, R. N., S. B. Heymsfield, S. Lichtman, J. Wang, and R. N. Pierson. Body composition in elderly people: the effect of criterion estimates on predictive equations. *Am. J. Clin. Nutr.* 53:1345–1353, 1991.
7. Baumgartner, R. N., S. B. Heymsfield, A. F. Roche, and M. Bernardino. Abdominal composition quantified by computed tomography. *Am. J. Clin. Nutr.* 48:936–945, 1988.
8. Baumgartner, R. N., R. L. Rhyne, P. J. Garry, and S. B. Heymsfield. Imaging techniques and anatomical body composition in aging. *J. Nutr.* 123:444–448, 1993.
9. Behnke, A. R., B. G. Feen, W. C. Wellman. The specific gravity of healthy men. *JAMA* 118:495–498, 1942.
10. Behnke, A. R., and J. H. Wilmore. *Evaluation and Regulation of Body Build and Composition.* Englewood Cliffs, NJ: Prentice Hall, 1974.
11. Birkenhager-Frenkel, C. H., P. Courpron, E. A. Hupscher, et al. Age-related changes in cancellous bone structure. *Bone Min.* 4:197–216, 1988.
12. Bittnerova, H. R., R. Rath, J. Svobodova, and J. Mosek. Total body water and sodium distribution space in women of different body weights. *Nutr. Abstr. Rev.* 39:2751, 1969
13. Borkan, G. A., D. E. Hults, S. G. Gerzof, and A. H. Robbins. Comparison of body composition in middle-aged and elderly males using computed tomography. *Am. J. Phys. Anthropol.* 66:289–295, 1985.
14. Borkan, G. A., S. G. Gerzof, A. H. Robbins, D. E. Hults, C. K. Silbert, and J. E. Silbert. Assessment of abdominal fat content by computed tomography. *Am. J. Clin. Nutr.* 36:172–177, 1982.

15. Borkan, G. A., and A. H. Norris. Fat redistribution and the changing body dimensions of the adult male. *Hum. Biol.* 49:494–514, 1977

16. Bouchard, C. Genetic factors in obesity. *Med. Clin. North Am.* 73:67–81, 1989.

17. Bouchard, C., A. Tremblay, J. Depires, et al. The response to long-term overfeeding in identical twins. *N. Engl. J. Med.* 322:1477–1482, 1990.

18. Brozek, J., F. Grande, J. T. Anderson, and A. Keys. Densitometric analysis of body composition: Revision of some quantitative assumptions. *Ann. N. Y. Acad. Sci.* 110:113–140, 1963.

19. Burr, M. L., and K. M. Phillips. Anthropometric norms in the elderly. *Br. J. Nutr.* 51:165–169, 1984.

20. Calloway, N. O., C. F. Foley, and P. Lagerbloom. Uncertainties in geriatric data. II. Organ size. *J. Am. Geriatr. Soc.* 13:20–29, 1965.

21. Cann, C. E., and H. K. Genant. Precise measurement of vertebral mineral content using computed tomography. *J. Comput. Assist. Tomogr.* 4:493–500, 1980.

22. Chien, S., M. T. Peng, K. P. Chen, T. F. Huang, C. Chang, and H. S. Fang. Longitudinal studies on adipose tissue and its distribution in human subjects. *J. Appl. Physiol.* 39:825–830, 1975.

23. Chumlea, W. C., and R. N. Baumgartner. Status of anthropometry and body composition data in elderly subjects. *Am. J. Clin. Nutr.* 50:1158–1166, 1989.

24. Chumlea, W. C., P. J. Garry, W. C. Hunt, and R. L. Rhyne. Serial changes in stature and weight in a healthy elderly population. *Hum. Biol.* 160:918–925, 1988.

25. Chumlea, W. C., A. F. Roche, and E. Rogers. Replicability for anthropometry in the elderly. *Hum. Biol.* 56:329–337, 1984.

26. Chumlea, W. C., A. F. Roche, and P. Webb. Body size, subcutaneous fatness and total body fat in older adults. *Int. J. Obesity* 8:311–317, 1984.

27. Clarys, J. P., A. D. Martin, and D. T. Drinkwater. Gross tissue weights in the human body by cadaver dissection. *Hum. Biol.* 56:459–473, 1984.

28. Cohn, S. H., K. J. Ellis, and D. Vartsky. Comparison of methods estimating body fat in normal subjects and cancer patients. *Am. J. Clin. Nutr.* 34:2839–2847, 1981.

29. Cohn, S. H., D. Vartsky, and S. Yasumura. Compartmental body composition based on total-body nitrogen, potassium, and calcium. *Am. J. Physiol.* 239:E524, 1980.

30. Cohn, S. H., A. N. Vaswani, S. Yasumura, K. Yuen, and K. J. Ellis. Improved models for determination of body fat by in vivo neutron activation. *Am. J. Clin. Nutr.* 40:255–259, 1984.

31. Dalsky, G. P., K. S. Stocke, A. A. Eshnai, E. Slatopolsky, W. C. Lee, and S. J. Birge. Weight-bearing exercise training and lumbar bone mineral content in postmenopausal women. *Ann. Intern. Med.* 108:824–828, 1988.

32. Delarue, J., T. Constans, D. Malvy, A. Pradignac, C. Couet, and F. Lamisse. Anthropometric values in an elderly French population. *Br. J. Nutr.* 71:295–302, 1994.

33. Després, J. P., D. Prud'homme, M. C. Pouliot, A. Tremblay, and C. Bouchard. Estimation of deep abdominal adipose-tissue accumulation from simple anthropometric measurements in men. *Am. J. Clin. Nutr.* 54:471–477, 1991.

34. Deurenberg, P., K. van der Kooij, P. Evers, and T. Hulshof. Is an adaptation of Siri's formula for the calculation of body fat percentage from body density in the elderly necessary? *Eur. J Clin. Nutr.* 43:559–567, 1989.

35. Deurenberg, P., K. van der Kooij, P. Evers, and T. Hulshof. Assessment of body composition by bioelectric impedance in a population aged >60 yr. *Am. J. Clin. Nutr.* 51:3–6, 1990.

36. Durnin, J. V. G. A., and J. Womersley. Body fat assessed from total body density and its estimation from skinfold thickness: measurements on 481 men and women aged from 16 to 72 yr. *Br. J. Nutr.* 32:77–97, 1974.

37. Ellis, K. J. Reference man and woman more fully characterized: Variations on the basis of body size, age, sex and race. *Biol. Trace Elem. Res.* 26–27:385–400, 1990.

38. Enzi, G., M. Gasparo, P. R. Biondetti, D. Fiore, M. Semisa, and F. Zurlo. Subcutaneous and visceral fat distribution according to sex, age, and overweight, evaluated by computed tomography. *Am. J. Clin. Nutr.* 44:739–746, 1986.

39. Fiatarone, M. A., E. C. Marks, N. D. Ryan, C. N. Meredith, L. A. Lipsitz, and W. J. Evans. High-intensity strength training in nonagenarians. *JAMA* 263:3029–3034, 1990.

40. Fidanza, F. A., A. Keys, and J. T. Anderson. Density of body fat in man and other animals. *J. Appl. Physiol.* 6:252–56, 1953.

41. Flynn, M. A., G. B. Nolph, A. S. Baker, and G. Krause. Aging in humans: A continuous 20-yr study of physiologic and dietary parameters. *J. Am. Coll. Nutr.* 11:660–672, 1992.

42. Flynn, M. A., G. B. Nolph, A. S. Baker, W. M. Martin, and G. Krause. Total body potassium in aging humans: a longitudinal study. *Am. J. Clin. Nutr.* 50:713–717, 1989.

43. Forbes, G. B. The adult decline in lean body mass. *Hum. Biol.* 48:161, 1976.

44. Forbes, G. B. *Human Body Composition: Growth, Aging, Nutrition and Activity.* New York: Springer-Verlag, 1987.

45. Forbes, G. B. Exercise and lean weight: the influence of body weight. *Nutr. Rev.* 50:157–161, 1992.

46. Forbes, G. B., A. R. Cooper, and H. H. Mitchell. The composition of the adult human body as determined by chemical analysis. *J. Biol. Chem.* 203:359–366, 1953.

47. Forbes, G. B., J. Gallup, and J. B. Hursh. Estimation of total body fat from potassium-forty content. *Science* 133:101–102, 1961.

48. Forbes, G. B., H. H. Mitchell, and A. R. Cooper. Further studies on the gross composition and mineral elements of the adult human body. *J. Biol. Chem.* 223:969, 1956.

49. Forbes, G. B., and J. C. Reina. Adult lean body mass declines with age: some longitudinal observations. *Metabolism* 9:653–663, 1970.

50. Friedl, K. E., J. P. DeLuca, L. J. Marchitelli, and J. A. Vogel. Reliability of body-fat estimations from a four-compartment model by using density, body water, and bone mineral measurements. *Am. J. Clin. Nutr.* 55:764–70, 1992.

51. Frontera, W. R., V. A. Hughes, K. J. Lutz, and W. J. Evans. A cross-sectional study of muscle strength and mass in 45 to 78 yr old men and women. *J. Appl. Physiol.* 71:644, 1991.

52. Fulop, T. Jr., I. Worum, J. Csongor, G. Foris, and A. Leovey. Body composition in elderly people. I. Determination of body composition by multiisotope methods and the elimination kinetics of these isotopes in healthy elderly subjects. *J. Gerontol.* 31:6–14, 1985.

53. Garn, S. M., C. G. Rohman, and P. Nolan, Jr. The developmental nature of bone changes during aging. JE Birren (ed). *Relations of Development and Aging.* Springfield, CT: Charles C Thomas, 1966.

54. Going, S. B., D. P. Williams, T. G. Lohman, and M. J. Hewitt. Aging, body composition, and physical activity: a review. *J. Aging Phys. Activity* 2:38–66, 1994.

55. Goran, M. I., and E. T. Poehlmann. Total energy expenditure and energy requirements in healthy elderly persons. *Metabolism* 41:744–753, 1992.

56. Grahame, R. A method for measuring human skin elasticity in vivo with observations on the effects of age, sex and pregnancy. *Clin. Sci.* 39:223–238, 1970.

57. Haarbo, J., U. Marslew, A. Gotfredsen, and C. Christiansen. Postmenopausal hormone replacement therapy prevents central distribution of body fat after menopause. *Metabolism* 40:1323–1326, 1991.

58. Hagberg, J. M., D. R. Seals, J. E. Yerg, et al. Metabolic responses to exercise in young and older athletes and sedentary men. *J. Appl. Physiol.* 65:900–908, 1988.

59. Hallfrisch, J., D. Muller, D. Drinkwater, J. Tobin, and R. Andres. Continuing diet trends in men: the Baltimore longitudinal study of aging (1961–1987). *J. Gerontol.* 45:M186–M191, 1990.

60. Hamdorf, P. A., R. T. Withers, R. K. Penhall, and J. L. Plummer. A follow-up study on the effects of training on the fitness and habitual activity patterns of 60- to 70- yr-old women. *Arch. Phys. Med. Rehabil.* 74:473–477, 1993.

61. Hankin, M. E., K. Munz and A. W. Steinbeck. Total body water content in normal and obese subjects. *Med. J. Australia* 2:533, 1976

62. Hansen, N. J., T. G. Lohman, S. B. Going, et al. Prediction of body composition in premenopausal females from dual-energy x-ray absorptiometry. *J. Appl. Physiol.* 75:1637–1641, 1993.

63. Heitmann, B. L. The effects of gender and age on associations between blood lipid levels and obesity in Danish men and women aged 35–65 yr. *J. Clin. Epidemiol.* 45:693–702, 1992.
64. Hertzog K. P., S. M. Garn and H. O. Hempy. Partitioning the effects of secular trend and aging on adult stature. *Am. J. Phys. Anthropol.* 31:111, 1969.
65. Hewitt, M. J., S. B. Going, D. P. Williams, and T. G. Lohman. Hydration of the fat-free mass in pre-pubescent children, young adults and older adults: Implications for body composition assessment. *Am. J. Physiol.* 265:E88–E95, 1993.
66. Heymsfield, S. B., Lichtman S, Baumgartner RN, et al. Body composition of humans: comparison of two improved four-compartment models that differ in expense, technical complexity, and radiation exposure. *Am. J. Clin. Nutr.* 52:52–58, 1990.
67. Heymsfield, S. B., and W. Waki. Body composition in humans: advances in the develop of multicompartment chemical models. *Nutr. Rev.* 49:97–108, 1991.
68. Heymsfield, S. B., J. Wang, S. Lichtman, Y. Kamen, J. Kehayias, and R. N. Pierson. Body composition in elderly subjects: a critical appraisal of clinical methodology. *Am. J. Clin. Nutr.* 50:1167–1175, 1989.
69. Heymsfield, S. B., Z. Wang, R. N. Baumgartner, F. A. Dilmanian, R. Ma, and S. Yasumura. Body Composition and aging: a study by in vivo neutron activation analysis. *J. Nutr.* 13:432–437, 1993.
70. Hoffman, N. Diet in the elderly. Needs and risks. *Med. Clin. North Am.* 77:745–756, 1993.
71. Huddleston, A. L., Rockwell, D., Kulund, D. N., and Harrison, R. B. Bone mass in lifetime athletes. *JAMA* 244:1107–1109, 1980.
72. Jackson, A. S., and M. L. Pollock. Practical assessment of body composition. *Physician Sports Med.* 13:76–90, 1985.
73. Jakicic, J. M., J. E. Donnelly, A. F. Jawad, D. J. Jacobsen, S. C. Gunderson, and R. Pascale. Association between blood lipids and different measures of body fat distribution: effects of BMI and age. *Int. J. Obesity* 17:131–137, 1993.
74. Johnson, R. K., M. I. Goran, and E. T. Poehlman. Correlates of over- and underreporting of energy intake in healthy older men and women. *Am. J. Clin. Nutr.* 59:1286–1290, 1994.
75. Keys A, and J. Brozek. Body fat in adult man. *Physiol Rev* 33:245–325, 1953.
76. Keys, A., H. L. Taylor, and F. Grande. Basal metabolism and age of adult man. *Metabolism* 22:579–587, 1973.
77. Knight, G. S., A. H. Beddoe, S. J. Streat, and G. L. Hill. Body composition of two human cadavers by neutron activation and chemical analysis. *Am. J. Physiol.* 250:E179–185, 1986.
78. Kohrt, W. M., M. T. Malley, G. P. Dalsky, and J. O. Holloszy. Body composition of healthy sedentary and trained, young and older men and women. *Med. Sci. Sports Exerc.* 24:832–837, 1993.
79. Krolner, B., Nielsen, and S. Pors. Bone mineral in the lumbar spine in normal and osteoporotic women: cross-sectional and longitudinal studies. *Clin. Sci.* 62:329–336, 1982.
80. Kuczmarski, R. J. Need for body composition information in elderly subjects. *Am. J. Clin. Nutr.* 50:1150–1157, 1989.
81. Larsson, B., P. Renstrom, K. Svardsudd, et al. Health and aging characteristics of highly physically active 65-yr old men. *Eur. Heart J.* 5(Suppl. E):31–35, 1984.
82. Lesser, G. T., and J. Markofsky. Body water compartments with human aging using fat-free mass as the reference standard. *Am. J. Physiol.* 236:R215–220, 1979.
83. Ley, C. J., B. Lees, and J. C. Stevenson. Sex- and menopause-associated changes in body-fat distribution. *Am. J. Clin. Nutr.* 55:950–954, 1992.
84. Lichtman, S. W., K. Pisarka, E. R. Berman, et al. Discrepancy between self-reported and actual caloric intake and exercise in obese subjects. *N. Engl. J. Med.* 327:1893–1898, 1992.
85. Lohman, T. G. Dual energy x-ray absoptiometry. Roche, A., T. G. Lohman, S. B. Heymsfield, (eds). *Body Composition Methods: A Reference Manual.* Champaign, IL: Human Kinetics, in press.
86. Lohman, T. G. *Advances in Body Composition Assessment.* Champaign, IL: Human Kinetics, 1992.

87. Lohman, T. G., and S. B. Going. Multicomponent models in body composition research: opportunities and pitfalls. K. J. Ellis and J. D. Eastman (eds). *Human Body Composition: In Vivo Methods, Models and Assessment.* New York: Plenum Press, 1993, pp. 53–58.

88. Lohman, T. G., S. B. Going, R. W. Pamenter, et al. Effects of resistance training on regional and total bone mineral density in premenopausal women: a randomized, prospective study. *J. Bone Mineral Res.* in press.

89. *Lunar DPX Technical Manual.* Madison, WI: Lunar Corporation, 1992.

90. Luthi, J. M., H. Howald, H. Claasen, K. Rosler, P. Vock, and H. Hoppeler. Structural changes in skeletal muscle tissue with heavy-resistance exercise. *Int. J. Sports Med.* 7:123–127, 1986.

91. Marcus, R. J. Kosek, A., Pfefferbaum, and Horning S. Age-related loss of trabecular bone in premenopausal women: a biopsy study. *Calcif. Tissue Int.* 35:406–409, 1983.

92. Martin, A. D., and D. T. Drinkwater. Variability in the measures of body fat, assumptions, or technique. *Sports Med.* 5:277–288, 1991.

93. Martin, A. D., W. D. Ross, D. T. Drinkwater, and J. P. Clarys. Prediction of body fat by skinfold caliper. Assumptions and cadaver evidence. *Int. J. Obesity* 9(Suppl. 1): 31–39, 1985.

94. Mazess R. B. On aging bone loss. *Clin. Orthop. Relat. Res.* 165:239–252, 1982.

95. Mazess, R. B., H. S. Barden, J. P. Bisek, and J. Hanson. Dual-energy x-ray absorptiometry for total body and regional bone-mineral and soft-tissue composition. *Am. J. Clin. Nutr.* 51:1106–1112, 1990.

96. Mazess, R. B., Barden, H. S., Drinka, P. J., Bauwens, S. F., Orwoll, E. S., and Bell, N. H. Influence of age and body weight on spine and femur bone mineral density in U.S. white men. *Bone Mineral* 5:645–652, 1990.

97. Mazess, R. B., H. S. Barden, M. Ettinger, et al. Spine and femur density using dual-photon absorptiometry in US white women. *Bone Mineral* 2:211–219, 1987.

98. Mazess, R. B., and Cameron, J. R. Bone mineral content in normal U.S. whites. Mazess, R. B. (ed). *International Conference on Bone Mineral Measurement* Washington, D.C.: U.S. Government Printing Office, 1974, pp. 228–237.

99. Mazess, R. B., W. W. Peppler, and M. Gibbons. Total body composition by dual photon (^{153}Gd) absorptiometry. *Am. J. Clin. Nutr.* 40:834–839, 1984.

100. McGandy, R. B., C. H. Barrows, A. Spanias, A. Meredith, J. L. Stone, and A. H. Norris. Nutrient intakes and energy expenditure in men of different ages. *J. Gerontol.* 21:581 587, 1966.

101. Mial W. E., M. T. Ashcroft, H. G. Lovell, and F. Moore. A longitudinal study of the decline in adult height with age in two Welsh communities. *Hum. Biol.* 39:445, 1967.

102. Minot, C. S. *The Problem of Age, Growth, and Death.* New York: Putnam, 1908.

103. Mitchell, H. H., T. S. Hamilton, F. R. Steggerda, and H. W. Bean. The chemical composition of the adult human body and its bearing on the biochemistry of growth. *J. Biol. Chem.* 158:625–637, 1945.

104. Montoye, H. J., E. L. Smith, D. F. Fardon, and E. T. Howley. Bone mineral in senior tennis players. *Scand. J. Sport Sci.* 2:26–32, 1980.

105. Moore, F. D., K. O. Olesen, J. D. McMurrey, H. V. Parker, M. R. Ball, and C. M. Boyden. *The Body Cell Mass and Its Supporting Environment.* Philadelphia: WB Saunders, 1963.

106. Morey, M. C., P. A. Cowper, J. R. Feussner, et al. Evaluation of a supervised exercise program in a geriatric population. *J. Am. Geriatr. Soc.* 37:348–354, 1989.

107. Muller, D. C., D. Elahi, R. E. Pratley, J. D. Tobin, and R. Andres. An epidemiological test of the hyperinsulinemia-hypertension hypothesis. *J. Clin. Endocrinol. Metab.* 76:544–548, 1993.

108. Najjar, M. F., and M. Rowland. *Anthropometric Reference Data and Prevalence of Overweight* Rockville, MD: National Center for Health Statistics, Vital and Health Statistics Series 11, 1987.

109. Noppa, H., M. Andersson, C. Gengtsson, A. Bruce, and B. Isaksson. Longitudinal studies of anthropometric data and body composition: the population of women in Goteborg, Sweden. *Am. J. Clin. Nutr.* 33:155–162, 1980.

110. Norris, A. H., T. Lundy, and N. W. Shock. Trends in selected indices of body composition in men between the ages of 30 and 80 yr. *Ann. N.Y. Acad. Sci.* 110:623–639, 1963.

111. Pace N. and E. N. Rathbun. Studies on body composition. III. The body water and chemically combined nitrogen content in relation to fat content. *J. Biol. Chem.* 158:685–691, 1945.

112. Pierson, R. N., D. H. Y. Lin, and R. A. Phillips. Total-body potassium in health: effects of age, sex, height, and fat. *Am. J. Physiol.* 226:206, 1974.

113. Pierson, R. N., J. Wang, E. W. Colt and P. Neumann. Body composition measurements in normal man: the potassium, sodium, sulfate and tritium spaces in 58 adults. *J Chronic Dis.* 35:419–428, 1982

114. Pierson, R. N., J. Wang, J. C. Thornton, T. B. Van Itallic, and E. W. D. Colt. Body potassium by four-pi ^{40}K counting: an anthropometric correction. *Am. J. Physiol.* 245:F234–239, 1984.

115. Poehlman, E. T., and E. Danforth. Endurance training increases metabolic rate and norepinephrine appearance rate in older individuals. *Am. J. Physiol.* 261:E233–E239, 1991.

116. Poehlman, E. T., A. W. Gardner, P. J. Arciero, M. I. Goran, and J. Calles-Escandon. Effects of endurance training on total fat oxidation in elderly persons. *J. Appl. Physiol.* 76:2281–2287, 1994.

117. Poehlman, E. T., and E. S. Horton. Regulation of energy expenditure in aging humans. *Annu. Rev. Nutr.* 10:255–275, 1990.

118. Poehlman, E. T., T. L. McAuliffe, D. R. Van Houten, and E. Danforth, Jr. Influence of age and endurance training on metabolic rate and hormones in healthy men. *Am. J. Physiol.* 259:E66–E72, 1990.

119. Pollock, M. L., C. Foster, D. Knapp, J. L. Rod, and D. H. Schmidt. Effect of age and training on aerobic capacity and body composition of master athletes. *J. Appl. Physiol.* 62:725–731, 1987.

120. Pratley, R., B. Nicklas, M. Rubin, et al. Strength training increases resting metabolic rate and norepinephrine levels in healthy 50- to 65-yr-old men. *J. Appl. Physiol.* 76:133–137, 1994.

121. Pruitt, L. A., R. D. Jackson, R. L. Bartels and H. J. Lehnhard. Weight-training effects on bone mineral density in early postmenopausal women. *J. Bone Mineral Res.* 7:179–185, 1992.

122. Reaven, P. D., J. B. McPhillips, E. L. Barrett-Connor, and M. H. Criqui. Leisure time exercise and lipid and lipoprotein levels in an older population. *J. Am. Geriatr. Soc.* 38:847–854, 1990.

123. Rico, H., M. Revilla, L. F. Villa, D. Ruiz-Contreras, E. R. Hernandez, and M. Alvarez de Buergo. The four-compartment models in body composition: Data from a study with dual-energy x-ray absorptiometry and near-infrared interactance on 815 normal subjects. *Metabolism* 43:417–422, 1994.

124. Rico, H., M. Revilla, R. Hernandez, J. M. Gonzalez-Riola, and L. F. Villa. Four-compartment model of body composition of normal elderly women. *Age Ageing* 22:265–268, 1993.

125. Riggs, B. L., H. W. Wahner, W. L. Dann, R. B. Mazess, and K. P. Offord. Differential changes in bone mineral density of the appendicular and axial skeleton with aging. *J. Clin. Invest.* 67:328–335, 1981.

126. Riggs, B. L., H. W. Wahner, L. J. Melton III, L. S. Richelson, H. L. Judd, and K. P. Offord. Rates of bone loss in the appendicular and axial skeletons of women: evidence of substantial vertebral bone loss before menopause. *J. Clin. Invest.* 7:1487–1491, 1986.

127. Rockwell, J. C., A. M. Sorensen, S. Baker, D. Leahey, J. L. Stock, J. Michaels, J., and D. T. Baran. Weight training decreases vertebral bone density in premenopausal women: a prospective study. *J. Clin. Endocrinol. Metab.* 71:988–992, 1990.

128. Roubenoff, R., J. J. Kehayias, B. Dawson-Hughes, and S. B. Heymsfield. Use of dual-energy x-ray absorptiometry in body composition studies: not yet a "gold standard." *Am. J. Clin. Nutr.* 58:589–591, 1993.

129. Schoeller DA. Changes in total body water with age. *Am. J. Clin. Nutr.* 50(Suppl.): 1176–1181, 1989.

130. Schoenborn, C. A. Health habits of US adults: the "Alameda 7" revisited. *Public Health Rep.* 101:571–580, 1986.

131. Schwartz, R. S., W. P. Shuman, V. L. Bradbury, et al. Body fat distribution in healthy young and older men. *J. Gerontol.* 45:M181–M185, 1990.

132. Schwartz, R. S., W. P. Shuman, V. Larson, et al. The effect of intensive endurance exercise training on body fat distribution in young and older men. *Metabolism* 40:545–551, 1991.

133. Seidell, J. C., A. Oosterlee, M. A. O. Thijssen, et al. Assessment of intraabdominal and subcutaneous abdominal fat: relation between anthropometry and computed tomography. *Am. J. Clin. Nutr.* 45:7–13, 1987.

134. Sheng, H. P., and R. A. Huggins. A review of body composition studies with emphasis on total body water and fat. *Am. J. Clin. Nutr.* 32:630–647, 1979.

135. Shephard, R. J., P. R. Kofsky, J. E. Harrison, K. G. McNeill, and A. Krondl. Body composition of older female subjects: new approaches and their limitations. *Hum. Biol.* 57:671–686, 1985.

136. Shimokata, H., R. Andres, P. J. Coon, D. Elahi, D. C. Muller, and J. D. Tobin. Studies in the distribution of body fat. II. Longitudinal effects of change in weight. *Int. J. Obes.* 13:455–464, 1988.

137. Shock, N. W., D. M. Watkin, and M. J. Yiengst. Age differences in the water content of the body as related to basal oxygen consumption in males. *J. Gerontol.* 18:1–8, 1963.

138. Silver, A. J., C. P. Guillen, M. J. Kahl, and J. E. Morley. Effect of aging on body fat. *J. Am. Geriatr. Soc.* 41:211–213, 1993.

139. Siri, W. E. The gross composition of the body. *Adv. Biol. Med. Physiol.* 4:239–280, 1956.

140. Siri, W. E. Body composition from fluid spaces and density: Analysis of methods. J. Brozek and A. Henschel (eds). *Techniques for Measuring Body Composition*. Washington, DC: National Academy of Science, 1961, pp. 223–244.

141. Smith, E. L., and S. W. Babcock. Effects of physical activity on bone loss in the aged. *Med. Sci. Sports* 5:68, 1973.

142. Smith, E. L., and W. G. Reddan. The effects of physical activity on bone in the aged. (1975). *Med. Sci. Sports* 7:84, 1975.

143. Smith, E. L., W. Reddan, and P. E. Smith. Physical activity and calcium modalities for bone mineral increase in aged women. *Med. Sci. Sports* 13:60–64, 1981.

144. Snead, D. B., S. J. Birge, and W. M. Kohrt. Age-related differences in body composition by hydrodensitometry and dual-energy X-ray absorptiometry. *J. Appl. Physiol.* 74:770–775, 1993.

145. Snow-Harter, C., and Marcus, R. Exercise, bone mineral density, and osteoporosis. *Exerc. Sport Sci. Rev.* 19:351–388, 1991.

146. Snyder, W. S., M. J. Cook, E. S. Nasset, L. R. Karhausen, G. P. Howels, and I. H. Tipton. *Report of the task group on reference man.* Oxford: Pergamon Press, 1984.

147. Sönnichsen, A. C., W. O. Richter, and P. Schwandt. Body fat distribution and serum lipoproteins in relation to age and body weight. *Clin. Chim. Acta* 202:133–140, 1991.

148. Steen, B. Body composition and aging. *Nutr. Rev.* 46:45–51, 1988.

149. Steen, B. Obesity in the aged. R. R. Watson (ed). *Handbook of Nutrition in the Aged, 2nd Ed.* Boca Raton, FL: CRC Press, 1994, pp. 3–10.

150. Steen, G. B., B. Isaksson, and A. Svanberg. Body composition at 70 and 75 yr of age: a longitudinal population study. *J. Clin. Exp. Gerontol.* 1:185–200, 1979.

151. Steen, B, B. K. Lundgren, and B. Isaksson. Body composition at age 70, 75, 79 and 81. A longitudinal population study. R. K. Chandra (ed). *Nutrition, Immunity, and Illness in the Elderly.* New York: Pergamon Press, 1985, pp. 49–52.

152. Stevens, J., R. G. Knapp, J. E. Keil, and R. R. Verdugo. Changes in body weight and girths in black and white adults studied over a 25 yr interval. *Int. J. Obes.* 15:803–808, 1991.

153. Svendsen, O. L., J. Haarbo, B. L. Heitmann, A. Gotfredsen, and C. Christiansen. Measurement of body fat in elderly subjects by dual-energy x-ray absorptiometry, bioelectrical impedance, and anthropometry. *Am. J. Clin. Nutr.* 53:1117–1123, 1991.
154. Svendsen, O. L., C. Hassager, I. Bergmann, and C. Christiansen. Measurement of abdominal and intra-abdominal fat in postmenopausal women by dual energy x-ray absorptiometry and anthropometry: comparison with computed tomography. *Int. J. Obes.* 17:45–51, 1993.
155. Trotter, M., G. E. Broman, and R. P. Peterson. Densities of bone of white and negro skeletons. *J. Bone Joint Surg.* 42:A58, 1960.
156. Trotter, M., and R. R. Petterson. Ash weight of human skeletons in percent of their dry, fat-free weight. *Anatomical Record* 23:341–358, 1955.
157. Tzankoff, S. P., and A. H. Norris. Longitudinal changes in basal metabolism in man. *J. Appl. Physiol.* 43:1001–1006, 1977.
158. Voorips, L. E., W. A. van Staveren, and J. G. A. J. Hautvast. Are physically active elderly women in a better nutritional condition than their sedentary peers? *Eur. J. Clin. Nutr.* 45:545–552, 1991.
159. Wang, J., S. B. Heymsfield, M. Aulet, J. C. Thorton, and R. N. Pierson. Body fat from body density: underwater weighing versus dual photon absorptiometry. *Am. J. Physiol.* 256:E829, 1989.
160. Wang, Z. M., R. N. Pierson, and S. B. Heymsfield. The five-level model: a new approach to organizing body-composition research. *Am. J. Clin. Nutr.* 56:19–28, 1992.
161. Watson, P. E., I. D. Watson, and R. D. Batt. Total body water volumes for adult males and females estimated from simple anthropometric measurements. *Am. J. Clin. Nutr.* 33:27–39, 1980.
162. Weits, T., E. J. van der Beek, M. Wedel, and B. M. ter haar Romeny. Computed tomography measurement of abdominal fat deposition in relation to anthropometry. *Int. J. Obes.* 12:217–225, 1987.
163. Weredin E. J. and L. H. Kyle. Estimation of the constancy of the density of fat-free body. *J. Clin. Invest.* 39:626–629, 1960.
164. White, M. K., R. B. Martin, R. A. Yeater, et al. The effects of exercise on the bones of postmenopausal women. *Int. Orthop.* 7:209–214, 1984.
165. Widdowson, E. M., R. A. McCance, and C. M. Spray. The chemical composition of the human body. *Clin. Sci.* 10:113–125, 1951.
166. Williams, D. P., S. B. Going, T. G. Lohman, M. J. Hewitt and A. E. Haber. Estimation of body fat from skinfold thicknesses in middle-aged and older men and women: a multiple component approach. *Am. J. Hum. Biol.* 4:595–605, 1992.
167. Williams, D. P., S. B. Going, L. A. Milliken, M. C. Hall, and T. G. Lohman. Practical techniques for assessing body composition in middle-aged and older adults. *Med. Sci. Sports Exerc.* 1994, in press.
168. Williams, D. P., S. B. Going, M. P. Massett, T. G. Lohman, L. A. Bare, andd M. J. Hewitt. Aqueous and mineral fractions of the fat-free body and their relation to body fat estimates in men and women aged 49–82 yr. K. J. Ellis and J. D. Eastman (eds). *Human Body Composition: In Vivo Methods, Models and Assessment.* New York: Plenum Press, 1993, pp. 109–113.
169. Williams, J. A., J. Wagner, R., Wasnich, et al. The effect of long-distance running upon appendicular bone mineral content. *Med. Sci. Sports Exerc. 16,* 223–227, 1984.
170. Womersley, J., J. V. G. A. Durnin, K. Boddy, and M. Mohoffy. Influence of muscular development, obesity and age on the fat-free mass of adults. *J. Appl. Physiol.* 41:223, 1976.
171. Yearick, E. S. Nutritional status of the elderly: anthropometric and clinical findings. *J. Gerontol.* 33:657–662, 1978.
172. Yiengst, M. J., C. H. Barrows, Jr., and N. W. Shock. Age changes in the chemical composition of muscle and liver in the rat. *J. Gerontol.* 14:400–404, 1959.
173. Young, C. M., J. Blondin, R. Tensuan, and J. H. Fryer. Body composition of "older" women. *J. Am. Diet Assoc.* 43:344–348, 1963.

15
Effects of Diving and Hyperbaria on Responses to Exercise*

KEIZO SHIRAKI, M.D., Ph.D.
JOHN R. CLAYBAUGH, Ph.D.

Humans exercising in water and the hyperbaric environment encounter several problems that differ from exercise in air, including (a) increased thermal conductivity; (b) reduced gravity, which induces redistribution of the body fluid; and (c) hydrostatic pressure. The hydrostatic pressure per se affects the human body during underwater exercise by changing physiological function of respiration (increased respiratory resistance and hypoxia) and circulation (increased vasomotor tone). Pressure also reduces the suit insulation and decreases the protective value of heat loss through the skin surface in cold water.

In relatively shallow dives, air can be breathed, but the diver is subjected to increasing partial pressures of oxygen and nitrogen as the depth increases. To achieve deeper dives, the composition of the ambient gases has to be altered to prevent harmful effects of too much oxygen and nitrogen narcosis. Lowering of these gas percentages with the addition of another gas, usually helium, alters the gas density and adds the unique effects of the specific gas including a modification of thermal balance of the body. The investigation of human workload tolerance and response to hyperbaria follows a historical course of the incorporation of these gas adjustments to the hyperbaric environment. Thus, earlier studies dealt considerably with the effects of hyperoxia and the potential for increased work tolerance, which remains an area of interest, whereas later studies have become more involved with sorting out the effects of increased oxygen and nitrogen, and of hydrostatic pressure per se. Only recently have other responses to exercise, specifically water and electrolyte and hormonal studies, been addressed.

THERMAL ASPECTS OF UNDERWATER EXERCISE

Water conducts heat from the human body about 25 times faster than air, and the heat capacity of water (density times specific heat) exceeds that of

---

*The opinions and assertions contained herein are the private views of the authors and are not to be construed as official or as reflecting the views of the Department of the Army or Department of Defense.

air by approximately 3,500 times. Because of these physical characteristics, human thermoregulatory mechanisms are incapable of preventing a decrease in internal body temperature during prolonged cold water exposure without additional insulation.

Traditionally, passive thermal insulation for the diver has taken one of two forms: thermal underwear covered by a dry suit, or a closed-cell foam-rubber wet suit. Dry suits usually provide satisfactory thermal protection for most cold water diving situations, but they often limit the diver's mobility and are subject to leakage. Wet suits provide greater mobility and adequate thermal protection for shallow and short cold water dives. However, the closed-cell foam is compressed significantly as hydrostatic pressure increases, resulting in a loss of insulation value at depth [48]. Therefore, a design for both dry and wet suits with effective thermal protection should be a high priority for divers' safety. It is also important to understand human heat exchanges and physiological defense mechanisms during cold water exposure.

The critical water temperature (defined as the temperature at which the tissue insulation becomes maximum due to maximal vasoconstriction) has been determined in human subjects with or without wet suits at various pressures. The effect of exercise on thermal balance at various water temperatures and pressures has also been determined. These studies indicate that humans in cool water are capable of maintaining body temperature to a certain extent by adjustment of the blood flow distribution between the proximal and distal parts of the body.

Basics of Thermoregulation

In normal humans, fluctuations of core body temperature are relatively slow and small in the face of large alterations in environmental temperature. By comparison, skin temperature varies more rapidly and widely with the environmental temperature. Body temperature represents a balance between heat production and heat dissipation. Heat loss in humans occurs mainly through the skin and partly through the respiratory tract. Heat loss through the skin occurs mostly by radiation, convection, and evaporation. However, the relative amounts of heat loss through these three pathways vary with environmental conditions. When a person is seated in a room of moderate temperature, both radiation and convection account for about 77% of total heat loss, and evaporation accounts for the remainder of total heat loss [19].

The range of ambient temperature between 28°C and 31°C is considered as the zone of vasomotor regulation of body temperature in an unclothed person, and this range is termed thermoneutral [21]. In this zone heat flux may be altered by changing cutaneous vascular tone, primarily in the limbs, and thermal equilibrium may be maintained without either sweating or increasing metabolism. Thus, skin blood flow is adjusted to control the flow of heat from the core to the periphery. An expression of the delivery of heat from core to surface is called "tissue conductance," and the reciprocal of conductance is defined as "tissue insulation." The lowest value of the zone of vasomotor regulation is called the "critical temperature." Below this temperature, core temperature cannot be maintained without increasing metabolic heat production (shivering). However, convective heat loss increases during shivering because of body movements, leading to increases in conductance and total heat loss.

Thermal Balance in Water

It is well recognized that the human body cools faster in water than in air of the same temperature. This is because the specific heat of water is roughly 1,000 times and thermoconductivity is 25 times greater than air. This direct loss of body heat in water is the dominant thermal problem for divers and, in fact, determines the duration of a diving work shift [36, 37].

HEAT TRANSFER COEFFICIENT OF WATER AND CRITICAL WATER TEMPERATURE. The primary pathways of heat transfer from the body surface to the surrounding water are convection and conduction. The combined heat transfer coefficient for convection and conduction varies from 38 kcal/(m^2·hr·°C) in still water to an average of 55 kcal/(m^2·hr·°C) in stirred water. Shivering in still water raises the heat transfer coefficient from 38 to 43 kcal/(m^2·hr·°C) [4]. According to Rapp [57], the conductive heat transfer coefficient is about 9 kcal/(m^2·hr·°C) regardless of the degree of stirring, whereas the convective heat transfer coefficient increases from 81 kcal/(m^2·hr·°C) in still water to 344 kcal/(m^2·hr·°C) at a swimming speed of 0.5 m/s. These values are 100–200 times higher than those in 1 atmospheres absolute (atm abs) air (1–2 kcal/(m^2·hr·°C)). Despite such marked differences in the convective heat transfer coefficient between air and water environments, the amount of heat loss in water has been estimated to be only about 2–5 times that in air at the same temperature. This indicates that heat loss in water is largely limited by core-to-skin tissue insulation and not by the skin-to-core heat transfer rate.

The range of neutral water temperature for a resting, unprotected man is between 33 and 35°C, and varies inversely with the thickness of subcutaneous fat [14, 66]. Moreover, the critical water temperature, 29–33°C, is also dependent upon the thickness of subcutaneous fat [58] (Fig. 1). Because typical diving water temperature is much lower than this neutral temperature range, it is obvious that divers are usually exposed to considerable cold water stress. Studies conducted on ama divers (professional breath-hold divers) in Japan and Korea [38, 63] demonstrated a loss of approximately 1,000 kcal/day attributable to diving.

PROTECTION BY WET SUITS. When the cold water stress is moderate (water temperature of 25–32°C), it is possible to maintain reasonable thermal equilibrium by increasing heat production with exercise [60]. For instance, a man can maintain his normal body temperature in water of 32°C when he is engaged in continuous underwater work that doubles oxygen consumption (2-met exercise, two-fold resting metabolic rate); and a 3-met exercise

FIGURE 1.

Relationship between critical water temperature and mean subcutaneous fat thickness in U.S. men and women and nondiving Korean men and women. Individual data obtained from unprotected subjects at 1 and 2 atmospheres absolute (atm abs) are also plotted in the figure. Note no pressure-dependent changes in critical water temperature (data from Ref. 24). Areas encompass range of values. Modified from Rennie [58].

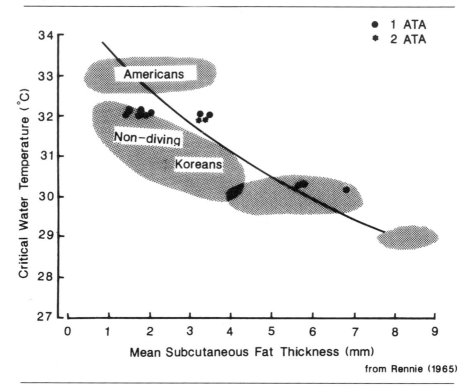

from Rennie (1965)

(three-fold resting metabolic rate) keeps body temperature normal in water temperature of 26°C [13, 60, and see below].

However, as the water temperature decreases below 24°C, heat loss becomes so great that it becomes virtually impossible to maintain thermal balance without wearing protective clothing. The most obvious difference between protected and unprotected divers was noted in the skin temperature (Fig. 2). Figure 2 also indicates changes in the core temperature (esophageal temperature) during immersion with and without protective suits. In all cases, core temperature decreased by the same amount, 0.2°C. However, in the fully protected subjects, the reduction in core temperature did not occur until the second hour. Wearing the jacket alone, the rate of fall in core temperature was about one-half of that observed without protection. In both experiments, the subject with the suit felt comfortable until the end of the 2-hour immersion [15].

Should One Exercise in Cold Water to Retard the Fall in Body Temperature?

WORK INTENSITY. Many factors have been reported to influence the rate at which people cool when they are immersed in cold water. These include subcutaneous fat thickness, surface area-to-mass ratio, and physical exercise [5, 8, 16, 39, 56]. The role of exercise, however, remains controversial. Several authors [7, 29, 40] have reported that exercise accelerates the rate of fall of core temperature, as compared with that seen during rest in cold

FIGURE 2.

Changes in the esophageal (Tes) and mean skin temperatures during immersion in water of 24°C with and without wet suits. Adapted from Craig and Dvorak [15].

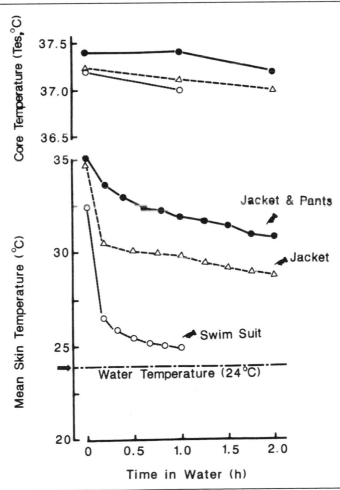

water. More specifically, Keatinge [41] reported that this is the case for water temperatures below 25°C. However, other investigators [12, 16, 47, 51] suggest that the intensity of exercise also influences core temperature response to cold water immersion; in fact, the performance of heavy exercise during immersion in water of 17–24°C can reduce the rate of fall of core temperature as compared with that observed during static immersion. Interestingly, the type of physical exercise also plays a role in determining core temperature response to cold water immersion. For instance, Toner et al. [70, 71] have reported that leg exercise is more effective than whole-body exercise in maintaining the esophageal temperature in water as cold as 18°C.

It thus appears that core temperature of humans immersed in water is determined by several factors such as exercise (intensity and type), subcutaneous fat thickness, and duration of immersion. Therefore, from the physiological point of view, it is important to establish the relationship between water temperature and the work intensity required to keep core body temperature unchanged in water. Sagawa et al. [60] have carried out such experiments in healthy male subjects, in which 30 minutes of rest in water of

FIGURE 3.

Time course of changes in the esophageal temperature at different work levels during immersion in water of critical temperature (31°C). Exercise 1, -2, and -3 refer to mean intensity of exercise at 2, 3, and 4 met, respectively.

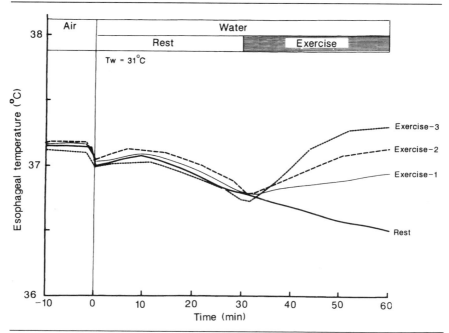

FIGURE 4.

Cumulative heat storage during rest and exercise in water of various temperatures. Adapted from Sagawa et al. [60].

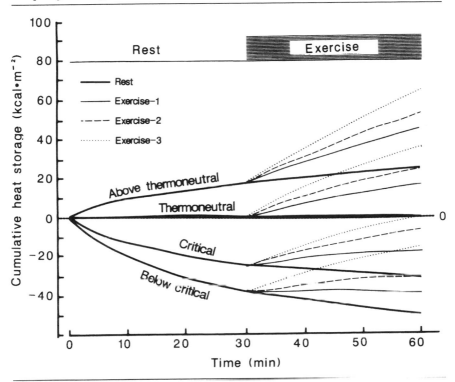

different temperatures was followed by a series of graded leg exercises (from 2 to 4 met) for 30 minutes. Four different water temperatures were used: (a) 2°C below critical water temperature (29°C), (b) critical water temperature (31°C), (c) thermoneutrality (34°C), and (d) 2°C above thermoneutrality (36°C). Figure 3 illustrates typical effects of leg exercise on core temperature (esophageal) at critical water temperature. During rest in water, esophageal temperature gradually decreased with time. However, during exercise, esophageal temperature increased to a higher level than at rest, and this rise in core temperature was in proportion to the work intensity. The time course of cumulative heat storage in water is shown in Figure 4. During the 30-minute rest period, cumulative heat storage was nearly eliminated at thermoneutrality, whereas it increased at above thermoneutrality, and decreased at below thermoneutrality. Leg exercise increased cumulative heat storage at all water temperatures, indicating that heat production during underwater exercise exceeds heat loss into the water. These results support the notion that leg exercise is effective in maintaining core temperature during cold water exposure, and the intensity of exercise should increase as water temperature decreases. In practice, work intensity more than 200 kcal/m²/hr (about 4 met) cannot be continued for a long period of time in water. The lowest water temperature in which humans can maintain body temperature with 4-met exercise is around 25°C, in agreement with the report of Keatinge [40].

Thus, 25°C may be the lowest water temperature in which an average unprotected person can continue to exercise without lowering core temperature, and is defined as "crucial water temperature." Below it, body temperature will continue to decrease even with continuous exercise. In contrast, the unprotected male ama of Japan lower their core body temperature in water of 27°C during diving with a metabolic heat production of 200 kcal·m⁻²·hr⁻¹ (4 met) for 1 hour [63]. This water temperature of 27°C is higher than the crucial water temperature of 25°C (see above). This disparity may be attributable to the fact that ama divers use both legs and arms during diving work. This type of exercise may accelerate body heat loss and lower body temperature, as reported by others [70]. Therefore the type of exercise in water is no doubt an important factor that modifies heat loss from the body (see below).

The finding that core temperature falls at a faster rate during static immersion [60] conflicts with earlier works [7, 29], because these latter authors concluded that exercise had an adverse effect on body heat conservation through increased whole-body conductance caused by the larger muscle blood flows during exercise and that the increase in heat production due to exercise was less than the increase in body heat loss, except when body insulation was much greater than normal. Their conclusion, however, was based on the observation of subjects engaged in whole body exercise (swimming or rowing) at a fixed intensity.

Classically, a close inverse relationship has been observed between the fall in core temperature and the skinfold thickness of subjects during immersion [8, 16, 56]. Veicsteinas et al. [73] have suggested that in cold water, the vasoconstricted muscle acts in series with fat and skin to provide additional tissue insulation. Rennie [59] has stated that the tissue insulation of resting subjects in cold water is made up of 75% vasoconstricted muscle and 25% subcutaneous fat and skin. During swimming or severe shivering, the "variable" insulation of muscle will be lost because of increased blood perfusion through exercising muscle, leaving only the "fixed" insulation of the subcutaneous fat and skin. If the conclusions of Rennie [59] are correct, then during static cold water immersion, one might expect the fall in core temperature of subjects to be more closely related to body weight (or muscle mass) than to subcutaneous fat thickness. On the other hand, during dynamic cold water immersion, when the variable insulation of muscle is lost, the fall in core temperature should be more closely related to subcutaneous fat thickness than to body weight [27].

TYPE OF EXERCISE. The results of the leg exercise study [60] suggest that the type of exercise is an important factor influencing core body temperature, as indicated by the fact that "leg-only" exercise resulted in smaller falls in core temperature when compared with static immersion [27]. Consideration of the results of the leg exercise [27, 60] and the arm exercise [71] studies suggests that the arms are an important source of heat loss during whole-body exercise in cold water.

Most recognized swimming strokes require a higher level of work from the arms than from the legs. Even at similar levels of work, the arms, because of their smaller muscle mass, will receive relatively higher blood flows per unit weight than the legs. This will result in a delivery by mass flow of more heat to the arms. In other words, the ability of the arms to retain heat is less than that of the legs because the arms have approximately twice the surface area-to-mass ratio of the legs [5] and the conductive pathway from the core to the surface of the limbs is shorter in the arms than in the legs.

SUMMARY. There are several factors that help to determine whether exercise during cold water immersion will accelerate or retard the fall in core temperature. These factors include water temperature, water agitation, fitness and fatness of the person, type of clothing worn (if any), and the intensity of exercise. In addition, the type of exercise performed also appears to be an important factor. Many of these factors interact; a leg exercise, for example, may only help maintain the core temperature when it is performed at high intensity. The number of possible interactions among the factors noted above make it very difficult to give general advice concerning whether or not people should exercise after accidental immersion in cold water.

Regional Heat Loss During Exercise in Water

The critical water temperature is considerably higher than the critical air temperature. Because maximal tissue insulation develops at this temperature [59], it is assumed that maximal vasoconstriction of the limbs and skin may be induced at a higher temperature in water than in air. Sagawa et al. [60] have measured regional body insulation during underwater exercise at various temperatures. They have confirmed that overall body insulation during rest is highest in water at critical temperature and decreases in water that is either colder or warmer than critical temperature. Tissue insulation decreases in water colder than critical temperature, presumably because of shivering and muscle vasodilation, whereas it decreases in warmer water because of an attenuation of vasoconstriction.

As stated above, it is generally agreed that tissue insulation significantly decreases during underwater exercise [53, 59]. As regards regional differences in tissue insulation during underwater exercise, Sagawa et al. [60] have observed that during immersion in water cooler than critical temperature (29°C), trunk insulation is less than that of the limbs. This is probably because of a longer conduction pathway in the limbs, an efficient countercurrent heat exchange in the limbs, and/or the predominance of shivering in the trunk. On the other hand, during immersion in water of neutral (34°C) or warmer (36°C) temperatures, limb insulation decreases more than in the trunk, probably because of an attenuated countercurrent heat exchange in the limbs. These findings of Sagawa et al. [60] are of prime importance because the results indicate that when water temperature is lower than thermoneutrality (<34°C) but above critical temperature, leg exercise facilitates heat loss from the limbs by releasing vasoconstrictor tone in skin vessels rather than by inducing active vasodilation of these regions. By contrast, exercise in water warmer than thermoneutrality (36°C) causes vasodilation in the trunk to facilitate heat loss into the water. This hypothesis is supported by experimental observation of greater increase in heat loss from the limbs than that from the trunk during exercise in water cooler than thermoneutrality. Interestingly, exercise in water cooler than thermoneutrality does not increase heat loss from the trunk as exercise intensity increases. If this observation applies to all dynamic immersions (immersion with exercise), it may be said that exercise-generated heat appears to be preserved more efficiently in the trunk than the limbs and also that the trunk keeps its maximum insulation during muscular exercise as well as at rest in cold water. By contrast, tissue insulation in the limbs is high during rest but decreases as the intensity of leg exercise increases. These findings suggest that most effective protection against heat loss during underwater exercise may be attained by preventing or minimizing heat loss from the limbs.

Thermal Balance in Wet-Suited Divers

SUIT INSULATION. The insulation provided by neoprene wet suits is due to the presence of trapped air [3]. Therefore, the volume of this trapped air, and thus suit insulation, will be inversely proportional to the depth of immersion (hydrostatic pressure). The apparent suit insulation is reduced by approximately 45% at 2 atm abs and 52% at 2.5 atm abs as compared with the one atm abs value [54] (Fig. 5, bottom panel). When this depth-insulation relation is extended to high pressure, suit insulation at 31 atm abs would be almost nil [64]. Fortunately, however, this is not the case in prolonged saturation dives, because the wet suits regain their original thickness in 24 hours by diffusion of environmental gas into the neoprene cells. Thus, the diver is able to perform an excursion dive at 31 atm abs in water of 25°C without encountering major thermal problems (unpublished observation). In a nonsaturation dive, such as a scuba dive, suit insulation decreases curvilinearly as the diving depth increases, and the diver loses heat even if the water temperature is not extremely low [54].

For open-sea divers who wear protective suits to minimize body heat loss, it is important to consider thermal problems associated with the wet, high-pressure environment. It may be said that the optimal thermal protective garment for divers (a) should have an adequate insulative layer that is unaffected by depth, (b) should not be significantly compromised by water

FIGURE 5.

Relationship between pressure and critical water (Tcw), esophageal (Tes) and mean skin (T̄sk) temperatures during immersion at 1, 2, and 2.5 atm abs (top), and mean wet-suit insulation (Isuit), total (tissue plus suits) insulation (Itotal), and mean body tissue insulation (Itissue) during immersion in water of critical temperature at 1, 2, and 2.5 atm abs (bottom). *P<0.05, and **P<0.001 compared with the corresponding value at 1 atm abs. Adapted from Park et al. [54].

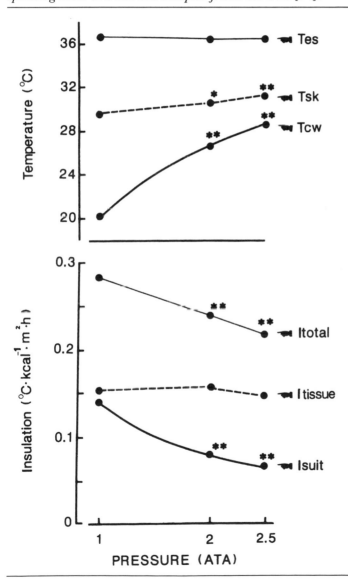

flow, and (c) should be provided with a gas layer that has an insulative value equivalent to that of air at 1 atm abs. For instance, a four-layer 1/4-inch unicellular neoprene foam wet suit at 1 atm abs provides 2.65 clo (0.48°C·kcal-1·m²·hr) of insulation to the diver. (Where clo is a unit of clothing; 1 clo is defined as the amount of insulation which maintains a man comfortable with a metabolic rate of 50 kcal per m² per hour in a room having an air velocity of 0.1 m per second, a temperature of 21°C, and a relative humidity of 50%). This is enough protection to maintain body heat in 5°C water for 5 hours. However, the suit is so bulky and ponderous as to effectively immobilize the diver [3]. Therefore it is necessary to develop an ideal suit that provides insulation equal to that provided by 1-inch-thick unicellular neoprene foam but without limiting mobility. This might be possible by adopting the concept of a rigid pressure suit, as conceived for the lunar landing garment of astronauts and proposed for adaptation to the deep-sea diver [3]. According to this concept, a rigid but maneuverable outer garment would permit divers to stay dry and work in a 1-atm abs air environment while diving in ambient pressures equivalent to many atmospheres.

RESPIRATORY HEAT LOSS. Another potentially critical problem associated with wet saturation dives is related to respiratory heat loss. According to a study conducted by the U.S. Navy, a diver engaged in heavy exercise with an oxygen consumption of 1 liter/min and breathing cold gas (7°C) at 3 atm abs loses 681 W through the respiratory system, which represents 65% of metabolic heat production [31]. At 31 atm abs, about 95% of this respiratory heat loss is from convection, and the rest is via evaporation for humidification of the inspired gas. At 1 atm abs air, however, the convective component accounts for only about 10% of the respiratory heat loss [49]. The respiratory heat loss of a diver in cold water at depth can lead to a severe negative heat balance. This problem can be eliminated only by heating the breathing gas [55].

CHANGES IN CRITICAL WATER TEMPERATURE AT VARIOUS PRESSURES. It is well established that tissue insulation is at its maximum in water at critical temperature at 1 atm abs; however, it is still not known whether this is also the case in the hyperbaric environment. Accordingly, it is important to know how the critical water temperature changes with depth (or pressure). Once we know the relationship between critical water temperature and depth, we can then determine whether the magnitude of maximum vasoconstriction at depth is the same as that at 1 atm abs. Iwamoto et al. [33] studied the effect of pressure on tissue insulation in unprotected subjects and observed that 2 atm abs pressure neither alters cutaneous vasomotor responses nor changes critical water temperature compared with 1 atm abs. However, Park et al. [54] observed changes in the critical water temperature in subjects wearing wet suits at 2 and 2.5 atm abs in comparison with 1 atm abs, with the average critical water temperature of wet-suited subjects being 22.3, 26.5, and 28.5°C at 1, 2, and 2.5 atm abs, respectively (Fig. 5, top panel). The reduction in wet suit insulation at pressure was exactly compensated for by increasing critical water temperature such that the suit heat loss remained similar at different pressures, resulting in a similar degree of skin cooling. Consequently, the vasomotor control to transfer the internal heat is identical at all pressures. These data clearly indicate that the increase in the critical water temperature of wet-suited subjects at high pressure is a simple consequence of changes in suit insulation and does not involve alterations in physiological mechanisms controlling body heat conservation.

Park et al. [54] also demonstrated that skin temperature in the hard and foot was significantly higher at pressure than at 1 atm abs (24.9, 27.3, and 28.6°C for 1, 2, and 2.5 atm abs, respectively, at the end of a 3-hour immersion). However, in other regions, the skin temperature did not significantly vary with pressure. It is not certain whether distal extremity skin temperature plays an important role in the determination of threshold skin temperature for the shivering response in wet-suited divers.

At present, the available data on critical water temperature at pressure (depth) are limited to a maximum of 2.5 atm abs because of technical difficulties. Measurements of critical water temperature during saturation dives will no doubt provide valuable information regarding the thermoregulatory responses of humans immersed in deeper water.

Regional Heat Loss and Insulation at Various Depths During Rest
A systematic evaluation of regional heat loss and its contribution to overall heat balance in subjects wearing wet suits in various water depths and temperatures is of prime importance. A precise knowledge of regional heat flow in wet-suited divers during cold water operations is required to design optimal protective devices.

Shiraki et al. [65] have measured regional heat exchange during a 3-hour exposure of 9 wet-suited exercising subjects immersed in water of critical temperature at 1, 2, and 2.5 atm abs. They made direct measurements of changes in regional heat loss from the skin (Htissue) and suit surface (Hsuit) concomitantly with core and skin temperatures. From these data, heat loss due to water convection under the suit (Hconv = Htissue − Hsuit) and thermal insulation of the tissue and wet suit have been estimated.

In all cases, large amounts of heat were lost from the whole body during the initial 30–40 minutes of immersion, with the chest losing the most. Later in the immersion period, trunk heat flux remained unchanged as compared with the initial level, but extremity flux declined with time. Suit insulation decreased as pressure increased, but tissue insulation remained virtually constant at all pressures tested (Fig. 5). Convection under the wet suits accounted for 11.5%, 3.6%, and 5.5% of total heat loss at 1, 2, and 2.5 atm abs, respectively. The heat lost by convection was mostly from the chest at all pressures.

Tissue insulation of the trunk increased slightly during the initial 20–40 minutes of immersion, after which it leveled off, whereas that of the limbs

FIGURE 6.

Changes in tissue insulation in various parts of the body during static immersion at critical temperature.

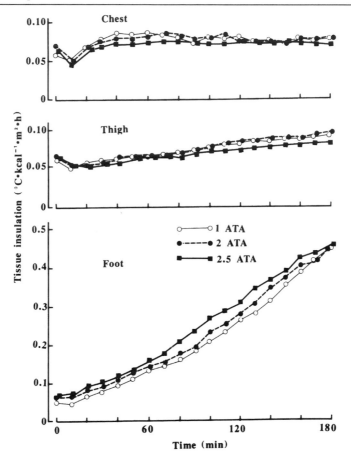

increased progressively over the entire course of immersion (Fig. 6). This indicates that in the wet-suited diver, maximum vasoconstriction is not attained in the limbs within 3 hours in water at critical temperature. In this respect immersion with wet suits is different from that without protection. These data clearly show that the capacity to increase tissue insulation is much greater in the extremities than in the trunk, in agreement with Cannon and Keatinge [7]. Perhaps, for this reason, heat flux can be extensively reduced in the extremities, but not in the trunk, during a prolonged immersion in cold water. Ferretti et al. [25] have observed that in naked subjects immersed in water at critical temperature, tissue heat loss in the limbs levels off after approximately 1 hour, suggesting that tissue insulation is maximal within 1 hour.

Because of the small surface area and extremely high tissue insulation of the hands and feet, heat loss through these regions of the body is relatively small (Table 1). Thus, the use of gloves and boots may have little practical value insofar as total body heat conservation is concerned during cold water immersion. However, the use of gloves is known to block sensory input from cold receptors in the distal extremities, which is particularly important in thermoregulation during immersion in cold water [10]. More studies are needed to define the overall merit of wearing gloves during cold water immersion.

Heat Loss During Exercise in Water of Various Pressures in Protected Divers

It has been reported that exercise greatly reduces the insulation of wet suits in cold water [75, 76]. This phenomenon has been attributed to convective heat flow underneath the wet suit [75] and/or increased effective surface area of the suit [76]. However, there is contradictory data showing that wet suit insulation calculated from directly measured heat flow from the skin and suits changes little during leg exercise in water at critical temperature (Table 2). This disagreement may be attributed to an overestimation [76] of convective heat dissipation from the water layer underneath the suit. In an other earlier report [76], suit insulation was calculated without accounting for the convection caused by the movement of the water layer between the skin and wet suit, leading to an overestimation of suit insulation during exercise.

Even if suit insulation is independent of workload, heat dissipation through the suit should increase in proportion to exercise intensity because the surface temperature gradient between the skin and wet suits becomes greater as the exercise intensity increases. Heat flow through the skin should also increase as work intensity increases in water at critical

TABLE 1

Regional Heat Flow during Static Immersion in Water in Critical Temperature at Different Pressures

	1 atm abs	2 atm abs	2.5 atm abs
Whole body, kcal·h⁻¹	98.6 ± 5.0	85.8 ± 2.7	81.8 ± 4.0
Chest, kcal·h⁻¹	21.1 ± 2.5	15.8 ± 1.0	16.1 ± 1.9
Back, kcal·h⁻¹	17.5 ± 1.0	18.7 ± 1.0	17.7 ± 1.0
Forearm, kcal·h⁻¹	5.8 ± 0.3	4.7 ± 0.3	4.8 ± 0.3
Hand, kcal·h⁻¹	10.4 ± 1.2	6.6 ± 0.4	5.9 ± 0.3
Thigh, kcal·h⁻¹	25.5 ± 1.5	23.8 ± 1.0	23.0 ± 1.5
Calf, kcal·h⁻¹	13.7 ± 0.7	12.3 ± 1.0	11.6 ± 0.6
Foot, kcal·h⁻¹	4.6 ± 0.5	3.8 ± 0.5	2.8 ± 0.3

Values are means ± SE of average values of last 15 minutes of immersion in water of critical temperature. atm abs, atmospheres absolute. Heat flow was calculated by multiplying measured regional heat flow (kcal·m⁻²hr-1) by the surface area (m²) of the corresponding body part.

TABLE 2
Wet Suit Insulation during Exercise in Water of Critical Temperature at Different Pressures

	Rest			2-met Exercise			3-met Exercise		
	1 atm abs	2 atm abs	2.5 atm abs	1 atm abs	2 atm abs	2.5 atm abs	1 atm abs	2 atm abs	2.5 atm abs
Whole body, °C·kcal-1·m²·hr									
	0.141 ±0.005	0.081 ±0.001	0.069 ±0.002	0.133 ±0.002	0.074 ±0.002	0.062 ±0.002	0.135 ±0.003	0.072 ±0.002	0.060 ±0.001
Chest, °C·kcal-1·m²·hr									
	0.228 ±0.032	0.114 ±0.005	0.114 ±0.015	0.252 ±0.022	0.128 ±0.011	0.109 ±0.016	0.231 ±0.023	0.134 ±0.017	0.125 ±0.021
Back, °C·kcal-1·m²·hr									
	0.213 ±0.004	0.117 ±0.005	0.091 ±0.002	0.193 ±0.005	0.111 ±0.004	0.093 ±0.003	0.194 ±0.005	0.111 ±0.003	0.092 ±0.006
Forearm, °C·kcal-1·m²·hr									
	0.110 ±0.003	0.065 ±0.002	0.049 ±0.003	0.099 ±0.003	0.057 ±0.003	0.044 ±0.003	0.106 ±0.006	0.056 ±0.003	0.050 ±0.003
Hand, °C·kcal-1·m²·hr									
	0.121 ±0.005	0.076 ±0.003	0.066 ±0.006	0.120 ±0.004	0.061 ±0.003	0.054 ±0.002	0.120 ±0.003	0.068 ±0.001	0.056 ±0.003
Thigh, °C·kcal-1·m²·hr									
	0.108 ±0.006	0.061 ±0.003	0.057 ±0.002	0.110 ±0.005	0.059 ±0.004	0.047 ±0.003	0.107 ±0.003	0.058 ±0.006	0.049 ±0.003
Calf, °C·kcal-1·m²·hr									
	0.100 ±0.003	0.052 ±0.002	0.041 ±0.002	0.097 ±0.003	0.058 ±0.002	0.043 ±0.002	0.110 ±0.006	0.054 ±0.003	0.043 ±0.003
Foot, °C·kcal-1·m²·hr									
	0.133 ±0.011	0.098 ±0.016	0.076 ±0.011	– –	0.081 ±0.061	0.107 ±0.239	– –	0.070 ±0.145	– –

Values are means ± SE of average values of last 15 minutes of immersion at critical temperature. atm abs, atmospheres absolute.

temperature, and the tissue insulation may decrease in contrast to a constant wet suit insulation. This may indicate that the increment of heat dissipation due to conduction is caused by an increase in temperature gradient between exercising muscle tissue and the skin surface, because blood flow in the skin does not change during exercise of intensity less than 3 met [59]. It is not practical to consider prolonged underwater exercise with work intensity higher than 4 met [60]. Therefore, we may assume that a wet-suited diver exposed to water at critical or below critical temperature is virtually always in a state of maximal vasoconstriction.

Increased heat generation in working muscles without a decrease in suit insulation during underwater exercise would retard the rate of core cooling in the protected diver working in cold deep water. Accordingly, it is suggested that dynamic immersion for wet-suited divers is advantageous for maintaining body temperature at depth as is the case in unprotected divers [60]. In other words, although wet suit insulation decreases as pressure increases, wet suits are thermally analogous to an increased thickness of the fat layer in the diver.

HYPERBARIA-INDUCED BRADYCARDIA AND EXERCISE

Of obvious importance to exercise performance is the ability of the heart to deliver adequate quantities of blood and O_2 to the muscles. Evans [22] cites the early recognition by Heller in 1897 of reduced heart rates in caisson workers exposed to hyperbaria of 2.5–3.6 atm abs, and subsequent studies by Dautrebande and Haldane in 1921 showing that breathing pure oxygen at 1 atm abs or 2 atm abs reduced heart rate. Therefore, it is not surprising that there is general agreement that increased inspired oxygen can play a role in the hyperbaria-induced bradycardia [22, 45].

In addition to hyperoxia, other factors are very important in the reduced heart rate during hyperbaria. These factors affect the heart rate response to exercise at both maximal and submaximal levels (representative data are summarized in Table 1). For instance, an investigation using eight subjects indicated that maintaining oxygen at normal levels, and increasing nitrogen to bring the pressure to 2 and then to 3.0 atm abs, progressively reduced maximal heart rate and oxygen consumption as determined with treadmill exercise [11]. Thus, the reduced maximal heart rate at pressure is probably not due entirely to hyperoxia. Similar conclusions were reached by Fagraeus [24]. He reasoned that if the inspired O_2 was the sole factor in the bradycardia associated with hyperbaria, the heart rate should be equally suppressed at 4.5 atm abs of air breathing compared with breathing 100% oxygen at 1 atm abs. He observed that heart rate was lower while breathing 100% O_2 at 1 atm abs compared with breathing air, but the heart rate was lowered further at 4.5 atm abs. This decrease in heart rate was evident at any given level of oxygen consumption. Similarly, Matsuda et al. [46] found a decrease in heart rate response to a submaximal workload of 500 kilopondmeters (kpm)/min at 7 atm abs where O_2 was 0.3 atm abs, as compared with air breathing at 1.2 atm abs. Thus, oxygen-independent factors that contribute to the hyperbaria-induced bradycardia also reduce the heart rate response to exercise. How these responses impact on the performance of exercise is dependent on the degree of hyperoxia and pressure.

The impact of hyperbaria-induced bradycardia on the ability to do work in this environment requires knowledge of cardiac output during exercise at hyperbaria. It was suggested from the experiments of Cook [11], and now several others (Table 1) that $\dot{V}O_2$max is reduced at hyperbaria. However, whether this is due to reduced O_2 delivery requires more experimentation. When O_2 pulse has been reported [11, 26, 52], it is usually not changed at maximal exercise (Table 1). Therefore, unless stroke volume is increased, maximal O_2 delivery must be compromised in hyperbaric environments because of the bradycardia. Dressendorpher et al. [18] assessed cardiac output by impedance cardiography and determined that despite the significant reduction in heart rate at maximal exercise performed either during slight hyperoxic or normoxic conditions at 18.6 atm abs there was no change in cardiac output. However, these experiments indicated that these subjects showed no decrement in $\dot{V}O_2$max, and a decrement may exist at saturation dives greater than at the 18.6 atm abs pressure they studied, as shown in Table 3.

The magnitude of the decrease in maximal heart rate at hyperbaria is not correlated to the depth of the dive. For instance, the decreases reported by Cook [11] and Fagraeus [24], at 2, 3, and 6 atm abs (see Table 1) were, respectively, average changes of 10, 21, and 9 beats per minute. Anthonisen et al. [1] reported no change in maximal heart rate at 4 and 6 atm abs, and at the deepest dives, heart rates reductions were similar to those at the lower pressures. Specifically, reductions of 8, 17, and 13 beats per minute were reported for the pressures of 18.6, 31, and 37.5 atm abs, respectively. Similarly, the decrements in $\dot{V}O_2$max are not correlated to depth. Of the four studies in Table 1 where average $\dot{V}O_2$max was decreased, the decrease was 5, 32, 13, and 9% with respect to ascending pressures of 3–37.5 atm abs, with no changes reported at pressures of 6–18.6 atm abs. Considering the data available, it would seem that with the exception of shallow dives, where hyperoxia may play a role (see below), $\dot{V}O_2$max either does not change, or with deeper saturation dives it may be slightly decreased. The small differences in $\dot{V}O_2$max between studies are not associated with differences in the composition of the inert gases, i.e., HeO_2 or trimix (1.3% O_2+5% N_2, balance He).

RESPIRATORY RESPONSES TO HYPERBARIA

Hyperbaric Hyperoxia and Exercise
Early studies by Hill et al. [30] showed rather convincingly that maximal oxygen consumption ($\dot{V}O_2$max) would be enhanced by breathing 50% O_2.

TABLE 3

Heart Rate (HR), Oxygen Consumption (V̇o₂), and Ventilatory (VE) Responses to Submaximal and Maximal Exercise

Reference		Workload	Direction of Change at Pressure				Pressure
			HR	V̇o₂	VE	O₂ pulse	
Submaximal							
Tauton et al.,	1970	1000–1800 kpm/min	→	←	→		2 atm abs (air)
Tauton et al.,	1970	1000–1800 kpm/min	→	←[a]	→		2 atm abs (O₂)
L'Huillier et al.,	1969	160 W	⇒	⇒	⇒		3 atm abs (air)
Fagraeus,	1974	150 W	⇒	⇐	⇒		4.5 atm abs (air)
Matsuda et al.,	1975	500 kpm/min	↕	←	↕	⇐	7 atm abs (He-O₂)
Dressendorfer,	1977	50% V̇o₂max	↕	⇐[a]	↕		18.6 atm abs (He-O₂)
Hamilton et al.,	1967	50% V̇o₂max	⇒	⇐	⇒		20 atm abs (He-O₂)
Salzano et al.,	1970	275–735 kpm/min	⇒	⇐	⇒[a]	⇐	31.3 atm. abs. (He-O₂)
Spaur et al.,	1977	150–300 kgm/min		⇐	⇒		49.5 atm abs (He-O₂)
Salzano et al.,	1984	0–1440 kpm/min	↕	↕	⇒		47–66 atm abs (Trimix)
Maximal							
Fagraeus et al.,	1973	Maximal	↕	⇐	⇒		1.4 atm abs (air)
Cook,	1970	Maximal	⇒	⇐	⇒	↕	2 atm abs (N₂-normox)
Cook,	1970	Maximal	⇒	⇐	⇒	⇒	3 atm abs (N₂-normox)
L'Huillier et al.,	1969	Maximal	⇒	⇒	⇒		3 atm abs (air)
Fagraeus,	1974	Maximal	↕	↕			6.0 atm abs (air)
Anthonisen et al.,	1976	Maximal	⇒	↕	⇒		4–6 atm abs (N₂-normox)
Dressendorfer,	1977	Maximal	⇒	↕	⇒	↕	18.6 atm abs (He-O₂)
Ohta et al.,	1981	Maximal	⇒	⇒	⇒	↕	31 atm abs (He-O₂)
Freund et al.,	1992	Maximal		⇒	⇒		37.5 atm abs (Trimix)

[a] Calculated value by original author, not measured directly.

This effect has also been shown at slightly elevated atmospheric pressure. For instance, Fagraeus et al. [23] demonstrated increased $\dot{V}O_2$max in subjects breathing 1.4 atm abs air, compared with 1 atm abs air (Table 1). These increases in $\dot{V}O_2$max were accompanied by increases in endurance time. However, no further increase in $\dot{V}O_2$max was associated with greater pressures in the air environment used [23]. In addition, as seen in Table 1, when the hyperoxic effects are removed, $\dot{V}O_2$max doesn't change or is decreased [1, 11, 18, 23, 26, 52]. The increases in $\dot{V}O_2$max associated with increased O_2 delivery would suggest that oxygen extraction from the blood by the working muscle is a limiting factor, and that by increasing the arterial O_2 content, one could increase muscle function. This point was addressed by Kaijser [35] in six subjects utilizing a spring-loaded hand ergometer and studying forearm arterial and venous O_2 contents. Work was performed in air at 1 atm abs, and at 3 atm abs of 100% O_2. Despite a calculated 15% reduction in forearm blood flow, the arterio-venous O_2 differences at exhaustion were the same in the two settings. Furthermore, although 3 of the subjects had extended times to exhaustion, 3 did not. The authors concluded, therefore, that limitation in oxygen consumption is not with O_2 delivery to the muscle cell, but the oxygen utilization system in the cell. Similar conclusions were reached by Welch et al. [74], where exercising leg muscle was studied under conditions of air breathing or while breathing 100% O_2 at 1 atm abs. These studies tend to contradict those of Hill [30] and Fagraeus [23]. However, more recently, Eiken et al [20] studied the functions of the quadriceps femoris in exercising human subjects while breathing air at 1 and 6 atm abs, and while breathing 100% O_2 at 1.3 atm abs. The latter two situations differed mainly in N_2, and the first and the last differed mainly in O_2. Exposure to 1.3 atm abs of O_2 was associated with greater peak torque, which was sustained over 60 contractions, compared with either of the other experimental conditions. The condition of 6 atm abs during air breathing, although initially producing similar values of peak torque as seen during the 1.3 atm abs of 100% O_2, gradually fell over the 60 contractions to levels nearly identical with the values obtained when the subjects were breathing air at 1.0 atm abs. Muscle biopsy results indicated that increased O_2 without the increased N_2 was associated with faster restoration of energy-rich phosphagens. It is clear that differences between the studies of the isolated muscle masses exist, yet a convincing explanation for the discrepancies between the reports on muscle performance is not available.

Lastly, previous exposure to increased O_2 may affect subsequent exercise during normal oxygen exposure. Cabric et al [6] recently reported findings from three groups of subjects who were compared for changes in work performance, $\dot{V}O_2$max, ventilation-oxygen uptake ratio, and blood lactate levels before and after exposure to 100% O_2 for 60 minutes at 2.8 atm abs. The groups differed by the amount of time after exposure allowed before the postexposure tests were performed. They were tested at 30 minutes, 3 hours, and 6 hours postexposure. Both the groups tested at 30 minutes and 3 hours postexposure showed increases in work capacity and $\dot{V}O_2$max and had longer treadmill times than the group tested 6 hours postexposure. Although measurements necessary for further determination of possible mechanisms were not made, the data provide an interesting observation that deserves further investigation.

Ventilatory Response

The reader is referred to reviews by Lamphier and Camporesi [43], Van Liew [72] and Anthonisen [2] for a more comprehensive coverage of the overall respiratory response to hyperbaria. A good summarizing experimental series demonstrating the effects of increased pressure on exercise induced respiratory changes was shown by Fagraeus [24] in a series of maximal exercise experiments in subjects at pressures of 1, 1.4, 2.0, 3.0, and 6.0 atm abs in air. Over the range of pressures, ventilation volume decreased by about 20% at 2 atm abs, about 35% at 3 atm abs, and to about 46% at 6 atm abs. As a consequence, $PACO_2$ steadily increased to an average increase of about 60% when maximum exercise was performed at 6 atm abs. In these same experiments, heart rate decreased about 5% and $\dot{V}O_2$max was slightly increased at 1.4 atm abs, but otherwise was unchanged. Thus, despite large reductions in VE, $\dot{V}O_2$ is only affected minimally. The results summarized in Table 1 indicate that hyperbaria reduces the minute ventilation of equivalent submaximal workloads as well as maximal exercise. This reduced ventilation is usually attributed to added resistance to flow resulting from the increased gas density, and usually results in evidence of CO_2 retention [1, 11, 24, 26, 28, 34, 61, 62, 67]. Furthermore, it is not uncommon to observe increased $\dot{V}O_2$ at submaximal exercise (Table 1), which most investigators have attributed to the added work of breathing. Clearly the resistance imposed by the breathing apparatus in these experiments will affect the results, and may account for some of the inconsistencies.

These observations of decreased VE during exposure to hyperbaria are predictable from the studies reviewed Lanphier and Camporesi [43]. By combining the work of several previous studies, a density-dependent decrease in maximum ventilatory volume (MVV) was described by the equation of MVVdepth = MVVo $\times$ $-$k (where MVVo is MVV measured at a density of 1.0, and k is a best-fit regression exponent). The square root of density (where k = 0.5) approximates this fit, but more recent estimates, possibly owing to lower resistance breathing equipment, estimate k to be 0.3–0.4. The lower the value of k the less MVV is reduced at depth according to this relationship. MVV may have some practical use in predicting VEmax at depth when the density is great enough to impair ventilation to an extent where mechanical ventilatory supply of ambient gas containing O_2 may be the limiting factor instead of cardiopulmonary limitations [43, 72].

The effect of gas density on respiratory and exercise parameters was specifically addressed in the predictive studies of Lambertsen et al. [42]. By taking advantage of the high density of Ne, gas densities equivalent to up to 5000 feet sea water (fsw) were studied by having divers breathe Ne, He and O_2 mixtures at a depth of 1200 fsw. In those studies subjects were able to exercise at approximately 80% of their sea level maximums at gas densities of about 22 times that of air at 1 atm abs (equivalent to 150 atm abs), with no evidence of dyspnea. However, these predictions may need some further interpretation because in the studies of Spaur et al. [67], severe dyspnea occurred at moderate workloads at 49.5 atm abs, gas density about 8 times that of air at 1 atm abs, when exercising during immersion. In contrast, however, Salzano et al. [61] report that dyspnea was a "rare occurrence" in saturation dives to 46.7 and 65.6 atm abs despite quite severe exercise. There was no significant dyspnea experienced by subjects during maximal exercise at 37.5 atm abs at dry saturation dive using trimix in a recent study by Freund et al. [26]. One major difference in the studies by Spaur et al. [67] and Salzano et al. [61] is that exercise was performed during immersion in the former studies. In upright exercise during immersion, hyperbaria was accompanied by a greater degree of hypoventilation when the hydrostatic pressure of the breathing apparatus was equilibrated at the level of the mouth as compared with the lungs [69]. In addition to the differences that immersion may contribute to dyspnea, there may also be effects of gas composition on the occurrence of dyspnea. In the studies by Salzano et al. [61], both HeO_2 and trimix (at both 5 and 10% N_2), were used in different dives, and a greater incidence of dyspnea was reported with HeO_2 breathing than with trimix.

It would appear, therefore, that hyperbaria has more profound effects on respiratory parameters than cardiovascular responses [72], but there are only modest effects on exercise performance and respiratory distress responses in pressure environments in the range of 31 atm abs in HeO_2 and 37.5 atm abs, using trimix. Furthermore, the predictive studies of Lambertsen et al. [42] and the deep saturation dives reported by Salzano et al. [61] clearly indicate the possibility of vigorous work at even greater pressures, but the lack of an explanation for the occurrence of dyspnea in other studies requires an awareness and caution to possibilities of dyspnea. Furthermore, considering that essentially all studies confirm approximately a 40% reduction in VE at maximal exercise over 18.6 atm abs, the reduced reserve capabilities must be acknowledged.

HORMONAL RESPONSES TO EXERCISE AT HYPERBARIA

Until recently most hyperbaric exercise studies focused on cardiovascular and respiratory measurements. Lately, however, results of studies on the interactions of exercise and fluid balance have been reported. The hyperbaric environment has profound and well-established effects on fluid balance [32]. By mechanisms not entirely understood, water balance is maintained during long periods of dry saturation dives at pressures of about 4 atm abs and greater by a maintained water input, decreased insensible water loss, and an increased urine output, and accompanying decreased urine osmolality. It is appropriate to consider, therefore, whether or not state of hydration would alter the exercise responses at hyperbaria. Doubt and Deuster [17] recently reported on exercise responses of immersed subjects who exercised in air at 1 atm abs and in HeO_2 at 5.5 atm abs. At each pressure the subjects exercised twice, once without a fluid load, and once with a fluid load. Drinking fluid while exercising in the immersed state did not change fluid balance, or thermal status, and there were only small changes in ventilation measurements when comparing responses between 1 atm abs and at 5.5 atm abs. Studies investigating the salt- and water-regulating hormonal responses to maximal exercise during a dry saturation dive to 37.5 atm was also recently reported [9]. The hyperbaric environment reduced basal levels of vasopressin and atrial natriuretic factor, and had no effect on aldosterone levels. Despite maximal exercise that achieved 90% of the sea level of maximum effort, vasopressin levels were not significantly elevated above baseline values, the atrial natriuretic factor values increased significantly, but the response was blunted compared with the sea level response, and aldosterone was similarly stimulated at both sea level and 37.5 atm abs. At 1 atm abs, vasopressin levels increased in response to maximal exercise approximately 5-fold to plasma levels of 4.3 $\mu U/mL$, compared with 0.9 $\mu U/mL$ at 37.5 atm abs. The inability of maximal exercise to stimulate vasopressin release is, indeed, remarkable, and demonstrates how greatly suppressed the vasopressin release is at hyperbaria. The consequences of these responses on the renal responses to exercise have not been reported.

In summary, exercise in hyperbaric environments has been an intensely studied topic of research for nearly a century, and the material presented here is not comprehensive in any one field. Therefore, reading of the reviews suggested is essential for complete coverage. The coverage given was intended to provide a starting place, and reasonably up-to-date information on the current status of cardiovascular, pulmonary, and hormonal responses to exercise and influences on workload tolerance.

REFERENCES

1. Anthonisen, N. R., G. Utz, M. H. Kryger, and J. S. Urbanetti. Exercise tolerance at 4 and 6 atm abs. *Undersea Biomed. Res.* 3:95–102, 1976.
2. Anthonisen, N. R. Physiology of diving. Respiration. In Shilling, C. W., C. B. Carlston, and R. A. Mathias (eds). *The Physician's Guide to Diving Medicine.* New York: Plenum Press, 1984, pp. 71–85.
3. Beckman, E. L. Thermal protective suits for underwater swimmers. *Mil. Med.* 132:195–209, 1967.

4. Boutelier, C., J. Colin, and J. Timbal. Détermination du coefficient d'échange thermique dans l'eau en écoulement turbulent. *J. Physiol. (Paris)* 63:207–209, 1971.

5. Burton, A. C. and Edholm O. G. *Man in a Cold Environment*. London: Edward Arnold, 1955.

6. Cabric, M., R. Medved, P. Denoble, M. Zivkovic, and H. Kovacevic. Effect of hyperbaric oxygenation on maximal aerobic performance in a normobaric environment. *J. Sports Med. Physical Fitness* 31:362–366, 1991.

7. Cannon, P., and W. R. Keatinge. The metabolic rate and heat loss of fat and thin men in heat balance in cold and warm water. *J. Physiol. (Lond.)* 154:329–344, 1960.

8. Carlson, L. D., A. C. L. Hsieh, F. Fullington, and R. W. Elsner. Immersion in cold water and body tissue insulation. *J. Aviat. Med.* 29:145–152, 1958.

9. Claybaugh, J. R., B. J. Freund, G. Luther, K. Muller, and P. B. Bennett. Effects of hyperbaria (360 MSW) on the hormonal response to maximal exercise in man. *FASEB J.* 6:A1461, 1992 (abstract 3042).

10. Choi, J. K., Y. S. Park, Y. H. Park, et al. Effect of wearing gloves on the thermal balance of Korean women wet-suit divers in cold water. *Undersea Biomed. Res.* 15:155–164, 1988.

11. Cook, J. C. Work capacity in hyperbaric environments without hyperoxia. *Aerospace Med.* 41:1133–1135, 1970.

12. Costill, D. L., P. J. Cahill, and D. Eddy. Metabolic resposes to submaximal exercise in three water temperatures. *J. Appl. Physiol.* 22:629–632, 1967.

13. Craig, A. B., Jr. Heat exchange between man and the water environment. In C. J. Lambertsen (ed). *Underwater Physiology VI*. Proceedings of the 4th Symposium on Underwater Physiology., New York: Academic Press, 1971, pp. 425–433.

14. Craig, A. B., Jr., and M. Dvorak. Thermal regulation during water immersion. *J. Appl. Physiol.* 21:1577–1585, 1966.

15. Craig, A. B., Jr., and M. Dvorak. Heat exchanges between man and the water environment. C. J. Lambertsen (ed.). *Underwater Physiology V. Proceedings of the 5th Symposium on Underwater Physiology*. Bethesda, MD: Fed. Am. Soc. Exp. Biol., 1976, pp. 765–773.

16. Craig, A. B., and M. Dvorak. Thermal regulation of man exercising during water immersion. *J. Appl. Physiol.* 25:29–35, 1968.

17. Doubt, T. J., and P. A. Deuster. Fluid ingestion during exercise in 25 degrees C water at surface and 5.5 atm abs. *Med. Sci. Sports Exerc.* 26:75–80, 1994.

18. Dressendorpher, R. H., S. K. Hong, J. F. Morlock. J. Pegg, B. Respicio, R. M. Smith, and C. Yelverton. Hana Kai II: a 17-day dry saturation dive at 18.6 atm abs. V. Maximal oxygen uptake. *Undersea Biomed. Res.* 4:283–296, 1977.

19. Dubois, E. F. The estimation of the surface area of the body. *Basal Metabolism in Health and Disease,* 3rd ed. Philadelphia: Lea & Febiger, 1936, pp. 125–144.

20. Eiken, O., C. M. Hesser, F. Lind, A. Thorsson, and P. A. Tesch. Human skeletal muscle function and metabolism during intense exercise at high O_2 and N_2 pressures. *J. Appl. Physiol.* 63:571–575, 1987.

21. Erikson, H., J. Krog, K. L. Andersen, and P. F. Scholander. The critical temperature in naked man. *Acta Physiol. Scand.* 37:35–39, 1956.

22. Evans, D. E. Physiology of diving, C. Cardiovascular effects. C. W. Shilling, C. B. Carlston, and R. A. Mathias (eds). *The Physician's Guide to Diving Medicine*. New York: Plenum Press, 1984, pp. 99–109.

23. Fagraeus, L., J. Karlsson, D. Linnarsson, and B. Saltin. Oxygen uptake during maximal work at lowered and raised ambient air pressures. *Acta Physiol. Scand.* 87:411–421, 1973.

24. Fagraeus, L. Cardiorespiratory and metabolic functions during exercise in the hyperbaric environment. *Acta Physiol. Scand. Suppl.* 414:1–40, 1974.

25. Ferretti, G., A. Veicsteinas, and D. W. Rennie. Regional heat flows of resting and exercising men immersed in cold water. *J. Appl. Physiol.* 64:1239–1248, 1988.

26. Freund, B. J., J. R. Claybaugh, J. Holthaus, G. Luther, and P. B. Bennett. Effects of hyperbaria on the cardiorespiratory responses to maximal exercise. *Med. Sci. Sports and Exerc.* 23:S156, 1992.

27. Golden, F. St. C. and Tipton, M. J. Human thermal responses during leg- only exercise in cold water. *J. Physiol. (Lond.)* 391:399–405, 1987.
28. Hamilton, R. W. Physiological responses at rest and in exercise during saturation at 20 atmospheres of He-O2. C. J. Lambertson, (ed). *Physiological Performance at Extreme Pressure.* Proceedings of the 3rd Symposium on Underwater Physiology. Baltimore: Williams & Wilkins, 1967, pp. 361–374.
29. Hayward, M. G., and Keatinge, W. R. Roles of subcutaneous fat and thermoregulatory reflexes in determining ability to stabilize body temperature in water. *J. Physiol. (Lond.)* 320:229–251, 1981.
30. Hill, A. V., C. N. H. Long, and H. Lupton. Muscular exercise, lactic acid and the supply and utilization of oxygen. Parts VII–VIII, *Proc. R. Soc. Edinburgh Section B: Biology.* 97:155–176, 1924.
31. Hoke, B., D. L. Jackson, J. M. Alexander, and E. T. Flynn. Respiratory heat loss and pulmonary function during cold-gas breathing at high pressure. C. J. Lambertsen (ed.). *Underwater Physiology V.* Proceedings of the 5th Symposium on Underwater Physiology. Bethesda, MD: Fed. Am. Soc. Exp. Biol., 1976, pp 725–740.
32. Hong, S. K., and J. R. Claybaugh. Hormonal and renal responses to hyperbaria. J. R. Claybaugh, and C. E. Wade (eds). *Hormonal Regulation of Fluid and Electrolytes: Environmental Effects.* New York: Plenum, 1989, pp. 117–146.
33. Iwamoto, J., S. Sagawa, F. Tajima, and K. Shiraki. Critical water temperature during water immersion at various atmospheric pressures in unprotected subjects. *J. Appl. Physiol.* 64: 2224–2228, 1988.
34. Jarrett, A. S. Alveolar carbon dioxide tension at increased ambient pressures. *J. Appl. Physiol.* 21:158–162, 1966.
35. Kaijser, L. Physical exercise under hyperbaric oxygen pressure. *Life Sciences.* 8:929–934, 1969.
36. Kang, B. S., S. H. Song, C. S. Suh, and S. K. Hong. Changes in body temperature and basal metabolic rate of the ama. *J. Appl. Physiol.* 18:483–488, 1963.
37. Kang, D. H., P. K. Kim, B. S. Kang, S. H. Song, and S. K. Hong. Energy metabolism and body temperature of ama. *J. Appl. Physiol.* 20:46–50, 1965.
38. Kang, D. H., Y. S. Park, Y. D. Park, et al. Energetics of wet-suit diving in Korean women breath-hold divers. *J. Appl. Physiol.* 54:1702–1707, 1983.
39. Keatinge, W. R. The effect of subcutaneous fat and of previous exposure to cold on the body temperature, peripheral blood flow and metabolic rate of men in cold water. *J. Physiol. (Lond.)* 153:166–178, 1960.
40. Keatinge, W. R. The effect of work and clothing on the maintenance of the body temperature in water. *Quat. J. Exp. Physiol.* 46:69–82, 1961.
41. Keatinge, W. R. *Survival in Cold Water.* Oxford: Blackwell, 1969.
42. Lambertson, C. J., R. Gelfand, R. Peterson, et al. Human tolerance to He, Ne, and N2 at respiratory gas densities equivalent to He-O2 breathing at depths to 1200, 2000, 3000, 4000, and 5000 feet of sea water (predictive studies III). *Aviat. Space Environ. Med.* 48:843–855, 1977.
43. Lanphier, E. H., and E. M. Camporesi. Respiration and exercise. P. B. Bennett, and D. H. Elliot (eds). *The Physiology and Medicine of Diving,* 3rd ed. San Pedro: Best, 1982, pp. 99–156.
44. L'Huillier, J., P. Varene, and C. Jacquemin. Exercise musculaire maximal en milieu hyperbare. *J. Physiologie.* 61(Suppl 1): 147, 1969.
45. Lin, Y. C., and K. K. Shida. Brief review: mechanisms of hyperbaric bradycardia. *Chin. J. Physiol.* 31:1–22, 1988.
46. Matsuda, M., H. Nakayama, A. Itoh, et al. Physiology of man during a 10-day dry heliox saturation dive (Seatopia) to 7 atm abs. I. Cardiovascular and thermoregulatory functions. *Undersea Biomed. Res.* 2:101–117, 1975.
47. Mcardle, W. D. J. R. Magel, R. J. Spina, R. J., Gergley, and M. M. Toner. Thermal adjustments to cold water exposure in exercising men and women. *J. Appl. Physiol.* 56:1572–1577, 1984.

48. Monji, K., K. Nakashima, Y. Sogabe, K. Miki, F. Tajima, and K. Shiraki. Changes in insulation of wet suits during repetitive exposure to pressure. *Undersea Biomed. Res.* 16:313–319, 1989.

49. Moore, T. O., J. F. Morlock, D. A. Lally, and S. K. Hong. Thermal cost of saturation diving: respiratory and whole body heat loss at 16.1 atm abs. C. J. Lambertson (ed). *Underwater Physiology V.* Proceedings of the 5th Symposium on Underwater Physiology. Bethesda, MD: Fed. Am. Soc. Exp. Biol., 1976, pp. 741–754.

50. Morrison, J. B., and J. T. Florio. Respiratory function during a simulated saturation dive to 1,500 feet. *J. Appl. Physiol.* 30:724–732, 1971.

51. Nadel, E. R., I. Holmer, U. Berg, P. O. Astrand, and J. A. J. Stolwijk. Energy exchanges of swimming man. *J. Appl. Physiol.* 36:465–471, 1974.

52. Ohta, Y., H. Arita, H. Nakayama, et al. Cardiopulmonary functions and maximal aerobic power during a 14-day saturation dive at 31 atm abs (Seadragon IV). A. J. Bachrach and M. M. Matzen (eds). *Underwater Physiology VII.* Proceedings of the 7th Symposium on Underwater Physiology. Bethesda, MD: Undersea Medical Society, 1981, pp. 209–221.

53. Park, Y. S., D. R. Pendergast, and D. W. Rennie. Decrease in body insulation with exercise in cool water. *Undersea Biomed. Res.* 11:159–168, 1984.

54. Park, Y. H., J. Iwamoto, F. Tajima, K. Miki, Y. S. Park, and K. Shiraki. Effect of pressure on thermal insulation in humans wearing wet-suits. *J. Appl. Physiol.* 64:1916–1922, 1988.

55. Piantadosi, C. Respiratory heat loss limits in helium-oxygen saturation diving. L. A. Kuehn (ed). *Thermal Constraints in Diving.* Bethesda, MD: Undersea Medical Society, 1981, pp. 45–54.

56. Pugh, L. G. C., and O. G. Edholm. The physiology of channel swimmers. *Lancet* 2:761–768, 1955.

57. Rapp, G. M. Convection coefficients of man in a forensic area of thermal physiology: heat transfer in underwater exercise. *J. Physiol. (Paris).* 63:392–396, 1971.

58. Rennie, D. W. Thermal insulation of Korean diving women and non-divers in water. H. Rahn, and T. Yokoyama (eds). *Physiology of Breath-Hold Diving and the Ama of Japan,* Washington, D.C.: National Academy of Sciences National Research Council 1965, pp. 315–324.

59. Rennie, D. W. Tissue heat transfer during exercise in water. K. Shiraki and M. K. Yousef (eds). *Man in Stressful Environments: Thermal and Work Physiology.* Springfield, IL: Charles C Thomas, 1987, pp. 211–223.

60. Sagawa, S., K. Shiraki, and M. K. Yousef. Water temperature and intensity of exercise in maintenance of thermal equilibrium. *J. Appl. Physiol.* 65:2413–2419, 1988.

61. Salzano, J. V., E. M. Compresi, B. W. Stolp, and R. E. Moon. Physiological responses to exercises at 47 and 66 atm abs. *J. Appl. Physiol.* 57:1055–1068, 1984.

62. Salzano, J., D. C. Rausch, and H. A. Saltzman, Cardio-respiratory responses to exercise at a simulated seawater depth at 1,000 feet. *J. Appl. Physiol.* 28:34–41, 1970.

63. Shiraki, K., S. Sagawa, N. Konda, Y. S. Park, T. Komatsu, and S. K. Hong. Energetics of wet-suit diving in Japanese male breath-hold divers. *J. Appl. Physiol.* 61:1475–1480, 1986.

64. Shiraki, K., N. Konda, S. Sagawa, and Y. S. Park. Diving pattern and thermoregulatory responses of male and female wet suit divers. C. E. G. Lundgren and M. Ferrigno (eds). *The Physiology of Breath-Hold Diving.* Bethesda, MD: Undersea and Hyperbaric Medicine Society, 1987, pp. 124–134.

65. Shiraki, K., Y. H. Park, J. Iwamoto, et al. Regional heat loss in wet-suited subjects at critical water temperature of different pressures. *FASEB J.* 2:1528, 1988.

66. Smith, R. M., and J. Hanna. Skinfolds and resting heat loss in cold air and water. *J. Appl. Physiol.* 39:93–102, 1975.

67. Spaur, W. H., L. W. Raymond, M. M. Knott, J. C. Crothers, W. R. Braithwaite, E. D. Thalmann, and D. F. Uddin. Dyspnea in divers at 49.5 atm abs; mechanical, not chemical in origin. *Undersea Biomed. Res.* 4:183–198, 1977.

68. Taunton, J. E., E. W. Banister, T. R. Patrick, P. Oforsagd, and W. R. Duncan. Physical work capacity in hyperbaric environments and conditions of hyperoxia. *J. Appl. Physiol.* 28:421–427, 1970.

69. Taylor, N. A. S., and J. B. Morrison. Effects of breathing-gas pressure on pulmonary function and work capacity during immersion. *Undersea Biomed. Res.* 17:413–428, 1990.

70. Toner, M. M., S. N. Sawka, and K. B. Pandolf. Thermal responses during arm and leg and combined arm-leg exercise in water. *J. Appl. Physiol.* 56:1355–1360, 1984.

71. Toner, M. M., S. N. Sawka, W. L. Holden, and K. B. Pandolf. Comparison of thermal responses between rest and leg exercise in water. *J. Appl. Physiol.* 59:284–253, 1985.

72. Van Liew, H. D. Mechanical and physical factors in lung function during work in dense environments. *Undersea Biomed. Res.* 10:255–264, 1983.

73. Veicsteinas, A., G. Ferretti, and D. W. Rennie. Superficial shell insulation in resting and exercising men in cold water. *J. Appl. Physiol. Respirat. Environ. Exerc. Physiol.* 52:1557–1564, 1982.

74. Welch, H. G., F. Bonde-Petersen, T. Graham, K. Klausen, and N. Secher. Effects of hyperoxia on leg blood flow and metabolism during exercise. *J. Appl. Physiol.* 42:385–390, 1977.

75. Wolff, A. H., S. R. K. Coleshaw, C. G. Newstead, and W. R. Keatinge. Heat exchange in wet suits. *J. Appl. Physiol.* 58:770–777, 1985.

76. Yeon, D. S., Y. S. Park, J. K. Choi, et al. Changes in thermal insulation during underwater exercise in Korean female wet-suit divers. *J. Appl. Physiol.* 62:1014–1019, 1987.

Index

References followed by t or f indicate tables or figures, respectively.

487